Radiographic Critique

Radiographic Critique

Kathy McQuillen-Martensen, RT(R)
Radiography Instructor
Program in Radiologic Technology
Department of Radiology
The University of Iowa Hospitals and Clinics
Iowa City, Iowa

W.B. SAUNDERS COMPANY
A Division of Harcourt Brace & Company
Philadelphia • London • Toronto • Montreal • Sydney • Tokyo

W.B. SAUNDERS COMPANY
A Division of
Harcourt Brace & Company

The Curtis Center
Independence Square West
Philadelphia, Pennsylvania 19106

Library of Congress Cataloging-in-Publication Data

McQuillen-Martensen, Kathy.

Radiographic critique/Kathy McQuillen-Martensen.—1st ed.

   p.   cm.

Includes bibliographical references and index.

ISBN 0–7216–4978–5

1. Radiography, Medical.   I. Title.

[DNLM: 1. Technology, Radiologic.   WN 160 1995]

RC78.M26 1995

616.07/572—dc20

DNLM/DLC   94–35039

RADIOGRAPHIC CRITIQUE   ISBN 0–7216–4978–5

Last digit is the print number: 9   8   7   6   5   4   3   2   1

PREFACE

Over the past 15 years, the field of radiography has made overwhelming advances while the basic information taught in positioning and radiographic critique classes has remained relatively the same, even though 30 to 40 percent of repeated radiographs are due to inaccurate patient positioning. While teaching the courses of radiographic positioning and critique I discovered that the instructional material available in positioning critique is limited and what is available is rather general. The material lacks one-to-one correlation between each aspect of patient positioning and the resulting radiograph; it rarely discusses how radiographic principles of part, film and beam alignment, and beam divergence relate to the positioning set-up procedure and how these principles affect the resulting radiograph; and it does not discuss how the procedural set-up should be adjusted if a less than adequate radiograph is produced. The weaknesses of this instructional material will affect the depth of student radiographers' education on this subject, since their understanding is then contingent on the instructor's knowledge of the subject and on the variety of inadequately positioned radiographs that can be found in the department's repeat bin. Poor instructional material will also affect students' ability to retain the subject, since it is difficult to retain information when there is no resource available for reinforcement. The staff technologists—and, inadvertently, patient care—are also affected when this information is not available, since there is no resource to assist technologists who wonders how the set-up procedure should be adjusted when a less than optimal radiograph is obtained.

The purpose of this book is to supply instructors, student radiographers, and technologists with increased information that will bridge the gap between patient positioning and the resulting radiograph. A basic course in anatomy is the only prerequisite to this book.

Chapter 1 begins by defining radiographic terminology and discussing how a radiograph should be properly hung on the view box. It then presents a radiographic critique form that lists all the aspects of a radiograph that should be evaluated and a discussion of the fundamentals under each of the items on the form, providing accurate and inaccurate example radiographs to supplement the concepts discussed. Included on the form are such headings as patient and hospital identification, film marking, patient and central ray positioning, collimation, radiation protection, recorded detail, distortion, film size and anatomical alignment, image receptor system, density, penetration, contrast, artifacts, and fulfillment of ordered procedure.

Chapters 2 through 10 focus on evaluating radiographs of the most commonly performed orthopedic procedures for accuracy in patient and central ray positioning and in the usage of technical factors. For each procedure, there are an accurately positioned radiograph with labeled anatomy, many examples of poorly positioned radiographs, photographs of a model demonstrating accurate patient positioning and demonstrating examples of patient mispositioning, and a radiographic evaluation criteria list. For each criterion in the list there is a discussion that correlates the evaluation criteria with the corresponding patient or central ray set-up procedure that defines how the resulting radiograph will appear if the correct patient or central ray set-up procedure is not followed, and that explains radiographic principles as they relate to the criterion. The radiographs for each procedure that demonstrate poor patient and central ray positioning are grouped together. Next to each of these radiographs is a synopsis discussing the anatomical structures that have been misaligned, how the patient or central ray was mispositioned, and how the patient or central ray should be repositioned to obtain an optimal radiograph. I used this arrangement to avoid requiring readers to flip through pages when comparing radiographs or when searching for a particular radiograph of interest. All the radiographs have labeled anatomical structures to help the reader identify anatomy that is without dimension and often magnified and distorted.

I designed the book to guide the reader in a systematic order through the body structures. It is not necessary to follow the text as it is written. One can freely skip from chapter to chapter or procedure to procedure and fully comprehend the material. In addition to this book, ancillary materials including a self-learning student workbook, instructor's manual, and slide set have been created. The workbook follows the same format as the book. For each chapter there are learning objectives and activities, study questions and poorly positioned radiographs to evaluate for every procedure, and a self-test. The instructor's manual provides a test bank of questions for each chapter and ideas on using the book. The slide set contains many of the radiographs from the book and can be used to complement lectures and supplement your radiograph file.

It is difficult to label this book as strictly a positioning or a radiographic critique text. I find that the two subjects cross each other closely. When I began teaching this material, I kept the classes of patient positioning and radiographic critique as two separate subjects, first teaching how the patient should be positioned and then focusing on how the resulting radiograph should appear. With experience I discovered that by simultaneously correlating the patient and central ray positioning procedure with the resulting radiograph and then presenting typical ways one could misposition the patient and associating it with the resulting radiograph, there was a growth in the students' ability to retain the information and to reliably predict radiographic outcomes. Each year since I have used this approach, I have found the courses on positioning and positioning critique are more exciting to teach and the students have enjoyed the interaction and problem-solving skills the classes have evoked.

Just as the methods of teaching a course are modified as new ideas are practiced in an attempt to increase the students' subject knowledge, I know this book is also anxiously awaiting modifications that will increase the readers' understanding of the subject. It is through your comments and suggestions that I can be made aware of which aspects of the book work well and which may need modification. Please feel free to contact me and in the meantime continue to "strive for perfection!"

KATHY MCQUILLEN-MARTENSEN, RT(R)

ACKNOWLEDGMENTS

Before I decided to write this book I received wonderful encouragement and support from my family, friends, and coworkers to take on the project. That encouragement and support never faltered throughout the years it has taken to finish the project. For that I am very thankful, for without it this book would never have existed.

Special thanks go to the following:

My mentor and friend, **Marilyn Holland,** RT, for being an influential figure throughout my career. You have always had faith in me and have given me support and encouragement on this project and others I have undertaken. Thank you for listening when I needed someone to bounce ideas off of.

Wilma Conner, RT, for the endless hours spent editing the text and radiographs. Conferring with you about the project always encouraged me to work harder.

Joan Radke, RT, **Sandra Woodfield,** RT, **Mary Dee Chamberlain,** RT, **Stephanie Setter,** RT, and **Shelley Matzen,** RT, for listening, testing, and questioning my positioning ideas; for the time spent reviewing the book; and for your unwavering support and friendship.

Sandy Mast, for your computer help, support, and friendship.

The University of Iowa's **Radiologic Technology Classes of 1988 to 1995,** for their challenging questions that caused me to search for answers and for their help in editing the book by using it before completion.

The **Staff Radiographers** at The University of Iowa Hospital and Clinics, for their professional expertise.

The **Radiology Department** at The University of Iowa Hospital and Clinics, for allowing me to use their beautiful facility for observation and photography.

Jim Olson, for advice on photography.

John Bartholomew, for advice and assistance with film copying.

Tracey Hess and **Jennifer Kronaizl** (soon to be RTs), for helping with photography and working as models. Your precise positioning skills and senses of humor made the time spent working on this project most productive and enjoyable.

Samantha Johnson, RT, and **Angie Holub,** RT, for assisting me with the knee cadaver study. Your positioning and organizational skills helped to ensure a successful study.

The professional staff at **W.B. Saunders Company,** for their work in the development of this book.

My children, **Nicole, Zachary,** and **Adam,** for being understanding when it seemed as if I was always working on "The Book."

And lastly, my husband, **Van,** for the constant love and support you have given me over the last three years as this book was being prepared. Know that even the littlest things you did did not go unnoticed.

KATHY MCQUILLEN-MARTENSEN, RT(R)

CONTENTS

CHAPTER **1**

Guidelines for Radiographic Critique 1

Terminology 1

Hanging Radiographs 3

Radiographic Evaluation: The Radiographic Critique Form 5

CHAPTER **2**

Radiographic Critique of the Chest and Abdomen 40

Chest 40

Abdomen 65

CHAPTER **3**

Radiographic Critique of the Upper Extremity 77

Finger 77

Thumb 87

Hand 95

Wrist 104

Forearm 126

Elbow 136

Humerus 154

CHAPTER **4**

Radiographic Critique of the Shoulder 165

Shoulder 165

Clavicle 184

Acromioclavicular (AC) Joint 189

Scapula 193

CHAPTER **5**

Radiographic Critique of the Lower Extremity 202

Toe 202

Foot 210

Calcaneus 224

Ankle 232

Lower Leg 244

Knee 251

Patella 272

Femur 278

CHAPTER **6**

Radiographic Critique of the Hip and Pelvis 290

Hip 290

Pelvis 303

Sacroiliac Joints 311

CHAPTER **7**

Radiographic Critique of the Cervical and Thoracic Vertebrae 316

Cervical Vertebrae 316

Cervicothoracic Vertebrae 337

Thoracic Vertebrae 341

CHAPTER **8**

Radiographic Critique of the Lumbar Vertebrae, Sacrum, and Coccyx **350**

    Lumbar Vertebrae **350**

    Sacrum **365**

    Coccyx **371**

CHAPTER **9**

Radiographic Critique of the Sternum and Ribs **376**

    Sternum **376**

    Ribs **383**

CHAPTER **10**

Radiographic Critique of the Cranium **393**

Posteroanterior Projection and Trauma Anteroposterior Projection **393**

Posteroanterior Projection (Caldwell Method) and Trauma Anteroposterior (Caldwell) Projection **398**

Anteroposterior Axial Projection (Towne Position) **402**

Lateral Position **406**

Submentovertex Projection (Basilar Position) **409**

Parietoacanthal Projection (Waters and Open-Mouth Waters Position) and Trauma Acanthoparietal Projection **412**

Bibliography **417**

Index **419**

Radiographic Critique

CHAPTER 1

Guidelines for Radiographic Critique

Through radiographic positioning and diagnostic exposure classes, we learned the skills needed to obtain optimal radiographs of all body structures. An optimal radiograph is one that demonstrates all the most desired features. It would demonstrate maximum recorded detail, perfect patient positioning, excellent penetration, contrast and density, and no motion or removable artifacts. Unfortunately, because of patient condition, equipment malfunction, or technologist error, such perfection is not obtained on every radiograph that is taken. A less than optimal radiograph should be thoroughly evaluated to determine the reason for error so the problem can be accurately corrected before the exam is repeated. A radiograph should never have to be taken a third time because the error was not accurately identified from the first mispositioned radiograph.

This book cannot begin to identify the standards of radiographic acceptability within all the different radiographic facilities. What might be an acceptable standard in one facility may not be in another. Even if a radiograph is not optimal but is still passable according to your facility's standards, it should be carefully studied to determine whether your skills can be improved before the next similar exam. Study the technical factors, such as placement of radiation protection, name identification plate and markers, or degree of collimation, to determine whether, on your next patient, you can improve the locations or can increase collimation. Closely studying the patient's positioning can reveal habits in positioning that you could correct in order to improve your radiographs. For example, if you believe you are positioning the femoral epicondyles perpendicular to the film for a lateral knee radiograph, but the radiographs you take consistently demonstrate the lateral condyle anterior to the medial condyle, you may learn to alter your positioning technique by increasing the anterior rotation of the patient by the distance usually demonstrated between the two condyles on your radiographs. This rotation should compensate for your error and should yield a radiograph with perpendicular alignment of the condyles.

As you study the radiographs in this book, you may find that many of them are acceptable within your facility, even though they do not meet optimal standards. The goal of this work is not to dictate to your facility what should be acceptable and unacceptable radiographs. It is to help you focus on improving your radiographic evaluation and positioning skills and to provide a guideline on how the patient or central ray was mispositioned for a radiograph containing an error.

TERMINOLOGY

Positioning and Anatomical Placement Terms

Many terms are used in radiography and in this book to describe the path of the x-ray beam, the patient's position, the precise location of an anatomical structure, where one anatomical structure is in reference to another, or how a certain structure will change its position as the patient moves in a predetermined direction. These terms can be used singly or in combinations. Familiarizing yourself with them will help you to understand statements made throughout this book and to converse professionally with others in the medical field. The combining form of each term is shown in parentheses.

Anterior (antero-): Refers to the front surface of the patient; used to express something that is situated at or directed toward the front: "The sternum is anterior to the vertebral column."
Distal (disto-): Refers to a structure of an extremity that is situated farther from the patient's torso; used when comparing the location of two extremity structures: "The foot is distal to the ankle."
Inferior (infero-): Refers to a structure within the patient's torso that is situated closer to the feet; used when comparing the location of two structures: "The symphysis pubis is inferior to the iliac crest."
Lateral (latero-): Refers to the patient's sides; used to express something that is directed or situated away from the patient's median plane or to express the outer side of an extremity: "The kidneys are lateral to the vertebral column." "Place the film against the lateral surface of the knee."
Lateral position: Refers to positioning of the patient so that the side of the torso or extremity being radiographed is placed adjacent to the film. When a lateral position of the torso, vertebrae, or cranium is defined, the term *right* or *left* is also included to state which side of the patient is placed closer to the film.

1

Medial (medio-): Refers to the patient's median plane; used to express something that is directed or situated toward the patient's median plane or to express the inner side of an extremity: "The sacroiliac joints are medial to the anterior superior iliac spines." "Place the film against the medial surface of the knee."

Oblique position: Refers to rotation of a structure away from an anteroposterior or posteroanterior projection. When obliquity of the torso, vertebrae, or cranium is defined, the terms *right* or *left* and *anterior* or *posterior* are used with the term *oblique,* to state the side of the patient placed closer to the film. A right anterior oblique (RAO) position states the patient was rotated so that the right, anterior surface was placed closer to the film. When obliquity of an extremity is defined, the term *medial* (internal) or *lateral* (external) is used with the term *oblique,* to state which way the extremity was rotated and which side of the extremity was positioned closer to the film. For a medial oblique position of the wrist, the medial side of the arm is placed closer to the film.

Posterior (postero-): Refers to the back of the patient; used to express something that is situated at or directed toward the back: "The knee joint is posterior to the patella."

Proximal (proximo-): Refers to a structure of an extremity that is situated closer to the patient's torso; used when comparing the location of two extremity structures: "The shoulder joint is proximal to the elbow joint."

Superior (supero-): Refers to a structure within the patient's torso that is situated closer to the head; used when comparing the location of two torso structures: "The thoracic cavity is superior to the peritoneal cavity."

The following list contains frequently used combinations of the preceding terms. You might recognize some of them as *projections* (term used to describe the entrance and exit points of the x-ray beam as it passes through the body when a radiograph is taken). The projections have been starred (*). In a projection, the path from the first location to the second must be straight.

anteroinferior	inferolateral	posterolateral
anterolateral	inferosuperior*	posteromedian
anteromedian	lateromedial*	posterosuperior
anteroposterior*	mediolateral*	superoinferior*
anterosuperior	posteroanterior*	superolateral
	posteroinferior	

Terms for Body Planes

Following are body planes that are used throughout this textbook. Becoming familiar with them will help you to better understand how the patient and central ray or film are positioned.

Coronal plane: An imaginary plane that passes through the body from side to side and divides it into two (not necessarily equal) sections, one anterior and one posterior.

Midcoronal plane: An imaginary plane that passes through the body from side to side and divides it into equal anterior and posterior sections, or halves.

Midsagittal or median plane: An imaginary plane that passes through the body anteroposteriorly or posteroanteriorly and divides it into equal right and left sections.

Sagittal plane: An imaginary plane that passes through the body anteroposteriorly or posteroanteriorly and divides it into right and left sections that are not necessarily equal.

Longitudinal or lengthwise: Refers to the long axis of the anatomical structure or object being discussed. A longitudinal axis on a 14 × 17 inch (35 × 43 cm) film would parallel the film's longer (17-inch or 43-cm) length. A longitudinal axis on a patient's thorax would parallel the midsagittal plane. To position the film lengthwise with the patient means to align the film's longitudinal axis with the patient's longitudinal axis.

Transverse, horizontal, or crosswise: Refers to a plane that is at a 90-degree angle from the longitudinal axis of the anatomical structure or object being discussed. The transverse axis of a 14 × 17 inch (35 × 43 cm) film would parallel the shorter (14-inch or 35-cm) length. The transverse axis on a patient's thorax would be perpendicular to the midsagittal plane.

General Terminology

Following are definitions of terms relating to patient or central ray positioning, anatomy alignment and identity, and technical procedures used throughout this book.

Abduct: To laterally draw an extremity away from the torso. The humerus is abducted when it is elevated laterally.

Adduct: To move an extremity toward the torso. The humerus is adducted when it is positioned closer to the torso after being abducted.

Align: To arrange in a line.

Articulation: A joint or place where two bones meet.

Artifact: An undesirable structure or substance that appears on the radiograph. It may or may not be covering information.

Caudal: The foot end of the patient. A caudally angled central ray is directed toward the patient's feet.

Cephalic: The head end of the patient. A cephalically angled central ray is directed toward the patient's head.

Concave: Curved or rounded inward.

Condyle: Rounded projection on a bone that often articulates with another bone.

Convex: Curved or rounded outward.

Cortical outline: The outer layer of a bone that is demonstrated on a radiograph as the white outline of an anatomical structure.

Depress: To lower or sink down, positioning at a lower level.

Detail: A part or item of the whole structure. The trabeculae are details in the femoral bone.

Deviate: To move away from the normal or routine.

Dorsiflex: To move the toes and forefoot upward.

Elongate: To make the long axis of an anatomical structure appear longer on the radiographic image. Angling the central ray proximally for a scaphoid position of the wrist elongates the image of the scaphoid.

Elevate: To lift up or raise, positioning at a higher level.

Extension: A movement that results in straightening of the structure. With extension of the elbow, the arm is straightened. Extension of the cervical vertebrae shifts the patient's head posteriorly in an attempt to separate the vertebral bodies.

Flexion: A movement that bends a structure. With flexion of the elbow, the arm is bent. Flexion of the cervical vertebrae shifts the patient's head forward in an attempt to bring the vertebral bodies closer.

Foreshorten: To make the long axis of an anatomical structure appear shorter on the radiographic image. Positioning the lower leg at a 45-degree angle with the film, while the central ray is perpendicular to the film, foreshortens the image of the lower leg on the radiograph.

Lateral (external) rotation: The act of turning the anterior surface of an extremity outward or away from the patient's torso midline.

Magnification: Increasing or enlarging both axes of a structure. The gonadal contact shield is magnified on the radiographic image if it is placed on top of the patient.

Medial (internal) rotation: The act of turning the anterior surface of an extremity inward or toward the patient's torso midline.

Object–image distance (OID): Distance from the object being radiographed to the film.

Palpate: Act of touching or feeling a structure through the skin.

Plantar flexion: The act of moving the toes and forefoot downward.

Profile: The outline of an anatomical structure. The glenoid fossa is demonstrated in profile on a Grashey method radiograph.

Project: The act of throwing the image of an anatomical structure forward. An angled central ray projects the anatomical part situated farther away from the film farther than the anatomical part situated closer to the film.

Pronate: To rotate or turn the upper extremity medially until the hand's palmar surface is facing posteriorly.

Protract: To move a structure forward or anteriorly. The shoulder is protracted when it is drawn forward.

Radiographic image: A close copy of the anatomical structures being radiographed that appears on the film's emulsion.

Radiolucent: Allows x-radiation to pass through. A radiolucent object appears dark on a radiograph.

Radiopaque: Prevents x-radiation from passing through. A radiopaque object shows up as a white image on a radiograph.

Recorded detail: A term used to describe the sharpness of structures that have been included on the radiographic image.

Retract: To move a structure backward or posteriorly. The shoulder is retracted when it is drawn backwards.

Source–image distance (SID): The distance from the anode's focal spot to the film.

Superimpose: To lie over or above an anatomical structure or object.

Supination: Rotating or turning the upper extremity laterally until the hand's palmar surface is facing anteriorly.

Symmetrical: Structures on opposite sides demonstrating the same size, shape, and position.

Trabecular pattern: The supporting material within cancellous bone. It is demonstrated radiographically as thin white lines throughout a bony structure.

HANGING RADIOGRAPHS

Prior to evaluation, a radiograph should be correctly hung on a view box. This section describes the proper hanging procedures for most radiographs. For any radiograph presented in the book but not listed here, the proper hanging procedure is described in the discussion of the radiograph, in the section on marker placement.

Radiographs of different parts, positions, and projections should be hung as follows:

- Torso, vertebral, cranial, shoulder, and hip radiographs: as if the patient is standing in an upright position.
- Finger, wrist, and forearm radiographs: as if the patient is hanging from the fingertips.
- Elbow and humerus radiographs: as if they are hanging from the patient's shoulder.
- Toe and AP and oblique foot radiographs: as if the patient is hanging from the toes.
- Lateral foot, ankle, lower leg, and femur radiographs: as if they are hanging from the patient's hip.
- Decubitus chest and abdominal radiographs: so that the side of the patient that was positioned upward when the radiograph was taken is upward on the hung radiograph.
- Axiolateral positions of the shoulder and hip: with the patient's anterior surface up and posterior surface down.

Which side (front or back) of the radiograph is placed against the view box is determined by the projection/position presented, as follows.

Anteroposterior (AP) and Posteroanterior (PA) Projections and Oblique Positions of the Torso, Vertebrae, and Cranium

Radiographs taken in an AP or PA projection or oblique position should be placed on the view box as if the viewer and the patient are facing each other. The right side of the patient's radiograph is on the viewer's left, and the left side of the patient's radiograph is on the viewer's right. Whenever AP projections or posterior oblique positions are taken, the R (right) or L (left) marker appears correct when the radiograph is accurately hung, as long as the marker was placed on the film correctly before the radiograph was taken (Fig. 1–1). When PA projections or anterior oblique positions are taken, the R or L marker appears reversed when the radiograph is accurately hung (Fig. 1–2).

Lateral Positions of the Torso, Vertebrae, and Cranium

The marker placed on a lateral radiograph of the torso, vertebrae, or cranium represents the side of the patient

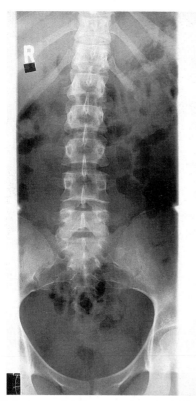

Figure 1-1. Accurately hung and marked AP projection.

positioned closer to the film. If the patient was positioned with the left side against the tabletop for a lateral lumbar vertebrae, a left marker should be placed on the film. If this marker is placed anteriorly (in front of the lumbar vertebrae), the radiograph can be hung in the same manner as an AP/PA projection, with the left marker placed on the

viewer's right side or the right marker placed on the viewer's left side (Fig. 1–3). In general, accurately hung laterally positioned radiographs demonstrate a correct marker as long as the marker was placed on the film correctly before the radiograph was taken. One exception to this guideline may be when left lateral chest radiographs are hung; often, reviewers prefer left lateral chest radiographs to be hung as if they were taken in the right lateral position.

Extremities

Extremity radiographs are hung as if the viewer's eyes are the x-ray beam going through the radiographic image in the same manner that the photons went through the extremity when it was radiographed. If a PA right hand radiograph is viewed, it should be hung so the thumb is positioned toward the viewer's left side (Fig. 1–4). If the viewer places his/her the right hand against the radiograph in a PA projection, it should be aligned like the image of the hand on a radiograph that has been accurately hung (i.e., the thumb and fingers should appear in the same order). For a lateral right-hand radiograph, the palmar side of the hand should be directed toward the viewer's left side. This indicates that the medial (ulnar) side of the hand was positioned closer to the film and that the x-ray beam went from the lateral side of the patient's hand to the medial side. As long as the R or L marker is placed on extremity films correctly before the radiograph is taken, it will be demonstrated accurately when the radiograph is correctly hung on the view box.

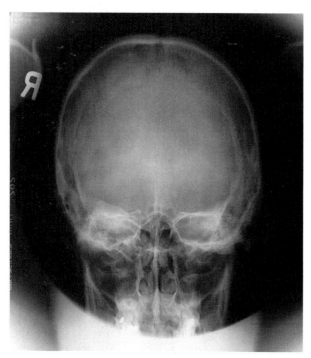

Figure 1-2. Accurately hung PA projection.

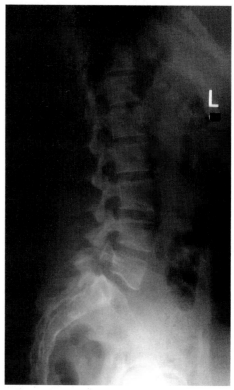

Figure 1-3. Accurately hung lateral position.

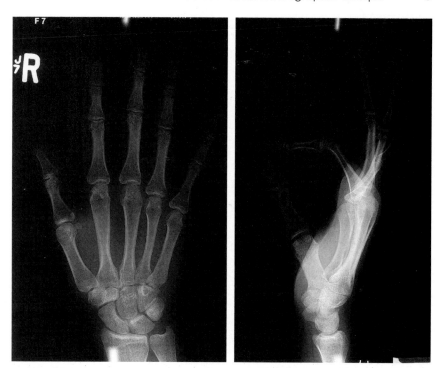

Figure 1-4. Accurately hung extremity radiograph.

RADIOGRAPHIC EVALUATION: THE RADIOGRAPHIC CRITIQUE FORM

Once a radiograph is correctly hung, it should be evaluated for positioning and technical accuracy. The evaluation should follow some consistent system or method, to ensure that all aspects of the radiograph are considered. The Radiographic Critique Form shown in Figure 1–5 contains a list of items that cover all the aspects of radiographic evaluation. For each item, several questions should be asked about a radiograph; these questions are presented and discussed in the remainder of this section. The answers to all the questions, when summarized, will determine whether the radiograph is acceptable. The form can be used as a checklist whenever you evaluate a radiograph.

The approach to radiographic evaluation outlined in Figure 1–5 is the approach taken in the "critique" sections of this book. You should take the time to review the general discussion of the critique items presented here, so as to understand the evaluation format used in the rest of the book. Each item listed in Figure 1–5, which represents a particular aspect of the evaluation, is shown here in **boldface**. It is followed by a list of the questions that should be asked about the radiograph in order to fully explore this aspect of the evaluation.

Facility's identification requirements—facility name, patient name and age, and examination time and date—are visualized on the radiograph.

1. Is the facility's name demonstrated on the radiograph?

Each radiograph should have the facility's name permanently photoflashed onto the film's emulsion. This information is routinely found within the identification (ID) plate and identifies ownership.

2. Are the patient's name and age visualized on the radiograph, and are they accurate?

The correct patient's name and age should be permanently photoflashed onto the film's emulsion. This information should be typed and legible. Evaluate all the radiographs within a routine series to ensure that the correct name has been exposed on each radiograph. Never assume that a radiograph has been correctly flashed. Always double-check. Flash cards can be easily switched or forgotten.

3. Are the examination time and date visualized on the radiograph?

The accuracy of exam time and date are necessary to distinguish the radiographs in a timed series and to match radiographs with their accompanying requisition and report.

4. Is the ID plate positioned so it does not obscure any anatomy of interest?

Evaluate the location of the ID plate on every radiograph. Has it obscured any anatomy of interest, or was it positioned in a place that is acceptable? By evaluating where the the ID plate is positioned on all radiographs taken, one can locate the best place to position the ID plate for future reference. When the film is positioned lengthwise, the ID plate is placed in the upper right or lower left corner. When the film is positioned crosswise, the ID plate is placed in the lower right or upper left corner. Some basic guidelines to follow when determining the best location to position the ID plate are: placing it outside the collimated field whenever possible, positioning it away from the direction the central ray is angled, and positioning it next to the narrowest anatomical structure.

RADIOGRAPHIC CRITIQUE FORM

Exam _____

_____ Facility's identification requirements—facility name, patient name, age, and hospital number, and exam time and date—are visualized on radiograph.

_____ Correct marker (e.g., R/L, arrow) is visualized on radiograph and demonstrates accurate placement.

_____ Required anatomy is present on radiograph.

_____ The relationships between the anatomical structures are accurate for the projection/position demonstrated.

_____ Maximum collimation efforts are evident on radiograph.

_____ Radiation protection is present on radiograph when indicated, and good radiation protection practices were used during procedure.

_____ Bony cortical outlines and/or soft tissue structures are sharply defined.

_____ Radiographic image is demonstrated without unwanted distortion.

_____ Correct film size has been used, and the film and anatomical structures have been accurately aligned.

_____ Correct image receptor system was used.

_____ Density and penetration are adequate to visualize the required bony and soft tissue structures.

_____ The radiographic contrast adequately visualizes the bony and soft tissue structures of interest.

_____ No preventable artifacts are present on the radiograph.

_____ The ordered procedure and the indication for the exam have been fulfilled.

_____ The requisition has been completed, and the repeat/reject analysis information has been provided as indicated by your facility.

Radiograph is: _____ **acceptable** _____ **unacceptable**

If radiograph is unacceptable, describe what measures should be taken to produce an acceptable radiograph. If radiograph is acceptable, but not optimal, describe any factors that could be adjusted to obtain an optimal radiograph.

Figure 1-5. Radiographic critique form.

Correct markers (R/L, arrow, etc.) are visualized on the radiograph and demonstrate accurate placement.

Lead markers are used to identify the patient's right and left sides, to indicate variations in the standard procedure, or to show the amount of time that has elapsed in timed procedures such as intravenous pyelography and small bowel studies. The markers are constructed of lead so as to be radiopaque (unable to be penetrated with x-radiation). Whenever a marker is placed on the cassette within the collimated light field, x-radiation will be unable to penetrate and fog the film. The result is a white image of the lead marker. To be consistent and to make the markers useful in hanging radiographs, place the markers on the cassette so they are correct and not reversed.

1. Is the marker visualized within the collimated field?

To ensure that the marker will be present on the radiograph, it must be positioned within the collimated light field so radiation will strike it. Place the markers on the cassette instead of on the tabletop or patient. This placement avoids marker distortion and magnification and prevents scattered radiation from crossing beneath the marker, fogging the area on the film where the marker would be visualized. It also prevents superimposition of the marker on the patient ID plate. Figure 1–6 demonstrates a marker that is undistorted and can be clearly seen as well as two examples of marker fogging, magnification, and distortion that resulted from placing the marker on the patient or tabletop instead of directly on the film.

When one is collimating within the size of the film used, it can be difficult to determine exactly where to place the marker on the cassette so it will remain within the collimated field and not obscure anatomical areas of interest. The best way of accomplishing this is to first collimate the desired amount and then use the collimator guide (Fig. 1–7) to determine how far from the film's midline to place the marker. Although different models of x-ray equipment have different collimator guides, the information displayed by all is identical. Each explains the film coverage one will have for the SID and amount of longitudinal and transverse collimation being used. If a 14 × 17 inch (35 × 43 cm) film is placed in the Bucky diaphragm at a set SID and the collimator guide indicates that you have collimated to an 8 × 17 inch (20 × 43 cm) field size, the marker should be placed 3.5 to 4 inches (10 cm) from the film's longitudinal midline in order to be included in the collimated field (Fig.

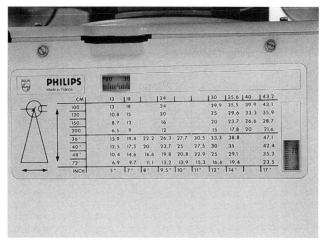

Figure 1-7. Collimator guide.

1–8). If the field was also longitudinally collimated, the marker would have to be positioned within this dimension as well. In the preceding example, if the collimator guide indicates that the longitudinal field is collimated to a 15-inch (38-cm) field size, the marker would have to be placed 7.5 inches (19 cm) from the film's transverse midline (see Fig. 1–8).

2. Is the marker positioned so it does not obscure areas of interest?

Usually, a film provides many areas in which to place the marker so it does not obscure needed information. Before taking a radiograph, you should imagine where the areas of interest will be located on it, and then situate the

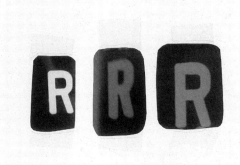

Figure 1-6. Marker magnification and distortion.

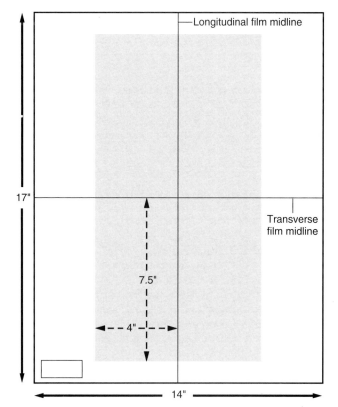

Figure 1-8. Marker placement for tightly collimated film.

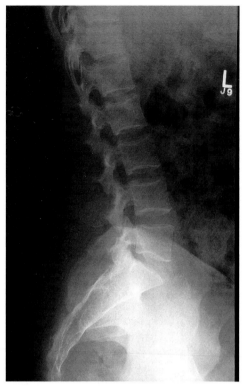

Figure 1-9. Marker placement for lateral position.

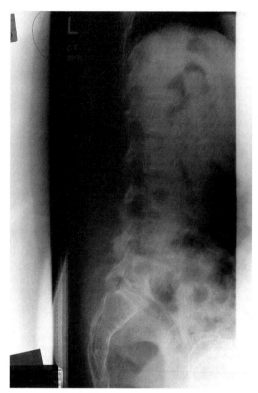

Figure 1-10. Poor marker placement in lateral position.

marker on the cassette where it is least likely to obscure anatomy of interest. Because the area of interest is most often located in the center of the collimated field, it is best to position markers as far away from the center of the film as possible.

3. Is the marker positioned in the best possible location for the projection/position being presented?

This question is best considered separately for each projection/position.

Anteroposterior and Posteroanterior Projections of the Torso, Vertebrae, and Cranium: For AP and PA projections, a right or left marker should be placed laterally within the collimated field on the side being marked. The patient's vertebral column is the dividing plane for the right and left sides. If you are marking the right side, position the R marker to the right of the vertebral column; if marking the left side, position the L marker to the left of the vertebral column (see Fig. 1-1).

Lateral Positions of the Torso, Vertebrae, and Cranium: When a patient is placed in a lateral position, the right or left marker placed on the cassette should indicate the side of the patient positioned closer to the radiographic film. If the patient's left side is positioned closer to the film for a lateral lumbar vertebrae, place an L marker on the cassette (Fig. 1-9). Whether the marker is placed anteriorly or posteriorly to the lumbar vertebrae does not affect the accuracy of the film's marking, although the images of markers placed posteriorly are often overexposed (Fig. 1-10).

Oblique Positions of the Torso, Vertebrae, and Cranium: In the oblique position, one side of the patient's body is situated closer to the film than the other

side. The marker placed on the cassette for the oblique position should identify the side of the patient that is positioned closer to the film and should be placed on the correct side of the patient. In a right anterior oblique (RAO) position, place an R marker on the cassette; for a left

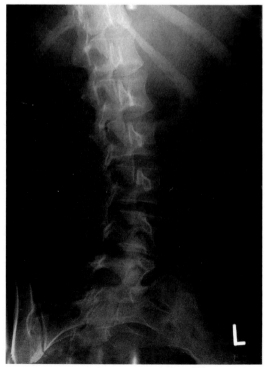

Figure 1-11. Marker placement for oblique position.

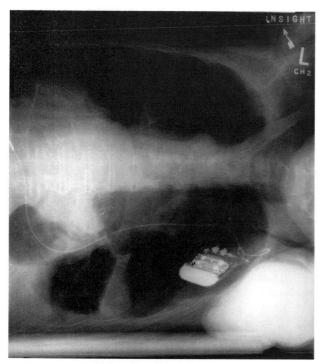

Figure 1-12. Marker placement for decubitus position.

posterior oblique (LPO) position, place an L marker on the cassette (Fig. 1–11). As with the AP/PA projections, the vertebral column is the plane used to divide the right and left sides of the body. For the right posterior oblique (RPO) position, place the R marker to the right of the vertebral column; for the left anterior oblique (LAO) position, place the L marker to the left of the vertebral column.

Lateral Decubitus Position of the Torso: Marking for the lateral decubitus position is identical to that for the AP/PA projection. Place an R marker to the right of the vertebral column when the right side is being identified, and an L marker to the left of the vertebral column when the left side is being identified. In this position, it is easier

to place the marker on the cassette and the marker will be better visualized if the side of the patient that is positioned up, away from the cart or tabletop the patient is lying on, is the side marked. Along with the right or left marker, use an arrow marker pointing up toward the ceiling to indicate which side of the patient is positioned away from the cart or tabletop (Fig. 1–12).

Projections and Positions of the Extremities: The marker placed on the cassette should identify the side of the patient being radiographed, an R marker to indicate the right side and an L marker to indicate the left side. When routine series of projections/positions for the fingers, hands, wrists, forearms, elbows, toes, feet, ankles, and lower legs are taken, more than one position is often placed on the same film. For such exams, it is necessary to mark only one of the positions placed on the film as long as they are all views of the same anatomical structure (Fig. 1–13). If positions of a right anatomical structure and its corresponding left are placed on the same film, mark both views with the correct R or L marker (Fig. 1–14). The only way to ensure that a marker will be demonstrated on the radiograph is to place it within the collimated light field and corresponding radiation field.

Projections and Positions of the Shoulder and Hips: The marker placed on the cassette for these radiographs should indicate the side of the patient being radiographed, an R marker for the patient's right side and an L marker to indicate the patient's left side (Fig. 1–15). It is best to place the marker laterally on AP/PA projections and oblique positions to prevent it from obscuring medial anatomical structures and to eliminate possible confusion about which side of the patient is being radiographed. Figure 1–16 demonstrates an AP hip radiograph with the marker placed medially. Because the marker is placed at the patient's midsagittal plane, the reviewer might conclude that the technologist was marking the other hip.

Lateral Cross-Table Radiography: When an exam is taken cross-table, as for a lateral shoulder or hip radiograph or to evaluate trauma to the vertebral column, position the marker anteriorly to prevent it from obscuring

Figure 1-13. Marker placement for unilateral extremity radiograph.

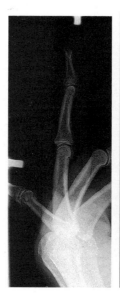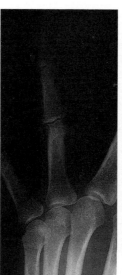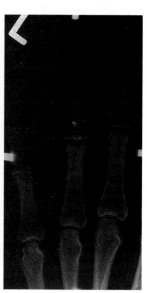

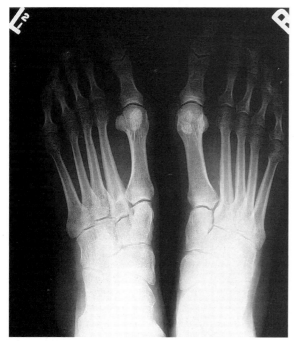

Figure 1-14. Marker placement for bilateral extremity radiograph.

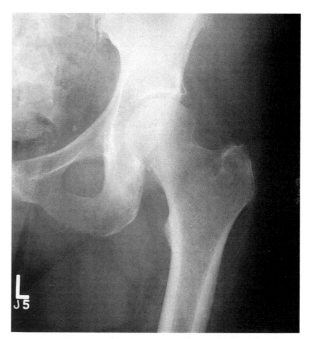

Figure 1-16. Poor marker placement on an AP projection of hip.

structures situated along the posterior edge of the film. The marker used should indicate the right or left side of the patient when the extremities, shoulder, or hip is radiographed (Fig. 1–17) and the side of the patient positioned closer to the film when the torso, vertebrae, or cranium is radiographed (see Fig. 1–9).

4. Double-check the marker for accuracy. Does the R or L marker correspond to the correct side of the patient?

Mismarking a radiograph can have many serious implications, including treatment of the incorrect anatomical structure. After a radiograph has been taken, evaluate it to determine whether the correct marker has been placed on

the radiograph. An R marker is visualized on the radiograph if the right side of the body was radiographed, and an L marker is visualized if the left side of the body was radiographed. This same evaluation should be done for the lateral position; is an R marker visualized if the right side of the patient was positioned closer to the film, or does an L marker visualize if the left side of the patient was placed closer to the film?

If both sides of the body are demonstrated on the same radiograph, as with an AP projection of the pelvis or abdomen, evaluate the film to ensure that an R marker is placed to the right of the vertebral column or an L marker is to the left of the vertebral column. This evaluation can be accomplished by using the patient ID plate. Begin by hanging the radiograph on the view box in the same manner as it was placed in the Bucky diaphragm. (For PA projections, hang the radiograph as if the patient's back is facing you. This is not the proper way to hang such a

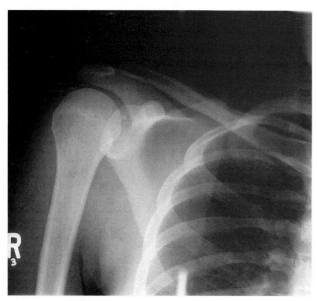

Figure 1-15. Marker placement for an AP projection of shoulder.

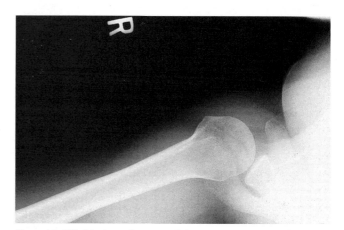

Figure 1-17. Marker placement for cross-table lateral radiograph.

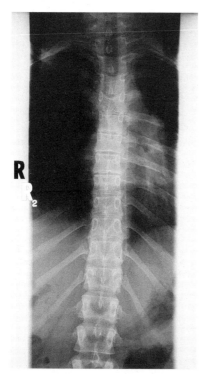

Figure 1-18. Faintly visible marker.

radiograph but is a method for determining marker accuracy.) The ID plate is in the lower right corner or the upper left corner on the radiograph. Then, position yourself as the patient was positioned in respect to the film. If the patient was in an AP projection, turn your back to the radiograph; if the patient was in a PA projection, face the radiograph. The marker on the radiograph should correspond to your right or left side: an R marker on your right side or an L marker on your left side.

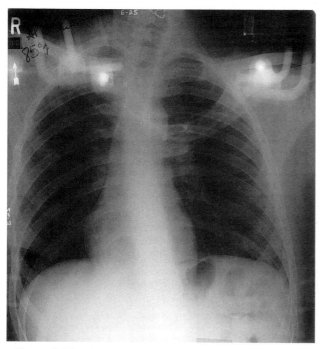

Figure 1-19. AP chest radiograph with accurate marking.

When a marker on a radiograph is only faintly visible, circle it and rewrite the information it displays next to it. *Do not* write the information over it (Fig. 1–18). If the R or L marker does not show up on the radiograph or the radiograph has been mismarked, it is best to repeat the radiograph. Do not guess or rely on what you may believe to be a ''sure'' sign. The heart shadow, which is normally located on the left side of the thorax, may be shifted toward the right because of a disease process (Fig. 1–19) or because the patient has situs inversus (total or partial reversal of the body organs).

When the radiographs presented in the critique sections of this book were photographed, the areas of importance were enlarged to better visualize the anatomy so positioning could be evaluated. Unfortunately, the enlargement often eliminated the markers that were placed on the radiographs. To prevent redundancy, I have not evaluated marker existence or placement on any of these radiographs, although this omission in no way is meant to decrease the importance of proper film marking. Use the guidelines presented in this section to evaluate marker placement on radiographs you critique.

Required anatomy is present on radiograph.

1. Is the anatomy required for this projection/position demonstrated on the radiograph?

For each projection/position a technologist radiographs, not only is the area of interest required on the radiograph, but a certain amount of the surrounding anatomy is also necessary. For example, because radiating wrist pain may be due to a distal forearm fracture, all wrist positions require that one fourth of the distal forearm be included with the wrist exam; a lateral ankle radiograph should include 1 inch (2.5 cm) of the fifth metatarsal base to rule out a Jones fracture. Become familiar with the anatomy to be included on each radiograph, as indicated in the critique section of this book, to avoid overcollimation or undercollimation and unnecessary repeats.

The relationships between the anatomical structures are accurate for the projection/position demonstrated.

1. Are the anatomical structures accurately displayed on the radiograph for the projection/position demonstrated, as indicated in the critique section of this book?

Evaluate each radiograph for proper anatomical alignment as defined in the radiographic critique sections of this book. Each projection/position that is described demonstrates a specific bony relationship, allowing a specific area of interest to be demonstrated. For example, an AP ankle radiograph demonstrates an open talotibial joint space (medial mortise), whereas the oblique view demonstrates an open talofibular joint space (lateral mortise), and the lateral view demonstrates the talar domes and soft tissue fat pads.

To align the anatomical structures correctly, it is necessary to demonstrate precise patient positioning and central ray alignment. How accurately the patient is placed in a true AP/PA, lateral, or oblique projection/position, whether the structure is properly flexed or extended, and how accurately the central ray is directed and centered in relation to the structure determines how properly the anatomy is aligned. Because few technologists carry protractors, there must be a method for them to determine whether the patient

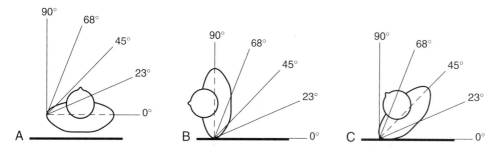

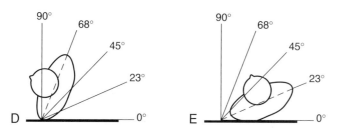

Figure 1-20. Estimating the degree of patient obliquity, viewing the patient's body from the top of the patient's head. See text for explanation.

is in a true AP/PA projection, lateral position, or specific degree of obliquity. For every projection/position described, an imaginary line (e.g., for the midsagittal or midcoronal plane, line connecting the humeral or femoral epicondyles) is given that can be used to align the patient with the film or tabletop. When the patient is in an AP/PA projection, the reference line should be aligned parallel (0-degree angle) with the film (Fig. 1–20A), and when the patient is in a lateral position, the reference line should be aligned perpendicular (90-degree angle) to the film (Fig. 1–20B). For a 45-degree oblique position, place the reference line halfway between the AP/PA projection and the lateral position (Fig. 1–20C); for a 68-degree oblique position, place the reference line halfway between the 45-degree and 90-degree angles (Fig. 1–20D); and for a 23-degree oblique position, place the reference line halfway between the 0-degree and 45-degree angles (Fig.1–20E). Even though these five angles are not the only angles used when a patient is positioned in radiography, they are easy to locate and can be used to estimate almost any other angle. For example, if a 60-degree oblique position is required, rotate the patient until the reference line is positioned at an angle slightly less than the 68-degree mark. I have used the torso to demonstrate this obliquity principle, but it can also be used for extremities. When an oblique position is required, always use the reference line to determine the amount of obliquity. Do not assume that a sponge will give you the correct angle. A 45-degree sponge may actually turn the patient more than 45 degrees if it is placed too far under the patient or if the patient's posterior or anterior soft tissue is thick.

For many exams, a precise degree of structure flexion or extension is required to adequately demonstrate the desired information. Technologists need to estimate the degree to which an extremity is flexed or extended when positioning the patient and when critiquing radiographs. When an extremity is in full extension, the degree of flexion is 0 (Fig. 1–21A), and when the two adjoining bones are aligned perpendicular to each other, the degree of flexion is 90

degrees (Fig. 1–21B). As described in the preceding discussion, the angle found halfway between full extension and 90 degrees is 45 degrees (Fig. 1–21C); the angle found halfway between the 45-degree and 90-degree angles is 68 degrees (Fig. 1–21D); and the angle found halfway between full extension and a 45-degree angle is 23 degrees (Fig. 1–21E). Because most flexible extremities flex beyond 90 degrees, the angles 113 and 135 degrees, as demonstrated in Figure 1–21F, should also be known.

Understanding how the central ray and the diverged x-ray beams shape the radiographic image is valuable knowledge that can be used to explain the causes of distortion. When the central ray is positioned perpendicular to the film and structure being radiographed, it is only at the center of the beam that the x-rays are aligned perpendicular. Away from the center of the beam, the x-rays that are used to record the image are diverged and expose the film at an angle (Fig. 1–22). The farther away from the central ray, the larger is the angle of divergence. Because of this beam shape, all anatomical structures that are aligned with the central ray are superimposed, whereas structures that are situated away from the central ray are distorted. The farther from the central ray the anatomical structures are placed, the more proximally (superiorly) or distally (inferiorly) they are projected (see Fig. 1–22).

To become familiar with all possibilities in positioning, it is best to study accurately and mispositioned radiographs simultaneously to correlate how patient and central ray positioning result in different anatomical relationships. Learn which structures lie anteriorly, posteriorly, medially, and laterally to one another, as well as the structures' movement capabilities. The more knowledgeable you become in this area, the easier it will be for you to determine how the patient or central ray mispositioning has resulted in a poorly positioned radiograph and how to prevent poor positioning under unusual circumstances.

2. How should the patient's positioning be adjusted before the radiograph is repeated?

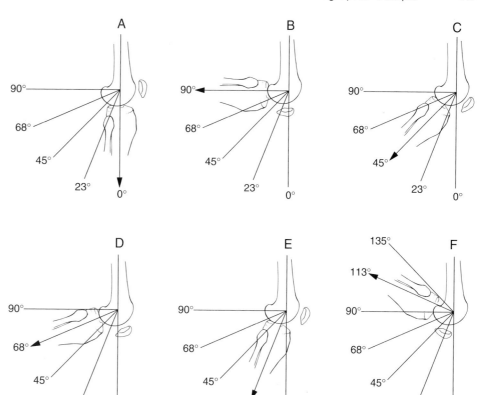

Figure 1-21. Estimating the degree of joint or extremity flexion. See text for explanation.

After it is determined that the relationships between the anatomical structures of the projection/position being evaluated are inaccurate, you must decide how the patient or central ray was mispositioned to obtain such a radiograph and how they should be adjusted to obtain accurate anatomical relationships. The guidelines and radiographs presented in the evaluation sections of this book for the projection/position being evaluated will help you in this decision. The most difficult structures to identify are those that are identical in shape and size, like the femoral condyles or talar domes. For these structures, three methods may be used to distinguish one of the structures from the other. The first method uses structures that surround the area of interest. For example, if a poorly positioned lateral ankle radiograph demonstrates inaccurate anteroposterior talar dome alignment and a closed tibiotalar joint space, one cannot view the joint space to determine which talar dome is anterior, but the relationship of the tibia and fibula can easily be used to deduce this information. The second method uses bony projections such as tubercles to identify one of the similar structures. For example, the medial femoral condyle can be distinguished from the lateral condyle on a lateral knee radiograph by locating the adductor tubercle that is situated on the medial condyle (Fig. 1–23). The third method of identifying a structure follows the rule that the anatomical structure situated farthest from the film is magnified the most (Fig. 1–24). On a left lateral chest radiograph, the right posterior ribs are situated posterior to the left because they are positioned farther from the film and are more magnified.

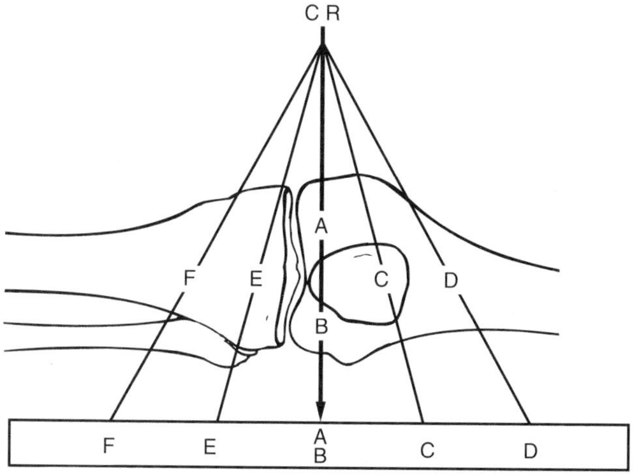

To reposition the patient for a repeat radiograph, begin by returning the patient to the original position; then adjust the patient the needed amount from this position. It is not wise to reposition the patient without starting at the original position, because to do so often results in too much or too little adjustment. Because you should start from the original position, it is important to pay close attention to the patient and central ray positioning prior to taking the initial radiograph. It is also best to use palpable anatomical structures to position the patient so that the same structures can be used to realign the patient if a repeat is required.

Figure 1-22. Effect of central ray placement on anatomical alignment.

3. How much adjustment from the patient's original position is needed?

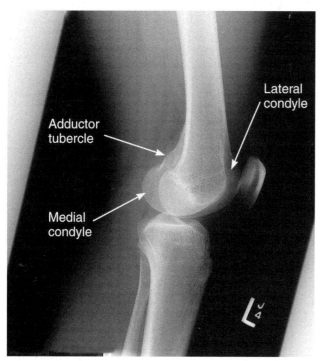

Figure 1-23. Poorly positioned lateral knee radiograph with the medial condyle posterior.

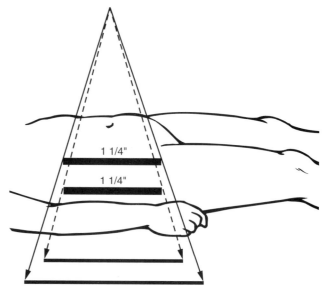

Figure 1-24. The part farthest from the film will magnify the most.

How much adjustment from the original position is needed depends on how far from accurate the anatomy is on the mispositioned radiograph. The most common adjustments are changing the patient's positioning and changing the degree of central ray angulation. When patient positioning needs to be adjusted, the amount of adjustment required is determined by the amount of distance demonstrated between specific anatomical structures and how these structures move toward or away from each other when the patient's position is adjusted.

If two structures are demonstrated without superimposition on a mispositioned radiograph, and if they should be superimposed on an accurately positioned radiograph of this projection/position, the amount of patient adjustment needed is half the distance demonstrated between the two structures that should be superimposed. For example, if on a mispositioned lateral knee radiograph, the femoral condyles are demonstrated with the lateral condyle situated anterior to the medial condyle, measure the distance between the anterior surfaces of the condyles to determine how much positioning adjustment is needed to properly superimpose the condyles (Fig. 1–23). To improve this misposition, rotate the patient's patella closer to the film, causing the medial condyle to rotate anteriorly and the lateral condyle to rotate posteriorly. Because the condyles rotate toward each other, the amount of adjustment needed is only half the distance that was demonstrated between the two condylar surfaces on the mispositioned radiograph.

If two structures are superimposed on a mispositioned radiograph and they should not be on an accurately positioned radiograph of this projection/position, the amount of patient adjustment needed to obtain accurate positioning is half the distance demonstrated between where the structures are and where they should be. For example, an

accurately positioned oblique ankle radiograph demonstrates the talus and fibula without superimposition and an open talofibular joint space. If the ankle is not rotated enough, the talus superimposes the fibula and obscures the talofibular joint space (Fig. 1–25). To determine how much to increase ankle obliquity from the original position in order to obtain an open talofibular joint, measure the amount of talar and fibular superimposition; then increase ankle obliquity by half of this measurement.

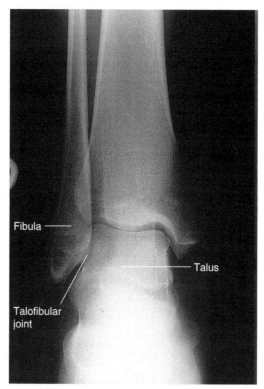

Figure 1-25. Poorly positioned oblique ankle radiograph with a closed talofibular joint.

When the central ray angulation needs to be adjusted to improve anatomical relationships on a mispositioned radiograph, the amount of adjustment needed depends on (1) the distance demonstrated between two structures that should be superimposed, (2) the amount of superimposition demonstrated between two structures that should be seen without superimposition, and (3) the object–image distances (OIDs) of the structures of interest. How much the central ray angulation will project two structures away from each other depends on the difference in the distances from the structures to the film. Note in Figure 1–26 that point A is farther from the film than point B. Even though point A is aligned with point B, an angled central ray used to record these two images would project point A farther inferiorly than point B. On an AP ''open-mouth'' projection of the dens, a 5-degree angulation moves the upper incisors in reference to the occipital bone about 1 inch (2.5 cm); on a lateral knee position, a 5-degree angulation moves the medial condyle in reference to the lateral condyle only 0.25 inch (0.6 cm). There is about 5 inches (12.5 cm) between the upper incisors and occipital skull base, but there is only about 2.5 inches (6.25 cm) between the medial and lateral condyles. When applicable, refer to the evaluation sections of this book for guidelines on the amount of angulation required to project structures a determined distance.

Maximum collimation efforts are evident on radiograph.

1. Is there evidence of a collimated border on all four sides of the image?

Good collimation practices are necessary to decrease the radiation dosage by limiting the amount of patient tissue exposed and to improve the visibility of recorded details and the radiographic contrast by reducing the amount of scattered radiation that reaches the film. As a general rule,

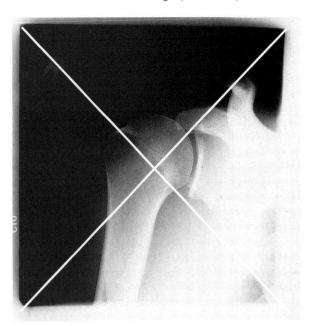

Figure 1–27. Using collimated borders to locate film center.

each radiograph should demonstrate a small collimated border around the entire image of interest. The only time this rule does not apply is when the entire film must be used to prevent clipping of needed anatomy, as in chest and abdominal radiography. This collimated border not only demonstrates good collimation practices but also can be used to determine the exact location of central ray placement. Make an imaginary X on the radiograph by diagonally connecting the corners of the collimated border (Fig. 1–27). The center of the X indicates the central ray placement for the radiograph.

Accurate placement of the central ray and alignment of the long axis of the part with the collimator's longitudinal light line are two positioning practices that will aid in obtaining tight collimation. When collimating, do not allow the collimator's light field to mislead you into believing you have collimated more tightly than you actually have. When the collimator's central ray indicator is positioned on the patient's torso and the collimator is set to a predetermined width and length, the light field demonstrated on the patient's torso does not represent the true width and length of the field set on the collimator. This is because x-rays (and the collimator light if the patient was not in the way) continue to diverge as they move through the torso to the film, increasing the field size as they do so (Fig. 1–28). The thicker the part being radiographed, the smaller the collimator's light field that appears on the patient's skin surface. On very thick patients, it is often difficult to collimate the needed amount when the light field appears so small, but on these patients, tight collimation demonstrates the largest improvement in the visibility of the recorded details.

Learn to use the collimator guide to determine the actual film coverage. For example, when an AP lumbar vertebrae radiograph is taken, the transversely collimated field should be reduced to an 8-inch (20-cm) field size. Because greater soft tissue thickness has nothing to do with an increase in the size of the skeletal structure, the transverse field should

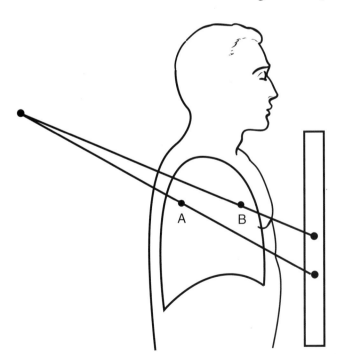

Figure 1–26. Upon angulation, the part farthest from the film is projected the most.

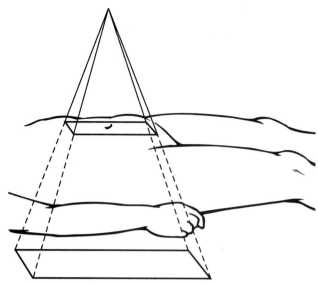

Figure 1-28. Collimator light field versus film coverage.

still be reduced when one is radiographing a thick patient. Accurately center the patient by using the centering light field, then set the transverse collimation length to 8 inches by using the collimator guide. Be confident that the film coverage will be sufficient even though the light field appears small.

2. Have you collimated to the patient's skin-line on all extremity, chest, and abdominal radiographs?

All extremity radiographs should demonstrate the colli-

mated borders positioned next to the skin-line of the thickest area of interest. Figure 1–29 shows an AP forearm radiograph. Note that the transversely collimated borders are adjacent to the elbow, the thickest area of the forearm.

Often, chest and abdominal radiographs show very little collimation because the entire film is needed to demonstrate the required anatomy. Whenever a small patient is radiographed, however, collimated borders should be demonstrated adjacent to the patient's skin-line (Fig. 1–30).

On some x-ray equipment, the collimator head can be rotated without rotating the entire tube column. This capability allows the technologist to increase collimation on anatomical structures such as the humerus and clavicle, which are not aligned directly with the longitudinal or transverse axes of the light field. Rotating just the collimator head does not affect the alignment of the beam with the grid; this alignment is affected only when the tube column is rotated.

3. Have you collimated to the specific anatomy desired on radiographs involving structures within the torso?

When radiographing a specific body structure within the torso, bring the collimated borders as close to the structure as possible. Use palpable anatomical structures around the area of interest to determine how close the borders are coming to the structure of interest. For the AP sacral radiograph shown in Figure 1–31, for example, the longitudinally collimated field was closed to the palpable symphysis pubis because the sacrum is located superior to the symphysis pubis on an accurately positioned sacral radiograph, and the transversely collimated field was closed to the palpable anterior superior iliac spines because the sacrum is located medial to them.

4. Are all required anatomical structures visualized on the radiograph?

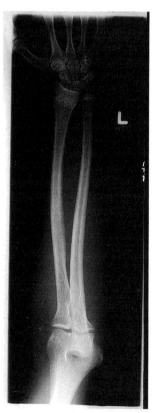

Figure 1-29. Proper "to skin-line" collimation on an AP forearm radiograph.

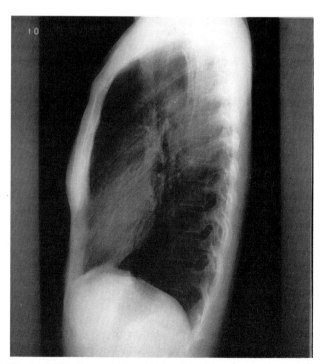

Figure 1-30. Proper "to skin-line" collimation on a lateral chest radiograph.

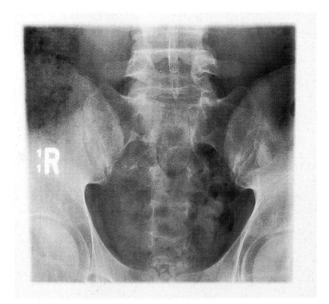

Figure 1-31. Proper collimation on an AP sacral radiograph.

Evaluate all radiographs to determine whether the required anatomical structures have been included. Poor centering or overcollimation can result in the clipping of required anatomy (Fig. 1–32).

Clipping of required anatomy can also result from overcollimation on a structure that is not placed in direct contact with the film, such as for a lateral third or fourth finger or lateral hand radiograph. Clipping occurs because the divergence of the x-ray beam has not been taken into consideration during collimation. To prevent clipping, view

the shadow of the object projected onto the cassette by the collimator light (Fig. 1–33). It will be magnified. This magnification is similar to the magnification the x-ray beam undergoes when creating the image. Allow the collimated field to remain open enough to include the shadow of the object, ensuring that the object will be shown in its entirety on the radiograph.

When the radiographs presented in the critique sections of this book were photographed, the areas of importance were enlarged to better visualize the anatomy so positioning could be evaluated. Unfortunately, this has eliminated the collimated borders. To prevent redundancy, I have not evaluated the collimation on any of these radiographs, but this decision in no way is meant to decrease the importance of proper collimation. Use the guidelines presented in this section to judge the adequacy of collimation on radiographs you evaluate.

Radiation protection is present on radiograph when indicated, and good radiation protection practices were used during procedure.

Proper gonadal shielding practices have proved to reduce radiation exposure of the female gonads by about 50 percent and of the male gonads by about 90 to 95 percent.[1] In spite of these statistics, children and adults are radiographed without proper shielding, even when its use would not cover information if properly applied. Gonadal shielding is often skipped because of the fear of mispositioning and covering up pelvic bone information. The assumption is that the patient will receive less radiation if the exam is taken without the shield than if it had to be repeated because the shield covered pelvic information. This is not a good argument. As professional technologists, we must always strive to improve our skills and to develop better ways to ensure good patient care in our facilities while obtaining good radiographs. All radiographs should be evaluated for the accuracy of gonadal shielding. It is by

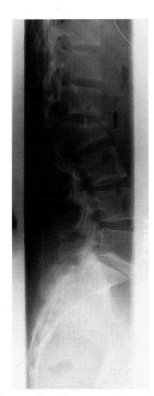

Figure 1-32. Poor collimation on a lateral lumbar vertebral radiograph.

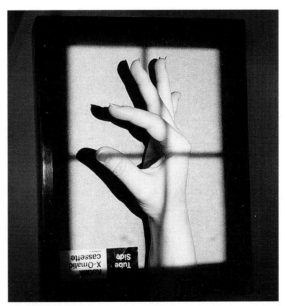

Figure 1-33. Viewing an object's shadow to determine proper collimation.

studying our shielding habits that we will learn to improve and perfect them.

1. Is gonadal shielding evident and accurately positioned on male and female patients when the gonads are within the primary beam and shielding is therefore indicated?

Gonadal Shielding in the AP Projection

Female Patient: Shielding the gonads of the female patient for an AP radiograph of the pelvis, hip, or lumbar vertebrae requires more precise positioning of the shield to prevent obscuring pertinent information. The first step in understanding how to properly shield an adult female is to know which organs should be shielded and their location. These organs are the ovaries, uterine (fallopian) tubes, and uterus. The uterus is found at the patient's midline, superior to the bladder. It is about 3 inches (7.5 cm) in length; its inferior aspect begins at the level of the symphysis pubis, and it extends anterosuperiorly. The uterine tubes are bilateral, beginning at the superolateral angles of the uterus and extending to the lateral sides of the pelvis. Tucked between the lateral side of the pelvis and the uterus and inferior to the uterine tubes are the ovaries. The exact level at which the uterus, uterine tubes, and ovaries are found varies from patient to patient.[2] Figures 1–34 and 1–35 show radiographs from two different hysterosalpingograms. Notice the variation in the location of the uterus, uterine tubes, and ovaries in these two patients. Because the location of these organs within the inlet pelvis cannot be determined with certainty, the entire inlet pelvis should be shielded to ensure that all the reproductive organs have been protected.

To properly shield the female gonad, use a flat contact shield made from at least 1 mm of lead and cut to the shape of the inlet pelvis (Fig. 1–36). Oddly shaped and male (triangular) shields do not effectively protect the female patient (Fig. 1–37). The dimensions of the shield used should be varied according to the amount of magnification the shield will demonstrate, which is determined by

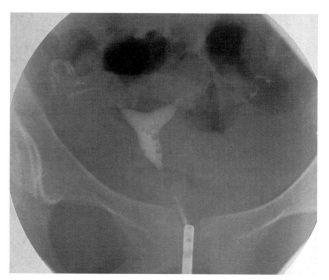

Figure 1-35. Hysterosalpingogram.

the OID, as well as the size of the patient's pelvis, which increases from infancy to adulthood. Each department should have different-sized contact shields for variations in female pelvic sizes for infants, toddlers, adolescents, and young adults.

To position the shield on the patient, place the narrower end of the shield just superior to the symphysis pubis, and allow the wider end of the shield to lay superiorly, over the reproductive organs. Side-to-side centering can be evaluated by placing an index finger just medial to each anterior superior iliac spine. The sides of the shield should be placed at equal distances from the index fingers. It may be wise to tape the shield to the patient. Patient motion such as breathing may cause the shield to shift to one side, inferiorly, or superiorly.

Male Patient: The reproductive organs that are to be shielded on the male are the testes, which are found within the scrotal pouch. The testes are located along the midsagittal plane inferior to the symphysis pubis. Shielding the testes of a male patient for an AP radiograph of the pelvis or hip requires more specific placement of the lead shield to avoid obscuring areas of interest. For these exams, a flat contact shield made from vinyl and 1 mm of lead should be cut out in the shape of a right triangle (one angle being 90 degrees). Round the 90-degree corner on this triangle. Place the shield on the adult patient with the rounded corner beginning about 1 to 1.5 inches (2.5 to 4 cm) inferior to the palpable superior symphysis pubis. When accurately positioned, the shield frames the inferior outlines of the symphysis pubis and inferior ramus and extends inferiorly until the entire scrotum is covered (Fig. 1–38). Each department should have different-sized male contact shields for the variations in male pelvic sizes for infants, youths, adolescents, and young adults.

Gonadal Shielding in the Lateral Position: Male and Female Patients:
When male and female patients are radiographed in the lateral position use gonadal shielding whenever (1) the gonads are within the primary radiation field and (2) shielding will not cover pertinent information. In the lateral position, male and female patients can be similarly shielded with a large flat contact

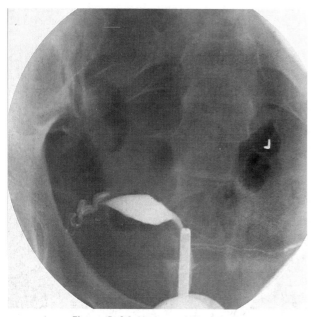

Figure 1-34. Hysterosalpingogram.

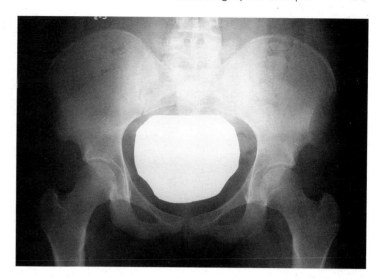

Figure 1-36. Proper gonadal shielding in the female.

shield or the straight edge of a lead apron. Begin by palpating the patient's coccyx and elevated anterior superior iliac spine (ASIS). Next, draw an imaginary line connecting the coccyx with a point 1 inch posterior to the ASIS, and position the longitudinal edge of a large flat contact shield or half-lead apron anteriorly against this imaginary line (Fig. 1–39). This shielding method can be safely used on patients being radiographed for lateral vertebral, sacral, or coccygeal radiographs without fear of obscuring areas of interest (Fig. 1–40).

2. Were radiation protection measures used for patients whose radiosensitive cells were positioned within 2.5 inches of the primary beam?

Shielding of radiosensitive cells should be done whenever they lie within 2.5 inches (5 cm) of the primary beam.[1] *Radiosensitive cells* are the eyes, thyroid, breasts, and gonads. To protect these areas, place a flat contact shield constructed of vinyl and 1 mm of lead or the straight edge of a lead apron over the area you want protected. Because the atomic number of lead is so high, radiation used in the diagnostic range will be readily absorbed within the shield.

3. Was tight collimation used?

Tight collimation reduces the radiation exposure of anatomical structures that are not required on the radiograph. Its use on chest radiography will reduce exposure of the patient's thyroid; on a cervical vertebral radiograph, it will reduce exposure of the eyes; on a thoracic vertebrae radiograph, it will reduce exposure of the breasts; and on a hip radiograph, it will reduce exposure of the gonads. Even when radiation protection efforts are not demonstrated on the radiograph, good patient care standards dictate their use.

4. Are any anatomical artifacts demonstrated on the radiograph?

Anatomical artifacts are anatomical structures of the patient or x-ray personnel that are demonstrated on the radiograph but should not be there. An example of such an artifact is shown in Figure 1–41. Notice how the patient's other hand was used to help maintain the position. This is not an acceptable practice. Many sponges and other positioning tools are available to adequately position and immobilize the patient. Whenever the hands of the patient

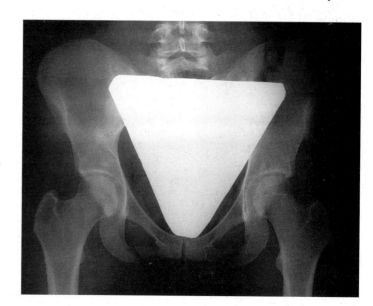

Figure 1-37. Poor gonadal shielding in the female.

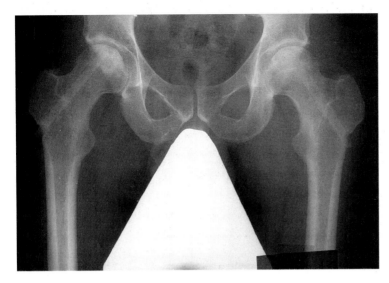

Figure 1-38. Proper gonadal shielding in the male.

or x-ray personnel must be within the radiation field, they must be properly attired with lead gloves.

5. *Were personnel who remained in the room during the exposure given protective clothing?*

All personnel and family members should be asked to leave the room before the radiographic exposure is made. If the patient cannot be left alone in the room during the exposure, lead protection clothing such as aprons, thyroid shields, glasses, and gloves should be worn by the personnel during any radiographic exposures. They should also be asked to stand as far from the primary beam as possible.

Bony cortical outlines and/or soft tissue structures are sharply defined.

1. *Was a small focal spot used when indicated?*

Using a small focal spot provides a radiograph with more recorded detail sharpness than using a large focal spot. A small focal spot should be used when small recorded details such as the bony trabecular patterns on extremities are of interest. Compare the trabecular patterns on the ankle radiographs in Figures 1–42 and 1–43. Figure 1–42 was taken using a large focal spot, and Figure 1–43 was taken using a small focal spot. Notice how utilizing a small focal spot increases the visibility of the bony trabeculae.

Today's radiographic equipment allows a small focal spot to be chosen for many high radiation exposures. On a phototimed exam the milliamperage (mA) used by the equipment is low when a small focal spot is chosen, resulting in the need for a long exposure time to obtain the

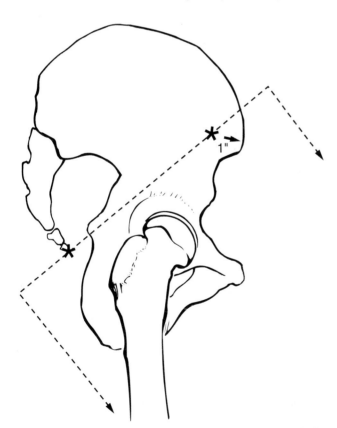

Figure 1-39. Gonadal shielding for the lateral position in both male and female.

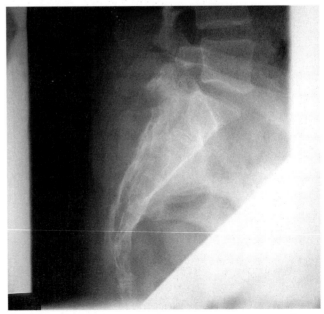

Figure 1-40. Proper gonadal shielding in the lateral position.

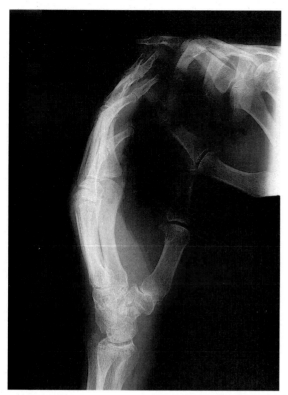

Figure 1-41. Poor radiation protection. See text for explanation.

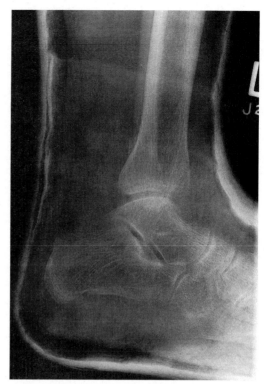

Figure 1-43. Recorded detail using small focal spot.

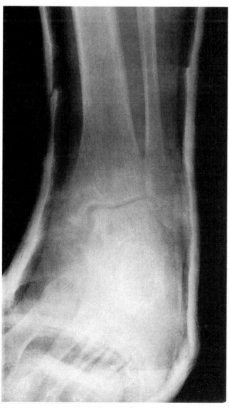

Figure 1-42. Recorded detail using large focal spot.

density required to adequately visualize the torso structures. Long exposure times often result in the demonstration of patient motion on the radiograph. One should weigh the expected exposure time and the possibility of motion against the advantages gained by choosing a small focal spot. If the patient's thickness measurement is large or the patient's ability to hold still is not reliable, you might consider choosing a large focal spot and high milliamperage.

2. Does the radiograph demonstrate signs of unwanted patient motion or unhalted respiration?

Motion on a radiograph is most often caused by patient movement during the exposure. This movement can be voluntary or involuntary. *Voluntary motion* is the patient's breathing or otherwise moving during the exposure. It can be controlled by explaining to the patient the importance of holding still, making the patient as comfortable as possible on the radiographic table, using the shortest possible exposure time, and employing immobilization devices. Radiographically, voluntary motion can be identified by blurred bony cortical outlines (Fig. 1– 44). *Involuntary motion* is movement the patient cannot control, such as peristaltic activity of the stomach and small or large intestine. The only means of decreasing the blur caused by involuntary motion is to use the shortest possible exposure time, which in some cases is not good enough. Radiographically, involuntary motion can be identified by sharp bony cortices and blurry gastric and intestinal gases (Fig. 1– 45). There are times when normal voluntary motions such as breathing or shaking can become involuntary motions. For example, an unconscious patient is unable to control breathing, and a patient with severe trauma may be unable to control shivering.

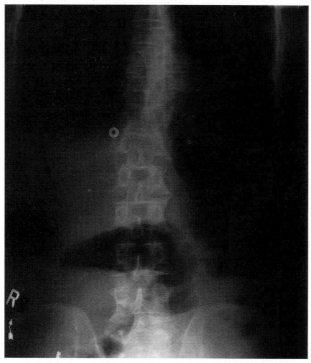

Figure 1-44. Voluntary patient motion during radiography.

second exposure. Another indication of a double-exposed radiograph is its density. Because the same film was exposed twice, the resulting radiographic density is higher than on a radiograph that was exposed only once.

3. Does the anatomy of interest demonstrate the least possible amount of magnification?

Magnification of an anatomical structure reduces its recognizability and blurs the recorded details. To prevent magnification, the anatomical structure of interest should always be positioned as close to the film as possible.

4. Was a detail screen used when indicated?

Departments often have more than one receptor system to choose from. A detail screen system should be used on all extremity work to increase the recognizability of the recorded details. Compare the trabecular patterns on the hand radiographs in Figures 1–47 and 1–48. Figure 1–47 was taken using a low-speed, detail screen, but Figure 1–48 was taken using a faster-speed, nondetail screen. Notice how utilizing a detail screen increased the visibility of the bony trabeculae.

5. Is there evidence of poor film-screen contact?

Poor film-screen contact will result if a foreign object was wedged between the film and the screen or if the cassette is damaged or warped. Radiographically, poor film-screen contact is demonstrated by a blurred image only in the area where the film and screen are not making direct contact. Figure 1–49 demonstrates an oblique hand radiograph. Note how the hand image is sharp everywhere except at the second and third digits. Because it would be impossible for these two fingers to move without causing the rest of the hand to also move, it can be concluded that this blurring is a result not of patient motion but of poor film-screen contact. The screen should be thoroughly cleaned and tested on a phantom. If the test radiograph does not demonstrate improved film-screen contact, the cassette should be replaced.

A double-exposed radiograph will also appear blurry and can easily be mistaken for patient motion (Fig. 1–46). When evaluating a blurry radiograph, look at the cortical outlines of bony structures that are lying longitudinally and transversely. Is there only one cortical outline to represent each bony structure, or are there two? Is one outline lying slightly above or to the side of the other? If one outline is demonstrated, the patient moved during the exposure, but if two are demonstrated, the radiograph was exposed twice, and the patient was in a slightly different position for the

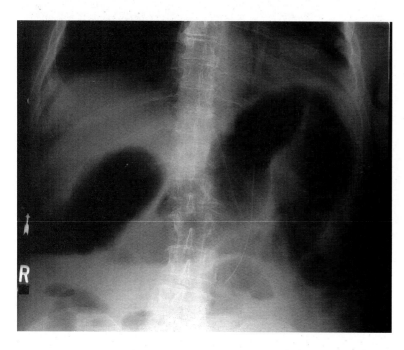

Figure 1-45. Involuntary patient motion during radiography.

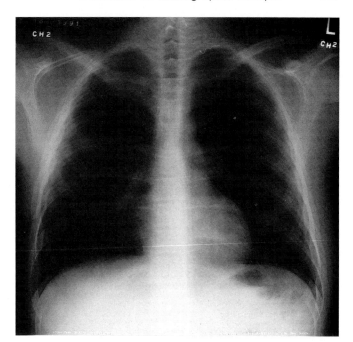

Figure 1-46. Double exposure of chest.

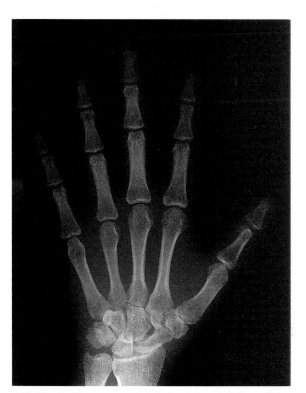

Figure 1-47. Recorded detail using a detail screen.

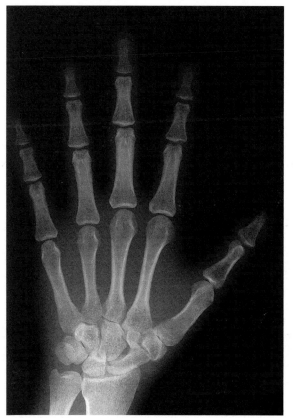

Figure 1-48. Recorded detail using a high-speed screen.

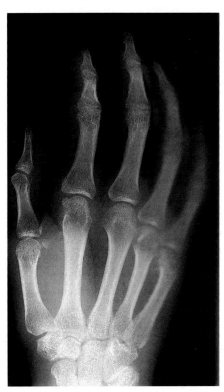

Figure 1-49. Poor film-screen contact.

Radiographic image is demonstrated without unwanted distortion.

1. Does your image demonstrate the structures as required in the critique sections of this book?

Because (1) no radiograph is taken with the part situated directly on the film, (2) no anatomical structure radiographed is flat, and (3) not all structures are radiographed with a straight beam, all radiographic images demonstrate some type of distortion. The distortion is either in size or in shape. The amount of size distortion, or magnification, depends on how far each structure is from the film. The farther away the part is situated, the more magnified the structure will be (see Fig. 1–24). *Size distortion* is represented when all axes of a structure have been equally magnified. Size distortion also results when the same structure, situated at the same OID, is radiographed at a different SID.

When an object is *shape distorted,* one of its axes has been elongated or foreshortened but the other has remained unaffected. Unwanted shape distortion can result from improper angling of the central ray, improper alignment of the part being radiographed with the film, or poor central ray placement.

Whether a distorted or nondistorted image is desired depends on what particular anatomical structure is being evaluated and how this structure is aligned with the surrounding structures. For example, to demonstrate the scaphoid without foreshortening, you must angle the central ray, thereby distorting the carpal bones that surround the scaphoid. To demonstrate the foramen magnum, dorsum sellae, and occipital bone in the AP axial projection of the cranium, you must distort the rest of the cranial and facial

bones. Yet you must not distort the acromioclavicular joints by positioning the central ray differently between the ''with weights'' and ''without weights'' radiographs, or a false diagnosis about separation may result. Refer to the evaluation sections of this book to determine whether your radiograph has demonstrated the desired anatomical structures properly.

Correct film size has been used, and the film and anatomical structures have been accurately aligned.

1. Was the film positioned crosswise (CW) or lengthwise (LW) correctly to accommodate required anatomy?

Evaluate your radiograph to determine whether all the required anatomy has been included. Deciding whether to place the film CW or LW is a simple matter of positioning it so that all the required anatomy can easily be demonstrated on the film. If the film is placed CW for an adult forearm radiograph, the film will not be long enough to accommodate the wrist and elbow joints on the same film. This is why adult forearm radiographs are taken with the film aligned lengthwise.

2. Was the film positioned CW or LW correctly to accommodate the patient's body habitus?

One needs to be aware of the three basic body types when positioning a patient for a PA/AP chest or AP abdominal radiograph: hypersthenic, sthenic, and asthenic. The *hypersthenic* patient has a wide, short thorax and a broad peritoneal cavity with a high diaphragm (Fig. 1–50). This body type requires the film to be placed CW for PA/AP chest radiographs in order to include the entire lung field and requires two CW films to be used for an AP abdominal radiograph in order to demonstrate the entire peritoneal cavity. The *asthenic* patient has a long, narrow thoracic cavity and a narrow peritoneal cavity with a lower diaphragm (Fig. 1–51). The *sthenic* body type is between the hypersthenic and asthenic body types (Fig. 1–52). Both the asthenic and sthenic body types require the film to be placed LW for the PA/AP chest and AP abdominal radiographs in order to include the entire lung field and peritoneal cavity, respectively.

3. Was the smallest possible film used, and were as many projections/positions as possible placed on the same film without overlap?

With the rising cost of health care, we must do whatever we can to reduce the cost of radiographic procedures. Choosing the correct film size for an exam and, when possible, placing more than one view on the same film are part of cost efficiency. How the film is placed (LW or CW) often dictates how many views can be placed on the film. For example, a 10 × 12 inch (24 × 30 cm) film placed crosswise can accommodate three views of the wrist, but the same size film placed lengthwise has space available for only two views.

Always evaluate the size of the film used and how you have chosen to place your radiographic series on a film to determine whether there is a more efficient way to use film space.

4. If more than one projection / position is placed on the same radiograph, were they all aligned in the same direction?

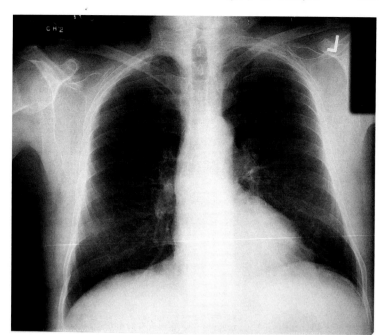

Figure 1-50. Chest radiograph of hypersthenic patient.

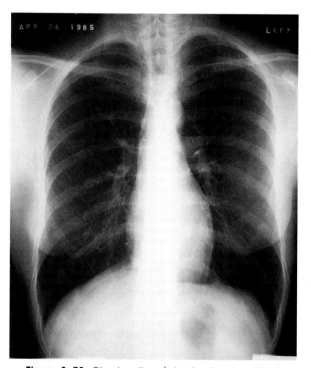

Figure 1-51. Chest radiográph of asthenic patient.

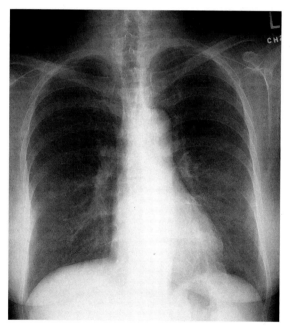

Figure 1-52. Chest radiograph of sthenic patient.

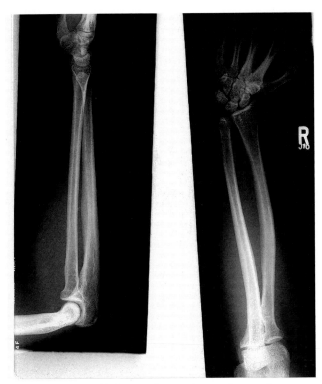

Figure 1-53. Proper film-anatomy alignment.

When you are radiographing an extremity and more than one projection/position is placed on the same radiograph, similar anatomical structures should be located at the same end of the radiograph. For example, when the AP and lateral views of the forearm are placed on the same 14 × 17 inch (35 × 43 cm) film, the elbows in the two views are to be demonstrated at the same end of the radiograph (Fig. 1–53). Failure to keep this alignment makes hanging and viewing of the radiograph difficult (Fig. 1–54).

Correct image receptor system was used.

1. Have you chosen the correct image receptor system for the body part being radiographed?

Receptor systems are chosen for their ability to demonstrate fine recorded details or for their speed. The more details a system can demonstrate, the less speed the system has, and consequently the more radiation exposure is needed to obtain adequate density.

Use low-speed, detail screen for most extremity exams. This system is for tabletop work only and should not be used when a grid is employed or when a thick body part is being radiographed. Use a medium-speed system when the detail capability provides little benefit. For example, hands and feet can have hairline fractures that may be visualized only on a detail screen; because a fracture of the femoral bone is very obvious, however, we do not need to see small details to identify it. Use a high-speed system on exams such as those taken for scoliosis, in which the bony cortical outlines are all that need to be visualized for measurements to be taken. Such a system should not be used when information about the structure itself is desired.

Density and penetration are adequate to visualize the required bony and soft tissue structures.

1. Does the radiograph adequately demonstrate the bony trabeculae and soft tissue structures of interest?

Study the area of interest on each radiograph to determine whether it demonstrates adequate density and penetration. Radiographic density is regulated primarily by the milliampere-seconds (mAs) used, whereas penetration is regulated by the kilovoltage peak (kVp) used. When adequate mAs is used, the bony trabecular patterns and soft tissue structures of interest are demonstrated. When the correct kVp is used, the bony cortical outlines are clearly visualized, the contrast scale is acceptable, and the amount of scattered radiation is not excessive.

To determine the amount of scattered radiation a radiograph has, inspect the area of the film directly outside the collimated borders. This area has no image, but fogging from the production of scattered radiation is present. Study radiographs of all anatomical structures that are adequately exposed and penetrated to familiarize yourself with the amount of scattered fogging that this area of the film routinely receives. Use this knowledge to identify when this area has excessive fogging. On extremity radiographs, there is very little if any fogging in this area, but radiographs of the torso and cranium demonstrate higher amounts of fogging.

2. Is the image on the radiograph overexposed or underexposed?

When a radiograph is *overexposed* (too much mAs used), it demonstrates density that is so dark the bony and soft tissue structures of interest are not well visualized. On such a radiograph, the radiographic contrast is acceptable, although on some overexposed radiographs, it is difficult to evaluate the contrast, because all the structures are too

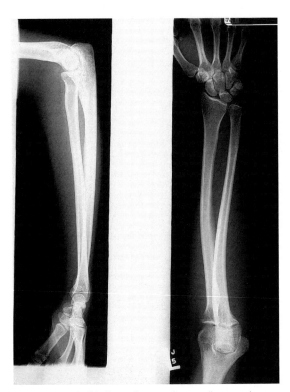

Figure 1-54. Poor film-anatomy alignment.

dark and the amount of scattered fogging demonstrated outside the collimated borders is what would be expected for that anatomical structure. Figure 1–55 demonstrates an overexposed AP sacral radiograph.

An *underexposed* radiograph (not enough mAs used) demonstrates density so light that the bony trabecular patterns cannot be evaluated. Usually on light radiographs, unless underexposure is extreme, the demonstration of the soft tissue structures is better. One way to distinguish whether a radiograph has been underexposed or underpenetrated is to study the bony cortical outlines of the structures of interest. On a radiograph that has been underexposed, the cortical outlines are visible, even though their density is light. Figure 1–56 demonstrates an underexposed AP thoracic vertebrae.

3. Is the image on the radiograph overpenetrated or underpenetrated?

A radiograph that has been adequately penetrated demonstrates the cortical outlines of the thinnest and thickest bony structures of interest with high contrast. If the anatomical structure of interest has been *overpenetrated* (too much kVp used), the radiograph demonstrates too much density, but in comparison with an overexposed radiograph, the cortical outlines of the thinnest parts of the structure are obscured and the thickest cortical outlines demonstrate a low contrast. Figure 1–57 demonstrates an overpenetrated distal forearm radiograph. An overpenetrated radiograph also shows a dramatic increase in the amount of scattered fogging outside the collimated borders.

If the anatomical structure of interest has been *underpenetrated* (not enough kVp used), the radiograph demonstrates too little density, but in comparison with an underexposed radiograph, the cortical outlines of the thickest

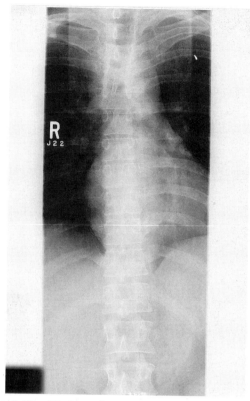

Figure 1-56. AP thoracic vertebrae radiograph underexposed by 2 times.

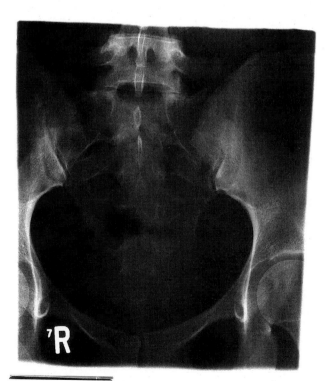

Figure 1-55. AP sacral radiograph overexposed by 2 times.

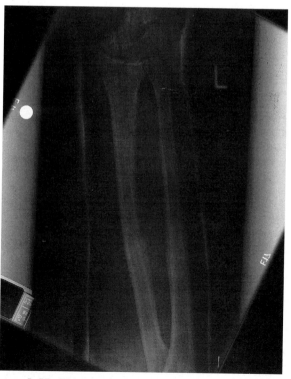

Figure 1-57. Distal forearm radiograph overpenetrated by 2 times.

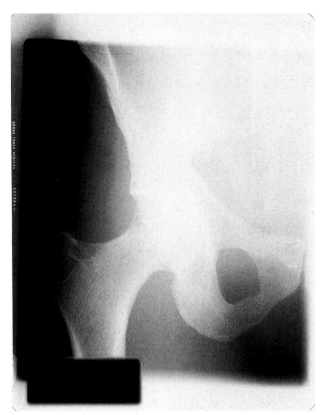

Figure 1-58. AP hip radiograph underpenetrated by 2 times.

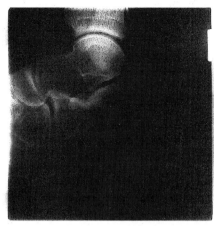

Figure 1-59. Lateral ankle radiograph overexposed by 3 or 4 times.

parts of the structure are not visualized. Figure 1–58 demonstrates an underpenetrated AP hip radiograph, showing the key difference between underexposed and underpenetrated radiographs. If the cortical outlines of the structure of interest can be seen even though the radiographic density is light, one can conclude that mAs needs adjusting; if the cortical outlines of the structure cannot be outlined and the radiographic density is light, a kVp adjustment is required.

4. How much adjustment in technique should be made for inadequate density or penetration?

Manually Set Exams: Before changing the technique and repeating a radiograph because it is too dark or light, evaluate all other factors that affect radiographic density. Was the SID set correctly? Did you read the technique chart correctly and set the kVp and mAs as stated on the technique chart? Was the patient measured correctly? Did you use the correct receptor system, and was the correct film placed in that system? Was a grid used if required? Only if these additional technical preparations were correct can one conclude that the film was dark or light because the mAs or kVp was inaccurately set.

If the radiograph needs to be repeated because it is overexposed, decrease the mAs at least 50 percent. (If the original mAs was 20, the new mAs will be 20 ÷ 2 = 10 mAs.) The kVp level should be the same as that used for the original radiograph. A radiograph should not be repeated for overexposure without making at least this much adjustment. What is more difficult to determine is the difference between an overexposed radiograph that requires the density to be cut in half (divided by 2) and one that requires the density to be decreased by 3 or 4 times (di-

vided by 3 or 4). When I teach exposure changes, I tell my students that the adjustment needed depends on the evaluation they make about the first radiograph. If the evaluation is something like "It's a little dark, maybe I could pass it, but I'd feel better if it was repeated," the change should be 2 times (Fig. 1–55). If the evaluation is more like "This is too dark. I definitely have to repeat it," the change should be 3 or 4 times. Figure 1–59 illustrates an overexposed lateral ankle radiograph.

If the radiograph has to be repeated because it was underexposed, increase the mAs at least 100 percent or 2 times. (If the original mAs was 20, the new mAs should be 20 × 2 = 40 mAs.) The kVp level should be the same as that used for the original radiograph. A radiograph should not be repeated for underexposure without making at least a 2 times change. When determining whether the radiograph is either 2 times or 3 to 4 times too light, use the same approach just described for the overexposed radiograph. If your evaluation is "It's a little light, maybe I could pass it, but I'd feel better if it was repeated," the change should be 2 times (Fig. 1–56). If the evaluation is more like "This is too light. It definitely needs repeating," the change should be 3 or 4 times. Figure 1–60 illustrates an underexposed lateral foot radiograph.

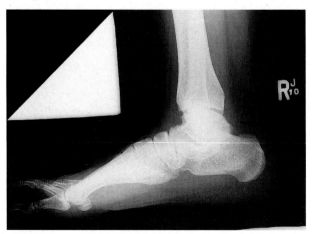

Figure 1-60. Lateral foot radiograph underexposed by 3 or 4 times.

Figure 1-61. Lateral knee radiograph overpenetrated by 3 or 4 times.

When a radiograph demonstrates a slightly less than optimal but still acceptable density, it should not be repeated unless another factor requires a repeat. Such factors include an artifact, patient motion, and mispositioning. For these radiographs, a 2 times density change would cause the repeated radiograph to be overexposed or underexposed, but a 30 percent change would improve the radiograph by providing a noticeable increase or decrease in density without overexposing or underexposing it. (To figure a 30 percent change, multiply the original mAs value by 0.3; then, add the result to the original mAs value to increase density, or subtract the result from the original mAs value to decrease the density.)

If the radiograph has to be repeated because it was overpenetrated, decrease the kVp by at least 15 percent. (If 80 kVp was used on the original radiograph, the new kVp is calculated by multiplying 80 by 0.15 and subtracting the result (12) from the original 80 kVp; the new kVp would be 68.) The mAs should be the same as that used on the original radiograph if the radiograph needs only a 2 times density change (Fig. 1–57). If, however, the radiograph is dark enough to indicate a required 3 or 4 times change in density and it is also overpenetrated, a combination kVp and mAs change might be indicated. Figure 1– 61 shows an overpenetrated lateral knee radiograph.

How many 15 percent kVp changes should be made when a radiograph is underpenetrated depends on your departmental standard for contrast. Generally, a change of more than 15 percent in kVp when the radiograph is overpenetrated may result in a radiograph with too short a contrast scale and, possibly, underpenetration. Use the optimal kVp (maximum kVp level that provides adequate penetration and contrast of radiographed structure) range for the anatomical structure being radiographed as a guideline for determining how much change should be made in kVp. First, calculate what the kVp level would be if decreased by 15 percent. Is this new kVp either at or no more than

slightly above the optimal level for the structure being radiographed? If so, you know there will be a significant penetration change, and any additional density adjustment should be made with mAs. Decreasing the kVp too far below optimum results in an underpenetrated radiograph, whereas if the kVp is too far above optimum for the structure being radiographed, a further 15 percent kVp change may be indicated.

If the radiograph has to be repeated because it was underpenetrated, increase the kVp by at least 15 percent. (If 50 kVp was used on the original radiograph, the new kVp is calculated by taking 50 × 0.15 and adding the result (7.5) to the original 50 kVp; the new kVp would be 57.5.) The mAs should be the same as that used on the original radiograph if the radiograph needs only a 2 times (100 percent) density change (see Fig. 1–58). If a radiograph is underpenetrated and light enough to require a 3 or 4 times density adjustment, a combination kVp and mAs change might be indicated. Figure 1–62 demonstrates an underpenetrated AP shoulder radiograph. How many 15 percent kVp changes should be made in this situation depends on your departmental standard for contrast and can be determined by using the optimal kVp level for the structure being radiographed as a guideline. First, calculate a 15 percent increase in the kVp level. Is this new kVp either at or no more than slightly above the optimal level for the structure being radiographed? If so, you know there will be a significant penetration change, and any additional density adjustment should be made with mAs. Increasing the kVp too far above optimum results in an overpenetrated radiograph, whereas if the kVp is too far below optimum for the structure being radiographed, a further 15 percent kVp change may be indicated.

Automatic Exposure (Phototimed) Exams: The kilovoltage peak is manually set for automatically exposed exams. Therefore, if a radiograph is obtained that is overpenetrated or underpenetrated, you should follow the guide-

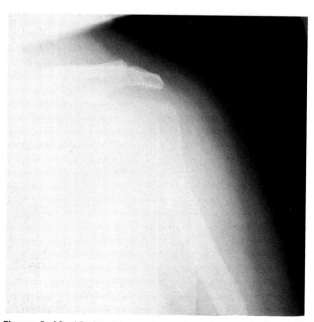

Figure 1-62. AP shoulder radiograph underpenetrated by 3 or 4 times.

lines described in the preceding discussion to evaluate penetration and make proper adjustments.

Overexposed or underexposed radiographs obtained using the automatic exposure controls are primarily a result of poor patient and ionizing chamber alignment. An overexposed radiograph results when the ionization chamber chosen is located beneath a structure that has a higher atomic number or is thicker or denser than the structure of interest. For example, when an AP abdomen radiograph is taken, the outside ionization chambers should be chosen and situated within the soft tissue, away from the lumbar vertebrae, to yield the desired abdominal soft tissue density. If the chamber situated under the lumbar vertebrae is used instead, the capacitor (device that stores energy) requires a longer exposure time to reach its maximum filling level and terminate the exposure. This is due to the high atomic number of bone and the higher number of photons that bone absorbs compared with soft tissue. The result will be a radiograph with adequate bone density but overexposed soft tissue. An underexposed radiograph results, however, when the ionization chamber chosen is located beneath a structure that has a lower atomic number or is thinner or less dense than the structure of interest. When an AP lumbar vertebrae radiograph is taken, the center ionization chamber is chosen and centered directly beneath the lumbar vertebrae. If one or both of the outside chambers or the center ionization chamber is off center, the radiograph is underexposed, because soft tissue, which has a lower atomic number than bone, is above the activated chamber.

An underexposed radiograph also results if a portion of the activated chamber has not been covered with body tissue, such as can happen when shoulder structures are

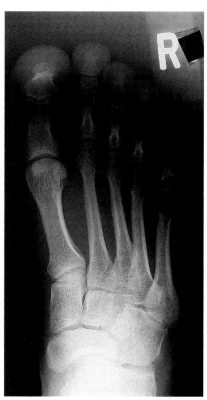

Figure 1-64. Compensating filter was used on toes.

radiographed. The part of the chamber not covered with tissue collects radiation so quickly that it will charge the capacitor to its maximum level, terminating the exposure before proper density of the shoulder structures has been reached. Premature termination of the exposure can also be avoided with tight collimation practices, because table and body scattered radiation will charge the capacitor.

An overexposed radiograph may result when the structure of interest is in close proximity to thicker structures and both are situated above the activated ionization chamber. For example, it is best not to use the automatic exposure controls on an AP "open-mouth" projection of the dens. On this exam, the upper incisors, occipital cranial base, and mandible add thickness to the areas superior and inferior to the dens and atlantoaxial joint. This added thickness causes the area of interest to be overexposed, because more time is needed for the capacitor to reach its maximum level as photons are absorbed in the thicker areas.

In most facilities, the automatic exposure thyristor (device used to set the maximum capacitor charge) is set to accommodate the most frequently used film/screen combination. If a higher-speed film/screen combination is used with this thyristor setting, the resulting radiograph is overexposed; if a lower-speed film/screen combination is used, the resulting radiograph is underexposed.

5. Has a compensating filter been used when indicated to obtain homogeneous density?

On some exams, when an exposure is set that will adequately demonstrate one structure of interest, other structures of interest are overexposed. This is due to the

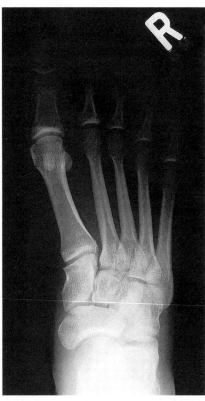

Figure 1-63. Compensating filter was not used on toes.

difference in body thickness between the two regions. AP projections of the shoulder, feet, and thoracic vertebrae are three exams that demonstrate this problem. To offset this thickness difference and obtain homogeneous density, place a compensating filter over or under the thinnest structure. Figures 1–63 and 1–64 show AP foot radiographs. The radiograph in Figure 1–63 was taken without using a compensating filter, whereas the radiograph in Figure 1–64 was taken with a compensating filter positioned over the distal metatarsals and phalangeal regions. Notice the better visualization of anatomical structures covered by the compensating filter.

The radiographic contrast adequately visualizes the bony and soft tissue structures of interest.

1. Does the radiographic contrast that is demonstrated adequately visualize the bony and soft tissue structures of interest?

On a radiograph that demonstrates good contrast, the gray scale is long enough to visualize the different bony and soft tissue structures. The contrast demonstrated on a radiograph is mainly controlled by the kVp level chosen for the radiograph. There is an optimum kVp level for every structure within the body that provides sufficient penetration and the best contrast for that body structure. There are, however, situations and different patient conditions in which this optimum kVp level does not provide the best contrast. In these cases, the kVp must be adjusted from the routinely used optimal level to obtain a scale of contrast that will better demonstrate the structures of interest.

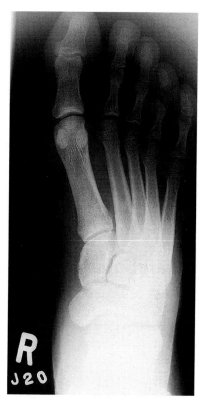

Figure 1-66. High-contrast radiograph.

If the contrast on a radiograph is very low (Fig. 1–65), very little difference is demonstrated between the shades of gray and the radiograph lacks a bright white shade. A low-contrast radiograph results when the kVp level is too high. If the contrast on the radiograph is too high (Fig. 1–66), the anatomical structures are demonstrated with black and white shades and very few if any gray shades. A high-contrast radiograph results when the kVp level is too low.

When the radiographic density on your film is adequate but the contrast level is not sufficient to adequately visualize all the anatomical structures, the contrast level can be adjusted by varying kVp, and the density can be maintained by counteracting the kVp adjustment with a comparable mAs adjustment. If you wish higher contrast, decrease the original kVp used by 15 percent and increase the mAs value used by 100 percent. For example, if the original technique was 80 kVp at 10 mAs, the new technique is 68 kVp at 20 mAs. If you wish lower contrast, increase the original kVp used by 15 percent and decrease the mAs value used by 50 percent. For example, if the original technique was 80 kVp at 10 mAs, the new technique would be 92 kVp at 5 mAs. In both of these situations, the radiographic density has remained the same as in the original radiograph, because the density adjustment made with kVp is offset by an equal mAs adjustment. The amount of adjustment one should make (2 times versus 3 or 4 times) depends on how dramatic a contrast change is desired. Be careful not to overpenetrate or underpenetrate the structure with too much adjustment.

2. Has the amount of scattered radiation produced been effectively controlled?

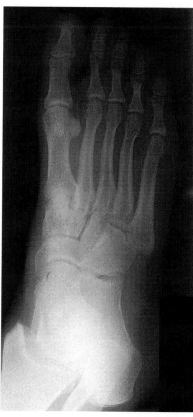

Figure 1-65. Low-contrast radiograph.

The contrast that a radiograph displays also depends on how much scattered radiation was allowed to reach the film. An increase in scattered radiation causes a decrease in radiographic contrast and a decrease in the visibility of details. Tight collimation and the use of a grid whenever the kVp is above 70 controls the amount of scattered radiation that reaches the film.

Flat contact shields can also be used to control the amount of scattered radiation that reaches the film. When anatomical structures are being examined that demonstrate an excessive amount of scattered fogging along the outside of the collimated borders, such as the lateral lumbar vertebrae, placing a large flat contact shield or the straight edge of a lead apron along the appropriate border greatly improves the visibility of the recorded details. Compare the lateral lumbar vertebral radiographs in Figures 1–67 and 1–68. Figure 1–67 was taken with a lead contact shield placed against the posterior edge of the collimator's light field. A contact shield was not used for Figure 1–68. Note the improvement in visualization of the lumbar spinous processes with use of the contact shield.

No preventable artifacts are present on the radiograph.

1. Are any artifacts visualized on the radiograph?

Artifacts are any undesirable structures recorded on the radiograph. They include (1) anatomical structures that obscure the area of interest or have no purpose for being there and that can be removed from the radiograph, (2) externally removable objects such as patient and or hospital possessions, (3) internal objects such as prostheses or monitoring lines, and (4) appearances that result from improper use of equipment.

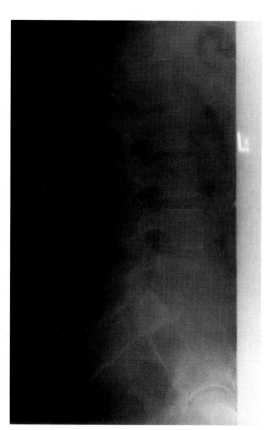

Figure 1-68. Contact shield was not used along posterior collimated border.

Before a radiograph is taken, it may be wise to have the patient change into a hospital gown and to ask whether any patient possessions are located in or around the area being radiographed. Because patients are often nervous and may forget to remove articles of clothing or for sentimental reasons may not remove jewelry pieces, you should re-check the area of interest even after the patient has changed into a gown. Once the patient is positioned and the film is ready to be exposed, take a last look to make sure all hospital possessions used are out of the radiographic field if possible and that those that are in the field, such as heart monitoring leads, have been shifted so they will superimpose the least amount of information.

2. Can you identify the artifact demonstrated on the radiograph?

It would be impossible to demonstrate in this book all the possible artifacts that can appear on a radiograph, but it is important for technologists to familiarize themselves with as many radiographic artifacts as possible. The more aware we are of what causes artifacts on the radiograph, the more careful patient and technical preparation procedures we learn to follow. It might be wise for your department to keep an envelope of radiographs that had to be repeated because of artifacts. From time to time, these can be studied to help keep all technologists current on the possibilities for facility-related artifacts.

Most possession-related artifacts are demonstrated on the radiograph as lighter densities than the anatomical structures that surround them. Artifacts that are related to

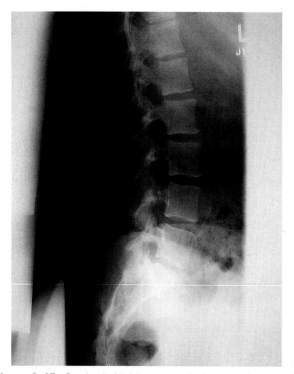

Figure 1-67. Contact shield was used along posterior collimated border.

poor film handling, such as film creases, static, and light leaks, most often exhibit greater density. The following discussion concerns different categories of radiographic artifacts and common examples of each.

Anatomical Structures: The most common anatomical artifact is the patient's own hand or arm. Figure 1–69 shows a supine abdominal radiograph in which the patient's hands are superimposing the upper abdominal region. More than likely, the patient was not positioned in this manner when the technologist left the room. Between this time and the time the exposure was taken, however, the patient found a more comfortable position. This example stresses the importance of explaining exams to patients so they understand the need to remain in the position the technologist places them in as well as the importance of rechecking each patient's position before the exposure is taken if much time has elapsed between positioning the patient and taking the radiograph. It is also not uncommon for a patient who is experiencing hip or lower back pain from lying on the radiographic table to place a hand beneath an affected hip. This will result in superimposition of the hip and hand on the radiograph. Remember that the patient does not know why repositioning because of discomfort is not acceptable.

Anatomical structures are considered artifacts even when they are not superimposing any area of interest but are still located within the collimated field and could easily have been excluded. Figure 1–70 shows such an artifact. This chest radiograph, produced with a portable x-ray machine, was taken with the patient's arms positioned tightly against the sides. Because humeri are not evaluated on a chest radiograph, there is no reason for them to be included, and

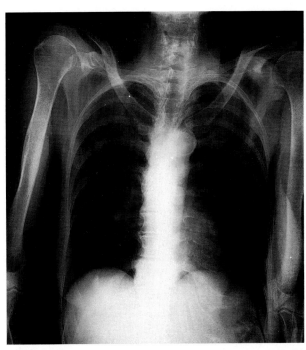

Figure 1-70. Anatomical artifact; patient's arms included in chest radiograph.

they could easily have been shifted out of the radiographic field.

External Artifacts: An external artifact is found outside the patient's body, such as a patient's possession that remained in a pocket or a hospital possession that was lying on top of or beneath the patient. The most common external artifacts are earrings, rings, necklaces, bra hooks, dental structures, hairpins, heart monitoring lines, and gown snaps (Fig. 1–71). Two external artifacts that are not as common

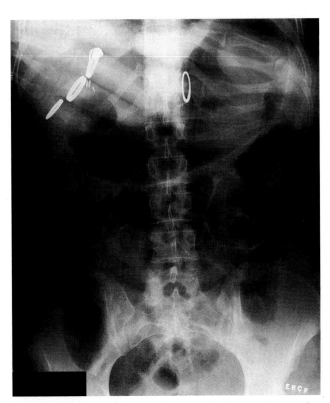

Figure 1-69. Anatomical artifact; patient's hands superimposed on supine abdominal radiograph.

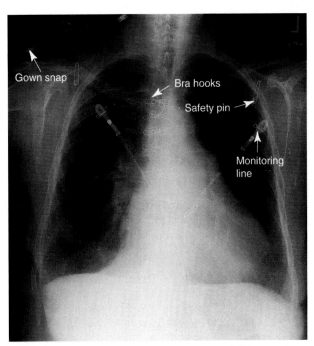

Figure 1-71. External artifacts from patient clothing and hospital monitoring equipment.

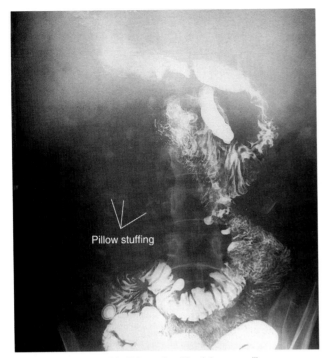

Figure 1-72. External artifact from a pillow.

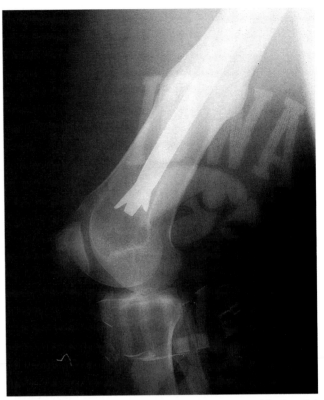

Figure 1-73. External and internal artifacts caused by imprint on patient clothing and leg prosthesis.

but do occasionally appear are caused by pillows (Fig. 1–72) and by the imprinted designs on shirts and pants (Fig. 1–73). Both of these artifacts can easily be avoided with proper patient preparation and positioning. Being aware of as many objects as possible that can create artifacts on the radiograph is the best way of preventing them.

Internal Artifacts: Internal artifacts are found within the patient. They cannot be removed and must be accepted. Examples of commonly seen internal artifacts are prostheses (Figs. 1–73 and 1–74) and pins, pacemakers (see Fig. 1–12), Swan-Ganz or central venous pressure lines, and nasogastric tubes.

If an artifact that is normally not found within the body is identified on a radiograph, it is the technologist's duty to discretely search and interview the patient or to consult the ordering physician to determine whether the artifact is locatable outside the patient's body. If it is not found, it may have been introduced into the patient through one of the body orifices. Your search and interview discoveries should be recorded on the patient's requisition. Figure 1–75 shows a pelvic radiograph of a patient who had swallowed several batteries.

Equipment-Related Artifacts: Grid lines that result from the use of stationary grids and improper use of grids are the most common equipment-related radiographic artifacts. They can be avoided by choosing a moving grid whenever possible and by properly aligning the central ray and grid. If a parallel grid was tilted or the central ray was angled toward the grid's lead strips, the radiograph demonstrates grid lines and a decrease in density on the side the central ray was angled toward (Fig. 1–76). If a focused grid was tilted or the central ray was angled toward the grid's lead strips, the radiograph demonstrates an overall decrease in density and grid lines across the radiograph

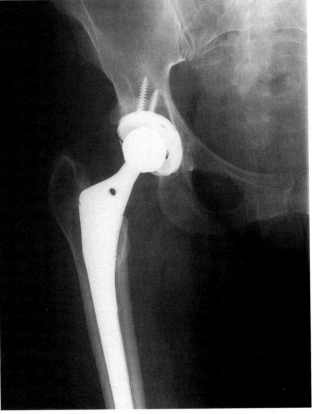

Figure 1-74. Internal artifact caused by prosthesis.

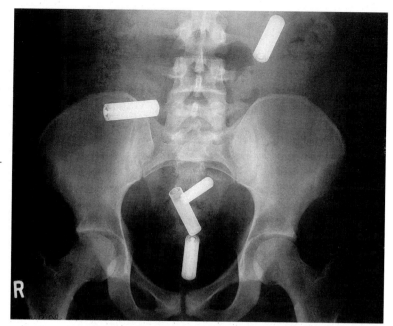

Figure 1-75. Internal artifact; patient has swallowed five batteries.

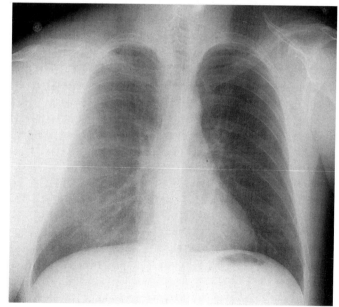

Figure 1-76. Equipment-related artifact. Either the parallel grid was tilted or the central ray was angled toward the grid lines.

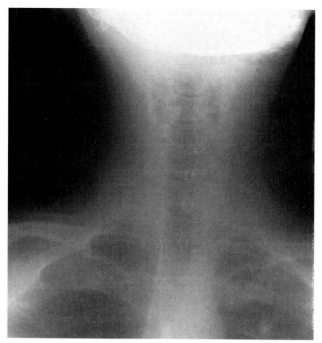

Figure 1-77. Equipment-related artifact. The focused grid was tilted or the central ray was angled toward the grid lines.

(Fig. 1–77). If a focused grid was inverted, the radiograph demonstrates the expected density in the center of the radiograph and a loss of density and grid lines on each side (Fig. 1–78).

Artifacts from Improper Film Handling and Processing: Improper film handling and processing can cause artifacts such as film creases, static (Fig. 1–79), fog, stains, scratches (Fig. 1–80), and hesitation marks (Fig.

1–81). They can be avoided by following a good quality control program for the darkroom, film storage, and processor.

3. What is the location of the artifact in respect to a palpable anatomical structure?

Whenever an external or an unidentifiable internal artifact is demonstrated on a radiograph, discretely search and interview the patient to determine the artifact's location. To pinpoint where to look for the artifact, study the radiograph to locate a palpable anatomical structure situated close to the artifact. This is the area where the search should begin.

4. Does the radiograph have to be repeated because of the artifact?

If an artifact that can be eliminated obscures any portion of the area of interest, the radiograph needs to be repeated. A gown snap that superimposes an area of the lungs on a chest radiograph could easily obscure a small lesion. A ring may easily obscure a hairline finger fracture.

If the artifact is located outside the field of interest, the radiograph does not need to be repeated, although the patient should be discretely searched and interviewed to determine whether the artifact is located externally or internally.

The ordered procedure and the indication for exam have been fulfilled.

1. Has the routine series been taken for the body structure ordered as determined by your facility?

One of the last steps to take before deciding whether a radiographic exam is acceptable is to make sure that you have taken all the radiographs that are recommended by your facility for the body part being radiographed. For

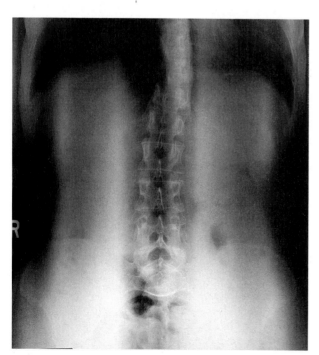

Figure 1-78. Equipment-related artifact. The focused grid was inverted.

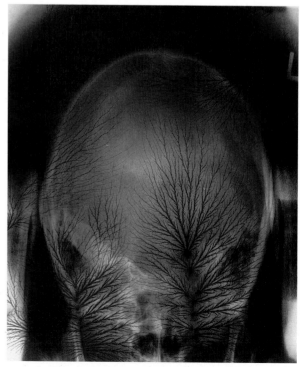

Figure 1-79. Film-handling artifact: static.

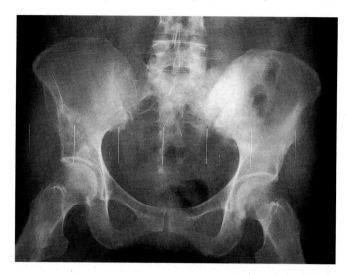

Figure 1-80. Film-handling artifact: scratches.

example, many facilities require that both an AP projection and a lateral position be taken whenever radiographs of the elbow are requested. This series of views provides the reviewer with the needed positions to accurately evaluate the patient's elbow.

2. Do the views in the routine series fulfill the indication for the exam, or must additional radiographs be taken?

Not only should the entire series be taken, but one should also determine whether the indication for the exam has been fulfilled. If an elbow exam is ordered and the indication of the exam was to evaluate or rule out a radial head fracture, an additional external oblique or radial head–capitulum position of the elbow may be needed to effectively rule out this fracture. Consult with the reviewer before allowing the patient to leave the radiographic department.

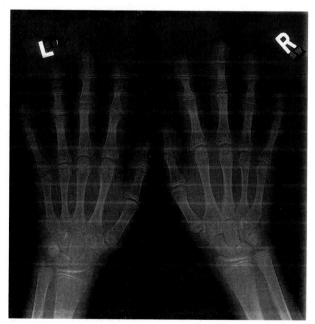

Figure 1-81. Film-handling artifact: hesitation marks.

The requisition has been completed, and the repeat / reject analysis information has been provided as indicated by your facility.

1. Has the requisition been completed?

The sections of the requisition that should be completed by the technologist are: the number and sizes of films that were used, the mAs, kVp, and distance used, the room number where the radiograph was taken, the technologist's name, the date and time of the procedure, and any additional patient history obtained from the patient-technologist interview (Fig. 1–82). Recording the number and sizes of films used on the requisition tells the reviewer how many radiographs there are to evaluate. The name(s) of the technologist(s) involved in the exam is valuable information if there is a question about the radiograph or patient, or if the patient was found to have a contagious disease and measures need to be taken to protect the technologist(s). Recording the same date and time of the procedure on the requisition that are visualized on the radiograph, as well as double-checking that the name of the patient is correct, provides a means of verifying that the requisition goes with a certain set of radiographs. The patient's history should be filled out by the ordering physician before the requisition arrives in the radiographic facility; any information the technologist has learned from interviewing and observing the patient that might assist the reviewer in the diagnosis should be added, however. This area of the form may also be used to note any situation requiring departure from the routine exam procedure. For example, if a hand radiograph was taken with the patient's ring still on the finger because the ring could not be removed, the technologist should record this fact in the patient history or note section of the requisition so that the reviewer understands why the ring appears on the radiograph.

2. Has the repeat/reject analysis information been supplied?

The facility's repeat/reject analysis card, an example of which is shown in Figure 1–83, should be filled out to indicate any positioning or technical errors that occurred during the procedure. This information provides your facility with a means of distinguishing areas where patient

PHYSICIAN ORDER FOR RADIOLOGIC/NUCLEAR MEDICINE
Consultation/Request for Procedure

Department of Radiology

DATE

HOSP. NO.

NAME

BIRTHDATE

ADDRESS

IF NOT IMPRINTED, PLEASE PRINT DATE, HOSP. NO., NAME AND LOCATION

Procedure Scheduled for Date _____ Time _____

Known Allergies _____

Female of Child-Bearing Age ☐ Yes ☐ No

Patient Transport ☐ Walk ☐ Cart ☐ Chair ☐ Isolette

Oxygen ☐ Yes ☐ No **Diabetic** ☐ Yes ☐ No

Pregnant ☐ Yes ☐ No **Lactating** ☐ Yes ☐ No

Isolation ☐ Strict ☐ Respiratory ☐ Protective
☐ Wound/Skin ☐ Enteric ☐ Blood ☐ Secretion/Excretion

☐ **Routine** ☐ **ASAP** ☐ **STAT** ☐ **Portable**
STAT Report ☐ Yes ☐ No
Phone _____ Pager No. _____

Imaging Specialty ☐ Ultrasound ☐ Magnetic Resonance Imaging ☐ Computed Tomography ☐ Nuclear Medicine

Procedure _____

Patient diagnosis _____

REASON FOR EXAM/CLINICAL FINDINGS _____

Physician's Signature _____ CLP No. _____ Date _____ **Return Report To** _____ Phone _____

Radiology use only

	KV	MAS	DIST
14 x 17			
11 x 14	PA		
10 x 12	LAT		
8 x 10			
9 x 9			
6 x 12			

Fluoro Time (min) _____

Room _____

Procedure _____

Physician _____

Notes _____

Actual Date of Proc. _____

Actual Time of Proc. _____

Technologist/ Sonographer _____

Contrast _____ Date _____

PHARMACEUTICALS AND AGENTS
Radiopharmaceuticals Administered _____ Amount _____ Time _____ By _____
Route of Administration ☐ I.V. ☐ Oral Other _____ Lot No. _____

Radiopharmaceuticals Administered _____ Amount _____ Time _____ By _____
Route of Administration ☐ I.V. ☐ Oral Other _____ Lot No. _____

IMAGING INSTRUCTIONS _____

PHYSICIAN'S RADIOPHARMACEUTICAL/ ADJUNCT DRUG PRESCRIPTIONS

☐ **Outpatient** ☐ **Inpatient**

_____

Technologist's Signature _____

Figure 1-82. The requisition form. The areas to be filled out by the technologist are shaded. (Courtesy of the University of Iowa Hospital and Clinics)

# OF EXAM FILMS	OVE	UNE	POS	PRO	ART	FOG	MOT	EQF	OTH
04 X 05	[ ]	[ ]	[ ]	[ ]	[ ]	[ ]	[ ]	[ ]	[ ]
06 X 12	[ ]	[ ]	[ ]	[ ]	[ ]	[ ]	[ ]	[ ]	[ ]
08 X 10	[ ]	[ ]	[ ]	[ ]	[ ]	[ ]	[ ]	[ ]	[ ]
09 X 09	[ ]	[ ]	[ ]	[ ]	[ ]	[ ]	[ ]	[ ]	[ ]
10 X 12	[ ]	[ ]	[ ]	[ ]	[ ]	[ ]	[ ]	[ ]	[ ]
11 X 14	[ ]	[ ]	[ ]	[ ]	[ ]	[ ]	[ ]	[ ]	[ ]
14 X 14	[ ]	[ ]	[ ]	[ ]	[ ]	[ ]	[ ]	[ ]	[ ]
14 X 17	[ ]	[ ]	[ ]	[ ]	[ ]	[ ]	[ ]	[ ]	[ ]
14 X 36	[ ]	[ ]	[ ]	[ ]	[ ]	[ ]	[ ]	[ ]	[ ]
14 X 51	[ ]	[ ]	[ ]	[ ]	[ ]	[ ]	[ ]	[ ]	[ ]
OTHER	[ ]	[ ]	[ ]	[ ]	[ ]	[ ]	[ ]	[ ]	[ ]

Figure 1-83. Example of a repeat/reject analysis card. OVE = overexposure; UNE = underexposure; POS = error in patient positioning; ART = artifact; FOG = film fog; MOT = patient motion; EQF = equipment failure; OTH = other. (Courtesy of the University of Iowa Hospital and Clinics)

service can be improved through in-service personnel training or equipment repair.

Radiograph is acceptable or unacceptable. If radiograph is unacceptable, describe what measures should be taken to produce an acceptable radiograph. If radiograph is acceptable but not optimal, describe factors that could be adjusted to obtain an optimal radiograph.

When a radiograph meets all the necessary requirements, it is considered an optimal radiograph, and it should not be repeated. When a radiograph is not optimal but may be acceptable, the question arises whether it is poor enough to repeat or whether the information needed can be obtained without exposing the patient to further radiation. Factors that should be considered when making this decision are:

- Your facility's standards
- The age and condition of the patient
- The conditions under which the patient was radiographed
- Whether obvious pathology is evident
- Whether the indications for the exam have been fulfilled.

Each facility has its own standards that will determine whether you should repeat a radiograph. If standards are low, your improving radiographic skills can raise them, thus increasing the accuracy of diagnosis. The age and condition of the patient as well as the situation under which the patient was radiographed have the largest weight in the decision to repeat a radiograph. Sometimes, a less than optimal radiograph must be accepted because repeating the radiograph is impossible, as in a surgery case; at other times, the patient cannot or will not cooperate. Whenever an exam is accepted that does not meet optimal standards, one should record on the requisition any information about the patient's condition or setup situation that resulted in acceptance of such an exam. A less than optimal radiograph may also be passed when the indication for exam is clearly fulfilled by the radiograph obtained. For example, if a lower leg exam was taken without the required knee joint, but the patient history states that the patient has a distal fibular fracture and the indication for the exam is to evaluate healing of the distal fibular fracture, it is obvious that the patient's knee is not being evaluated. As long as the distal fibula is included in its entirety on the original radiograph, it should not be repeated.

It is important that all unacceptable radiographs and those less than optimal radiographs that have been accepted are studied carefully to determine whether the situation(s) that caused them could be eliminated on future exams. When a radiograph is repeated, the overall radiation dosage to the patient increases and the cost of patient care rises, because a repeat requires more technologist time, film, supplies, and equipment use.

References

1. Statkiewicz MA, Viconti PJ, Ritenour RE. Radiation Protection in Medical Radiography, ed 2. St. Louis: CV Mosby Co, 1993, pp 173–174.
2. Clemente CD (ed). Gray's Anatomy, ed 30. Philadelphia: Lea & Febiger, 1985, pp 1566–1575.

CHAPTER 2

Radiographic Critique of the Chest and Abdomen

CHEST

Posteroanterior Projection

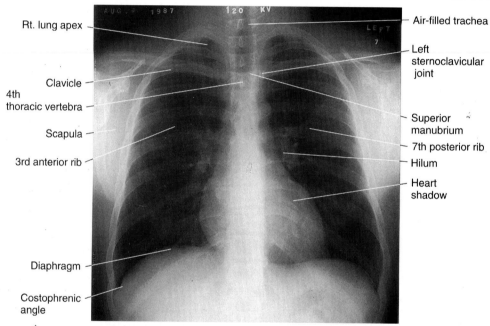

Rt. lung apex

Clavicle

4th thoracic vertebra

Scapula

3rd anterior rib

Diaphragm

Costophrenic angle

Air-filled trachea

Left sternoclavicular joint

Superior manubrium

7th posterior rib

Hilum

Heart shadow

Figure 2-1. Accurately positioned PA chest radiograph.

Radiographic Evaluation

Facility's identification requirements are visualized on radiograph.
- These requirements are facility name, patient name, age, and hospital number, and exam time and date.
- Position the name ID plate superiorly, to prevent it from obscuring a costophrenic angle.

A right or left marker, identifying correct side of patient, is present on radiograph and does not superimpose anatomy of interest.
- Place the marker laterally in the upper shoulder region.

There is no evidence of preventable artifacts, such as undergarments, necklaces, and gown snaps.

- It is recommended that the patient be instructed to remove all clothing above the waist and to change into a snapless hospital gown prior to the procedure.

Contrast and density are adequate to demonstrate vascular lung markings throughout the lung field and to visualize fluid levels or the presence of air within the pleural cavity.
- Vascular lung markings are scattered throughout the lungs and are evaluated for changes that may indicate pathology. A pneumothorax (presence of air in pleural cavity) or pneumectomy (removal of lung) may be indicated if no lung markings are present, whereas excessive lung markings may suggest lesions such as fibrosis, interstitial or alveolar edema, or compression of the lung tissue.[1] To demonstrate precise fluid levels,

40

chest radiographs should be taken with the patient upright and the x-ray beam horizontal. In this position, the air rises and the fluid gravitates to the lowest position, creating an air-fluid line or separation. This separation can be identified as a decrease in density on the radiograph wherever the denser fluid is present in the lung field. The erect PA chest radiograph is also an excellent method of discerning the presence of free intraperitoneal (within abdominal cavity) air beneath the diaphragm.

Beam penetration is sufficient to faintly demonstrate the thoracic vertebrae and posterior ribs through the heart and mediastinal structures.
- An optimal 100 to 130 kVp technique sufficiently penetrates the heart shadow and visualizes the thoracic vertebrae as well as provides the long scale of contrast necessary to visualize the lung details. A grid should be used to absorb the scattered radiation produced by the thorax, reducing fog.

The lung markings, diaphragm, heart borders, and bony cortical outlines are sharply defined.
- Sharply defined recorded details are obtained when patient respiration and body movements are halted and when the least amount of object–image distance (OID) is maintained. A 72-inch (183-cm) source–image distance (SID) is used to decrease the magnification of the heart and lung details.

The seventh thoracic vertebra is at the center of the collimated field. The apices, lateral lungs, and costophrenic angles are included within the field.
- Centering a perpendicular central ray to the midsagittal plane, at a level about 7.5 inches (18 cm) inferior to the vertebra prominens (seventh cervical spinous process), places the seventh thoracic vertebra in the center of the radiograph. The seventh thoracic vertebra is identified on the radiograph by counting down the vertebral column from the first thoracic vertebra, which is located just superior to the lung field and is the first vertebra that demonstrates rib attachment. This central ray placement also centers the lung field on the radiograph, allowing tight collimation on all sides of the lungs.
- ***Film Size and Direction:*** A 14 × 17 inch (35 × 43cm) film should be large enough to include all the required anatomical structures. The direction of film placement (crosswise versus lengthwise) must also be considered to ensure full lung coverage. For the average sthenic patient and the asthenic patient, whose lung fields are long and narrow, position the film lengthwise. For the hypersthenic patient, whose lung field is short and wide, position the film crosswise.
- ***Change in Lung Dimensions Upon Inspiration:*** Along with body type, consider how the lung expands on deep inspiration when choosing film size and placement. Upon inspiration, the lungs expand in three dimensions: transversely, anteroposteriorly, and vertically. Evaluate the transverse and vertical dimen-

sions to determine how the film should be placed. When a patient takes a deep breath, will the costophrenic angles still be included on the radiograph? Determine this by placing a hand along the patient's side at the level of the costophrenic angles, then asking the patient to inhale. If your hands remain within the film's boundaries on inspiration, the film is wide enough to accommodate the patient. If your hands move outside the film's boundaries on inspiration, consider using a larger film or placing the film crosswise. It is the vertical dimension that will demonstrate the greatest expansion. During high levels of breathing, as when we coax a patient into deep inspiration for a chest radiograph, the vertical dimension can increase by as much as 4 inches (10 cm). This full vertical lung expansion is necessary to demonstrate the entire lung field. Radiographing the patient in an upright position and encouraging a deep inspiration demonstrates the greatest amount of vertical lung field. Circumstances that may prevent full lung expansion include disease processes, advanced pregnancy, excessive obesity, being seated in a slouching position, and confining abdominal clothing.[2]

A true PA projection is demonstrated. The distances from the vertebral column to the sternal (medial) ends of the claviculae are equal, the air-filled trachea is aligned with the vertebral column, and a small amount of the heart shadow is visualized on the right side of the patient's thoracic vertebrae.
- To avoid chest rotation, position the patient's shoulders and arms at equal distances from the film, and instruct the patient to distribute body weight evenly on both feet and to face forward (Fig. 2–2). A rotated chest radiograph demonstrates distorted mediastinal structures and may create an uneven density between the lateral borders of the chest. This density difference occurs because the x-ray beam traveled through less tissue on the chest side positioned away from the film

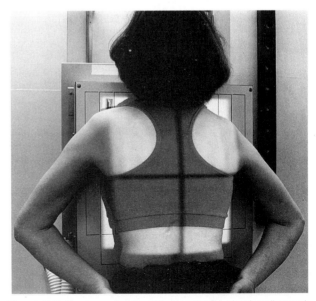

Figure 2-2. Proper patient positioning for PA chest radiograph.

than on the side positioned closer to the film. It may be detected when the chest has been rotated as little as 2 or 3 degrees.³ Because any variation in structural relationships or density may represent a pathological condition, the importance of providing nonrotated PA chest radiographs cannot be overemphasized.

- **Detecting Rotation:** Rotation is effectively detected on a PA chest radiograph by evaluating the distance between the vertebral column and the sternal ends of the claviculae or the sternoclavicular (SC) joints. When the distances between the sternal ends of the claviculae and the vertebral column are unequal, the SC joint that demonstrates the lesser amount of vertebral column superimposition represents the side of the chest that is positioned farther from the film (see Rad. 1). The opposite is true for an AP projection; the side of the chest positioned closer to the film demonstrates the SC joint superimposing the least amount of the vertebral column.

- **Distinguishing Scoliosis from Rotation:** You can distinguish scoliosis from rotation by comparing the distance from the vertebral column to the SC joints and the distance from the costophrenic angles to the lateral soft tissue outline. These distances are routinely equal in a patient with scoliosis but are different in a rotated patient (see Rad. 1). If the patient's shoulders and arms were positioned with the same degree of anterior rotation, the scapulae appear symmetrical if the patient has scoliosis, but demonstrate increased scapular body and thorax superimposition on the side of the patient positioned farthest from the film if the patient was rotated.

Claviculae are positioned on the same horizontal plane.

- The lateral ends of the claviculae are positioned on the same horizontal plane as the medial clavicle ends by depressing the patient's shoulders. Accurate clavicle positioning lowers the lateral claviculae, positioning the middle and lateral claviculae away from the apical chest region and providing better visualization of the apical lung field. When a PA chest radiograph is taken without depressing the shoulders, the lateral ends of the claviculae are elevated, causing the middle and lateral claviculae to be demonstrated within the apical chest region (see Rad. 3).

- **Poor Midcoronal Plane versus Poor Shoulder Positioning:** When a PA chest radiograph is taken with the patient's upper midcoronal plane tilted toward the film, the claviculae are not demonstrated horizontally but are seen vertically (see Rad. 4). One can distinguish poor shoulder positioning from poor mid-coronal plane positioning by measuring the amount of lung field visualized superior to the claviculae. A radiograph with poor shoulder positioning demonstrates decreased lung field superior to the claviculae, whereas a radiograph with poor midcoronal plane positioning demonstrates increased lung field superior to the claviculae.

The humeri are abducted away from the chest, and the scapulae are located outside the lung field.

- Placing the back of the patient's hands on the hips

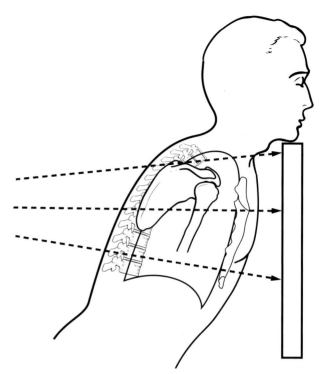

Figure 2–3. Chest foreshortening.

draws the humeri away from the chest. This positioning also allows the patient to easily rotate the elbows and shoulders anteriorly in order to place the scapulae outside the lung field. When the scapulae are accurately positioned, the superolateral portion of the lungs is better visualized. If a chest radiograph is taken without anterior rotation of the elbows and shoulders, the scapulae are seen superimposing the superolateral lung field (see Rad. 1).

The manubrium is superimposed by the fourth thoracic vertebra with about 1 inch (2.5 cm) of the apical lung field visualized above the claviculae, and the lungs and heart are demonstrated without foreshortening.

- The tilt of the midcoronal plane determines the relationship of the manubrium to the thoracic vertebrae, the amount of apical lung field seen above the claviculae, and the degree of lung and heart foreshortening. When the midcoronal plane is vertical, the manubrium is projected at the level of the fourth thoracic vertebra, about 1 inch (2.5 cm) of the apices are visualized above the claviculae, and the lungs and heart are demonstrated without foreshortening. If the superior midcoronal plane is tilted forward, however, as demonstrated in Figure 2–3, the lungs and heart are foreshortened, the manubrium is situated at the level of the fifth thoracic vertebra or lower, and more than 1 inch (2.5 cm) of apices is demonstrated above the claviculae (see Rad. 4). Conversely, if the superior midcoronal plane is tilted backwards, as demonstrated in Figure 2–4, the lungs and heart are foreshortened, the manubrium is situated at a level between the first and third thoracic vertebrae, and less than 1 inch (2.5 cm) of apices is demonstrated above the claviculae (see Rad. 5).

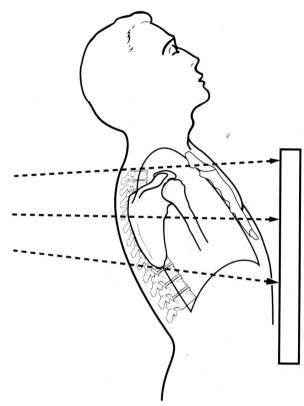

Figure 2-4. Chest foreshortening.

Ten to 11 posterior ribs are demonstrated above the diaphragm, indicating full lung aeration.

- To obtain maximum lung aeration, take the exposure with the patient in an upright position and after the second full inspiration. When the patient is positioned upright, the abdominal organs and diaphragm shift inferiorly, providing more space for maximum vertical lung expansion.
- A study by Crapo and associates[4] found that total lung capacity is best obtained when the patient is coaxed into a deep inspiration. In practice, this is accomplished by taking the radiograph after the patient's *second* full inspiration. If fewer than 10 posterior ribs are demonstrated, the lungs were not fully inflated. Before repeating the radiograph, attempt to obtain a deeper inspiration and determine whether a patient condition might have caused the poor inhalation. Chest radiographs that are taken on expiration may also demonstrate a decrease in radiographic density, because a decrease in air volume increases the concentration of pulmonary tissues.
- ***Expiration Chest Radiograph:*** Abnormalities such as a pneumothorax or foreign body may indicate the need for an expiration chest radiograph. For such a radiograph, all evaluation requirements listed for a PA chest radiograph should be met except the number of ribs demonstrated above the diaphragm. On an expiration chest, as few as nine posterior ribs may be demonstrated, the lungs are denser, and the heart shadow is broader and shorter[1] (see Rad. 6). It may be necessary to increase the exposure (mAs) when a PA chest projection is taken on expiration and lung details are of interest.

Critiquing Radiographs

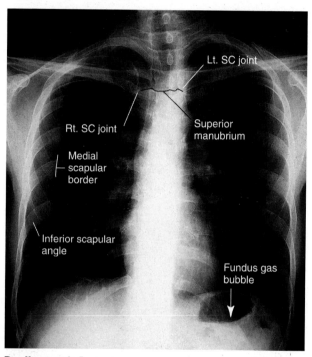

Radiograph 1.

Critique: The right SC joint is visualized without vertebral column superimposition, and the vertebral column is superimposing the left SC joint; the patient was slightly rotated, with the left side of the chest positioned closer to the film than the right. (This is a left anterior oblique position.) The medial borders of the scapulae are demonstrated within the superolateral lung field; the shoulders and elbows were not anteriorly rotated.

Correction: To offset chest rotation, position the right-shoulder closer to the film. The shoulders should be at equal distances from the film. Rotate the elbows and shoulders anteriorly, to draw the scapulae out of the lung field.

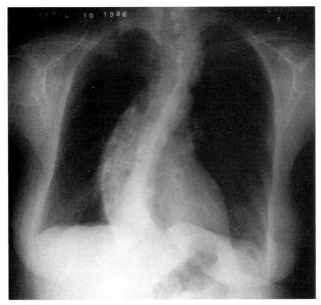

Radiograph 2.

Critique: The thoracic vertebrae demonstrates scoliosis, giving a rotated appearance to the chest.
Correction: No correction movement is required. A PA chest radiograph on a patient with scoliosis will appear rotated.

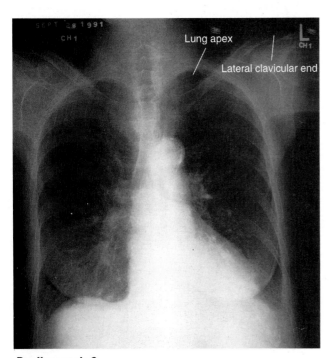

Radiograph 3.

Critique: The claviculae are not horizontal, and the lateral ends of the claviculae are elevated, obscuring the apices; the patient's shoulders were not depressed.
Correction: Depress the patient's shoulders.

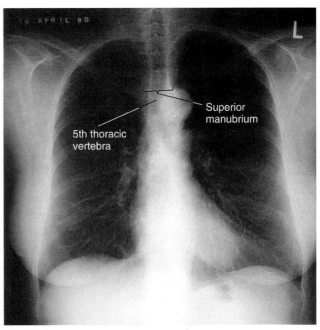

Radiograph 4.

Critique: The manubrium is situated at the level of the fifth thoracic vertebra, and more than 1 inch (2.5 cm) of the apices is demonstrated superior to the claviculae; the upper midcoronal plane was tilted toward the film (see Fig. 2–3).
Correction: Move the patient's upper thorax away from the film until the midcoronal plane is vertical.

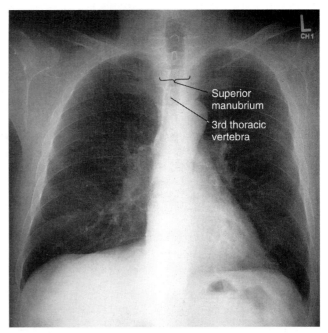

Radiograph 5.

Critique: The manubrium is situated at the level of the second thoracic vertebra, and less than 1 inch (2.5 cm) of the apices is demonstrated superior to the claviculae; the upper midcoronal plane was tilted away from the film (see Fig. 2–4).
Correction: Move the patient's upper thorax toward the film until the midcoronal plane is vertical.

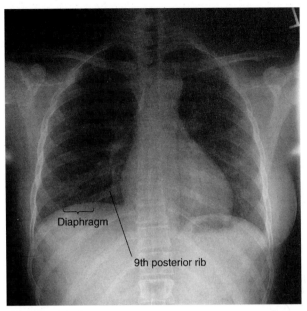

Radiograph 6.

Critique: Only a small portion of the ninth posterior rib is demonstrated above the diaphragm; the radiograph was taken at the end of expiration. The medial borders of the scapulae are demonstrated within the superolateral lung field; the shoulders and elbows were not anteriorly rotated.
Correction: If an expiration PA chest radiograph is desired, no change in respiration is required. If an inspiration PA chest radiograph is desired, repeat the radiograph, making the exposure after the second full inspiration. Rotate the elbow and shoulders anteriorly, to draw the scapulae out of the lung field.

Chest: Left Lateral Position

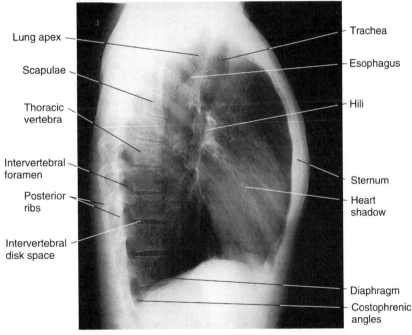

Figure 2-5. Accurately positioned lateral chest radiograph.

Radiographic Evaluation

Facility's identification requirements are visualized on radiograph.
- These requirements include facility name, patient name, age, and hospital number, and exam time and date.
- Position the name ID plate superiorly, to prevent it from obscuring any portion of the lung field.

A left marker, identifying side of patient positioned closer to film, is present on radiograph and does not superimpose anatomy of interest.
- Place a left marker anterosuperiorly in the light field.

There is no evidence of preventable artifacts, such as undergarments, necklaces, and gown snaps.

- It is recommended that the patient be instructed to remove all clothing above the waist and to change into a snapless hospital gown prior to the exam.

Contrast, density, and penetration are adequate to demonstrate the vascular lung markings throughout the lung field. The soft tissue outlines of air-filled trachea, heart shadow, and hilus as well as the cortical outlines of the posterior ribs, sternum, and thoracic vertebrae are visualized.

- Vascular lung markings are scattered throughout the lung field and are evaluated for changes that may indicate pathology. An optimal 100 to 130 kVp technique sufficiently penetrates the heart shadow and demonstrates the lung markings located beneath it as well as provides the long scale of contrast necessary to visualize the lung details. A grid should be used to absorb the scattered radiation produced by the thorax, reducing fog and increasing the visibility of details.

The lung markings, diaphragm, heart borders, and bony cortical outlines are sharply defined.

- Sharply defined recorded details are obtained when patient respiration and body movements are halted and when the least amount of object–image distance (OID) is maintained. A 72-inch (183-cm) source–image distance (SID) is used to decrease the magnification of the heart and lung details.

The midcoronal plane, at the level of the eighth thoracic vertebra, is at the center of the collimated field. The lung apices, sternum, posterior ribs, diaphragm, and costophrenic angles are included within the field.

- Centering a perpendicular central ray to the midcoronal plane, at a level about 8.5 inches (21 cm) inferior to the vertebra prominens, places the central ray at the level of the eighth thoracic vertebra. This lower centering, compared with that for the PA chest radiograph, is needed to include the right costophrenic angle on the radiograph. Because the right costophrenic angle is positioned at a long OID and the central ray is centered superior to it, the costophrenic angle is projected inferiorly.
- Positioning the midcoronal plane vertically prevents forward or backward leaning, which may result in clipping of the sternum or posterior ribs. Open the transversely collimated field to the closest anterior or posterior skin-line. For most adult lateral chest radiographs, the full film length is needed, although you should collimate to the film's upper and lower borders.
- A 14 × 17 inch (35 × 43 cm) lengthwise film should be adequate to include all the required anatomical structures.

The chest demonstrates no rotation when the posterior and the anterior ribs are nearly superimposed—demonstrating no more than a 0.5-inch (1-cm) space between them—the sternum is in profile, and the intervertebral foramina of the thoracic vertebrae are open.

- To avoid chest rotation align the shoulders, the posterior ribs and the posterior pelvic wings perpendicular to the film (Fig. 2–6). This alignment, which nearly

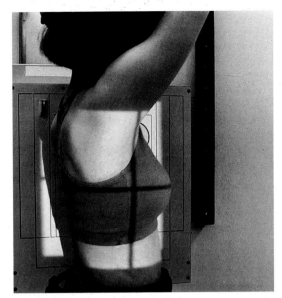

Figure 2–6. Proper patient positioning for lateral chest radiograph.

superimposes each pair, is accomplished by resting an extended flat hand against each, respectively, then adjusting the patient's rotation until the hand is positioned perpendicular to the film. Because the right lung field and ribs are positioned at a greater OID than the left lung field and ribs, the right lung field and ribs are more magnified. This magnification prevents the posterior and anterior ribs from being directly superimposed. Routinely, about a 0.5-inch (1-cm) separation is demonstrated between the right and left posterior ribs, with the right posterior ribs projecting behind the left. When the posterior ribs are directly superimposed, this separation is demonstrated between the anterior ribs (see Rad. 7).

- **Detecting Chest Rotation:** Chest rotation is effectively detected on a lateral chest radiograph by evaluating the degree of posterior rib and anterior rib superimposition. When more than 0.5 inch (1 cm) of space exists between the right and left anterior ribs or between the right and left posterior ribs, the chest was rotated for the radiograph. A rotated lateral chest radiograph obscures portions of the lung field and distorts the heart and hilum shadows.
- **Distinguishing the Right and Left Lungs:** When a rotated lateral chest radiograph has been obtained, determine how to reposition the patient by identifying the hemidiaphragms and therefore the lungs. There are many ways in which this can be accomplished, but not all may be demonstrated on each lateral chest radiograph. The first and easiest method of discerning the hemidiaphragm is to identify the *gastric air bubble.* On an upright patient, gas in the stomach rises to the fundus (superior section of stomach), which is located just beneath the left hemidiaphragm (see Rad. 8). If this gastric bubble is visualized on the radiograph, you know that the left hemidiaphragm is located directly above it.

The second method of distinguishing one lung from the other uses the heart shadow. Because the heart

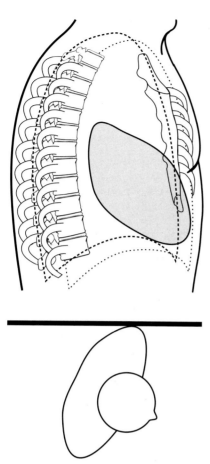

Figure 2-7. Rotation—left lung anterior.

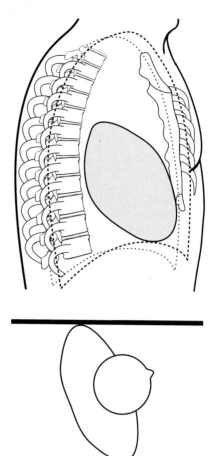

Figure 2-8. Rotation—right lung anterior.

shadow is located in the left chest cavity and extends anteroinferiorly to the left hemidiaphragm, outlining the *superior heart shadow* enables you to recognize the left lung. As demonstrated in Figure 2–7, if the left lung is positioned anteriorly, the outline of the superior heart shadow continues beyond the sternum and into the anterior lung (see Rad. 9). Figure 2–8 demonstrates the opposite rotation; the right lung is positioned anteriorly. Note how the superior heart shadow does not extend into the anterior situated lung but ends at the sternum (see Rad. 10). It is most common on rotated lateral chest radiographs for the left lung to be rotated anteriorly and the right lung rotated posteriorly.

Another method of identifying the right lung from the left is to follow the *inferior border of the heart shadow* to the left hemidiaphragm. This method is recommended only when the inferior heart shadow border is clearly defined, as on Radiograph 11. Because the heart shadow is located on the left side of the chest, when the inferior heart shadow extends below the superior hemidiaphragm—as demonstrated in Radiograph 11—the left lung is the inferior lung. When the left lung is the superior lung, it is difficult to clearly distinguish the inferior heart shadow because it is obscured by lung markings.

- ***Repositioning the Rotated Patient:*** Once the lungs have been identified, reposition the patient by rotating the thorax. When the left lung was anteriorly positioned on the original radiograph, rotate the left thorax posteriorly, and when the right lung was anteriorly positioned, rotate the right thorax posteriorly. Because both lungs move simultaneously, the amount of adjustment should be only half of the distance demonstrated between the posterior ribs.

- ***Distinguishing Scoliosis from Rotation:*** On radiographs of patients with spinal scoliosis, the lung field may appear rotated owing to the lateral deviation of the vertebral column (see Rad. 12). The anterior ribs are superimposed but the posterior ribs demonstrate differing degrees of separation, depending on the severity of scoliosis. View the accompanying PA chest radiograph to confirm this patient condition. Familiarizing yourself with the lateral radiograph obtained on a patient with scoliosis prevents unnecessary repeats.

The lungs are demonstrated without foreshortening, with nearly superimposed hemidiaphragms.

- To obtain a lateral chest radiograph without lung foreshortening, position the midsagittal plane parallel with the film. When radiographing a patient with broad shoulders and narrow hips, it is essential to place the hips away from the film to maintain a parallel midsagittal plane. In ninety percent of persons the right lung and diaphragm are situated at a slightly higher elevation than the left lung and diaphragm.[5] This elevation is caused by the liver, which is situated

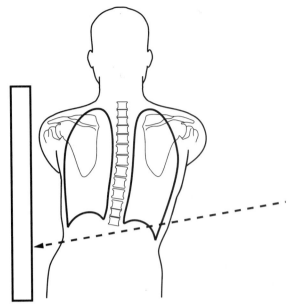

Figure 2-9. Chest foreshortening.

directly below the right diaphragm. Because the right diaphragm is elevated, one might expect it to be demonstrated above the left diaphragm when the patient is radiographed from the side, but this is not true when the midsagittal plane is correctly positioned. Because the anatomical part positioned farthest from the film diverges and magnifies the most, the right lung will be projected and magnified more than the left lung. The resulting radiograph demonstrates near superimposition of the two hemidiaphragms. It is when the midsagittal plane has not been positioned parallel with the film that lung foreshortening and poor hemidiaphragm positioning occur.

- ***Poor Midsagittal Plane Positioning:*** Figure 2–9 demonstrates a common misposition. The patient's shoulders and hips were both resting against the film, causing the inferior midsagittal plane to tilt toward the film. This positioning projects the right hemidiaphragm inferior to the left on the radiograph (see Rad. 13). When such a radiograph has been obtained, determine how the patient was mispositioned by using one of the methods described previously to distinguish the right lung from the left lung. Before repeating a lateral chest radiograph because of foreshortening, scrutinize the patient's accompanying PA projection radiograph to determine whether the patient is one of the 10 percent of persons whose hemidiaphragms are at the same height or whether a pathological condition is causing the left hemidiaphragm to be projected above the right.

- ***Right versus Left Lateral Chest Radiograph:*** There are two distinct differences between a left lateral chest radiograph and a right lateral chest radiograph, the size of the heart shadow and the superimposition of the hemidiaphragms. Both differences are a result of a change in OID and magnification. For a right lateral chest radiograph, the right thorax is positioned closer to the film. In this position, any anatomical structures located in the right thorax are

magnified less than structures located in the left thorax, because of the difference in OID. Radiographically, the heart shadow is more magnified, and the left hemidiaphragm projects lower than the right hemidiaphragm (see Rad. 14). One advantage of performing a right rather than left lateral chest radiograph is the increase in right lung radiographic detail that results from positioning of the right lung closer to the film.

There is no superimposition of humeral soft tissue over the anterior lung apices.

- Positioning humeri vertically and instructing the patient to cross the forearms above the head prevent superimposition of the humeral soft tissue over the anterior lung apices (see Rad. 8). Many dedicated chest units provide holding bars for the patient's arms. When using them, make sure the humeri are placed high enough to prevent this soft tissue overlap. If the holding bars cannot be raised high enough, position the patient's arms as just described.

The anteroinferior lung and the heart shadow are well defined.

- This area is most clearly defined when the patient is radiographed in a standing position. If the patient is seated and leaning forward, the anterior abdominal tissue is compressed, obscuring the anteroinferior lung and the heart shadow; this is especially true in an obese patient (see Rad. 15). Consideration of patient condition dictates how the radiograph will be taken. To best demonstrate this region on the seated patient, have the patient lean back slightly, allowing the anterior abdominal tissue to relax. Do not lean the patient so far back, however, that the posterior lungs are left off the radiograph.

The 11th thoracic vertebra is entirely superimposed by lung field, with the hemidiaphragms visualized inferior to it, indicating full lung aeration.

- To obtain maximum lung aeration, take the exposure after the second full inspiration with the patient in an upright position. When a lateral chest radiograph demonstrates a portion of the 11th thoracic vertebra inferior to the hemidiaphragms and a patient condition does not exist to have caused such a radiograph, full lung aeration has not been accomplished (see Rad. 16). Repeat the radiograph with a deeper patient inspiration. The lungs must be inflated to evaluate lung markings. Chest radiographs that are taken on expiration may also demonstrate a decrease in radiographic density, because a decrease in air volume increases the concentration of pulmonary tissues.

- ***Identifying the 11th Thoracic Vertebra:*** You can identify the 11th thoracic vertebra by locating the 12th thoracic vertebra—which has the last rib attached to it—and counting up one. To confirm this finding, evaluate the curvature of the posterior aspect of the thoracic and lumbar bodies. The thoracic curvature is kyphotic (forward curvature), and the lumbar curvature is lordotic (backward curvature). Follow the posterior vertebral bodies of the lower thoracic and upper lumbar vertebrae, watching for the subtle change in

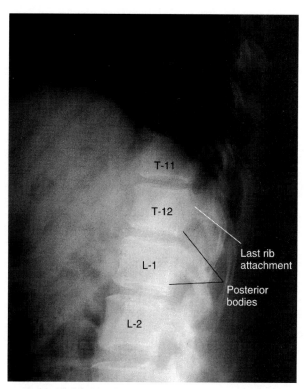

Figure 2-10. Identifying the 12th thoracic vertebra.

curvature from kyphotic to lordotic. The 12th thoracic vertebra is located just above this change (Fig. 2–10). You will find that on most fully aerated adult lateral chest radiographs, the diaphragms are demonstrated dividing the body of the 12th thoracic vertebra.

Critiquing Radiographs

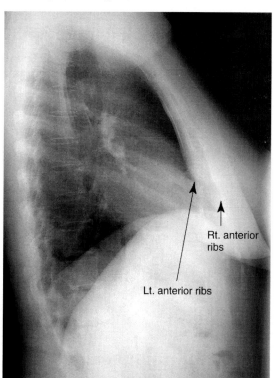

Radiograph 7.

Critique: Posterior ribs are directly superimposed, and there is about 0.5 inch (1 cm) of space between the right and left anterior ribs.
Correction: No correction movement is required. The superimposition is due to the increased magnification of the right lung over the left lung, as a result of the greater OID.

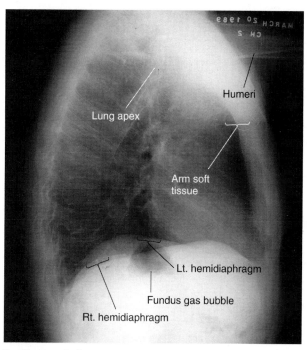

Radiograph 8.

Critique: The humeri soft tissue shadows are superimposing the anterior lung apices.
Correction: Have the patient raise the arms until the humeri are vertical, removing them from the field.

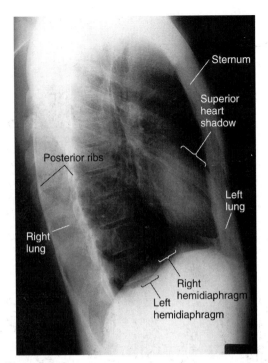

Radiograph 9.

Critique: The right and left posterior ribs are separated by more than 0.5 inch (1 cm), indicating that the chest was rotated. The gastric bubble has not been demonstrated, but the superior heart shadow is seen extending beyond the sternum and into the anteriorly situated lung, verifying that it is the left lung. The patient was positioned with the left thorax rotated anteriorly and the right thorax rotated posteriorly.

Correction: Position the right thorax slightly anteriorly. The amount of movement should be only half the distance between the posterior ribs. For this patient, the movement should be approximately 1 inch (2.5 cm).

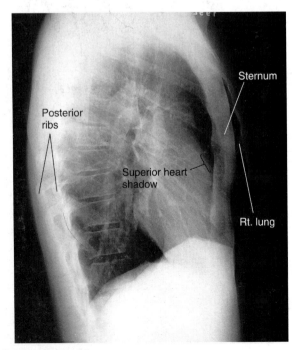

Radiograph 10.

Critique: The right and left posterior ribs are separated by more than 0.5 inch (1 cm), indicating that the chest was rotated. The superior heart shadow does not extend beyond the sternum, verifying that the right lung is situated anterior to the sternum, and the left lung posteriorly. The patient was positioned with the right thorax rotated anteriorly and the left thorax rotated posteriorly.

Correction: Position the right thorax posteriorly.

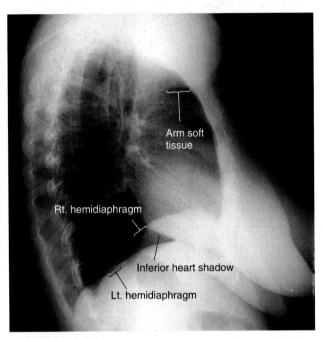

Radiograph 11.

Critique: The right and left posterior ribs are separated by more than 0.5 inch (1 cm), indicating that the chest was rotated. The inferior heart shadow extends to the inferiorly located hemidiaphragm, verifying that the left lung is situated inferiorly, and the right lung superiorly. By using this information and following the hemidiaphragm, you also find that the right lung is situated posterior to the left lung. The patient was positioned with the left thorax rotated anteriorly and the right thorax rotated posteriorly.

Correction: Position the right thorax anteriorly.

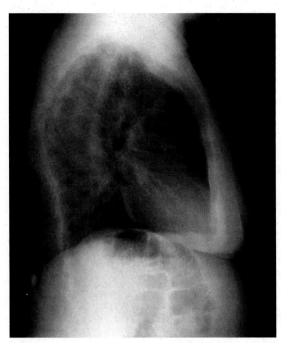

Radiograph 12.

Critique: The right and left posterior ribs demonstrate differing degrees of separation. The patient has scoliosis. Evaluate the patient's accompanying PA projection radiograph to confirm this finding.

Correction: No correction movement is required. A lateral chest radiograph on a patient with scoliosis demonstrates uneven posterior rib separation.

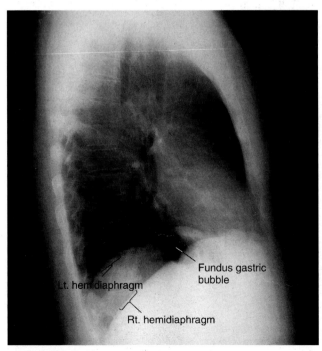

Radiograph 13.

Critique: The left hemidiaphragm is superior to the right hemidiaphragm. This is verified by the visualization of the gastric bubble below the left hemidiaphragm and by the outline of the posterior heart shadow, which ends at the superior hemidiaphragm. The patient's lower thorax was situated closer to the film than the upper thorax (see Fig. 2–9).

Correction: Before repeating the radiograph, scrutinize the patient's accompanying PA projection radiograph carefully. Determine whether the hemidiaphragms are at the same height or whether there is a pathological condition that could have caused the left diaphragm to be projected above the right. If no such condition is evident repeat the radiograph; shift the patient's hips away from the film until the midsagittal plane is placed parallel with the film.

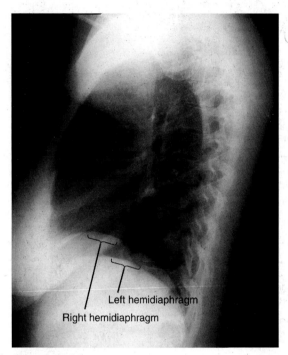

Radiograph 14.

Critique: This is a right lateral chest radiograph. The right hemidiaphragm is situated superior to the left hemidiaphragm, and the heart shadow is enlarged.

Correction: If a right lateral chest radiograph is desired, no correction is needed. Otherwise, a left lateral chest radiograph should be obtained.

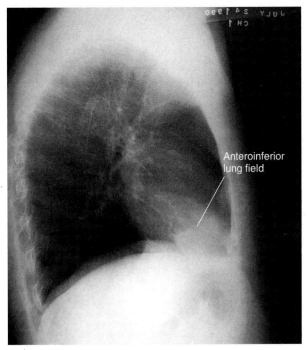

Radiograph 15.

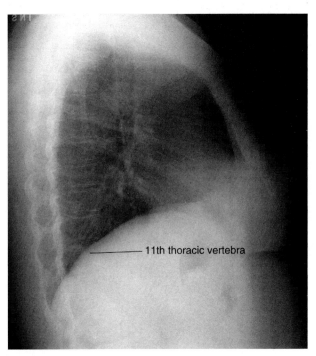

Radiograph 16.

Critique: The anterior abdominal tissue is pressing against the anteroinferior lung and heart shadows, preventing their clear visualization. The patient was leaning forward in a seated position.

Correction: Allow patient to lean back slightly, relaxing the abdominal tissue. Do not lean the patient so far back, however, that the posterior lungs are left off the radiograph.

Critique: A portion of the 11th thoracic vertebra is demonstrated inferior to the hemidiaphragms. The radiograph was not taken after full inspiration.

Correction: Coax the patient into taking a deeper inspiration.

Chest: Anteroposterior Projection
(Supine or With Portable X-Ray Unit)

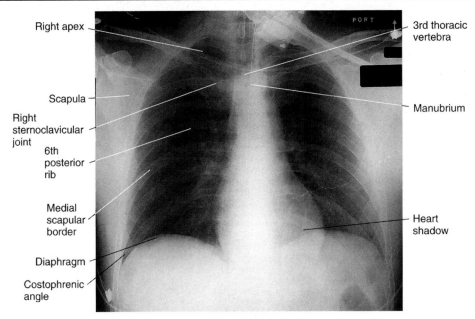

Figure 2-11. Accurately positioned AP chest radiograph.

Radiographic Evaluation

Facility's identification requirements are visible on radiograph.
- These requirements are the facility name, patient name, age, and hospital number, exam time and date.
- Position the name ID plate superiorly, to prevent it from obscuring a costophrenic angle.

A right or left marker, identifying correct side of patient, is present on radiograph and does not superimpose anatomy of interest.
- Place the marker laterally, in the upper shoulder region. Indicate on radiograph and requisition the time of the exam and the degree of patient elevation. Writing the time of day on the radiograph is especially important if the patient's progress is being followed and multiple chest radiographs are to be taken on the same day. Knowledge of the degree of elevation helps the reviewer determine the exact amount of fluid in the patient's lungs. To demonstrate precise air-fluid levels, chest radiographs should be taken with the patient upright and the x-ray beam horizontal. In this position, the air rises and the fluid gravitates to the lowest position, creating an air-fluid separation. This separation is identified as a decrease in density on the radiograph wherever the dense fluid is present in the lung field. If the patient is positioned only partially upright, the fluid line will slant, like water in a tilted jar. The true amount of fluid cannot be discerned on a radiograph unless the fluid is level, in the slanted position, the chest may appear to have more fluid than it actually does. When the patient is supine, the fluid is evenly spread throughout the lung field, preventing visualization of fluid levels.

There is no evidence of preventable artifacts, such as undergarments, necklaces, gown snaps, and patient monitoring lines.
- All patient monitoring lines that can be removed or shifted out of the lung field should be.
- When patient monitoring lines remain within the lung field, they may obscure lung details (see Rad. 17).

Contrast, density, and penetration are adequate to demonstrate vascular lung markings throughout lung field. Soft tissue outlines of the air-filled trachea, the heart shadow, and the cortical outline of posterior and anterior ribs are visualized.
- A grid is not employed in portable radiography, because it is difficult to ensure that the grid and central ray are aligned accurately, preventing grid cutoff. When no grid is used, a lower (65 to 75) kVp technique is needed to prevent excessive scattered radiation from reaching the film and hindering contrast. Although the lower kilovoltage peak will sufficiently penetrate the lung field, it seldom provides enough penetration to visualize structures within and behind the heart shadow.
- *Heart Penetration on Portable Chest Radiographs:* When a chest radiograph is used to evaluate the placement of apparatus positioned within the mediastinal region, such as a Swan-Ganz catheter, central venous pressure line, or endotracheal tube, the heart shadow should be penetrated. The accurate placement of these lines cannot be evaluated without heart penetration. Accomplish this penetration by increasing the kVp. The resulting radiograph will visualize a penetrated heart shadow with the thoracic vertebrae, posterior ribs, and chest lines, such as Swan-Ganz catheter or central venous pressure lines, clearly demonstrated through it. The amount of scattered radiation reaching the film will also increase, resulting in overall lower radiographic contrast (see Rad. 19).

The lung markings, diaphragm, heart borders, and bony cortical outlines are sharply defined.
- Sharply defined recorded details are obtained when patient respiration and body movements are halted and when the least amount of object–image distance (OID) is maintained. A 40 to 50 inch (102 to 127 cm) source–image distance (SID) is used. This SID is lower than that used for routine chest radiography and demonstrates greater heart magnification owing to the increase in x-ray divergence.

The seventh thoracic vertebra is at the center of the collimated field. The apices, lateral lungs, and costophrenic angles are included within the field.
- Centering the central ray to the midsagittal plane at a level about 4 inches (10 cm) inferior to the jugular notch places the seventh thoracic vertebra in the center of the radiograph. This central ray placement also centers the lung field on the radiograph, permitting tight collimation on all sides of the lungs. A 14 × 17 inch (35 × 43 cm) film should be adequate to include all the required anatomical structures.
- *Film Size and Direction for Portable Chest Radiography:* The direction of film placement (crosswise versus lengthwise) must also be considered to ensure full lung coverage. For the average sthenic patient and for the asthenic patient whose lung fields are long and narrow, position the film lengthwise. For the hypersthenic patient, whose lung field is short and wide, position the film crosswise. Upon inspiration, the lungs expand in three dimensions: transversely, anteroposteriorly, and vertically. Evaluate the transverse dimension to determine the direction the film should be placed. View the lateral side of the chest during deep inspiration to determine whether the lateral margins of the chest will remain within the film boundaries. If the lateral chest margins move outside the film boundaries during inspiration, consider placing the film crosswise. It is safe to position the film crosswise on most patients for portable chest radiography, because the vertical dimension does not fully expand in a recumbent or seated patient.

The chest demonstrates no rotation: The distances from the vertebral column to the sternal ends of the claviculae are equal, the air-filled trachea is aligned with the vertebral column, and a small amount of the heart shadow is visualized on the right side of the patient's thoracic vertebrae.

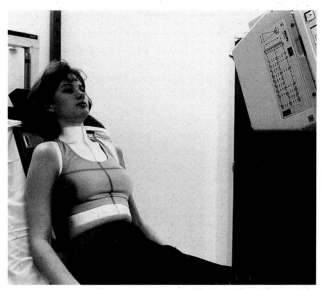

Figure 2-12. Proper patient positioning for AP chest radiograph.

- To avoid chest rotation, place the patient's shoulders and pelvis on a straight plane, and position the film parallel with the bed (Fig. 2–12). On beds with special padding, it may be necessary to place a sponge beneath one side of the film to keep it level and parallel. Because the patient's chest and film move simultaneously, if the film is not level, the chest is rotated. On a rotated chest radiograph, mediastinal structures are distorted and there is uneven density between the lateral borders of the chest.
- ***Detecting Chest Rotation on a Portable Radiograph:*** You can detect poor film balance and, consequently, chest rotation by evaluating the distance between the vertebral column and the sternal ends of the claviculae or the sternoclavicular (SC) joints. When the distances between the sternal (medial) ends of the claviculae and the vertebral column are unequal, the SC joint that superimposes the least amount of the vertebral column represents the side of the chest and film border positioned closer to the bed (see Rad. 17).

The claviculae are positioned on the same horizontal plane.

- When the patient's condition allows, position the lateral ends of the claviculae on the same horizontal plane as the medial ends by depressing the patient's shoulders. Accurate positioning of the claviculae lowers the lateral ends of the claviculae, positioning the middle and lateral claviculae away from the apical chest region and improving visualization of the apical lung field. If the patient is unable to depress the shoulders, the middle and lateral ends of the claviculae will be seen in the apical chest region.
- ***Poor Shoulder Positioning versus Poor Central Ray Alignment:*** When an AP chest radiograph is taken with the central ray angled too caudally, the claviculae are not demonstrated horizontally but are seen vertically (see Rad. 18). One can distinguish poor shoulder positioning from poor central ray align-

ment by measuring the amount of lung field demonstrated superior to the claviculae. A radiograph with poor shoulder positioning demonstrates decreased lung field superior to the claviculae, whereas a radiograph with poor central ray alignment demonstrates increased lung field superior to the claviculae.

The scapulae are demonstrated within the lung field. The distal humeri have been abducted out of the radiographic field.

- To position the scapulae outside the lung field, place the back of the patient's hands on the hips, and rotate the elbows and shoulders anteriorly. Most patients who require a portable or supine chest radiograph are incapable of positioning their arms in this manner, resulting in a radiograph with the scapulae positioned in the lung field. For this situation, at least abduct the patient's arms to place the humeri outside the radiographic field.

The manubrium superimposes the fourth thoracic vertebra with about 1 inch (2.5 cm) of the apices demonstrated above the claviculae, and the posterior ribs demonstrate a gentle downward contour.

- The alignment of the central ray with respect to the patient determines the relationship of the manubrium to the thoracic vertebrae, the amount of apical lung field seen above the claviculae, and the contour of the posterior ribs. For accurate alignment of this anatomy, position the central ray perpendicular to the film and the patient's chest. Inaccurate central ray angulation misaligns this anatomy and elongates or foreshortens the heart and lung structures. Angling the central ray caudally projects the manubrium inferior to the fourth thoracic vertebra, demonstrating more than 1 inch (2.5 cm) of lung apices above the claviculae, and changes the posterior rib contour to vertical. A caudal angle also elongates the heart and lung structures (see Rad. 18). Angling the central ray cephalically projects the manubrium superior to the fourth thoracic vertebra, demonstrating less than 1 inch (2.5 cm) of lung apices above the claviculae, and changes the posterior rib contour to horizontal. A cephalic angle also foreshortens the heart and lung structures (see Rad. 19). The more the angulation is mispositioned, either caudally or cephalically, the more distorted the anatomy.
- ***Patient with Spinal Kyphosis:*** On the supine or portable chest radiograph of a patient with spinal kyphosis (excess convexity of the thoracic vertebrae), the position of the manubrium and claviculae and the contour of the posterior ribs may appear similar to those on a chest radiograph for which the central ray was angled caudally. Also, if the patient is unable to elevate the chin, it may superimpose the apical chest region (Fig. 2–13); compensate for this patient condition by using a *slight* (5 to 10 degrees) cephalic angulation.
- ***Supine Patient:*** For the supine AP chest radiograph, the patient's shoulders and upper thorax are naturally extended posteriorly, resulting in an upward lift of the manubrium, claviculae, and superior ribs. This upward lift of the thorax can be offset with a 5-degree caudal central ray angulation.

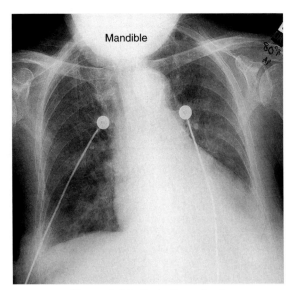

Figure 2-13. Kyphotic patient.

Nine to ten posterior ribs are demonstrated above the diaphragm, indicating full lung aeration for the non-erect chest radiograph.

- In a supine or seated patient, the diaphragm is unable to shift to its lowest position, because the abdominal organs are compressed and push against the diaphragm. As a result, the lungs are not fully aerated, and only nine to ten posterior ribs are demonstrated above the diaphragm. To obtain maximum lung aeration for a patient who is able to follow instructions, take the exposure after the second full inspiration. For the unconscious or ventilated patient, observe chest motion or ventilator indicators during respiration, and take the exposure when the chest is most expanded.

Critiquing Radiographs

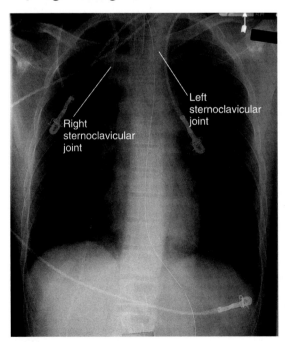

Radiograph 17.

Critique: There are many patient monitoring lines superimposing the lung field. The right SC joint is visualized away from the vertebral column, whereas the left SC joint is superimposing the vertebral column. The film was not positioned parallel with the bed. The right side of the patient and the right film boundary were positioned closer to the bed than the left side and boundary.

Correction: If monitoring lines can be removed, do so. If the lines cannot be removed, shift them to overlie the least amount of lung field. Place a sponge beneath the right film border to position the film parallel with the bed.

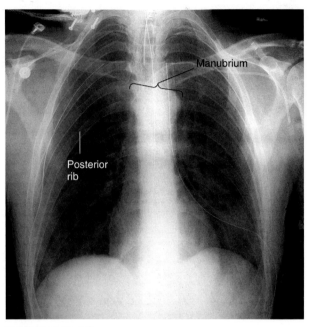

Radiograph 18.

Critique: The manubrium is superimposing the fifth thoracic vertebra, more than 1 inch (2.5 cm) of apical lung field is visualized above the claviculae, and the lateral clavicular ends are elevated. The posterior ribs demonstrate a vertical contour. All are indications that a caudal angulation was used.

Correction: To improve this radiograph, the central ray needs to be adjusted cephalad until it is aligned perpendicular to the film.

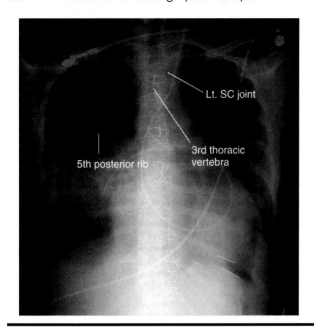

Radiograph 19.

Critique: The manubrium is superimposing the third thoracic vertebra, and less than 1 inch (2.5 cm) of apical lung field is visualized above the claviculae. The posterior ribs demonstrate a horizontal contour. The central ray was angled cephalically.
Correction: To improve this radiograph, the central ray needs to be adjusted caudally until it is aligned perpendicular to the film.

Chest: Lateral Decubitus Position

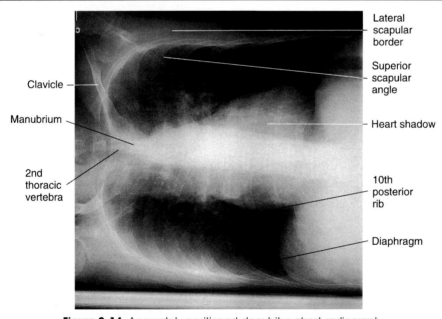

Figure 2-14. Accurately positioned decubitus chest radiograph.

Radiographic Evaluation

Facility's identification requirements are visible on radiograph.
- These requirements are facility name, patient name, age, and hospital number, and exam time and date.
- Position the name ID plate toward the patient's shoulders so it does not obscure any portion of the lungs.

A right or left marker identifying correct side of patient and an arrow or similar marker identifying side of patient positioned up and away from tabletop or cart are present on radiograph. Markers do not superimpose anatomy of interest.
- Place a right or left marker laterally and an arrow or word marker, indicating side of patient that is positioned away from the table or cart, within collimated light field. Do not superimpose any portion of the lung field with the marker.

There is no evidence of preventable artifacts, such as undergarments, necklaces, and gown snaps.

• It is recommended that patient be instructed to remove all clothing from the waist up and to change into a snapless hospital gown prior to the procedure.

Contrast and density are adequate to demonstrate vascular lung markings throughout lung field and to visualize air or fluid levels within the pleural cavity. There is sufficient beam penetration to faintly demonstrate the thoracic vertebrae and posterior ribs through the heart and mediastinal structures.

• An optimal 100 to 130 kVp technique sufficiently penetrates the heart shadow and provides the long scale of contrast necessary to visualize lung details. A grid should be used to absorb the scattered radiation produced by the thorax, reducing fog and increasing the visibility of details.

• ***Positioning to Demonstrate Pleural Air or Fluid:*** The lateral decubitus position is primarily used to confirm the presence of air (pneumothorax) or fluid (pleural effusion) in the pleural cavity. To best demonstrate the presence of air, position the affected side of the thorax away from the tabletop or cart so that the air rises to the highest level in the pleural cavity. If the affected side were placed against the tabletop or cart, the air might be obscured by the mediastinal structures. To best demonstrate fluid in the pleural cavity, position the affected side against the tabletop or cart. This positioning allows the fluid to gravitate to the lowest level of the pleural cavity, away from the mediastinal structures.

• ***Techniques to Demonstrate Pleural Air or Fluid:*** Along with positioning efforts, the technique factors chosen are also very important factors in identifying a pneumothorax or pleural effusion radiographically. When a pneumothorax is suspected, demonstration of lung markings is necessary. Radiographically, the absence of such markings indicates a pneumothorax. The lung markings are best demonstrated when the radiograph is neither overexposed nor overpenetrated. A darker density radiograph is acceptable, however, when pleural effusion is suspected. Because fluid is more dense than lung tissue, it presents a distinct underexposed, level area on a darker radiograph.

When selecting the exposure (mAs) and kVp to be used for a decubitus chest radiograph, evaluate the patient's records carefully to determine whether the technique factors should be set to demonstrate the presence of air or fluid. If a pneumothorax is suspected, decrease the kVp 8 percent from the routinely used setting. If pleural effusion is suspected, increase the mAs by 35 percent over the routinely used setting.[6]

The lung markings, diaphragm, heart borders, and cortical outlines are sharply defined.

• Sharply defined recorded details are obtained when patient respiration and body movements are halted and when the least amount of object–image distance (OID) is maintained. A 72-inch (183-cm) source–image distance (SID) is used to decrease the magnification of the heart and lung details.

The seventh thoracic vertebra is centered within the collimated field. The entire lung field, showing the apices, lateral lungs, and costophrenic angles, is included within the field.

• Centering a perpendicular central ray to the midsagittal plane at a level about 7.5 inches (18 cm) inferior to the vertebra prominens for the PA projection and 4.5 inches (11 cm) inferior to the jugular notch for the AP projection places the seventh thoracic vertebra in the center of the radiograph. This central ray placement also centers the lung field on the radiograph, allowing tight collimation on all sides of the lungs. A 14 × 17 inch (35 × 43 cm) film should be adequate to include all the required anatomical structures. For most patients, it is acceptable to use the dedicated chest unit, which will position the film crosswise to the patient and still include the entire lung field on the radiograph. In a recumbent patient, the diaphragm is unable to move to its lowest position on inspiration, preventing full vertical lung expansion. Because the lungs are unable to expand fully, a crosswise film will provide adequate lung coverage. To be certain the lateral borders are included on the radiograph, center the film and the central ray to the midsagittal plane.

The chest demonstrates a true AP or PA projection, without rotation. The air-filled trachea is aligned with the vertebral column. A small amount of heart shadow is demonstrated on the right side of the patient's thoracic vertebrae. The distance from the vertebral column to the sternal end of the clavicle is the same on each side.

• The decubitus chest radiograph can be taken in either an AP or a PA projection. In the AP projection, it is easier for the patient to maintain a true projection, without rotation, because the knees can be flexed. It is also easier for the patient to move closer to the film and raise the arms when in an AP position. To avoid chest rotation, align the shoulders, the posterior ribs, and the posterior pelvic wings perpendicular to the cart the patient is lying on (Fig. 2–15). This alignment

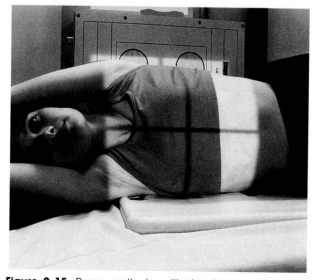

Figure 2–15. Proper patient positioning for decubitus chest radiograph.

positions the patient's shoulders and lungs at equal distances from the film. Accomplish posterior rib and pelvic wing alignment by resting your extended flat hand against each, respectively, then adjusting the patient's rotation until your hand is positioned perpendicularly to the cart. It is most common for a patient to lean the elevated shoulder, lung, and pelvic wing anteriorly when rotated. A pillow placed between the patient's knees may help to eliminate this forward rotation.

- **Detecting Chest Rotation:** Rotation is readily detected on an AP or PA decubitus chest radiograph by evaluating the distances between the vertebral column and the sternal ends of the claviculae or the sternoclavicular (SC) joints. On a nonrotated decubitus chest radiograph, the distances from the vertebral column to the SC joints should be equal. When the chest is rotated, this distance is no longer equal; one of the SC joints moves toward the vertebral column and the other moves away. On a rotated AP projection, the SC joint that superimposes the vertebral column represents the side of the chest positioned farther from the film (see Rad. 20). The opposite is true for a PA projection. For this projection, the SC joint on the side of the chest positioned farther from the film shows less vertebral column superimposition (see Rad. 21).

- **AP versus PA Chest Radiographs:** One can determine whether a chest radiograph was taken in an AP or PA projection by analyzing the appearance of the sixth and seventh cervical vertebrae and the first thoracic vertebra. In the AP projection, these vertebral bodies and their intervertebral disk spaces are demonstrated without distortion (Fig. 2–16). In the PA projection, the vertebral bodies are distorted, the intervertebral disk spaces are closed, and the spinous processes and laminae of these three vertebrae are well visualized (Fig. 2–17). The reason for these variations

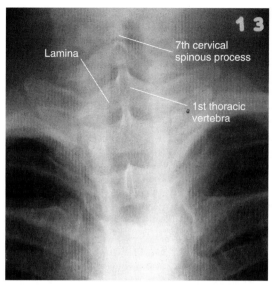

Figure 2-17. PA projection.

is related to the divergence of the x-ray beam used to radiograph these three vertebrae and to the anterior convexity of the cervical and upper thoracic vertebrae.[7]

The arms, mandible, and lateral borders of the scapulae are situated outside the lung field, and the lateral aspect of clavicle is projected upward.

- The lateral borders of the scapulae are drawn away from the lung field when the patient's arms are positioned above the head. This positioning also draws the lateral ends of the clavicle superiorly. If the arms are not positioned in this manner, the arms and the lateral borders of the scapulae are demonstrated within the upper lung field (see Rad. 20).

- Position the patient with the chin elevated, because otherwise it may superimpose the lung apices on the radiograph, especially in the PA projection (see Rad. 21).

The manubrium and the third or fourth thoracic vertebrae are superimposed.

- The tilt of the midcoronal plane determines the level at which the manubrium superimposes the thoracic vertebrae. When the midcoronal plane is parallel with the film on the AP projection, the manubrium and the third thoracic vertebra are superimposed. When the midcoronal plane is parallel with the film on the PA projection, the manubrium is superimposed by the fourth thoracic vertebra. The difference in thoracic vertebrae and manubrium superimposition between the AP and PA projections is due to the effect of beam divergence on the anatomical part positioned farther from the film.

- When the upper coronal plane is tilted toward or away from the film, the relationship between the manubrium and thoracic vertebrae is changed, and the lung field is distorted. When the upper coronal plane is tilted toward the film for the AP projection, which is the most common error, the manubrium moves superiorly (see Rad. 22). This poor positioning is obtained when

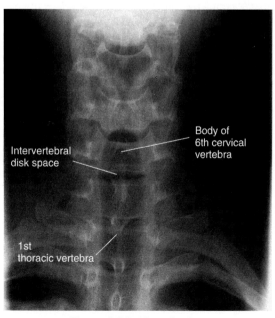

Figure 2-16. AP projection.

the upper thoracic vertebrae are straightened in an attempt to place the shoulders and lower cervical vertebrae directly against the cassette, resulting in a lordotic appearance. When the upper coronal plane is tilted away from the film for the AP projection, the manubrium moves inferiorly. The opposite is true for a PA decubitus radiograph: On forward tilting, the manubrium is inferior to the fourth thoracic vertebra, and on backward tilting, the manubrium is superior to the fourth thoracic vertebra.

Nine to ten posterior ribs are demonstrated above the diaphragm.

- In a recumbent position, the diaphragm is unable to shift to its lowest position owing to pressure from the peritoneal cavity. As a result, the lungs are not fully aerated, and only nine to ten posterior ribs are demonstrated above the diaphragm. To obtain maximum lung aeration, the exposure should be taken after the second full inspiration.

The lung field positioned against the cart is demonstrated without superimposition of the cart pad.

- Elevating the patient on a radiolucent sponge or on a hard surface such as a cardiac board prevents the chest from sinking into the cart pad. When the patient's body is allowed to sink into the cart pad, artifact lines are seen superimposing the lateral lung field of the side down (see Rad. 20). Because fluid in the pleural cavity gravitates to the lowest level, it is in this area that the fluid will be demonstrated, and superimposition of the cart pad and the lower lung field may obscure fluid that has settled in the lowest level.

Critiquing Radiographs

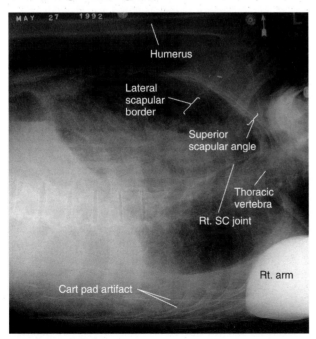

Radiograph 20.

Critique: This radiograph demonstrates numerous positioning problems. First, the patient has been rotated, as indicated by the superimposition of the right SC joint over the vertebral column. Because this radiograph was taken in an AP projection, as indicated by the sixth and seventh cervical vertebrae, the patient's right side was positioned farther from the film. Second, the arms have not been positioned above the patient's head. The right arm is positioned at a 90-degree angle with the body. Note the underexposed area next to the right lung apex. The left arm is resting against the patient's side, resulting in the visualization of the entire left scapula within the lung field. Cart pad artifacts are superimposing the lateral aspect of the right lung, because the patient was not elevated on a cardiac board or radiolucent sponge.

Correction: Rotate the patient's right side toward the film until the patient's shoulders, posterior ribs, and posterior pelvic wing are aligned perpendicular to the cart. Position the patient's arms above the head, and elevate the chest on a cardiac board or radiolucent sponge.

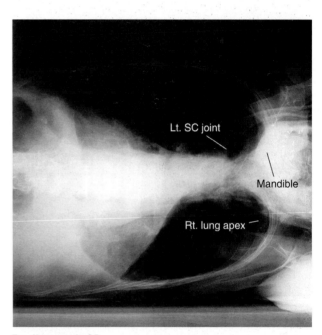

Radiograph 21.

Critique: This radiograph demonstrates two positioning problems. First, the chest has been rotated, as indicated by the superimposition of the vertebral column over the right SC joint. Because this radiograph was taken in a PA projection, as indicated by the cervical vertebrae that can be seen above the mandible, the patient's right side was positioned closer to the film. Second, because the chin was not elevated, the mandible is obscuring the apical lung region.

Correction: Rotate the patient's right side away from the film, aligning the shoulders, posterior ribs, and posterior pelvic wings perpendicular to the cart, and elevate the patient's chin.

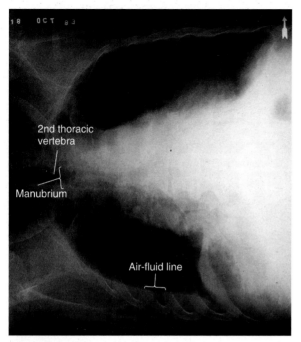

Radiograph 22.

Critique: An AP chest projection demonstrates undistorted lungs when the manubrium is situated at the level of the third thoracic vertebra. On this AP radiograph, the manubrium is situated at the level of the second thoracic vertebra. The midcoronal plane was not parallel with the film, and the upper thorax was tilted toward the film.

Correction: Shift the upper thorax away from the film until the midcoronal plane is parallel with the film.

Chest: AP Lordotic Projection

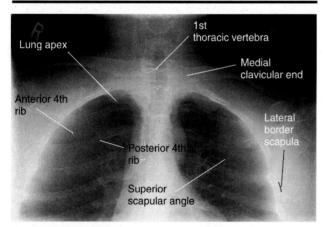

Figure 2-18. Accurately positioned lordotic chest radiograph.

Radiographic Evaluation

Facility's identification requirements are visible on radiograph.

- These requirements are facility name, patient name, age, and hospital number, and exam time and date.
- Position the name ID plate superiorly, to prevent it from obscuring a costophrenic angle.

A right or left marker, identifying correct side of patient, is present on radiograph and does not superimpose anatomy of interest.

- Place the marker laterally in the upper shoulder region.

There is no evidence of preventable artifacts, such as undergarments, necklaces, and gown snaps.

- It is recommended that the patient be instructed to remove all clothing above the waist and to change into a snapless hospital gown prior to the exam.

Contrast, density, and penetration are adequate to demonstrate vascular lung markings throughout lung field. Cortical outlines of clavicle, superior thoracic vertebrae, and posterior and anterior ribs are visualized.

- Overlying soft tissues, clavicle, and upper ribs often obscure the apical lung markings on a PA projection of the chest. The anterior ends of the first ribs may project a suspicious-looking shadow in the apices. The lordotic view is taken to visualize areas of the apical lungs obscured on the PA projection and to provide a different anatomical perspective that can be used to evaluate suspicious areas. An optimal 100 to 130 kVp technique sufficiently penetrates the mediastinal structures and provides the long scale of contrast that is needed to visualize the lung details. A grid should be used to absorb the scattered radiation produced by the thorax, reducing fog.

The lung markings and bony cortical outlines are sharply defined.

- Sharply defined recorded details are obtained when patient respiration and body movements are halted and the least amount of object–image distance (OID) is maintained. A 72-inch (183-cm) source–image distance (SID) is used to decrease the magnification of the heart and lung details.

The superior lung field is centered within the collimated field. The clavicle, the apices, and two thirds of the lung field are included within the field.

- Centering the central ray to the midsagittal plane halfway between the manubrium and the xiphoid positions the superior lung field at the center of the radiograph. Because the lung field is foreshortened, this centering will include most of the lung field on the radiograph. A higher centering is required if only the lung apices are desired. Lung foreshortening also creates the need for tight vertical collimation to prevent unnecessary exposure of abdominal and cervical vertebral tissue.
- A 14 × 17 inch (35 × 43 cm), lengthwise film should be adequate to include all the required anatomical structures.

The medial ends of the claviculae are projected superior to the lung apices onto the first thoracic vertebra. The heart shadow can be outlined, although it is foreshortened and wider than on a corresponding PA chest radiograph. The posterior and anterior portions of the first through fourth ribs lie horizontally and are nearly superimposed.

- The claviculae are projected above the apices, and the upper ribs are superimposed by positioning the patient

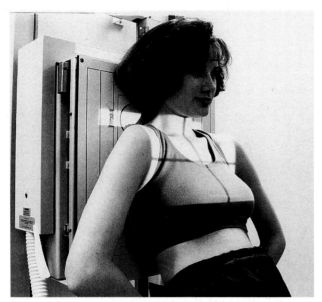

Figure 2-19. Proper patient positioning for lordotic chest radiograph—no central ray angle.

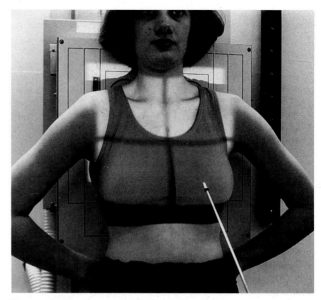

Figure 2-20. Proper patient positioning for lordotic chest radiograph—central ray angled.

using one of two methods. First, the patient's back can be arched, leaning the upper thorax and shoulders toward the film, as demonstrated in Figure 2–19. The correct amount of arching is accomplished when the patient's feet are placed about 12 inches (30 cm) away from the film before the back is arched. The angle formed between the midcoronal body plane and film should be approximately 45 degrees. Second, the patient remains upright, and a 15-degree cephalic central ray angulation is used to shift the claviculae (Fig. 2–20). With both of these methods, the claviculae and the anterior ribs are displaced superiorly. The claviculae are projected above the apices onto the first thoracic vertebra, and the anterior ribs are projected onto their corresponding posterior ribs. Inspiration also aids in obtaining this accurate positioning. When the patient inhales, the anterior ends of the first two ribs, the claviculae, and the manubrium move superiorly.

- **_Poor Patient or Central Ray Positioning:_** Inadequate back extension or central ray angulation is identified on a radiograph when the claviculae are not projected above the lung apices and when the anterior and posterior ribs are not superimposed. When the patient's back is not arched enough, or more cephalic angulation is needed, the claviculae superimpose the lung apices, and the anterior ribs are demonstrated inferior to their corresponding posterior rib (see Rad. 23). If a radiograph is obtained in which lung fields have been so foreshortened that the apices are obscured and the posterior ribs are superimposed and

cannot be distinguished, the patient's back was arched too much or the cephalic angle was too extreme (see Rad. 24).

The lateral borders of the scapulae are drawn away from the lung field, and the superior angles of the scapulae are demonstrated away from lung apices.

- The lateral borders and the superior angles of the scapulae are drawn away from the lung field by placing the back of the patient's hands on the hips and rotating the elbows and shoulders anteriorly. This position allows visualization of the lung apices without scapular obstruction.
- When the elbows and shoulders are not rotated anteriorly, the lateral borders of the scapulae are demonstrated in the lung field, and the superior scapular angles are projected into the lung apices (see Rad. 25).

The chest demonstrates no signs of rotation when the distances from the vertebral column to the sternal ends of the claviculae are equal.

- The patient's shoulders should be equal distances from the film to prevent rotation. Chest rotation can be identified on an AP lordotic radiograph by evaluating the distance between the vertebral column and the sternal ends of the claviculae or the sternoclavicular (SC) joints. When the distance between the sternal claviculae and the vertebral column are unequal, the SC joint that superimposes the least of the vertebral column is the side of the chest that was positioned closer to the film.

Critiquing Radiographs

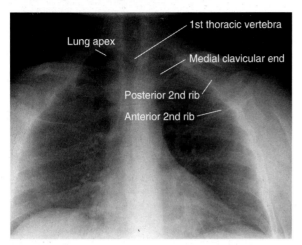

Radiograph 23.

Critique: The claviculae are superimposing the lung apices, and the anterior ribs are demonstrated inferior to their corresponding posterior rib. Either the patient's back was not arched enough or the central ray was not angled enough cephalically.

Correction: If the patient's back was arched to obtain this radiograph, increase the amount of arch or add a cephalic angulation. If this exam was obtained by using a cephalic angulation, as demonstrated in Figure 2–20, increase the degree of central ray angulation.

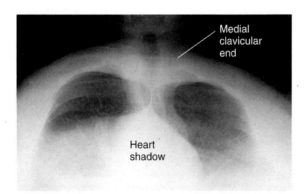

Radiograph 24.

Critique: The lung field demonstrates excessive foreshortening, and the individual ribs cannot be identified. Either the patient's back was arched too much or the central ray was angled too cephalically.

Correction: If the patient's back was arched to obtain this radiograph, decrease the amount of arch. If this exam was obtained by using a cephalic angulation, as demonstrated in Figure 2–20, decrease the degree of central ray angulation.

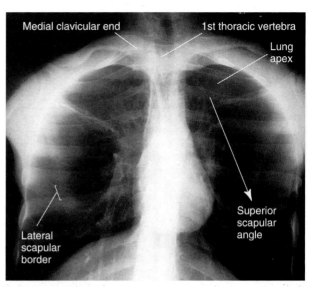

Radiograph 25.

Critique: The lateral borders of the scapulae are demonstrated within the lung field, and the superior scapular angles are demonstrated within the apical region. The patient's elbows and shoulders where not rotated anteriorly.

Correction: Place the backs of the patient's hands on the hips, and rotate the elbows and shoulders anteriorly.

Chest: Anterior Oblique Positions
(RAO and LAO)

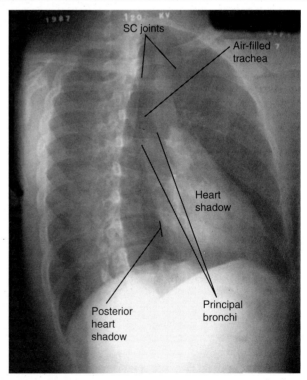

Figure 2–21. Accurately positioned 45-degree RAO chest radiograph.

Radiographic Evaluation

Facility's patient identification requirements are visible on radiograph.

- These requirements are facility name, patient name, age, and hospital number, and exam time and date.
- Position the name ID plate superiorly, to prevent it from obscuring a costophrenic angle.

A right or left marker, identifying side of patient positioned closer to the film, is present on radiograph and does not superimpose anatomy of interest.

- Place the right or left marker laterally in the light field at the upper shoulder region.

There is no evidence of preventable artifacts, such as undergarments, necklaces, and gown snaps.

- It is recommended that patient be instructed to remove all clothing above the waist and to change into a snapless hospital gown prior to the procedure.

Contrast, density, and penetration are adequate to demonstrate vascular lung markings throughout lung field. Soft tissue outlines of the air-filled trachea and heart shadow and cortical outlines of posterior and anterior ribs and thoracic vertebrae are visualized.

- Vascular lung markings are scattered throughout the lung field and are evaluated for changes that may indicate pathology. On the anterior oblique chest radiograph, the lung positioned farther from the film should demonstrate clear vascular markings. The air-filled trachea should also be demonstrated in the lung field positioned farther from the film. An optimal 100 to 130 kVp technique penetrates the heart shadow and mediastinal structures enough to visualize the vascular lung markings and air-filled trachea as well as provides the long scale of contrast necessary to visualize the lung details. A grid should be used to absorb the scattered radiation produced by the thorax, reducing fog.

The lung markings, diaphragm, heart borders, and bony cortical outlines are sharply defined.

- Sharply defined recorded details are obtained when patient respiration and body movements are halted. A 72-inch (183-cm) source–image distance (SID) is used to decrease the magnification of the heart and lung details.

The right and left principal bronchi are at the center of the collimated field. The apices, costophrenic angles, and lateral chest walls are included within the field.

- Centering a perpendicular central ray at a level about 7.5 inches (18 cm) inferior to the vertebra prominens places the central ray at the level of the bronchi. Accurate transverse positioning is obtained when the same amount of film distance is present on either side of the patient. A 14 × 17 inch (35 × 43 cm) film should be adequate to include all the required anatomical structures. The direction of film placement (crosswise or lengthwise) must also be considered to ensure full lung coverage. For the sthenic and asthenic patient, turn the film lengthwise; for the hypersthenic patient, turn the film crosswise.

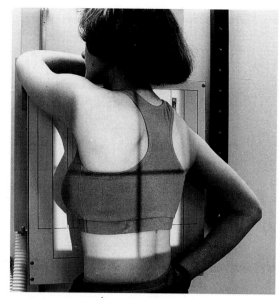

Figure 2-22. Proper patient positioning for RAO chest radiograph.

About twice as much lung field is demonstrated on one side of the thoracic vertebrae as on the other side, and the sternoclavicular (SC) joints are demonstrated without spinal superimposition, indicating that a 45-degree obliquity has been obtained.

- Rotating the patient until the midcoronal plane is aligned 45 degrees with the film (Fig. 2–22) provides the reviewer with an additional perspective of the lungs, which will assist in the detection of pulmonary diseases or artifacts. The lung field better demonstrated on an anterior oblique view is the one positioned farther from the film. A right anterior oblique (RAO) position demonstrates the left lung, whereas a left anterior oblique (LAO) position demonstrates the right lung.

- ***Verifying Accuracy of Obliquity:*** When evaluating a radiograph, you can be certain that a 45-degree obliquity has been obtained if (1) twice as much lung field is demonstrated on one side of the thoracic vertebrae as on the other side, and (2) the SC joints, air-filled trachea, and principal bronchi are demonstrated without spinal superimposition. The heart shadow is also demonstrated without spinal superimposition on an RAO chest radiograph, whereas a portion of the heart shadow superimposes the thoracic vertebrae on an LAO chest radiograph. Because the heart is located more to the left of the thoracic vertebrae, a 60-degree patient obliquity is necessary to visualize the heart shadow without spinal superimposition on the LAO.

  Figure 2–23 demonstrates a 45-degree LAO chest radiograph. Note that the lung field on one side is twice as large as on the other and that there is slight superimposition of the thoracic vertebrae and heart shadow. Compare this radiograph with the 60-degree LAO chest radiograph shown in Figure 2–24. Note that there is more than two times as much lung field on one side of the thoracic vertebrae as the other in Figure 2–24, and that the heart shadow and thoracic

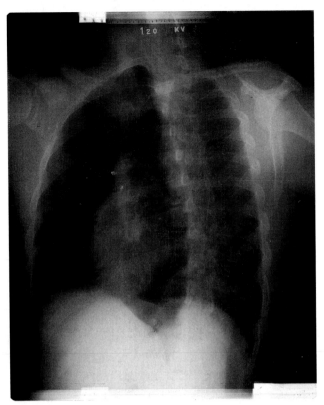

Figure 2-23. Accurately positioned 45-degree LAO chest radiograph.

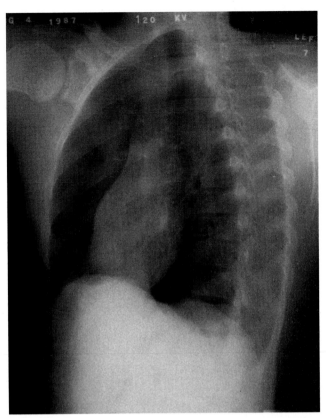

Figure 2-24. Accurately positioned 60-degree LAO chest radiograph.

vertebrae are not superimposed. How much obliquity should be obtained depends on the exam indications. When the exam is being performed to evaluate the lung field, a 45-degree oblique radiograph is required; when the outline of the heart is of interest, a 60-degree oblique view is required.

- ***Repositioning the Inaccurately Rotated Patient:*** If the desired 45-degree obliquity is not obtained on a chest radiograph, compare the amount of lung field demonstrated on either side of the thoracic vertebrae. If the radiograph demonstrates more than two times the lung field on one side of the thoracic vertebrae than on the other side, the patient was rotated more than 45 degrees. If less than two times the lung field is demonstrated on one side of the thoracic vertebrae than the opposite side, the patient was not rotated enough (see Rad. 26).

To determine repositioning movements for the 60-degree LAO radiograph, evaluate the heart shadow and thoracic vertebrae superimposition. With adequate obliquity, the heart shadow is positioned just to the right of the thoracic vertebrae. If the oblique position is less than 60 degrees, the heart shadow superimposes the thoracic vertebrae, as on a 45-degree LAO chest radiograph. Excess obliquity produces a radiograph similar to a rotated lateral chest radiograph.

- ***Posterior Oblique Chest Radiographs:*** Routinely, anterior oblique radiographs are performed for oblique chest radiography because they position the heart closer to the film. When posterior oblique (RPO and LPO) chest radiographs are taken, however, the preceding evaluation corresponds in the following way. The LPO position demonstrates the lung situated closer to the film, which is the left lung. To review this position, use the RAO evaluation previously described. For the RPO position, the right lung is of interest, and the LAO evaluation should be followed. A 45-degree obliquity is required in the LPO radiograph to rotate the heart away from the thoracic vertebrae, but a 60-degree obliquity is needed for the RPO position.

Ten to 11 posterior ribs are demonstrated above the hemidiaphragms, indicating full lung aeration.

- To obtain maximum lung aeration, take the exposure after the second full inspiration. If fewer than ten posterior ribs are demonstrated, the lungs were not fully inflated. Determine whether a patient condition hindered full aeration. If not, repeat the radiograph following full inspiration.

Critiquing Radiographs

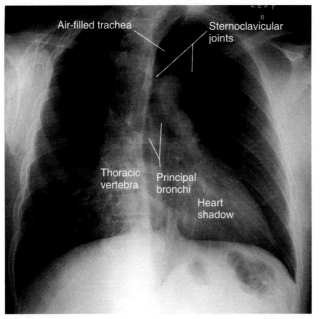

Radiograph 26.

Critique: This radiograph was taken with the patient in an RAO position. Less than two times the lung field is demonstrated on the left side of the thoracic vertebrae than on the right side. The thoracic vertebrae are superimposing a portion of the heart shadow and the air-filled trachea. The obliquity was less than 45 degrees.

Correction: Increase the degree of patient obliquity until the midcoronal plane is placed at a 45-degree angle with the film.

ABDOMEN

Anteroposterior Projection (Supine and Upright)

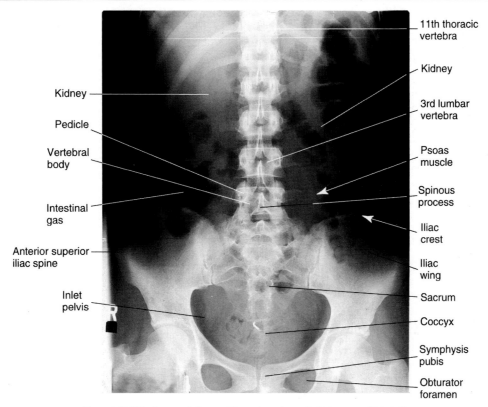

Figure 2-25. Accurately positioned supine abdomen radiograph.

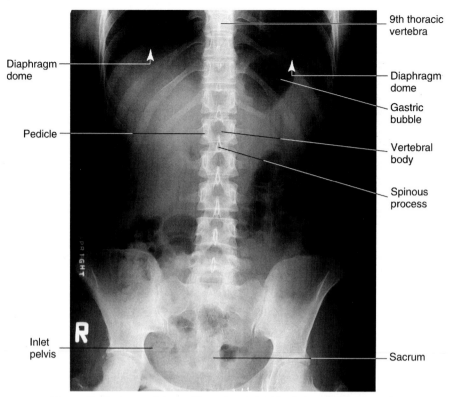

Diaphragm dome

Pedicle

Inlet pelvis

R

9th thoracic vertebra

Diaphragm dome

Gastric bubble

Vertebral body

Spinous process

Sacrum

UPRIGHT R

Figure 2-26. Accurately positioned upright AP abdomen radiograph.

Radiographic Evaluation

Facility's identification requirements are visible on radiograph.

- These requirements are facility name, patient name, age, and hospital number, and exam time and date.
- Position the name ID plate inferiorly, to prevent it from obscuring the soft tissue structures in the upper left quadrant.

A right or left marker identifying correct side of patient is present on radiograph. *Upright Radiograph:* **An arrow marker points upward or another type of marker indicates that this radiograph was taken with the patient in an upright position. The markers do not superimpose anatomy of interest.**

- Place marker(s) laterally in lower corner of film to avoid superimposing any portion of the peritoneal cavity.

There is no evidence of preventable artifacts, such as buttons and zippers.

- The patient should be instructed to remove outer clothing and any underclothes containing artifacts, then to change into a snapless hospital gown before the procedure.

Contrast and density are adequate to demonstrate the collections of fat that outline the psoas muscles and kidneys as well as the bony structures of the lumbar vertebrae. Penetration is sufficient to visualize the bony trabecular patterns and cortical outlines of the lumbar

vertebrae and pelvis without overpenetrating the abdominal tissues.

- An optimal 65 to 75 kVp technique sufficiently penetrates the soft tissue and bony structures of the abdomen. This kVp setting enhances the subtle radiation absorption differences among the fat, gas, muscles, and solid organs, which mainly consist of water. Because soft tissue abdominal structures are similar in atomic number and density, whether two soft tissue structures that border each other are visible or not depends on their arrangement with respect to the gas and fat collections that lie next to them, around them, or within them. These same gas and fat collections are used to identify diseases and masses within the abdomen. The presence or absence of gas, as well as its amount and location within the intestinal system, may indicate a functional, metabolic, or mechanical disease, whereas routinely seen collections of fat may be displaced or obscured with organ enlargement or mass invasion.[8] Use a high-ratio grid to reduce the scattered radiation that reaches the film, thereby reducing fog and increasing the visibility of the recorded details, and providing a higher-contrast radiograph.
- **Abdominal Anatomy:** The soft tissue structures that can be outlined if appropriate radiographic density and contrast have been obtained on an abdominal radiograph are the lateral psoas muscles and kidneys. The psoas muscles are located lateral to the lumbar vertebrae. They originate at the first lumbar vertebra on each side and extend to the corresponding lesser trochanter. Radiographically, the psoas muscles are

visualized on an AP abdominal radiograph as long triangular soft tissue shadows on each side of the vertebral bodies. The kidneys are found in the posterior abdomen and are identified on the radiograph as bean-shaped densities located on each side of the vertebral column 3 inches (7.5 cm) from the midline. The upper kidney poles lie on the same transverse level as the spinous process of the eleventh thoracic vertebra, and the lower poles lie on the same transverse level as the spinous process of the third lumbar vertebra. The right kidney is usually demonstrated about 1 inch (2.5 cm) inferior to the left kidney because of its location beneath the liver.[9] Occasionally, a kidney may be displaced inferior (nephrotosis) to this location, because it is not held in place by adjacent organs or its fat covering; this condition is most often seen in thin patients.[10]

- **Techniques to Compensate for Specific Patient Conditions:** The routine technique obtained from the anteroposterior body measurement of patients with suspected large amounts of *bowel gas* may overexpose areas of the abdomen that are overlaid with gas (see Rad 27). (The patient measures the same whether gas or dense soft tissue causes the thickness.) This increased radiographic density is due to the low density (number of atoms per given area) characteristic of gas. As the radiation passes through the patient's body, fewer photons are absorbed where gas is located than where there is dense soft tissue. To compensate for this situation, decrease the exposure (mAs) 30 to 50 percent or the kVp 5 to 8 percent from the routinely used technique before the radiograph is taken.[6]

An underexposed radiograph may result on patients with suspected *ascites* (invasion of fluid in peritoneal cavity), *obesity, bowel obstructions, or soft tissue masses.* This is because sections of the abdomen that normally contain gas or fat do not, resulting in an increase in the density of the soft tissue. To compensate for this situation, increase the exposure (mAs) 30 to 50 percent or the kVp 5 to 8 percent from the routinely used technique before the radiograph is taken.[6]

When an upright abdominal radiograph is taken on a patient with *excessive abdominal soft tissue,* the soft tissue often drops down and forward. This movement results in a larger anteroposterior measurement at the lower abdominal level than at the upper abdominal level. For such patients, use two crosswise films to include all the abdominal structures, and take measurements of the lower *and* upper abdominal areas to ensure that accurate radiographic density of each area will be obtained.

The cortical outlines of the posterior ribs, lumbar vertebrae, and pelvis and the gases within the stomach and intestines are sharply defined.

- Sharply defined recorded details are obtained when patient motion is controlled, respiration is halted, a short exposure time is used, and a short object–image distance (OID) is maintained.
- **Voluntary versus Involuntary Motion:** Two kinds of motion may be evident on an abdominal

radiograph: voluntary and involuntary. Voluntary motion is caused by breathing or moving during the exposure. It can be controlled by explaining to the patient the importance of holding still, making the patient as comfortable as possible on the radiographic table, and using the shortest possible exposure time. Radiographically, voluntary motion can be identified as blurred bony cortices and gastric and intestinal gases (see Fig. 1–44, page 22).

Involuntary motion is caused by the peristaltic activity of the stomach or small or large intestine. This movement is considered involuntary because the patient cannot control this movement as with breathing. The only means of decreasing the blur caused by involuntary motion is to use the shortest possible exposure time, and in some cases, this is not good enough. Radiographically, involuntary motion can be identified as sharp bony cortices and blurry gastric and intestinal gases (see Fig. 1–45, page 22).

The abdomen demonstrates an AP projection. The spinous processes are aligned with the midline of the vertebral bodies, and the distance from the pedicles to the spinous processes is the same on both sides. The sacrum is centered within the inlet of pelvis and is aligned with the symphysis pubis.

- To obtain an AP *supine* abdominal radiograph, place the patient supine on the radiographic table. Position the shoulders and anterosuperior iliac spines at equal distances from the tabletop to prevent rotation, and draw the patient's arms away from the abdominal area to prevent them from superimposing the abdominal region (Fig. 2–27).
- An AP *upright* abdominal radiograph is obtained by placing the patient against an upright radiographic tabletop. Position the shoulders and anterosuperior iliac spines at equal distances from the tabletop to prevent rotation, and draw the patient's arms away

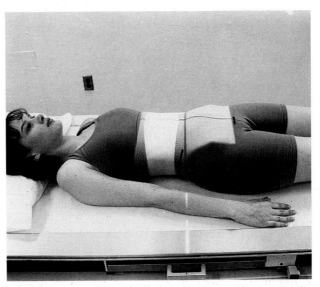

Figure 2-27. Proper patient positioning for supine abdomen radiograph.

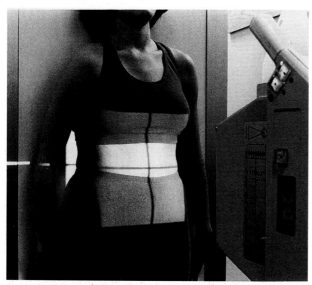

Figure 2–28. Proper patient positioning for upright AP abdomen radiograph.

from the abdominal area to prevent them from superimposing the abdominal region (Fig. 2–28).

- **Demonstrating Intraperitoneal Air:** To best demonstrate intraperitoneal air, the patient should be positioned upright for 10 to 20 minutes before the radiograph is taken.[11] This allows enough time for the air to move away from the soft tissue abdominal structures and rise to the level of the diaphragms. If a patient has come to the radiographic department for a supine and upright abdominal series, begin with the upright radiograph if the patient was ambulatory (able to walk) or transported by wheelchair. An ambulatory or wheelchair patient has been upright long enough for the air to rise, so does not have to wait for the radiograph to be taken.

- **Detecting Abdominal Rotation:** Rotation of an abdominal radiograph can decrease the visualization of fat lines that surround abdominal structures. For example, the lateral psoas muscles are outlined because of the fat that lies next to them. When the patient is rotated to one side, this fat shifts from lateral to anterior or posterior with respect to the muscle. The shift eliminates the subject contrast difference that exists when the muscle and fat are separated, hindering the usefulness of the psoas muscles as diagnosing indicators.

    The upper and lower lumbar vertebrae can demonstrate rotation independently or simultaneously, depending on which section of the body is rotated. If the patient's thorax was rotated but the pelvis remained in an AP projection, the upper lumbar vertebrae and abdominal cavity demonstrate rotation. If the patient's pelvis was rotated but the thorax remains in an AP projection, the lower vertebrae and abdominal cavity demonstrate rotation. If the patient's thorax and pelvis were rotated simultaneously, the entire lumbar column and abdominal cavity demonstrate rotation.

    Rotation is effectively detected on an AP abdominal radiograph by comparing the distance from the pedi-

cles to the spinous processes on each side and by evaluating the centering of the sacrum within the inlet pelvis. If the distance from the pedicles to the spinous processes is greater on one side of the vertebrae than on the other, or if the sacrum is rotated toward one side of the inlet, pelvic rotation is present (Rad. 28). The side with the smaller distance between the pedicles and spinous processes and toward which the sacrum is rotated is the side of the patient positioned farther from the tabletop and film.

- **Distinguishing Abdominal Rotation from Scoliosis:** In patients with scoliosis, the lumbar bodies may appear rotated owing to the lateral twisting of the vertebrae. Scoliosis of the vertebral column can be very severe, demonstrating a large degree of lateral deviation, or it can be subtle, demonstrating only a small degree of deviation. Severe scoliosis is very obvious and is seldom mistaken for patient rotation, whereas subtle scoliotic changes can be easily mistaken for patient rotation (see Rad. 29). Although both demonstrate unequal distances between the pedicles and spinous processes, there are clues that can be used to distinguished subtle scoliosis from rotation. The long axis of a rotated vertebral column remains straight, whereas the scoliotic vertebral column demonstrates lateral deviation. When the lumbar vertebrae demonstrate rotation, it has been caused by the rotation of the upper or lower torso. The middle lumbar vertebrae (L3–4) cannot rotate unless the lower thoracic vertebrae or upper or lower lumbar vertebrae are also rotated. On the scoliotic radiograph, the middle lumbar vertebrae may demonstrate rotation without corresponding upper or lower vertebral rotation. Familiarity with the difference between a rotated lumbar vertebral column and a scoliotic one will prevent unnecessary repeats on patients with spinal scoliosis.

The long axis of the lumbar vertebral column is aligned with the long axis of the collimated field.

- Aligning the long axis of the lumbar vertebral column with the long axis of the collimated field ensures that the lateral abdominal cavity will not be clipped. To obtain proper upper abdominal alignment, align the xiphoid with the collimator's longitudinal light line. To obtain proper lower abdominal alignment, find the point halfway between the patient's palpable anterior superior iliac spines; then align this point with the collimator's longitudinal light line. Do not assume that the patient's navel is positioned directly above the vertebral column. Often it is shifted to one side.

The radiograph was taken on expiration, and the diaphragm dome is located superior to the 11th thoracic vertebra.

- From full inspiration to expiration, the diaphragm position moves from an inferior to a superior position. This movement also changes the pressure placed on the abdominal structures. On full expiration, the right side of the diaphragm dome is at the same transverse level as the eighth or ninth thoracic vertebrae, whereas on inspiration, it may be found at the same transverse level as the 11th thoracic vertebra. If the abdominal radiograph is taken on inspiration, the inferior placement of the diaphragm places pressure on the abdominal organs, resulting in less space in the peritoneal cavity and greater abdominal denseness.[9]

Supine Position: **The fourth lumbar vertebra is centered within the collimated field. The spinous process of the 11th thoracic vertebra, the lateral body soft tissues, the iliac wings, and the obturator foramina are included within the field.**

- Including the spinous process of the 11th thoracic vertebra ensures that the kidneys, tip of liver, and spleen, which all lie inferior to it, will be present on the radiograph. Including the obturator foramina ensures that the inferior border of the peritoneal cavity is included on the radiograph (see Rad. 30).
- To position the fourth lumbar vertebra in the center of the collimated field, use a 40 to 48 inch (102 to 122 cm) source–image distance (SID). Center a perpendicular central ray with the patient's midsagittal plane at the level of the iliac crest for the female patients and at a level 1 inch (2.5 cm) inferior to the iliac crest for male patients, to allow for the difference in size and longitudinal dimension between the female and male pelvises.
- ***Centering the Central Ray in Males versus Females:*** The centering determination measurements for male patients were taken from several male and female pelvic radiographs, because (1) the patient is positioned in the same manner for a pelvic radiograph as for an AP abdominal radiograph, (2) the magnification factors (SID and OID) are identical to those used for an AP abdominal radiograph, and (3) all pelvic anatomy was included and could be easily measured. The only difference in setup procedure between AP pelvis and AP abdominal radiographs is the centering of the central ray. Although the superior centering used for the AP abdominal radiograph projects the anteriorly located pelvic structures slightly more inferiorly than they appear on an AP pelvis radiograph, the influence is the same on all abdominal films and affects the male and female pelvises in the same manner. A measurement of each pelvis radiograph was taken from the most superiorly located surface of the right iliac crest to the most inferior aspect of the right obturator foramen. Although slight variations of about 0.25 inch (0.6 cm) did exist within each gender, the average female measurement was 8.5 inches (21 cm) and the average male measurement was 9.5 inches (24 cm). Because the film length used for AP abdominal radiographs is 17 inches (43 cm) and the pelvis is to fit on the lower half, one can see why accurate central ray placement is important to include the needed structures.
- ***Film Size and Direction:*** A 14 × 17 inch (35 × 43 cm) lengthwise film should be adequate to include all the required anatomical structures on *sthenic* and *asthenic* patients.

  If the spinous process of the 11th thoracic vertebra is not included on this radiograph, take a second radiograph using an 11 × 14 inch (28 × 35 cm) crosswise film. It is necessary for the second radiograph to include about 2 to 3 inches (5 to 7.5 cm) of the same transverse section of the peritoneal cavity imaged on the first radiograph, to ensure that no middle peritoneal information has been excluded. The top of the film should extend to the patient's xiphoid (which is at the level of the tenth thoracic vertebra) to make sure that the spinous process of the 11th thoracic vertebra is included. The longitudinal collimated field should remain fully open for both films. Transversely, collimate to the patient's lateral skinline.

  Use two 14 × 17 inch (35 × 43 cm) crosswise films on *hypersthenic* patients to include all the necessary anatomical structures. Take the first radiograph with the central ray centered to the midsagittal plane at a level 1 inch (2.5 cm) inferior to the anterior superior iliac spines. Position the bottom of the second film so it includes 2 to 3 inches (5 to 7.5 cm) of the same transverse section of the peritoneal cavity imaged on the first radiograph to ensure that no middle peritoneal information has been excluded. The top of the film should extend to the patient's xiphoid (which is at the level of the tenth thoracic vertebra) to make sure that the spinous process of the 11th thoracic vertebra is included. Open the longitudinal and transversely collimated fields to the full 14 × 17 inch (35 × 43 cm) field size for both films.

- ***Gonadal Shielding:*** Use gonadal shielding for supine radiographs on all male patients and on female patients if two films are required and the upper abdomen is being radiographed. Do not shield female patients if the lower abdomen is being radiographed, because the shield may obscure needed information.

Upright Position: **The third lumbar vertebra is centered within the collimated field. Included within the field are the diaphragm, the ninth thoracic vertebra, the lateral body soft tissue, and the iliac wings.**

- The upright abdominal position is most often used to evaluate the peritoneal cavity for intraperitoneal air. To demonstrate intraperitoneal air, the diaphragm must be included in its entirety, because the air would be located directly inferior to the domes of the diaphragm (see Rad. 31). When the radiograph is taken on expiration, including the ninth thoracic vertebra will ensure visualization of the diaphragm. To place the ninth thoracic vertebra at the top of the radiograph and to center the third thoracic vertebra to the center of the collimated field, place the top of the film (*not* the top of the collimator's light field) at a level 2.5 inches (6.25 cm) superior to the xiphoid. Use a 40 to 48 inch (102 to 122 cm) SID. Center a perpendicular central ray with the midsagittal plane and film center.
- ***Film Size and Direction:*** A 14 × 17 inch (35 × 43 cm) lengthwise film is adequate to include all the required anatomical structures on the average *sthenic* and *asthenic* patient. Open the longitudinal and transversely collimated fields the full 14 × 17 inch (35 × 43 cm) field size.

  Use two 14 × 17 inch (35 × 43 cm) crosswise films on *hypersthenic* patients to include all the necessary anatomical structures. Take the first radiograph with the top of the film placed at a level 2.5 inches (6.25 cm) superior to the xiphoid. Place the top of the second film so it will include 2 to 3 inches (5 to 7.5 cm) of the same transverse section of the peritoneal cavity imaged on the first radiograph, to ensure that no middle peritoneal information has been excluded. Center the central ray to the midsagittal plane for both radiographs, and open the longitudinal and trans-

versely collimated fields to the full 14 × 17 inch (35 × 43 cm) field size for both films.

- **Gonadal Shielding:** Use gonadal shielding for upright radiographs on all male patients and on female patients if two films are required and the upper abdomen is being radiographed. Do not shield female patients when the lower abdomen is radiographed, because the shield may obscure needed information.

Critiquing Radiographs

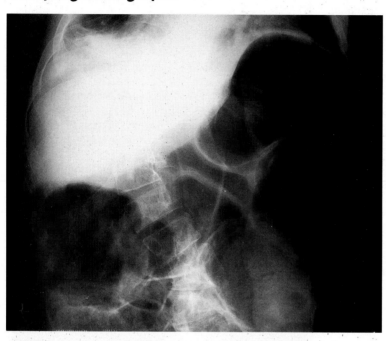

Radiograph 27.

Critique: This abdominal radiograph was taken on a hypersthenic patient who had an excessive amount of bowel gas. In an attempt to demonstrate the areas superimposed with bowel gas, the exposure (mAs) was decreased. The decrease resulted in an underexposed area beneath the right diaphragm.

Correction: If this abdominal area is of importance, a second radiograph should be taken with increased exposure. If the indication for the exam is to evaluate bowel gas, the radiograph is acceptable.

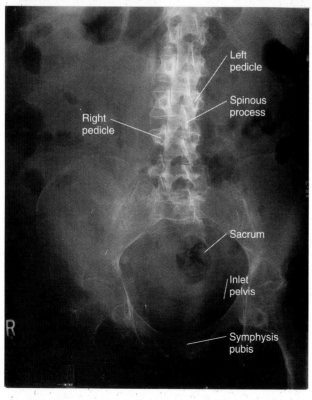

Radiograph 28.

Critique: The sacrum is not aligned with the symphysis pubis, and the distance from the left pedicles to the spinous processes is less than the distance from the right pedicles to the spinous processes. The patient was rotated onto the right side (RPO). The lateral soft tissue is not included.

Correction: Rotate the patient toward the left side until the shoulders and anterior superior iliac spines are positioned at equal distances from the film. Use two crosswise films.

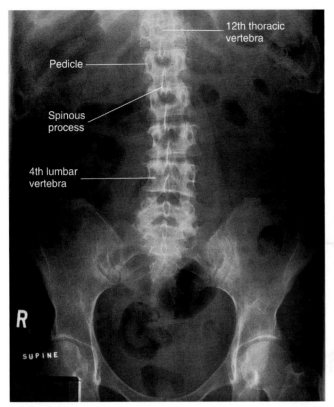

Radiograph 29.

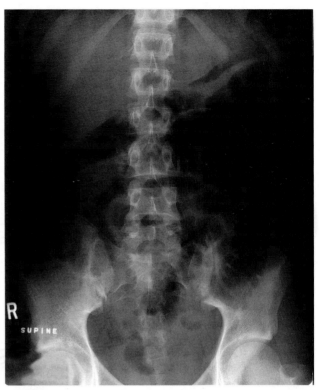

Radiograph 30.

Critique: The vertebral column deviates laterally at the level of the second through fourth lumbar vertebrae, the sacrum is centered within the inlet pelvis, and the distances from the pedicles to the spinous processes of the 12th thoracic vertebra and fifth lumbar vertebra are equal. The obturator foramina are not entirely demonstrated. The vertebral column demonstrates subtle spinal scoliosis and the central ray and film were centered too superiorly.

Correction: No correction movement is required for scoliosis. An AP abdominal radiograph of a patient with scoliosis appears rotated. Position the central ray and film 1 inch (2.5 cm) inferiorly.

Critique: This is a supine abdominal radiograph. The symphysis pubis, obturator foramina, and inferior peritoneal cavity are not included on the radiograph. The central ray was centered too superiorly.

Correction: Because this is a male patient, center the central ray 1 inch (2.5 cm) inferior to the iliac crest.

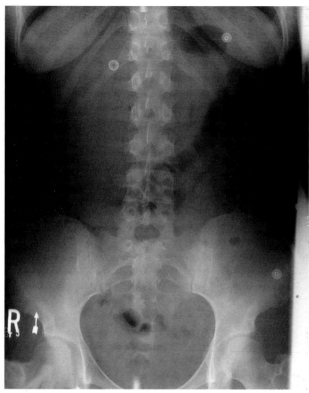

Radiograph 31.

Critique: This is an upright AP abdominal radiograph. The domes of the diaphragm are not included on the radiograph. The central ray was centered too inferiorly. Also, three gown snap artifacts are present on the radiograph.

Correction: Center the central ray about 2 inches (5 cm) superiorly, and either shift the gown snaps away from the abdominal areas or have the patient change into a snapless hospital gown.

Abdomen: Left Lateral Decubitus
Position (Anteroposterior Projection)

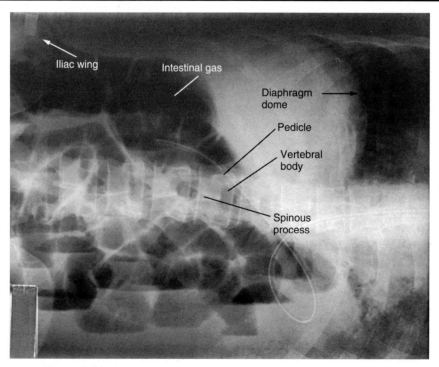

Figure 2-29. Accurately positioned decubitus abdominal radiograph.

Radiographic Evaluation

Facility's identification requirements are visible on radiograph.

- These requirements are facility name, patient name, age, and hospital number, and exam time and date.
- Position the name ID plate inferiorly, to prevent it from obscuring the soft tissue structures in the upper left quadrant.

A right marker, identifying the right side of patient, and an arrow or similar marker, indicating that the right side of patient was positioned up and away from the tabletop or cart, are present on radiograph and do not superimpose anatomy of interest.

- Place a right marker and an arrow or word marker indicating which side of the patient was positioned away from the tabletop or cart and the film. Do not allow the markers to superimpose any portion of the right upper peritoneal cavity or lung field, or the right lateral iliac wing region. It is in these areas that intraperitoneal air, if present, will be visualized.

There is no evidence of preventable artifacts, such as buttons and zippers.

- The patient should be instructed to remove outer clothing and any underclothes containing artifacts, and then to change into a snapless hospital gown before the procedure.

Contrast and density are adequate to demonstrate the collections of fat that outline the psoas muscles and kidneys, as well as the bony structures of the lumbar vertebrae. Penetration is sufficient to visualize the bony trabecular patterns and cortical outlines of the lumbar vertebrae and pelvis without overpenetrating the abdominal tissues.

- An optimal 65 to 75 kVp technique sufficiently penetrates the soft tissue and bony structures of the abdomen. This kVp setting enhances the subtle radiation absorption differences that exist among fat, gas, muscles, and solid organs, which mainly consist of water. Because soft tissue abdominal structures are similar in atomic number and density, whether two soft tissue structures that border each other are visible or not depends on their arrangement with respect to the gas and fat collections that lie next to them, around them, or within them.[8] Use a high-ratio grid to reduce the scattered radiation that reaches the film, thereby reducing fog, increasing the visibility of the recorded details, and providing a higher-contrast radiograph.
- ***Abdominal Anatomy:*** The soft tissue structures that one should be able to outline, if appropriate radiographic density and contrast have been obtained on an abdominal radiograph, are the lateral psoas muscles and the kidneys. The psoas muscles are located lateral to the lumbar vertebrae. They originate at the first lumbar vertebra on each side and extend to the corresponding lesser trochanter. Radiographically, the psoas muscles are visualized on an AP abdominal radiograph as long triangular soft tissue shadows on either side of the vertebral bodies. The kidneys are found in the posterior abdomen and are identified on the radiograph as bean-shaped densities located on each side of the vertebral column, 2 to 3 inches (5 to 7.5 cm) from the midline.

- ***Techniques to Compensate for Specific Patient Conditions:*** The routine technique obtained from the anteroposterior body measurement of patients with suspected large amounts of *bowel gas* may overexpose areas of the abdomen overlaid with gas. This is because gas absorbs fewer photons than soft tissue. To compensate for this situation, decrease the exposure (mAs) 30 to 50 percent or the kVp 5 to 8 percent from the routinely used technique before the radiograph is taken.[6]

  An underexposed radiograph may result on patients with suspected *ascites, obesity, bowel obstructions,* or *soft tissue masses.* This is because sections of the abdomen that normally contain gas or fat do not, resulting in greater soft tissue density and photon absorption. To compensate for this, increase the exposure (mAs) 30 to 50 percent or the kVp 5 to 8 percent from the routinely used technique before the radiograph is taken.[6]

- ***Using a Wedge-Compensating Filter:*** When a decubitus abdominal radiograph is taken on a patient with *excessive abdominal soft tissue,* the soft tissue often drops toward the tabletop or cart. This movement results in a smaller anteroposterior measurement at the elevated right side than at the left side, which is positioned closer to the tabletop or cart. To compensate for this thickness difference, a wedge-compensating filter may be used. The wedge filter absorbs some of the x-ray photons before they reach the patient, thus decreasing the number of photons exposing the film where the filter is located. The thick end of the wedge filter absorbs more photons than the thin end. When a wedge-compensating filter is used, attach it to the x-ray collimator head with the thick end positioned toward the patient's right side and the thin end toward the left side. The collimator light projects a shadow of the compensating filter onto the patient. Position the shadow of the thin end at the level of the thickest part of the abdomen, allowing the thick end to extend toward the right side. Then set a technique that will accurately expose the thickest abdominal region. The wedge-compensating filter should absorb the needed photons to prevent overexposure of the thinner abdominal region. When the filter has been accurately positioned, radiographic density is uniform throughout the abdominal structures. Positioning the filter too close to or too far away from the thickest part of the abdomen results in an overexposed or underexposed area on the radiograph, respectively.

The cortical outlines of the posterior ribs, lumbar vertebrae, and pelvis, and the gases within the stomach and intestines are sharply defined.

- Sharply defined recorded details are obtained when patient motion is controlled, respiration is halted, a short exposure time is used, and a short object–image distance (OID) is maintained.

- ***Motion:*** A decubitus abdominal radiograph can demonstrate voluntary or involuntary motion. Radiographically, voluntary motion can be identified by blurred cortices and gastric and intestinal gases. It can be controlled by explaining to the patient the importance of holding still, making the patient as comfortable as possible on the radiographic table, and using the shortest possible exposure time. Involuntary motion can be identified radiographically as sharp bony cortices and blurry gastric and intestinal gases. The only means of decreasing the blur caused by involuntary motion is to use the shortest possible exposure time, and this, in some cases, is not good enough.

The abdomen demonstrates an AP projection. The spinous processes are aligned with the midline of the vertebral bodies, and the distance from the pedicles to the spinous processes is the same on both sides.

- A decubitus abdominal radiograph is obtained by placing the patient in a left lateral recumbent position on the tabletop or cart with the back resting against a grid cassette or the upright film holder. Because intraperitoneal air migrates to the elevated diaphragm, the left lateral position is chosen to position the gastric bubble away from where the intraperitoneal air will migrate. To avoid rotation, align the shoulders, the posterior ribs, and the posterior pelvic wings perpendicular to the tabletop or cart (Fig. 2–30). Accomplish this alignment by resting your extended flat hand against each, respectively, and then adjusting the patient's rotation until your hand is positioned perpendicular to the tabletop or cart. It is most common for a patient to rotate the elevated thorax and pelvic wing anteriorly. A pillow placed between the patient's knees may help to eliminate this forward rotation.

- ***Demonstrating Intraperitoneal Air:*** The lateral decubitus position is primarily used to confirm

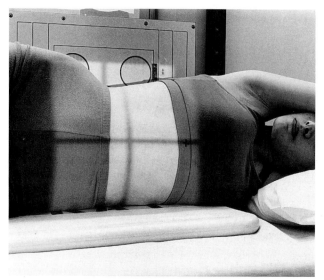

Figure 2-30. Proper patient positioning for decubitus abdomen radiograph.

the presence of intraperitoneal air. To best demonstrate intraperitoneal air, the patient should be left in this position for 10 to 20 minutes before the radiograph is taken, allowing enough time for the air to move away from the soft tissue abdominal structures and rise to the level of the right diaphragm. To eliminate long waiting periods for patients who are candidates for a decubitus abdomen, have them transported to the radiography department in the left lateral decubitus position.[11]

- ***Detecting Abdominal Rotation:*** The upper and lower lumbar vertebrae can demonstrate rotation independently or simultaneously, depending on which section of the body is rotated. If the patient's thorax is rotated but the pelvis remains in an AP projection, the upper lumbar vertebrae and abdominal cavity demonstrate rotation. If the patient's pelvis is rotated but the thorax remains in an AP projection, the lower vertebrae and abdominal cavity demonstrate rotation. If the patient's thorax and pelvis are rotated simultaneously, the entire lumbar column and abdominal cavity demonstrate rotation.

  Rotation is effectively detected on an AP abdominal radiograph by comparing the distance from the pedicles to the spinous processes on each side and evaluating the position of the sacrum within the inlet pelvis. If the distance from the pedicles to the spinous processes is greater on one side of the vertebrae than on the other side, the side with the smaller distance between the pedicles and spinous processes was the side of the patient positioned farther from the film. If the sacrum is not centered within the inlet pelvis but is rotated toward one side of the pelvis, the side toward which the sacrum is rotated is the side of the patient positioned farther from the film (see Rad. 32).

- ***Distinguishing Rotation from Scoliosis:*** On patients with spinal scoliosis, the lumbar bodies may appear rotated owing to the lateral twisting of the vertebrae. A radiograph on a patient with spinal scoliosis and a rotated decubitus abdomen demonstrates unequal distances between the pedicles and spinous processes. There are clues that can be used to distinguish scoliosis from rotation. The long axis of a rotated vertebral column remains straight, whereas the scoliotic vertebral column demonstrates lateral deviation. When the lumbar vertebrae demonstrate rotation, it has been caused by the rotation of the upper or lower torso. The middle lumbar vertebrae (L3–4) cannot rotate unless the lower thoracic vertebrae or the upper or lower lumbar vertebrae are also rotated. On the scoliotic radiograph, the middle lumbar vertebrae may demonstrate rotation without corresponding upper or lower vertebral rotation. Familiarity with the difference between a rotated lumbar vertebral column and a scoliotic one will prevent unnecessary repeats on patients with spinal scoliosis.

The radiograph was taken on expiration. The diaphragm domes are located superior to the 11th thoracic vertebra.

- From full inspiration to expiration, the diaphragm position moves from an inferior to a superior position.

This movement also changes the pressure placed on the abdominal structures. On full expiration, the superior portion of the right upper diaphragm dome is at the same transverse level as the eighth or ninth thoracic vertebrae, whereas on inspiration, it may be found at the same transverse level as the 11th thoracic vertebra. The left diaphragm is about 0.5 inch (1.25 cm) lower than the right diaphragm on both inspiration and expiration. When the decubitus abdominal radiograph is taken on expiration, there is less pressure on the peritoneal contents and greater space in the peritoneal cavity. If the decubitus position is taken on inspiration, the inferior placement of the diaphragm puts pressure on the abdominal organs, resulting in less space in the peritoneal cavity and greater abdominal density.[11, 12]

The third lumbar vertebra is centered within the collimated field. The right hemidiaphragm, ninth thoracic vertebra, right lateral soft tissues, and iliac wing are included within the field.

- The decubitus abdominal position is most often used to evaluate the peritoneal cavity for intraperitoneal air. To demonstrate intraperitoneal air, the right hemidiaphragm or iliac wing must be included. In the left lateral decubitus position, any intraperitoneal air rises to the highest level. On most patients, the intraperitoneal air moves to the right upper quadrant just below the diaphragm, between the liver and abdominal wall. One exception to this placement of intraperitoneal air occurs in women with wide hips, whose highest level within the peritoneal cavity is just over the iliac bone.[8]
- ***Film Size and Direction:*** A 14 × 17 inch (35 × 43 cm) film positioned lengthwise should be adequate to include all the anatomical structures in asthenic and sthenic patients. To place the ninth thoracic vertebra at the top of the radiograph and to center the third thoracic vertebra within the center of the collimated field, place the top of the film at a level 2.5 inches (6.25 cm) superior to the xiphoid (see Rad. 33). Center a horizontal central ray with the midsagittal plane. Open the longitudinally and transversely collimated fields to the full 14 × 17 inch (35 × 43 cm) size. If the right lateral soft tissue does not appear to be included with this positioning, use two crosswise films instead of one lengthwise.

  Use two 14 × 17 inch (35 × 43 cm) films positioned crosswise in respect to the patient to include all the necessary anatomical structures in the hypersthenic patient. Take the first radiograph with the top of the film placed at a level 2.5 inches (6.25 cm) superior to the xiphoid. Position the top of the second film so it includes about 2 to 3 inches (5 to 7.5 cm) of the same transverse section of the peritoneal cavity imaged on the first radiograph, to ensure that no middle peritoneal information has been excluded. For both radiographs, center a horizontal central ray with the midsagittal plane. Open the longitudinally and transversely collimated fields to the full 14 × 17 inch (35 × 43 cm) field size.
- ***Gonadal Shielding:*** Use gonadal shielding on all male patients and on female patients if two films are required and the upper abdomen is being radiographed. Do not shield a female patient if the lower abdomen is radiographed, because the shield may obscure needed information.

Critiquing Radiographs

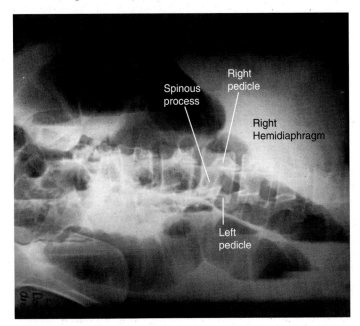

Radiograph 32.

Critique: The sacrum is not centered within the pelvic inlet, and the distance from the left pedicles to the spinous processes is less than the distance from the right pedicles to the spinous processes. The patient's right side was positioned closer to the film than the left side. The right diaphragmatic dome is included on this radiograph, although it is very close to the film's upper edge.

Correction: Rotate the patient's right side away from the film until the shoulders and the anterior superior iliac spines are positioned at equal distances from the film, and shift the film and central ray 1 inch (2.5 cm) superiorly.

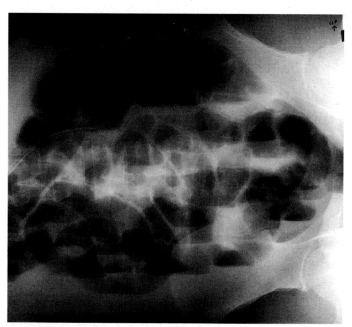

Radiograph 33.

Critique: The right hemidiaphragm is not included in the radiograph. The film and central ray were positioned too inferiorly.

Correction: Move the film and central ray superiorly. Place the top of the film at a level 2.5 inches (6.25 cm) superior to the xiphoid, and center the central ray with the midsagittal plane and film center.

References

1. Pearce DJ, Rau JL. (1984). Understanding Chest Radiographs. Denver, CO:Multi-Media Publishing, 1984, pp 34–36.
2. Anagnostakos NP, Tortora GJ. Principles of Anatomy and Physiology, ed 6. New York: Harper & Row, 1990, pp 702–704.
3. Fraser RG, Paré JAP, Paré PD, et al. Diagnosis of Diseases of the Chest, ed 3. Philadelphia: WB Saunders, 1988, pp 282–285.
4. Armstrong J, Crapo RO, Montague T. Inspiratory lung volume achieved on routine chest films. Invest Radiol 14:137–140, 1979.
5. Esinberg RL. Gastrointestinal Radiology: A Pattern Approach, ed 2. Philadelphia: JB Lippincott, pp 151–153.
6. Carroll QB. Fuch's Radiographic Exposure, Processing and Quality Control, ed 5. Springfield, IL: Charles C Thomas, 1993, pp 158–162.
7. Kattan KR, Wiot JF. How was this chest roentgenogram taken, AP or PA? Am J Roentgenol 117:843–845, 1973.
8. Baker SR. The Abdominal Plain Film. Norwalk, CT: Appleton & Lange, 1990, pp 6–13, 74–75.
9. Clemente CD (ed). Gray's Anatomy, ed 3. Philadelphia: Lea & Febiger, 1985, pp 94, 482.
10. Anagnostakos NP, Tortora GJ. Principles of Anatomy and Physiology, ed 6. New York: Harper & Row, 1990, pp 826–828.

CHAPTER 3

Radiographic Critique of the Upper Extremity

FINGER (2nd through 5th digits)

Posteroanterior Projection

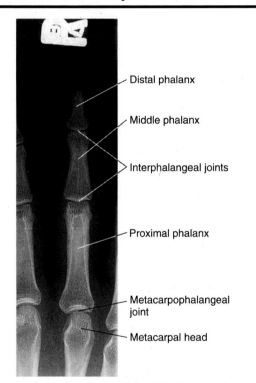

Distal phalanx

Middle phalanx

Interphalangeal joints

Proximal phalanx

Metacarpophalangeal joint

Metacarpal head

Figure 3-1. Accurately positioned PA finger radiograph.

Radiographic Evaluation

Facility's identification requirements are visible on radiograph.
- These requirements are facility name, patient name, age, and hospital number, and exam time and date.
- The patient ID plate does not obscure any anatomy of interest.

A right or left marker, identifying correct hand, is present on radiograph and does not superimpose anatomy of interest.
- Place the marker within the collimated light field so that it does not superimpose any portion of the af-

fected finger. It may be necessary to open the collimated field to include the marker within the light field.
- When more than one view of the finger is placed on the same film, only one of the views needs to be marked.

There is no evidence of preventable artifacts, such as rings, bandages, and splints.
- If the patient's condition prevented ring removal, shift the ring away from the affected area of the fingers, and indicate the situation on the requisition.
- Consult with the ordering physician and the patient about whether bandages or splints can be removed.

Contrast and density are adequate to demonstrate the surrounding soft tissue and bony structures of the affected digit. Penetration is sufficient to visualize the bony trabecular patterns and cortical outlines of the phalanges and metacarpal.
- An optimal 50 to 60 kVp technique sufficiently penetrates the bony and soft tissue structures of the finger and provides high radiographic contrast.

The bony trabecular patterns and cortical outlines of the phalanx are sharply defined.
- Motion is the most common cause of poor definition on a radiograph. It can be controlled by explaining the procedure so the patient is aware of what is expected, by making the patient as comfortable as possible during the exam, and by utilizing a short exposure time. When the patient is unable to control hand and finger movement, immobilization props may be needed. The sharpness of details can also be increased by using a detail screen and a small focal spot as well as by maintaining a short object–image distance (OID).

The finger demonstrates a true PA projection. The soft tissue width and the midshaft concavity are the same on both sides of the phalanges.
- Finger rotation is controlled by the amount of palm supination. A true PA projection is accomplished when the palm is positioned flat against the cassette (Fig. 3–2).

77

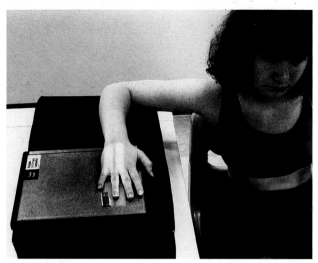

Figure 3-2. Proper patient positioning for PA finger radiograph.

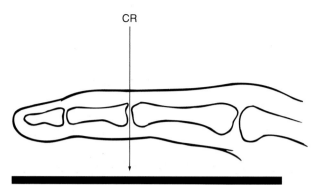

Figure 3-3. Accurate alignment of joint space and central ray *(CR)*.

of the collimator's longitudinal light line enables you to collimate tightly without clipping the distal phalanx or distal metacarpal.

- **Detecting Finger Rotation:** Because the thumb prevents the hand from rotating laterally, medial rotation is the most common rotation error. Take a few minutes to study a finger skeleton and note how the midshafts of the phalanges have equal concavity in a PA projection. As the skeleton is rotated internally or externally, the amount of concavity increases on the side rolled away from the film, whereas the side closer to the film demonstrates less concavity. The same observations can be made about the soft tissue that surrounds the phalanges. More soft tissue width is evident on the surface that is rolled away from the film than on the surface closer to the film. Look for this midshaft concavity and soft tissue width variation to indicate rotation on a finger radiograph (see Rad. 1).

  Note on a hand skeleton that the second metacarpal is the longest of the finger digits and that the length decreases with each adjacent metacarpal. This knowledge can be used to determine whether the patient's finger was internally or externally rotated for a mispositioned PA finger radiograph. If the finger was externally rotated, the aspect of the phalanges demonstrating the greater midshaft concavity faces the longer metacarpal (see Rad. 1). If the finger is internally rotated, the aspect of the phalanges demonstrating the greater midshaft concavity faces the shorter metacarpal.

- **AP Projection Finger Rotation:** If a finger is radiographed in an AP projection but demonstrates rotation on the radiograph, the aspect of the phalanx that demonstrates the greater midshaft concavity and soft tissue width is positioned closer to the film, a situation opposite to that in the PA projection.

The long axis of the affected digit is aligned with the long axis of the collimated field.

- Aligning the long axis of the finger with the long axis

There is no soft tissue overlap from adjacent digits.

- Spreading the fingers slightly prevents soft tissue overlapping from adjacent fingers. It is difficult to evaluate the soft tissue of an affected finger when superimposition of other soft tissue is present.

The interphalangeal (IP) and metacarpophalangeal (MP) joints are demonstrated as open spaces, and the phalanges are not foreshortened.

- The IP and MP joint spaces are open and the phalanges are not foreshortened if the finger is fully extended and the central ray is perpendicular and centered to the proximal IP (PIP) joint. This finger positioning and central ray placement align the joint spaces parallel with the central ray and perpendicular to the film, as demonstrated in Figure 3–3, resulting in open joint spaces. It also prevents foreshortening of the phalanges, because their long axes are aligned parallel with the film and perpendicular to the central ray. The alignment of the central ray and film with the joint spaces and phalanges changes when the finger is flexed. Note, in Figure 3–4, how finger flexion causes the phalanges to foreshorten and superimpose into the joint spaces (see Rad. 2).

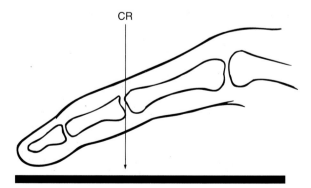

Figure 3-4. Poor alignment of joint space and central ray *(CR)*.

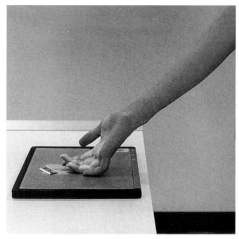

Figure 3-5. Patient positioning for AP flexed finger radiograph.

- ***Positioning the Unextendable Finger:*** If the patient is unable to extend the finger, it may be necessary to use an AP projection to demonstrate open IP and MP joint spaces and to visualize the phalanges without foreshortening. In this case, carefully evaluate the requisition to determine the phalanx and joint space of interest. Then supinate the patient's hand into an AP projection, elevating the proximal metacarpals until the phalanx of interest is parallel with the film and the joint space of interest is perpendicular to the

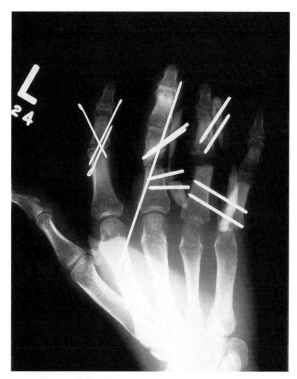

Figure 3-7. AP projection with flexed fingers.

film (Fig. 3–5). Figures 3–6 and 3–7 demonstrate how patient positioning determines the anatomy that is visualized. For Figure 3–6, the patient was radiographed in a PA projection with fingers arched. For Figure 3–7, the same patient was radiographed in an AP projection with the proximal metacarpals elevated to place the affected proximal phalanges parallel with the film. Note the difference in visualization of the joint spaces and proximal phalanx fractures.

The proximal interphalangeal (PIP) joint is at the center of the collimated field. The distal, middle, and proximal phalanges and half of the metacarpal are included within the field.

- Centering a perpendicular central ray to the PIP joint places the joint in the center of the radiograph. Open the longitudinal collimation to include the distal phalanx and the distal half of the metacarpal. Transverse collimation should be to the finger skin-line.

- One third of an 8 × 10 inch (18 × 24 cm) film placed crosswise should be adequate to include all the required anatomical structures.

- Some facilities request that an unaffected adjacent digit be included on the radiograph for comparison purposes. For a finger being radiographed for the first time, some facilities want the entire metacarpal to be visualized on the radiograph.

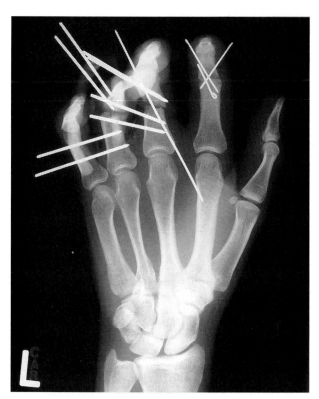

Figure 3-6. PA projection with flexed fingers.

Critiquing Radiographs

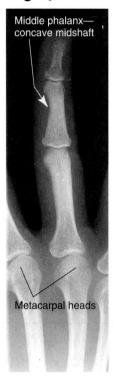

Radiograph 1.

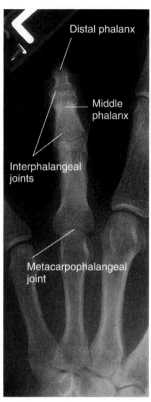

Radiograph 2.

Critique: The soft tissue width and the concavity of the phalangeal midshafts on either side of the phalanx are not equal; the finger was rotated for the radiograph. Because the side of the phalanges with the greater concavity is facing the long metacarpal, the finger was rotated externally for the radiograph.

Correction: Place the finger in a true PA projection by rotating the finger slightly internally. The hand should be flat against the cassette.

Critique: The IP and MP joints are closed, and the distal and middle phalanges are foreshortened; the patient's finger was flexed.

Correction: Extend the patient's finger, and place the palm flat against the cassette. If the patient is unable to extend the finger, radiograph it in an AP projection, elevating the proximal metacarpals until the affected phalanx is parallel with the film or the affected joint space is perpendicular to the film (see Fig. 3–5).

Finger: Oblique Position

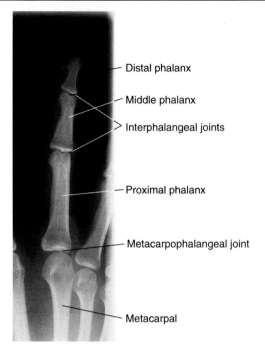

— Distal phalanx

— Middle phalanx

> — Interphalangeal joints

— Proximal phalanx

— Metacarpophalangeal joint

— Metacarpal

Figure 3–8. Accurately positioned oblique finger radiograph.

Radiographic Evaluation

Facility's patient identification requirements are visible on radiograph.
- These requirements usually are facility name, patient name, age, and hospital number, and exam time and date.
- The patient ID plate does not obscure any anatomy of interest.

A right or left marker, identifying the correct hand, is present on radiograph and does not superimpose anatomy of interest.
- Place the marker within the collimated field, so that it does not superimpose any portion of the affected finger. It may be necessary to open the collimated field to include the marker.
- When more than one view of the finger is placed on the same film, only one of the views needs to be marked.

There is no evidence of preventable artifacts, such as rings, bandages, and splints.
- If the patient's condition prevented ring removal, the situation should be indicated on the requisition.
- Consult with the ordering physician and the patient about whether bandages or splints can be removed.

Contrast and density are adequate to demonstrate the surrounding soft tissue and bony structures of the affected digit. Penetration is sufficient to visualize the bony trabecular patterns and cortical outlines of the phalanges and metacarpal.
- An optimal 50 to 60 kVp technique sufficiently pene-

trates the bony and soft tissue structures of the finger and provides high radiographic contrast.

The bony trabecular patterns and cortical outlines of the phalanges are sharply defined.
- Patients who are comfortable and understand what is expected of them are less likely to move during the exposure. Use immobilization props when necessary to control a moving finger. Sharpness of details is also increased by using a detail screen and a small focal spot as well as by maintaining a short object–image distance (OID).

The digit has been placed in a 45-degree oblique position. Twice as much soft tissue width is demonstrated on one side of the digit as on the other side, and more concavity is demonstrated on one aspect of the phalangeal midshafts than on the other.
- An oblique finger position is accomplished by rotating the affected finger 45 degrees from the PA projection (Fig. 3–9). It is most common and comfortable for a patient to rotate the finger and hand into a medially oblique position for an oblique finger radiograph, although a lateral oblique position may be taken when radiographing the second digit, to prevent a long OID.
- Examine a finger skeleton in a PA projection and in anterior oblique and lateral positions. Note how the phalangeal midshaft concavity varies as the digit is rotated. In a PA projection, the midshaft concavity is the same on the two sides. In an oblique position, the midshaft concavity is greater on the side rolled away from the film than on the side positioned closer to the film. In a lateral position, the anterior aspect of the digit is concave, whereas the posterior aspect demonstrates a slight convexity. Similar observations can be made about the soft tissue that surrounds the phalanx. More soft tissue width is evident on the surface that demonstrates greater midshaft concavity and is rotated away from the film.

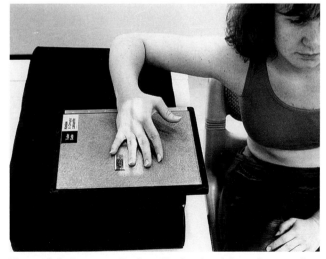

Figure 3–9. Proper patient positioning for oblique finger radiograph.

- **Assessing Accuracy of Oblique Positioning:** Study the amount of phalangeal midshaft concavity and soft tissue width demonstrated on oblique finger radiographs to verify the accuracy of rotation and to determine the proper repositioning movement needed when an oblique digit radiograph shows too much or too little obliquity. A 45-degree oblique digit radiograph demonstrates more phalangeal midshaft concavity and soft tissue width on the side positioned away from the film.

  Use the soft tissue width to assess the degree of digital obliquity. If there is twice as much soft tissue width on one side of the digit as on the other, a 45-degree oblique position has been obtained. If the phalangeal midshaft concavity and soft tissue width on either side of the digit are more nearly equal, the finger was not rotated enough for the radiograph (see Rad. 3). If the soft tissue width on one side of the digit is more than twice as much as on the other, and when one aspect of the phalangeal midshaft is concave but the other aspect is convex, the angle of obliquity was more than 45 degrees (see Rad. 4).

The long axis of the affected digit is aligned with the long axis of the collimated field.

- Aligning the long axis of the finger with the long axis of the collimation field enables you to collimate tightly without clipping the distal phalanx or distal metacarpal.

There is no soft tissue overlap from adjacent digits.

- Slightly spread the patient's fingers to prevent overlapping of the adjacent finger's soft tissue onto the affected finger's. Superimposition of these soft tissues makes it difficult to evaluate the soft tissue of the affected finger (see Rad. 5).

The interphalangeal (IP) and metacarpophalangeal (MP) joints are visualized as open spaces, and the phalanges are not foreshortened.

- The IP and MP joint spaces are open and the phalanges are not foreshortened if the finger is fully extended and positioned parallel with the film and perpendicular to the central ray. When the hand and fingers are positioned obliquely, some of the fingers are no longer placed against the cassette but are positioned at varying OIDs. In this position, the distal phalanges naturally tilt toward the film.

  To keep the affected finger parallel with the film and to maintain open joint spaces, it may be necessary to place a sponge beneath the distal phalanx. This is especially true when the third and fourth digits are radiographed, for they are at the greatest OID.

  It is also necessary to center a perpendicular central ray to the PIP joint to maintain open joint spaces. Failure to position the affected finger parallel with the film and perpendicular to the central ray foreshortens the phalanges and closes the joint spaces (see Rad. 6).

The proximal interphalangeal (PIP) joint is at the center of the collimated field. The distal, middle, and proximal phalanges and half of the metacarpal of the affected digit are included within the field.

- Centering the central ray to the PIP joint places the joint in the center of the radiograph. Open the longitudinal collimation to include the distal phalanx and the distal half of the metacarpal. Transverse collimation should be to the finger skin-line.
- One third of an 8 × 10 inch (18 × 24 cm) film placed crosswise should be adequate to include all the required anatomical structures.
- Some facilities require an unaffected adjacent digit to be included on the radiograph for comparison purposes. Also, for a finger being radiographed for the first time, some facilities want the entire metacarpal to be visualized on the radiograph.

Critiquing Radiographs

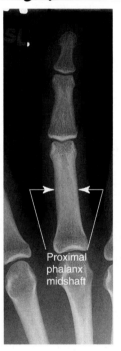

Radiograph 3.

Critique: On either side of the phalanx, there is nearly equal soft tissue width and midshaft concavity; the patient's finger was positioned at less than 45 degrees of obliquity for the radiograph.
Correction: Increase the finger obliquity to 45 degrees. Keep the finger parallel with the film.

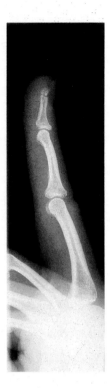

Radiograph 4.

Critique: There is more than two times as much soft tissue width on one side of the phalanges as on the other. One aspect of the midshafts of the phalanges is concave, and the other aspect is slightly convex. Obliquity was more than 45 degrees for this radiograph.

Correction: Decrease the finger obliquity to 45 degrees.

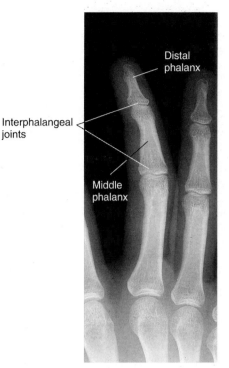

Radiograph 6.

Critique: The IP joint spaces are closed, and the distal and middle phalanges are foreshortened; the finger was not positioned parallel with the film.

Correction: Position the finger parallel with the film. It may be necessary to position a radiolucent sponge beneath the distal phalanx to maintain accurate finger positioning.

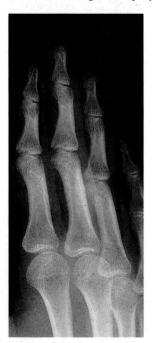

Radiograph 5.

Critique: Soft tissue from an adjacent digit is superimposing the affected digit's soft tissue; fingers were not spread apart.

Correction: Spread the fingers until the adjacent fingers are positioned away from the affected finger.

Finger: Lateral Position

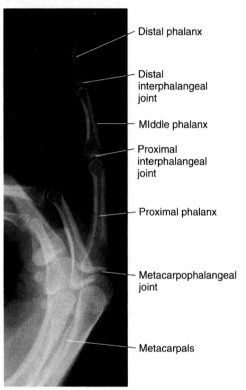

Distal phalanx

Distal interphalangeal joint

Middle phalanx

Proximal interphalangeal joint

Proximal phalanx

Metacarpophalangeal joint

Metacarpals

Figure 3–10. Accurately positioned lateral finger radiograph.

Radiographic Evaluation

Facility's patient identification requirements are visible on radiograph.

- These requirements usually are facility name, patient name, age, and hospital number, and exam time and date.
- The patient ID plate does not obscure any anatomy of interest.

A right or left marker, identifying correct hand, is present on radiograph and does not superimpose anatomy of interest.

- Place the marker within the collimated light field so that it does not superimpose any portion of the affected finger. It may be necessary to open the collimated field to include the marker within the light field.
- When more than one view of the finger is placed on the same film, only one of the views needs to be marked.

There is no evidence of preventable artifacts such as rings, bandages, and splints.

- If patient's condition prevented ring removal, the situation should be indicated on the requisition (see Rad. 7). Consult with the ordering physician and the patient about whether bandages or splints can be removed.

Contrast and density are adequate to demonstrate the surrounding soft tissue and bony structures of the af-
fected digit. Penetration is sufficient to visualize the bony trabecular patterns and cortical outlines of the phalanges and metacarpal.

- An optimal 50 to 60 kVp technique sufficiently penetrates the bony and soft tissue structures of the finger and provides high radiographic contrast.

The bony trabecular patterns and cortical outlines of the phalanges are sharply defined.

- Patients who are comfortable and understand what is expected of them are less likely to move during the exposure. Use immobilization props when necessary to control a moving finger. Recorded detail sharpness is also increased by using a detail screen and a small focal spot as well as by maintaining a short object–image distance (OID).

The digit of interest is in a true lateral position with no signs of rotation. The anterior aspect of the middle and proximal phalanges demonstrates midshaft concavity, and the posterior aspects of the phalanges show slight convexity.

- A lateral finger position is accomplished by rotating the affected finger 90 degrees from the PA projection (Fig. 3–11). Whether the hand is rotated internally or externally to obtain this goal depends on which finger is being radiographed. When the second and third fingers are being radiographed, rotate the hand internally. When the fourth and fifth fingers are being radiographed, rotate the hand externally.
- ***Distinguishing Lateral Position from Rotated Position:*** To understand the difference between a truly lateral digit position and one that is rotated, study a finger skeleton in lateral and anterior oblique positions. Note how the midshaft concavity of the middle and proximal phalanges varies as the digit is rotated. In a lateral position, the anterior aspect of these phalanges is concave, but the posterior aspect demonstrates slight convexity. In an oblique position, both sides of the middle and proximal phalangeal midshafts demonstrate concavity, but the side rolled

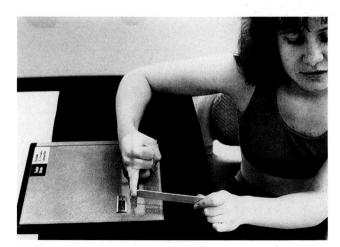

Figure 3–11. Proper patient positioning for lateral finger radiograph.

away from the film shows a greater degree of concavity than the side positioned closer to the film. The soft tissue width at either side of the phalanx also changes in the lateral and oblique positions. More soft tissue is present on the side of the phalanges that demonstrates greater midshaft concavity (see Rad. 8).

The long axis of the affected digit is aligned with the long axis of the collimated light field.
- Aligning the long axis of the finger with the long axis of the collimated field enables you to collimate tightly without clipping the distal phalanx.

There is no soft tissue overlap from adjacent digits.
- Flex the unaffected fingers into a tight fist, allowing the finger of interest to remain extended. To visualize the proximal phalanx, it may be necessary to extend the affected finger with an immobilization prop or to tape the unaffected fingers away from affected finger. If the unaffected fingers are not drawn away from the proximal phalanx of the affected finger, they will superimpose the area, preventing adequate visualization (see Rad. 7).

The interphalangeal (IP) joints are visualized as open spaces, and the phalanges are not foreshortened.
- The IP joints are open and the phalanges are demonstrated without foreshortening as long as the finger was positioned parallel with the film and the central ray was perpendicular to and centered with the proximal IP (PIP) joint.
- When the third and fourth digits are radiographed, they are positioned at a greater OID than the second and fifth digits. To keep the third and fourth digits parallel with the film, it may be necessary to place a sponge beneath their distal phalanges. When a finger is not positioned parallel with the film and perpendicular to the central ray, the IP joint spaces are closed and the phalanges are foreshortened.

The PIP joint is at the center of the collimated field. The distal, middle, and proximal phalanges and the metacarpal head of the affected digit are included within the field.
- Centering the central ray to the PIP joint places the joint in the center of the radiograph. Open the longitudinal collimation to include the distal phalanx and the metacarpal head. Transverse collimation should be to the finger skin-line.
- One third of an 8 × 10 inch (18 × 24 cm) film placed crosswise should be adequate to include all the required anatomical structures.

Critiquing Radiographs

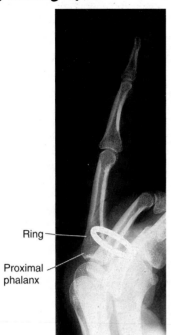

Radiograph 7.

Critique: The unaffected fingers were not flexed enough to prevent soft tissue or bony superimposition of the affected digit's proximal phalanx. An unaffected finger has a ring artifact that is superimposing the digit of interest.

Correction: Tightly flex the unaffected fingers away from the affected finger. It may be necessary to tape fingers to help the patient hold the position. Hyperextending the affected finger with an immobilization prop may also help to increase demonstration of the proximal phalanx. Remove the ring if possible.

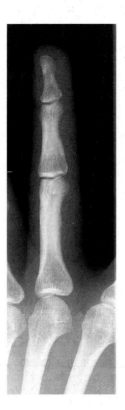

Radiograph 8.

Critique: Concavity is demonstrated on both sides of the middle and proximal phalangeal midshafts, indicating that the finger was slightly rotated for this radiograph.

Correction: Rotate the finger into a lateral position.

THUMB (1st Digit)

Anteroposterior Projection

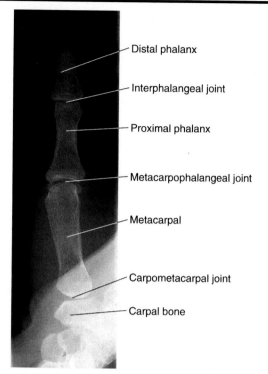

— Distal phalanx

— Interphalangeal joint

— Proximal phalanx

— Metacarpophalangeal joint

— Metacarpal

— Carpometacarpal joint

— Carpal bone

Figure 3-12. Accurately positioned AP thumb radiograph.

Radiographic Evaluation

Facility's patient identification requirements are visible on radiograph.
- These requirements usually are facility name, patient name, age, and hospital number, and exam time and date.
- The patient ID plate does not obscure any anatomy of interest.

A right or left marker, identifying the correct hand, is present on radiograph and does not superimpose anatomy of interest.
- Place the marker within the collimated light field so that it does not superimpose any portion of the thumb. When more than one view of the thumb is placed on the same film, only one of the views needs to be marked.

There is no evidence of preventable artifacts, such as bandages and splints.
- Consult with the ordering physician and the patient about whether bandages or splints can be removed.

Contrast and density are adequate to demonstrate the surrounding soft tissue and bony structures of the affected digit. Penetration is sufficient to visualize the bony trabecular patterns and cortical outlines of the phalanges and metacarpal.

- An optimal 50 to 60 kVp technique sufficiently penetrates the bony and soft tissue structures of the thumb and provides high radiographic contrast.

The bony trabecular patterns and cortical outlines of the metacarpal and phalanges are sharply defined.
- Sharply defined recorded details are obtained when patient movement is halted, a detail screen and small focal spot are used, and a short object–image distance (OID) is maintained.

The first digit demonstrates a true AP projection. The soft tissue width and concavity are the same on both sides of the phalangeal and metacarpal midshafts.
- A true AP projection is accomplished by internally rotating the patient's hand until the thumb is positioned in an AP projection (Fig. 3–13). The thumbnail can be used as a reference to determine when the thumb is truly positioned AP. The nail should be positioned directly against the cassette and not visible on either side of the thumb. A nonrotated AP thumb radiograph demonstrates equal concavity on either side of the phalangeal and metacarpal midshafts as well as equal soft tissue width on either side of the phalanges.
- ***Detecting Thumb Rotation:*** When the thumb is rotated away from an AP projection, the amount of midshaft concavity decreases on the side rolled away from the film and increases on the side rolled closer to the film. The same observation can be made about the soft tissue surrounding the phalanges when the thumb is rotated. Less soft tissue width is evident on the surface farther from the film than on the surface closer to the film. If the hand is internally rotated too far, causing the thumbnail to face away from the fingers, the resulting radiograph demonstrates more phalangeal and metacarpal midshaft concavity on the side of the thumb next to the fingers (see Rad. 9).

  If the hand has been insufficiently rotated, the thumbnail faces the fingers, and the resulting radiograph demonstrates more phalangeal and metacarpal midshaft concavity on the side of the thumb opposite the fingers. Often, this latter positioning error results

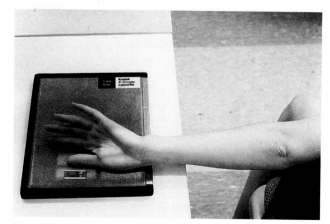

Figure 3-13. Proper patient positioning for AP thumb radiograph.

in superimposition of the fourth and fifth metacarpals onto the first metacarpal, obscuring its visualization.

The long axis of the thumb is aligned with the long axis of the collimated field.

- Aligning the long axis of the thumb with the long axis of the collimator's longitudinal light line enables you to collimate tightly without clipping the distal phalanx or proximal metacarpal (see Rad. 10).

The interphalangeal (IP), metacarpophalangeal (MP), and carpometacarpal (CM) joints are visualized as open joint spaces, and the phalanges are not foreshortened.

- The IP, MP, and CM joint spaces are open and the phalanges are demonstrated without foreshortening as long as the thumb was fully extended and the central ray was perpendicular to and centered with the MC joint space. This positioning aligns the joint spaces parallel with the central ray and perpendicular to the film, and positions the long axis of the phalanges perpendicular to the central ray and parallel with the film. These relationships change when the thumb is flexed for the radiograph. Thumb flexion foreshortens the phalanges and superimposes them over the joint spaces (see Rad. 11).

Superimposition of the medial palm soft tissue over the proximal first metacarpal and the carpometacarpal joint is minimal.

- When the thumb is in an AP projection, the medial palm soft tissue superimposes the proximal first metacarpal and the CM joint. Only a small amount of this soft tissue overlap occurs when the medial palm surface is drawn away from the thumb. It may be necessary to use the patient's other hand as an immobilization device to maintain good positioning of the medial palmar surface. If the medial surface of the palm is not drawn away from the thumb, the soft tissue and possibly the fourth and fifth metacarpals obscure the proximal first metacarpal and CM joint (see Rad. 12).

- ***Evaluating a PA Thumb Radiograph:*** The principles of AP thumb radiographic evaluation can be used to evaluate a PA projection thumb radiograph (Fig. 3–14), with the following modifications. First, if the thumb was rotated away from a true PA projection,

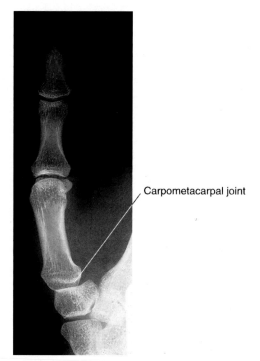

Carpometacarpal joint

Figure 3-14. Accurately positioned PA thumb radiograph.

the phalangeal and metacarpal midshafts demonstrate more concavity on the side rolled away from the film than on the side positioned closer to the film. Second, the medial palm soft tissue does not overlap the proximal first metacarpal and CM joint. Third, on a PA projection, the CM joint is closed.

The metacarpophalangeal (MP) joint is at the center of the collimated field. The distal and proximal phalanges, the metacarpal, and the carpometacarpal (CM) joint are included within the field.

- Centering the central ray to the MP joint, which is located where the palm's interconnecting skin attaches to the thumb, places the joint in the center of the radiograph. Open the longitudinal collimation to include the distal phalanx and CM joint. Transverse collimation should be to the thumb skin-line.

- One third of an 8 × 10 inch (18 × 24 cm) film placed crosswise should be adequate to include all the required anatomical structures.

Critiquing Radiographs

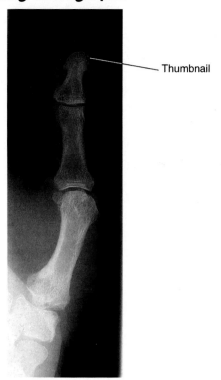

Thumbnail

Radiograph 9.

Critique: The soft tissue width and the concavity of the phalangeal and metacarpal midshafts are not the same on either side. The side next to the fingers demonstrates more concavity. The soft tissue shadow of the thumbnail is visualized facing away from the fingers. The hand was internally rotated too far, demonstrating the thumb in an oblique position.

Correction: Decrease the internal hand rotation until the thumb is in a true AP projection. The thumbnail should be resting against the cassette and should not be visible on either side of the thumb.

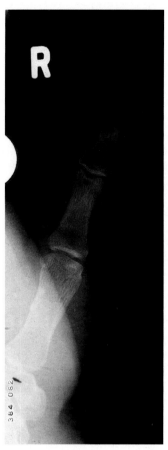

Radiograph 10.

Critique: The long axis of the thumb is not aligned with the long axis of the collimated field. Note that the proximal metacarpal and the CM joint are clipped.

Correction: Align the long axis of the thumb with the long axis of the collimated field.

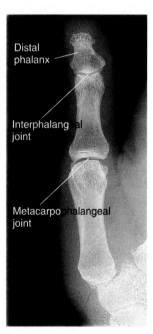

Distal phalanx

Interphalangeal joint

Metacarpophalangeal joint

Radiograph 11.

Critique: The distal phalanx is foreshortened, and the distal interphalangeal (DIP) joint space is closed. The thumb was flexed.
Correction: Fully extend the thumb.

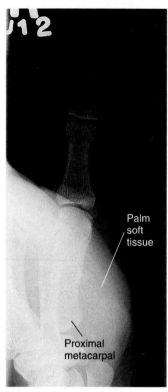

Radiograph 12.

Critique: The fifth metacarpal and the medial palm soft tissue are superimposing the proximal first metacarpal and CM joint. The medial metacarpal and palmar surface have not been drawn away from the thumb.
Correction: Using the patient's other hand or another immobilization device, draw the medial side of hand and palmar surface away from the thumb. Make sure that the thumb does not rotate away from a true AP projection with this movement.

Thumb (1st digit): Lateral Position

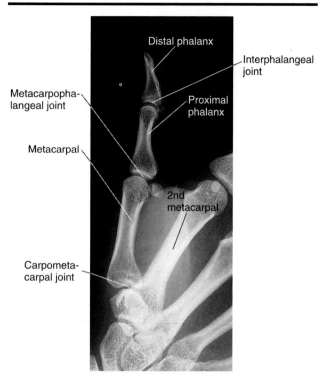

Figure 3-15. Accurately positioned lateral thumb radiograph.

Radiographic Evaluation

Facility's patient identification requirements are visible on radiograph.
- These requirements usually are facility name, patient name, age, and hospital number, and exam time and date.
- The patient ID plate does not obscure any anatomy of interest.

A right or left marker, identifying the correct hand, is present on the radiograph and does not superimpose anatomy of interest.
- Place the marker within the collimated light field so that it does not superimpose any portion of the thumb.

There is no evidence of preventable artifacts, such as bandages and splints.
- Consult with the ordering physician and the patient about whether bandages or splints can be removed.

Contrast and density are adequate to demonstrate the surrounding soft tissue and bony structures of the affected digit. Penetration is sufficient to visualize the bony trabecular patterns and the cortical outlines of the phalanges and metacarpal.
- An optimal 50 to 60 kVp technique sufficiently penetrates the bony and soft tissue structures of the thumb and provides high radiographic contrast.

The bony trabecular patterns and cortical outlines of the phalanges and metacarpal are sharply defined.

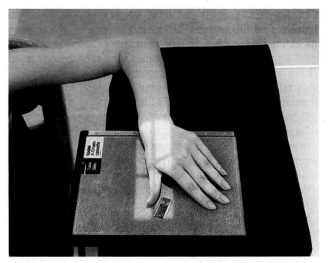

Figure 3-16. Proper patient positioning for lateral thumb radiograph.

- Sharply defined recorded details are obtained when patient motion is halted, a detail screen and a small focal spot are used, and a short object–image distance (OID) is maintained.

The thumb demonstrates a true lateral position. The anterior aspect of the proximal phalanx and metacarpal demonstrates midshaft concavity, and the posterior aspect of the phalanx and metacarpal demonstrates slight convexity.

- To accomplish lateral thumb positioning, place the patient's hand flat against the cassette; then flex the hand and fingers only until the thumb naturally rolls into a lateral position (Fig. 3–16). Overflexion causes superimposition of the second and third proximal metacarpals onto the proximal first metacarpal, obscuring it (see Rad. 13). When the hand and fingers are accurately flexed and the thumb is in a lateral position, the midshaft of the proximal phalanx and metacarpal demonstrates concavity on their anterior aspects and convexity on their posterior aspects. If the patient's hand is not rotated enough to place the thumb in a lateral position, the posterior and the anterior aspects of these midshafts show some degree of concavity (see Rad. 14).

The long axis of the first digit is aligned with the long axis of the collimated field.

- Aligning the long axis of the thumb with the long axis of the collimator's longitudinal light line enables you to collimate tightly without clipping the distal phalanx or proximal metacarpal.

The interphalangeal (IP), metacarpophalangeal (MP), and carpometacarpal (CM) joints are visualized as open spaces, and the phalanges are not foreshortened.

- The IP, MP, and CM joints are open and the phalanges are not foreshortened if the entire thumb was resting against the cassette and was positioned parallel with the film and if the central ray was centered with the MP joint.

The proximal first metacarpal is only slightly superimposed by the proximal second metacarpal.

- Whenever possible, the anatomical part of interest should be demonstrated without superimposition. For a lateral thumb radiograph, the proximal metacarpal can be demonstrated with only a very small amount of superimposition if the thumb is abducted away from the palm. Failure to abduct the thumb results in a significant amount of first and second proximal metacarpal overlap and obstruction of the CM joint (see Rad. 15).

The first metacarpophalangeal (MP) joint is at the center of the collimated field. The distal and proximal phalanges, the metacarpal, and the carpometacarpal (CM) joint are included within the field.

- Centering the central ray to the MP joint, which is located where the palm's interconnecting skin attaches to the thumb, places the joint in the center of the radiograph. Open the longitudinal collimation to include the distal phalanx and CM joint. Transverse collimation should be to the thumb skin-line.
- One third of an 8 × 10 inch (18 × 24 cm) film placed crosswise should be adequate to include all the required anatomical structures.

Critiquing Radiographs

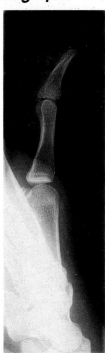

Radiograph 13.

Critique: The second and third proximal metacarpals are superimposing the first proximal metacarpal. The hand was overflexed.
Correction: Abduct the thumb away from the hand, and decrease the hand flexion while maintaining a lateral thumb position.

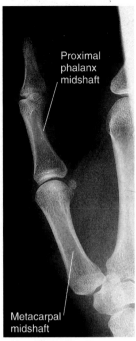

Radiograph 14.

Critique: The thumb is not in a true lateral position. The anterior and posterior aspects of the proximal phalanx and metacarpal midshafts demonstrate concavity, indicating that the hand was not adequately flexed.
Correction: Increase the degree of hand flexion until the thumb rolls into a true lateral position.

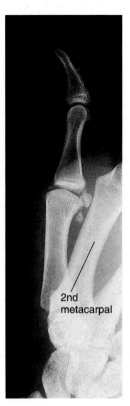

Radiograph 15.

Critique: The proximal metacarpal is superimposed by the proximal second metacarpal. The thumb was not abducted.
Correction: Abduct the thumb.

Thumb (1st Digit): Lateral Oblique Position

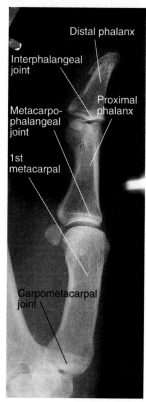

Figure 3-17. Accurately positioned oblique thumb radiograph.

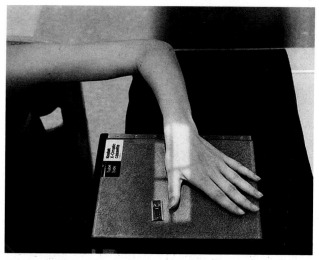

Figure 3-18. Proper patient positioning for oblique thumb radiograph.

Radiographic Evaluation

Facility's patient requirements are visible on radiograph.

- These requirements usually are facility name, patient name, age, and hospital number, and exam time and date.
- The patient ID plate does not obscure any anatomy of interest.

A right or left marker, identifying the correct hand, is present on the radiograph and does not superimpose anatomy of interest.

- Place the marker within the collimated light field so that it does not superimpose any portion of the thumb.

There is no evidence of preventable artifacts, such as bandages and splints.

- Consult with the ordering physician and the patient about whether bandages or splints can be removed.

Contrast and density are adequate to demonstrate the surrounding soft tissue and bony structures of the affected digit. Penetration is sufficient to visualize the bony trabecular patterns and the cortical outlines of the phalanges and metacarpal.

- An optimal 50 to 60 kVp technique sufficiently penetrates the bony and soft tissue structures of the thumb and provides high radiograph contrast.

The bony trabecular patterns and cortical outlines of the phalanges are sharply defined.

- Sharply defined recorded details are obtained when patient motion is halted, a detail screen and small focal spot are used, and a short object–image distance (OID) is maintained.

The thumb has been positioned obliquely at 45 degrees. There is twice as much soft tissue and more phalangeal and metacarpal midshaft concavity on the side of the thumb next to the fingers than on the other side.

- When the hand is extended and the palmar surface is placed flat against the cassette, the thumb is rotated into a 45-degree lateral oblique position (Fig. 3–18). In this position, there is more midshaft concavity on one side of the phalanges and metacarpal than on the other side. If the hand is not placed flat against the cassette, the thumb rolls toward a lateral position. The more flexed the fingers are, the closer the thumb is to a lateral position. Such positioning can be identified on a radiograph by noting the concavity of the anterior aspect and the convexity of the posterior aspect of the proximal phalanx and metacarpal (see Rad. 16).

The long axis of the thumb is aligned with the long axis of the collimated field.

- Aligning the long axis of the thumb with the long axis of the collimation light field enables you to collimate tightly without clipping the distal phalanx or proximal metacarpal (see Rad. 17).

The interphalangeal (IP), metacarpophalangeal (MP), and carpometacarpal (CM) joints are visualized as open joint spaces, and the phalanges are not foreshortened.

- The IP, MP, and CM joint spaces are open and the metacarpal and phalanges are not foreshortened when the first proximal metacarpal palmar surface remains flat against the cassette. If the hand is medially obliqued, the palmar surface is lifted off the cassette, causing the thumb to tilt downward. The downward tilt closes the IP and MP joint spaces and foreshortens the phalanges (see Rad. 18).

The first metacarpophalangeal joint is at the center of the collimated field. The distal and proximal phalanges, metacarpal, and carpometacarpal joint are included within the field.

- Centering the central ray to the MP joint, which is located where the palmar interconnecting skin attaches to the thumb, places the joint in the center of the radiograph. Open the longitudinal collimation to include the distal phalanx and CM joint. Transverse collimation should be to the thumb skin-line.
- One third of an 8 × 10 inch (18 × 24 cm) film placed crosswise should be adequate to include all the required anatomical structures.

Critiquing Radiographs

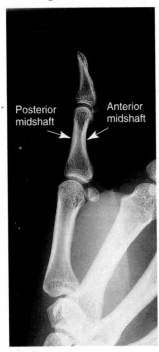

Radiograph 16.

Critique: The midshafts of the proximal phalanx and metacarpal demonstrate slight convexity on their anterior surfaces and concavity on their posterior surfaces. The thumb was positioned at more than 45 degrees of obliquity. The patient's palm was not placed flat against the cassette.
Correction: Extend the patient's hand and place the palm flat against the cassette.

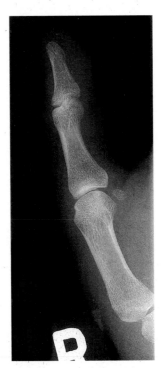

Radiograph 17.

Critique: The long axis of the thumb is not aligned with the long axis of the collimated field. Note that the proximal metacarpal and the CM joint are partially clipped.
Correction: Align the long axis of the thumb with the long axis of the collimation field.

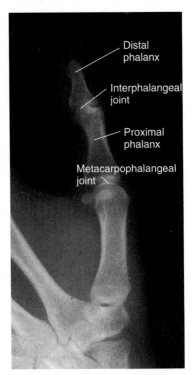

Radiograph 18.

Critique: The IP and MP joints are closed, and the phalanges are foreshortened. The first proximal metacarpal palmar surface was not positioned against the cassette, and the thumb was tilting down toward the cassette.
Correction: Place the palmar surface and thumb against the cassette.

HAND

Posteroanterior Projection

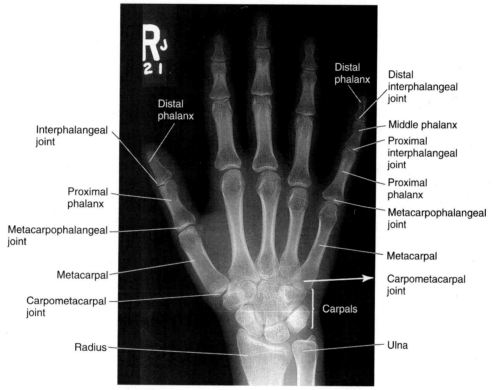

Figure 3-19. Accurately positioned PA hand radiograph.

Radiographic Evaluation

Facility's patient identification requirements are visible on radiograph.
- These requirements usually are facility name, patient name, age, and hospital number, and exam time and date.
- The patient ID plate does not obscure any anatomy of interest.

A right or left marker, identifying the correct hand, is present on the radiograph and does not superimpose anatomy of interest.
- Place the marker within the collimated light field so that it does not superimpose any portion of the hand.
- When more than one view of the hand is placed on the same film, only one of the views needs to be marked.

There is no evidence of preventable artifacts, such as rings, bracelets, watches, bandages, and splints.
- If the patient's condition prevents ring removal, the situation should be indicated on the requisition.
- Consult with the ordering physician and the patient about whether bandages or splints can be removed.

Contrast and density are adequate to demonstrate the surrounding metacarpal and digital soft tissue and bony structures of the hand. Penetration is sufficient to visualize the bony trabecular patterns and the cortical outlines of the phalanges, metacarpals, and carpal bones.
- A high-contrast, optimal 50 to 60 kVp technique sufficiently penetrates bony and soft tissue structures and enhances the natural subject contrast of the hand.

The bony trabecular patterns and cortical outlines of the phalanges, metacarpals, and carpal bones are sharply defined.

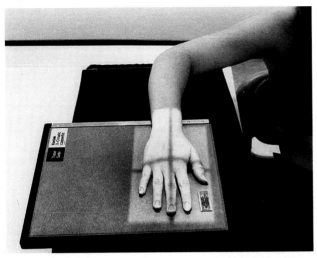

Figure 3-20. Proper patient positioning for PA hand radiograph.

- Sharply defined recorded details are obtained when patient motion is halted, a detail screen, and a small focal spot are used and a short object–image distance (OID) is maintained.

The digits and metacarpals demonstrate a true PA projection. The soft tissue outlines of the second through fifth phalanges are uniform, there is equal distance between the metacarpal heads, and the same midshaft concavity is demonstrated on either side of the phalanges and metacarpals of the second through fifth digits.

- A true PA projection of the hand is obtained when the patient fully extends the hand and rests the palmar surface (pronation) flat against the cassette (Fig. 3–20).
- ***True PA versus Medial Oblique Hand Position:*** If the hand is not fully extended but is slightly flexed, it often relaxes into a medial oblique position when it is resting against the cassette. Radiographically, a medial oblique position is signified by slight superimposition of the third through fifth metacarpal heads and unequal soft tissue thickness and midshaft concavity on the sides of the phalanges. The metacarpals also show unequal midshaft concavity and spacing (see Rad. 19). Abducting the patient's arm and placing the forearm and humerus on the same horizontal plane, with the elbow flexed 90 degrees, assists in preventing a medial oblique position. When the

patient has been positioned in this manner, the ulnar styloid appears in profile on the radiograph. Internal rotation of the hand is seldom a problem, because the thumb prevents this movement.

The long axes of the third digit and metacarpal are aligned with the long axis of the collimated field.

- Align the collimator's longitudinal light line with the long axis of the third finger and metacarpal. This alignment allows you to obtain tight collimation.

There is no soft tissue overlap of adjacent digits.

- Fingers should be spread slightly to prevent soft tissue overlapping (Rad. 19).

The interphalangeal (IP), metacarpophalangeal (MP), and carpometacarpal (CM) joints are visualized as open spaces, and the phalanges and metacarpals are not foreshortened. The thumb is visualized in a 45-degree oblique position.

- The IP, MP, and CM joint spaces are open and the phalanges and metacarpals are not foreshortened when the hand and fingers are fully extended and when the central ray is perpendicular to and centered with the third MP joint space.
- When the hand is flexed, the joint spaces are no longer in alignment, and the phalanges and metacarpals are no longer perpendicular to the central ray. This results in closed joint spaces and foreshortening of the phalanges and metacarpals (Rad. 20). The position of the first digit also changes when the radiograph is taken with the hand flexed, because flexion rotates the first digit into a lateral position.

The third metacarpophalangeal (MP) joint is at the center of the collimated field. The distal, middle, and proximal phalanges, the metacarpals, the carpals, and approximately 1 inch (2.5 cm) of the distal radius and ulna are included within the field.

- Centering the central ray to the third MP joint places it in the center of the collimated light field. This MP joint is situated just slightly distal to the head of the third metacarpal. Once the central ray is centered, open the longitudinal collimation to include the distal phalanx and the distal forearm. Transverse collimation should be to the skin-line of the first and fifth fingers.
- Either one half of a 10 × 12 inch (24 × 30 cm) film placed crosswise or a single 8 × 10 inch (18 × 24 cm) film placed lengthwise should be adequate to include all the required anatomical structures.

Critiquing Radiographs

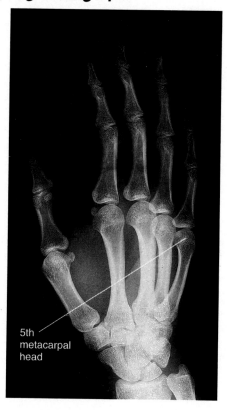

5th
metacarpal
head

Radiograph 19.

Critique: This radiograph demonstrates numerous positioning problems. First, the hand was externally rotated (in a medial oblique position), as indicated by the superimposition of the third through fifth metacarpal heads and by the unequal midshaft concavity on either side of the phalanges and metacarpals. Second, the digital soft tissue is overlapping, signifying that the fingers were not adequately spread apart. Finally, the interphalangeal joint spaces are closed and the distal and middle phalanges are foreshortened, because the fingers were not positioned parallel with the film.

Correction: Fully extend the hand and fingers; then position the palm flat against the cassette. Next, slightly spread the fingers to prevent soft tissue overlap.

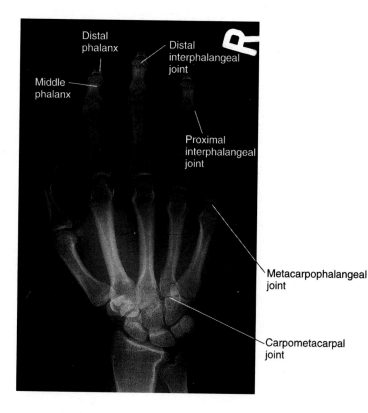

Distal
phalanx

Middle
phalanx

Distal
interphalangeal
joint

Proximal
interphalangeal
joint

Metacarpophalangeal
joint

Carpometacarpal
joint

Radiograph 20.

Critique: The IP and CM joints are closed and the phalanges and metacarpals are foreshortened. The first digit demonstrates a lateral position. The hand and fingers were flexed for this radiograph.

Correction: Fully extend the patient's hand and fingers, then place them flat against the cassette.

Hand: Medial Oblique Position
(External Oblique Position)

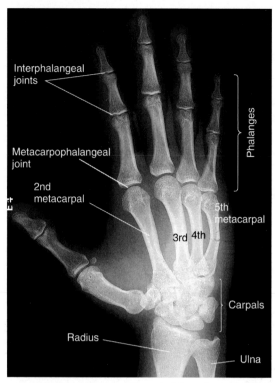

Figure 3–21. Accurately positioned oblique hand radiograph.

Radiographic Evaluation

Facility's patient identification requirements are noticeable on radiograph.

- These requirements usually are facility name, patient name, age, and hospital number, and exam time and date.
- The patient ID plate does not obscure any anatomy of interest.

A right or left marker, identifying the correct hand, is present on the radiograph and does not superimpose anatomy of interest.

- Place the marker within the collimated light field so it does not superimpose any portion of the hand.
- When more than one view of the hand is placed on the same film, only one of the views needs to be marked.

There is no evidence of preventable artifacts, such as rings, bracelets, watches, bandages, and splints.

- If the patient's condition prevents ring removal, the situation should be indicated on the requisition.
- Consult with the ordering physician and the patient about whether bandages or splints can be removed.

Contrast and density are adequate to demonstrate the surrounding metacarpal and digital soft tissue and bony

structures of the hand. There is sufficient penetration to visualize the bony trabecular patterns and the cortical outlines of the phalanges, metacarpals, and carpal bones.

- A high-contrast, optimal 50 to 60 kVp technique sufficiently penetrates the bony and soft tissue structures and enhances the natural subject contrast of the hand.

The bony trabecular patterns and the cortical outlines of the phalanges, metacarpals, and carpal bones are sharply defined.

- Sharply defined recorded details are demonstrated when patient motion is halted, a detail screen and small focal spot are used, and a short object–image distance (OID) is maintained.

The hand has been obliqued 45 degrees medially (externally). Each of the second through fifth metacarpal midshafts demonstrates more concavity on one side than on the other and have varying amounts of space between them. The first and second metacarpal heads are not superimposed, and the third through fifth metacarpal heads are slightly superimposed.

- To accomplish a medial oblique hand position, begin with the hand in a PA projection. Then, externally rotate the hand until it forms a 45-degree angle with the film (Fig. 3–22).
- To confirm the 45-degree angle, it is best to view the hand and not the wrist. The wrist often appears to be more oblique than the hand, so using the wrist can result in a miscalculation of the amount of obliquity. This is especially true if the humerus and forearm have not been placed on the same horizontal plane. When the patient has been positioned with the arm on the same horizontal plane, the ulnar styloid is demonstrated in profile medially on the radiograph. A radiolucent sponge can be used to help maintain this position.

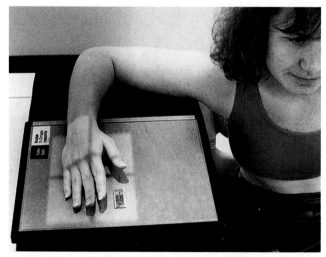

Figure 3-22. Proper patient positioning for oblique hand radiograph with extended fingers.

- **_Verifying Oblique Hand Position:_** A 45-degree oblique hand position can radiographically be recognized by the amount of metacarpal midshaft and metacarpal head superimposition. If the hand has not been rotated enough, the metacarpal relationship is similar to that demonstrated on a PA projection radiograph of the hand: The midshafts of the metacarpals are nearly evenly spaced, and the metacarpal heads are not superimposed (see Rad. 21). If the hand is rotated more than the required 45 degrees, the third through fifth metacarpal midshafts are superimposed on the radiograph (see Rad. 22).

The long axes of the third digit and metacarpal are aligned with the long axis of the collimated field.

- Align the collimator's longitudinal light line with the long axis of the third finger and metacarpal.

There is no soft tissue overlap of adjacent digits.

- Fingers should be spread slightly to prevent soft tissue overlapping (see Rad. 23).

The interphalangeal (IP) and metacarpophalangeal (MP) joints are visualized as open spaces, and the phalanges are demonstrated without foreshortening. The thumb's position may vary from a lateral to an oblique position.

- The IP and MP joint spaces are open and the phalanges are not foreshortened when the hand and fingers are fully extended and aligned parallel with the film. A radiolucent sponge should be used to help the patient maintain this positioning.
- **_Disadvantages of Using Fingers as Props:_** A common positioning error in oblique hand radiography is to use the patient's fingers instead of a sponge to maintain the oblique position. For this positioning, the fingers are flexed until the fingertips touch the film to prop the hand for the oblique position (Fig. 3–23). Such positioning closes the IP joint spaces and foreshortens the phalanges (see Rad. 24). In some

facilities, using the fingers as props is acceptable when the metacarpals are of interest and no attention is to be given to the patient's phalanges.

The third MP joint is at the center of the collimated field. The distal, middle, and proximal phalanges, the metacarpals, the carpals, and approximately 1 inch (2.5 cm) of the distal radius and ulna are included within the field.

- Centering the central ray to the third MP joint places it in the center of the collimated light field. The MP joint is situated just slightly distal to the head of the third metacarpal. Once the central ray is centered, open the longitudinal collimation to include the distal phalanges and the distal forearm. Transverse collimation should be to the closest skin-line of the first and fifth fingers.
- Either one half of a 10 × 12 inch (24 × 30 cm) film placed crosswise or a single 8 × 10 inch (18 × 24 cm) film placed lengthwise should be adequate to include all the required anatomical structures.

Critiquing Radiographs

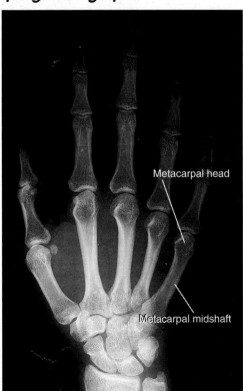

Radiograph 21.

Critique: The metacarpal heads demonstrate no superimposition, the metacarpal midshaft concavities are uniform, and the spaces between the metacarpal midshafts are nearly equal. The hand was not rotated enough.
Correction: Externally rotate the hand until the metacarpals and the film form a 45-degree angle.

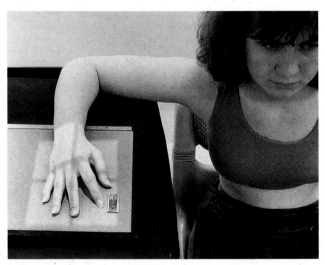

Figure 3-23. Proper patient positioning for oblique hand radiograph with flexed fingers.

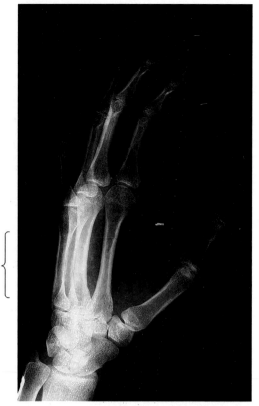

Metacarpal midshafts

Radiograph 22.

Critique: The midshafts of the third through fifth metacarpals are superimposed. The patient's hand was placed at more than 45 degrees of obliquity.

Correction: Internally rotate the hand until the metacarpals and the film form a 45-degree angle.

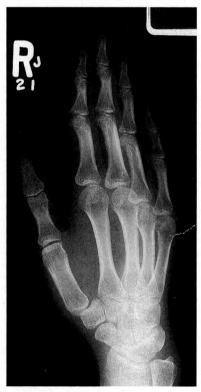

Radiograph 23.

Critique: There is soft tissue overlap of each digit onto the adjacent digit. The fingers were not spread apart.
Correction: Spread all fingers enough to prevent soft tissue overlap.

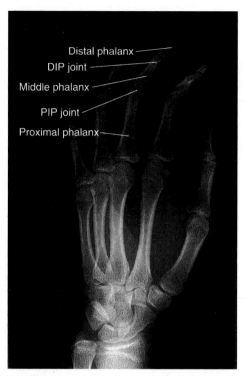

Distal phalanx
DIP joint
Middle phalanx
PIP joint
Proximal phalanx

Radiograph 24.

Critique: The distal and middle phalanges are foreshortened, and the IP joint spaces are closed. The fingers were not positioned parallel with the film, but were instead used to prop the hand (see Fig. 3–23).
Correction: Extend the fingers and place them parallel with the film. It may be necessary to situate a radiolucent sponge beneath the fingers to maintain this positioning.

Hand: Lateromedial Projection
(``Fan'' Lateral Position)

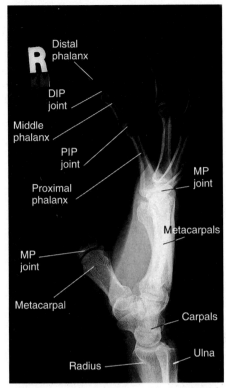

Figure 3–24. Accurately positioned lateral hand radiograph.

Radiographic Evaluation

Facility's patient identification requirements are noticeable on radiograph.
- These requirements usually are facility name, patient name, age, and hospital number, and exam time and date.
- The patient ID plate does not obscure any anatomy of interest.

A right or left marker, identifying the correct hand, is present on the radiograph and does not superimpose anatomy of interest.
- Place the marker within the collimated light field so it does not superimpose any portion of the hand.
- When more than one view of the hand is placed on the same film, only one of the views needs to be marked.

There is no evidence of preventable artifacts, such as rings, bracelets, watches, bandages, and splints.
- If the patient's condition prevents ring removal, the situation should be indicated on the requisition.
- Consult with the ordering physician and the patient about whether bandages or splints can be removed.

Contrast and density are adequate to demonstrate the surrounding metacarpal soft tissue and bony structures of the hand. Penetration is sufficient to visualize the
bony trabecular patterns and the cortical outlines of the phalanges, metacarpals, and carpal bones.
- A high-contrast, optimal 50 to 60 kVp technique sufficiently penetrates the bony and soft tissue structures and enhances the natural subject contrast of the hand.
- For the "fan" lateral hand radiograph, it is difficult to simultaneously demonstrate the phalanges and the metacarpals with optimal density, because of the difference in thickness between the two body parts when the fingers are separated. Evaluate the requisition to determine what anatomy of the hand is of interest so the mAs can be adjusted to obtain optimal density in that area.

The bony trabecular patterns and cortical outlines of the phalanges, metacarpals, and carpal bones are sharply defined.
- Sharply defined recorded details are obtained when patient motion is halted, a detail screen and small focal spot are used, and a short object–image distance (OID) is maintained.

The second through fifth digits are separated, demonstrating little superimposition of the proximal bony or soft tissue structures. The thumb is demonstrated without superimposition of the other digits. Its position may vary from a PA projection to a slightly oblique position.
- For a lateral hand position, place the medial hand surface resting against the film; then fan or spread the fingers as far apart as possible without superimposing the thumb. The fingers are fanned most effectively by drawing the second and third fingers anteriorly and the fourth and fifth fingers posteriorly. The amount of finger separation obtained will depend on the patient's mobility (Fig. 3–25). Immobilization sponges are available to help maintain proper positioning. When the fingers are fanned, they can be individually studied. If the fingers are not adequately separated, they superimpose each other on the radiograph (see Rad. 25).

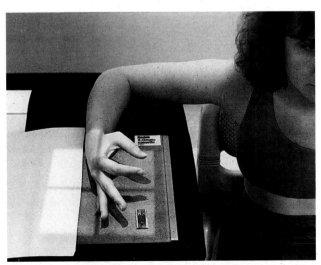

Figure 3–25. Proper patient positioning for lateral hand radiograph.

The second through fifth metacarpals are superimposed.

- Superimpose the second through fifth metacarpals by palpating the patient's knuckles and placing them directly on top of one another.
- ***Verifying a True Lateral Hand Position:*** On a "fan" lateral radiograph, a true lateral wrist position—represented by superimposition of the ulna and radius—is not always accomplished when the metacarpal midshafts are superimposed. Instead, the ulna is demonstrated slightly posterior to the radius. Because of this variation, a true lateral position of the hand should be determined by judging the degree of superimposition of the second through fifth metacarpal midshafts. If the metacarpal midshafts are not superimposed and the fifth metacarpal is demonstrated anterior to the second through fourth metacarpal, the hand was slightly externally rotated or supinated (see Rad. 25). The fifth metacarpal can be identified by its length; it is the shortest. If the metacarpal midshafts are not superimposed and the second metacarpal is demonstrated anterior to the third through fifth metacarpal, the hand was slightly internally rotated or pronated (see Rad. 26). The second metacarpal can also be identified by its length; it is the longest.

The long axes of the metacarpals and carpal bones are aligned with the long axis of the collimated field.

- Align the collimator's longitudinal light line with the long axis of the metacarpals.

The interphalangeal (IP) joints are open, and the phalanges are not foreshortened.

- The IP joint spaces are open and the phalanges are not foreshortened when the phalanges are positioned parallel with the film (see Rad. 26). It may be necessary to depress the proximal thumb to place the thumb parallel with the film.

The metacarpophalangeal (MP) joints are at the center of the collimated field. The distal, middle, and proximal phalanges, the metacarpals, the carpals, and about 1 inch (2.5 cm) of the distal radius and ulna are included within the field.

- Centering the central ray to the second MP joint places it in the center of the collimated light field. Once the central ray is centered, open the longitudinal collimation to include the distal phalanges and the distal forearm. Transverse collimation should be to the skinline of the first and fifth fingers.
- Either one half of a 10 × 12 inch (24 × 30 cm) film placed crosswise or a single 8 × 10 inch (18 × 24 cm) film placed lengthwise should be adequate to include all the required anatomical structures.

OPTIONAL DIGIT POSITIONING

Lateral Hand in Extension
The second through fifth digits are fully extended and superimposed. Density of the second through fifth digits and metacarpals is uniform, but the first metacarpal density is overexposed. The positioning evaluation for the metacarpals and distal forearm is the same as for the "fan" lateral radiograph.

- Extending the hand and fingers until they are aligned on the same plane places the hand in extension (see Rad. 27). It has been suggested that foreign bodies of the palm can be better localized when the lateral hand radiograph is taken in extension.[1]

Lateral Hand in Flexion
The second through fifth digits are flexed and superimposed. Density of the second through fifth digits and metacarpals is uniform, but the first metacarpal density is overexposed. The positioning for the metacarpals and distal forearm is the same as for the "fan" lateral radiograph.

- Flex the second through fifth fingers until they meet the first finger but do not superimpose it (see Rad. 28). It has been suggested that this position of the lateral hand is taken to distinguish the degree of anterior or posterior displacement of a fractured metacarpal.[1]

Critiquing Radiographs

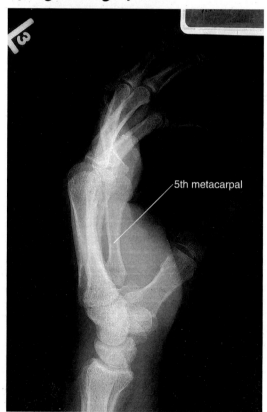

5th metacarpal

Radiograph 25.

Critique: The second through fifth metacarpal midshafts are not superimposed, and the shortest (fifth) metacarpal is anterior to the third through fourth metacarpals. The hand was externally rotated or supinated. The second through fifth digits are nearly superimposed, indicating that the patient's fingers were not adequately fanned.

Correction: Internally rotate or pronate the patient's hand until the metacarpals are superimposed. If patient mobility allows, increase the amount of finger separation.

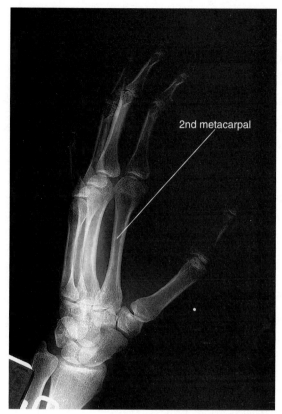

2nd metacarpal

Radiograph 26.

Critique: The second through fifth metacarpal midshafts are not superimposed, and the longest (second) metacarpal is anterior to the third through fifth metacarpals. The hand was internally rotated or pronated. The middle and distal phalanges are foreshortened, and the IP joint spaces are closed, indicating that the second through fourth digits were not positioned parallel with the film.

Correction: Externally rotate or supinate the patient's hand until the metacarpals are superimposed. Place the second through fifth digits parallel with the film. It may be necessary to use a radiolucent sponge beneath the proximal fingers to maintain position.

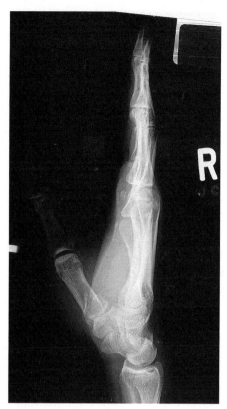

R

Radiograph 27.

Critique: The digits are superimposed. This radiograph was taken with the hand and fingers in full extension.

Correction: If an extension lateral hand radiograph is desired, no correction is required. If a "fan" lateral hand radiograph is desired, fan or spread the fingers as far apart as possible by drawing the second and third fingers anteriorly and the fourth and fifth fingers posteriorly.

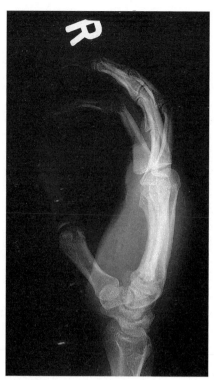

Radiograph 28.

Critique: The digits are superimposed. This radiograph was taken with the hand and fingers flexed.

Correction: If a flexed lateral hand radiograph was desired, no correction is required. If a "fan" lateral hand was desired, fan or spread the fingers as far apart as possible by drawing the second and third fingers anteriorly and the fourth and fifth fingers posteriorly.

WRIST

Posteroanterior Projection

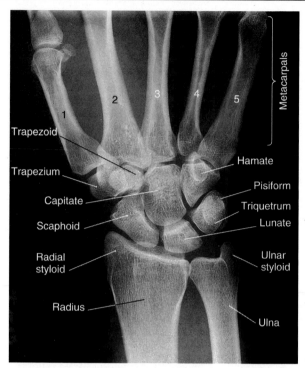

Figure 3-26. Accurately positioned PA wrist radiograph.

Radiographic Evaluation

Facility's patient identification requirements are visible on radiograph.
- These requirements usually are facility name, patient name, age, and hospital number, and exam time and date.
- The patient ID plate does not obscure any anatomy of interest.

A right or left marker, identifying the correct wrist, is present on the radiograph and does not superimpose anatomy of interest.
- Place the marker within the collimated light field so it does not superimpose any portion of the affected wrist. It may be necessary to open the light field to include the marker.
- When more than one view of the wrist is placed on the same radiograph, only one of the views needs to be marked.

There is no evidence of preventable artifacts, such as bracelets, watches, bandages, and splints.
- Consult with the ordering physician and the patient about whether bandages or splints can be removed.

Contrast and density are adequate to demonstrate the scaphoid fat stripe and the surrounding soft tissue and bony structures of the wrist. Penetration is sufficient to

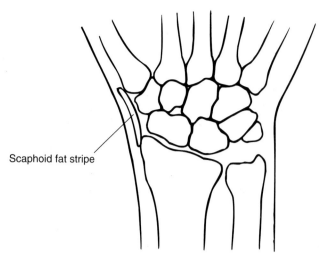

Figure 3–27. Location of scaphoid fat stripe. (Courtesy Educational Reviews, Inc.) (Reproduced with permission from Martensen K. II. Radiographic Positioning and Evaluation of the Wrist. (In-Service Reviews in Radiologic Technology, vol 16, no 5.) Birmingham, AL: Educational Reviews, Inc., 1992.)

visualize the bony trabecular patterns and the cortical outlines of the carpal bones.

- A high-contrast, low (50 to 60) kVp technique best enhances the soft tissue and bony structures of the wrist.
- **Significance of the Scaphoid Fat Stripe:** The scaphoid fat stripe is one of the soft tissue structures that should be visualized on all PA wrist radiographs (Fig. 3–27). It is convex and is located just lateral to the scaphoid in a noninjured wrist. A change in the convexity of this stripe may indicate to the reviewer the presence of joint effusion or of a radial side fracture of the scaphoid, radial styloid process, or proximal first metacarpal.[2, 3]

The bony trabecular patterns and cortical outlines of the carpal bones are sharply defined.

- Sharply defined radiographic details are obtained when patient motion is controlled, a detail screen and a small focal spot are used, and a short object–image distance (OID) is maintained.

The wrist is positioned in a true PA projection. The radial and ulnar styloids are at the extreme lateral and medial edges, respectively, of each bone. The radioulnar articulation is open, and superimposition of the metacarpal bases is limited.[4, 5]

- Rotation of the wrist and forearm is controlled by the position of the hand, elbow, and humerus. A PA projection is accomplished by abducting the humerus until it is positioned parallel with the film and the elbow is in a lateral position. The hand is then pronated, placing the wrist in a PA projection (Fig. 3–28).
- **Detecting Wrist Rotation and Styloid Position:** Rotation of the wrist and forearm will result from hand, humerus and elbow movements. When the hand and wrist are rotated externally into a medial oblique position, the carpal bones and the metacarpal

bases located on the medial aspect of the wrist are superimposed, whereas those located laterally are not. The lateral interconnecting carpal and metacarpal joint spaces are also demonstrated (see Rad. 29).

Internal rotation (or lateral oblique position) of the hand and wrist causes the laterally located carpal bones and the metacarpal bases to superimpose and increases visualization of the pisiform and hamate hook (see Rad. 30).

External and internal hand and wrist rotation also cause the radial styloid to rotate out of profile, closing the radioulnar articulation.

When the humerus and elbow are mispositioned, the placement of the ulna is changed. Positioning the elbow in a lateral position with the humerus parallel with the film brings the ulnar styloid in profile medially. The ulna and radius cross each other if the humerus is not abducted but is allowed to remain against the patient's side with the hand pronated. This inaccurate positioning can be identified on a tightly collimated PA wrist radiograph by viewing the ulnar styloid, which is rotated anteriorly and is no longer demonstrated in profile (see Rad. 36).

The distal radius is demonstrated without foreshortening. The anterior and posterior carpal articulating margins of the radius are nearly superimposed.

- The distal radial carpal articular surface is concave and slants approximately 11 degrees from posterior to anterior.[6] Because the forearm is positioned parallel with the film for a PA wrist radiograph, the slant of the distal radius causes the posterior radial margin to project slightly (0.25 inch or 0.6 cm) distal to the anterior radial margin, obscuring the radiocarpal joints.
- **Distal Radioulnar Articulation:** If a radiograph is obtained that demonstrates an excessive amount of the radial articulating surface, or if open radioscaphoid and radiolunate joint spaces are desired, view the distal radioulnar articulation to determine the correct-

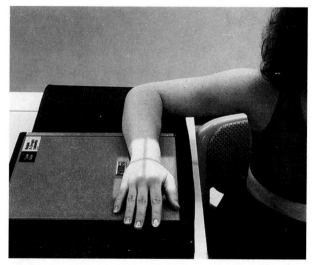

Figure 3–28. Proper patient positioning for PA wrist radiograph.

ing movement. The posterior edge of this surface is blunt, whereas the anterior edge is rounded. Study the distal end of a radial skeletal bone to better familiarize yourself with this difference.

If a radiograph is obtained that demonstrates the posterior radial margin distal to the anterior margin, the proximal forearm was elevated higher than the distal forearm (see Rad. 31). If the anterior radial margin is demonstrated distal to the posterior margin, the proximal forearm was positioned lower than the distal forearm. To superimpose the distal radial surfaces and to demonstrate radioscaphoid and radiolunate joints as open spaces (see Rad. 30), the proximal aspect of the forearm should be positioned slightly (5 to 6 degrees from horizontal) lower than the distal forearm.

- **_Positioning Patient with Thick Proximal Forearm:_** On a patient with a large muscular or thick proximal forearm, it may be necessary to allow the proximal forearm to hang off the film or table in order to position the forearm parallel with the film. If the patient is not positioned in this manner, the radius will be foreshortened, demonstrating an excessive amount of radial articular surface, and superimposition of the scaphoid and lunate onto the radius will be greater (see Rad. 31).

The second through fifth carpometacarpal (CM) joint spaces are open. The scaphoid is only slightly foreshortened, and the lunate is trapezoidal.

- When the wrist is placed in a neutral, nonflexed position, these three radiographic appearances are achieved.
- To place the wrist in a neutral position, curl the patient's fingers, flexing the hand until the metacarpals are angled to about 10 to 15 degrees with the film.
- **_Effect of Flexion and Extension on Carpal Bones:_** View your own wrist in a PA projection with the hand extended flat against a hard surface. Note how the wrist is slightly flexed. Next, begin slowly flexing your hand and notice how the wrist moves from a flexed to an extended position with increased hand flexion.

To understand how carpal bone position varies with wrist flexion and extension, study the drawings of the scaphoid, capitate, and lunate bones in Figure 3–29. Note how the positions of these carpals change with each movement. Also study the position of the CM joint space in reference to a perpendicular central ray.

Radiographs 32 and 33 demonstrate a PA wrist in flexion (the hand was extended) and extension (the hand was overflexed), respectively. Compare these radiographs with the properly positioned wrist radiograph in Figure 3–26. Wrist flexion resulted in obscured fourth and fifth CM joint spaces, a foreshortened scaphoid that has taken a signet ring configuration (a large circle with a smaller circle within it), and a triangular lunate. Wrist extension has resulted in foreshortened metacarpals, closed second and third CM joint spaces, an elongated scaphoid, and a triangular lunate.[7]

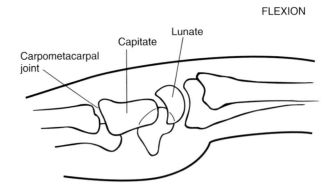

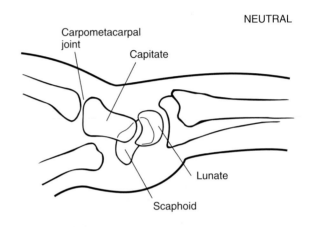

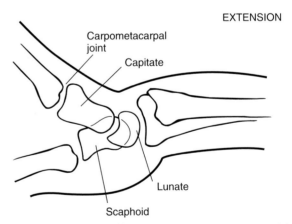

Figure 3–29. Lateral wrist in flexion (*top*), neutral position (*middle*), and extension (*bottom*). (Courtesy Educational Review, Inc.) (Reproduced with permission from Martensen K. II. Radiographic Positioning and Evaluation of the Wrist. (In-Service Reviews in Radiologic Technology, vol 16, no 5.) Birmingham, AL: Educational Reviews, Inc., 1992.)

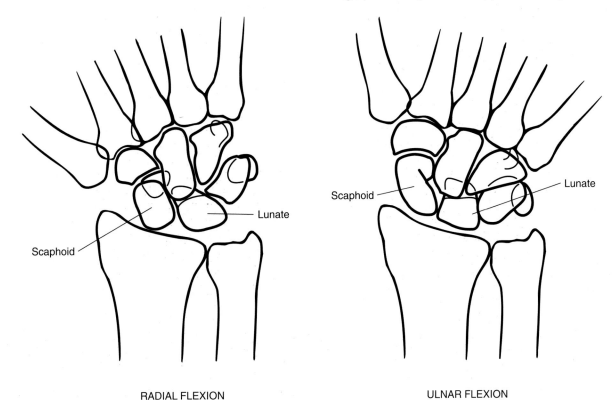

RADIAL FLEXION   ULNAR FLEXION

Figure 3-30. PA wrist in radial flexion *(left)* and ulnar flexion *(right)*. (Courtesy Educational Reviews, Inc.) (Reproduced with permission from Martensen K. II. Radiographic Positioning and Evaluation of the Wrist. (In-Service Reviews in Radiologic Technology, vol 16, no 5.) Birmingham, AL: Educational Reviews, Inc., 1992.)

The long axes of the third metacarpal and the radius are aligned with the long axis of the collimated light field. The scaphoid and half of the lunate are positioned distal to the radius.

- If the long axes of the third metacarpal and the midforearm are aligned with the long axis of the collimated light field, the patient's wrist has been placed in a neutral position. If a neutral position is not maintained for a PA projection wrist radiograph, the shapes of the scaphoid and the position of the lunate are altered (Fig. 3-30 and Rads. 34 and 35). Radial flexion of the wrist causes the distal scaphoid to shift anteriorly (toward the palmar surface) and to be foreshortened, forming a signet ring configuration. The lunate will shift medially, toward the ulna. In ulnar flexion, the distal scaphoid tilts posteriorly (dorsally) and is elongated, and the lunate shifts laterally, toward the radius.[7] Radial flexion and ulnar flexion views of the wrist may be specifically requested to demonstrate wrist joint mobility.

The carpal bones are at the center of the collimated field. The carpal bones, one fourth of the distal ulna and radius, and half of the proximal metacarpals are included within the field.

- The wrist joint is located at a level just distal to the palpable ulnar styloid. To obtain an image of the carpal bones with the least amount of distortion, a perpendicular central ray should be placed at this level and centered to the midwrist area. Open the longitudinal collimation to include half of the metacarpals. Transverse collimation should be to the wrist skin-line.

- Either one half of an 8 × 10 inch (18 × 24 cm) film or one third of a 10 × 12 inch (24 × 30 cm) film placed crosswise should be adequate to include all the required anatomical structures.

- ***Wrist Exam Taken to Include More Than One Fourth of the Forearm:*** When a wrist exam is requested to include more than one fourth of the distal forearm, the central ray should remain on the wrist joint, and the collimation field should be opened to demonstrate the desired amount of forearm. This method will result in an extended, unneeded radiation field distal to the metacarpals. A lead strip placed over this extended radiation field protects the patient's phalanges and prevents backscatter from reaching the film. The advantage of this method over centering the central ray proximal to the wrist joint is an undistorted demonstration of the carpal bones.

EFFECT OF UPPER EXTREMITY MOVEMENTS ON BONY COMPONENTS OF THE WRIST

The wrist is a very complex joint with numerous bony components and movement possibilities. In an attempt to simplify the effect that different upper extremity movements have on the bony components, I will summarize some of them. The positions of the elbow and hand affect forearm and wrist rotation and can be identified by the positions of the ulnar and radial styloid, respectively. When the elbow is in a lateral position, the ulnar styloid is in profile. When the hand is in a true PA projection, the radial styloid is in profile.

It is the hand position that varies the shape of the scaphoid. If the wrist is flexed as a result of hand extension or is radial flexed, the scaphoid is foreshortened. If the wrist is extended as a result of hand flexion or is ulnar flexed, the scaphoid is elongated.

The shape and location of the lunate also vary with the position of the wrist and hand. It becomes triangular with hand extension and flexion and changes position in reference to the distal radius with radial and ulnar flexion. In radial flexion, the lunate is positioned distal to the radioulnar articulation, whereas in ulnar flexion, it is positioned distal to the radius.

Because the shapes of the scaphoid and lunate can be changed with more than one positioning movement, it is necessary to evaluate mispositioned radiographs carefully to determine which movement is causing the misposition. It is also possible for two corrections to be needed simultaneously to obtain accurate positioning. Hand flexion and extension are easily identified by evaluating the CM joints. Hand and wrist deviations are identified by evaluating the alignment of the third metacarpal with the radius.

Critiquing Radiographs

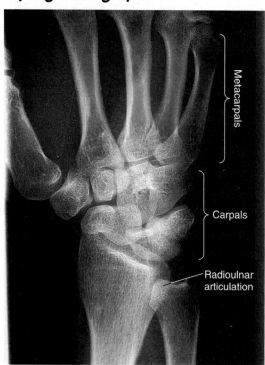

Radiograph 29.

Critique: The medially located carpal bones and metacarpals are superimposed, whereas the laterally located carpal and metacarpal joint spaces are open. The radioulnar articulation is closed, and the radial styloid is not in profile. The wrist was externally rotated (in a medial oblique position). The ulnar styloid is in profile, indicating that the elbow and humerus were accurately positioned.

Correction: Internally rotate the hand until the wrist is in a true PA projection.

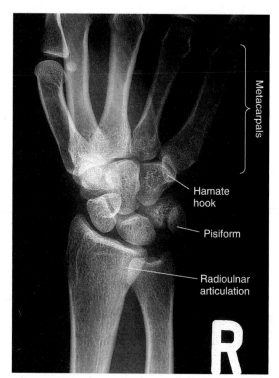

Radiograph 30.

Critique: The laterally located carpals and metacarpals are superimposed, and the pisiform and hamate hook are visualized. The radioulnar articulation is closed. The wrist was internally rotated (in a lateral oblique position). The ulnar styloid is in profile, indicating accurate elbow and humerus positioning, and the distal radial articular surface is directly superimposed, demonstrating open radiolunate and radioscaphoid joint spaces. The proximal forearm was positioned slightly lower than the distal forearm.

Correction: Rotate the hand externally until the wrist is in a true PA projection.

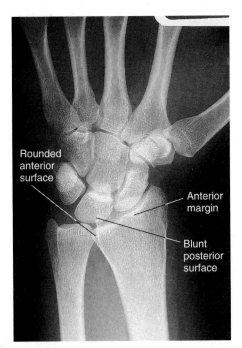

Radiograph 31.

Critique: The posterior margin of the distal radius is too far distal to the anterior margin. The posterior margin can be identified by the blunt, posterior ulnar articulating edge. The forearm was foreshortened, with the proximal forearm positioned higher than the distal forearm.

Correction: Lower the proximal forearm until it is parallel with the film. If you desire a superimposed distal radial articular surface, which will demonstrate open radio-lunate and radioscaphoid joint spaces, position the proximal forearm slightly (5 to 6 degrees from horizontal) lower than the distal forearm. For a patient with a thick proximal forearm, allow the proximal forearm to hang off the film or table.

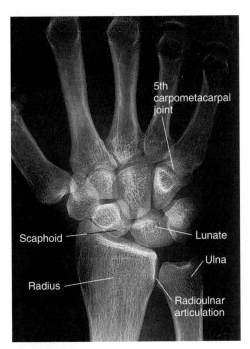

Radiograph 32.

Critique: The scaphoid is foreshortened and has a signet ring configuration, the CM joints are obscured, and the lunate is triangular but is properly positioned distal to the radius. Two hand mispositions will cause this scaphoid shape, radial flexion and hand extension. Because the lunate is properly positioned distal to the radius, radial flexion can be eliminated as the positional problem. Hand extension (wrist flexion) is the cause of this mispositioning.

Correction: Curl the patient's fingers, flexing the hand until the metacarpals are angled at about 10 to 15 degrees with the film.

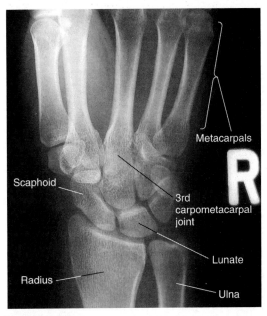

Radiograph 33.

Critique: The scaphoid is elongated, and the second through fourth metacarpals are superimposing the CM joints. The lunate is triangular but is properly positioned distal to the radius. Two hand mispositions will cause this scaphoid shape, ulnar flexion and hand overflexion (metacarpals angled at more than 10 to 15 degrees with the film). Because the lunate is properly positioned distal to the radius, ulnar flexion can be eliminated as the positional problem. Hand overflexion (wrist extension) is the cause of this misposition.

Correction: Extend fingers and hand until the metacarpals are angled at 10 to 15 degrees with the film.

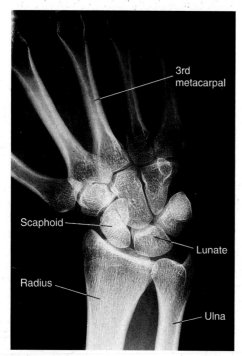

Radiograph 34.

Critique: The scaphoid is foreshortened, the lunate is positioned mostly distal to the ulna, and the third metacarpal is not aligned with the long axis of the radius. Because the scaphoid foreshortens with both hand extension and radial flexion, you can determine the correct repositioning movement for this radiograph by evaluating the position of the third metacarpal and the openness of the CM joint spaces. The third metacarpal is not aligned with the radius and the scaphoid is foreshortened, so you can conclude that the patient was in radial flexion. Because the CM joint spaces are open, the hand was properly flexed.

Correction: Ulnar-flex the wrist until the third metacarpal and the midforearm are aligned, placing the hand and wrist in a neutral deviated position. If a radial flexion wrist radiograph is desired to evaluate patient mobility, no correction movement is required.

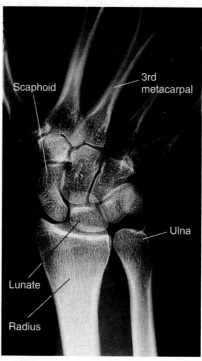

Radiograph 35.

Critique: The scaphoid is elongated, the lunate is entirely positioned distal to the radius, and the third metacarpal is not aligned with the long axis of the radius. All of these positioning points indicate that the wrist was in ulnar flexion for the radiograph. Because the CM joint spaces are open, you can conclude that the hand was accurately flexed.

Correction: Radial-flex the wrist until the third metacarpal is aligned with the midforearm, placing the hand and wrist in a neutral deviated position. If an ulnar flexion wrist radiograph is desired to evaluate patient mobility, no correction movement is required.

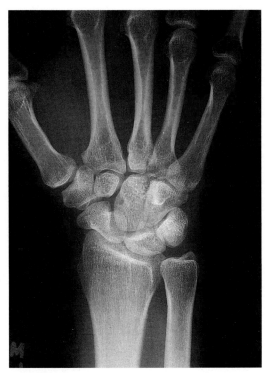

Radiograph 36.

Critique: This radiograph has many positioning problems. First, neither the radial nor ulnar styloid is in profile, indicating that the hand and the humerus were mispositioned. Next, the distal radius is foreshortened. Note how the articulating surface is demonstrated with the posterior margin far too distal to the anterior margin. The proximal forearm was positioned higher than the distal forearm. Finally, the scaphoid is foreshortened, and the fourth and fifth CM joints are obscured. The radiograph was taken with the wrist in slight external rotation, with the fourth and fifth metacarpals resting against the cassette, although the second and third distal metacarpals were elevated accurately.

Correction: Flex the elbow and abduct the humerus 90 degrees, placing the entire arm on the same horizontal plane. Internally rotate the hand and wrist until they are positioned in a true AP projection. Curl the fingers, flexing the hand until the metacarpals are angled at 10 to 15 degrees with the film.

Wrist: Medial Oblique Position
(External Oblique Position)

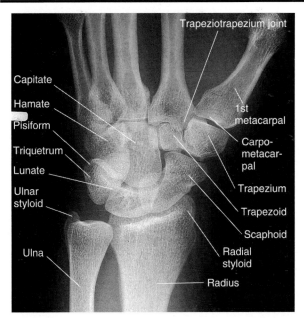

Figure 3-31. Accurately positioned oblique wrist radiograph.

Radiographic Evaluation

Facility's patient identification requirements are visible on radiograph.
- These requirements usually are facility name, patient name, age, and hospital number, and exam time and date.
- The patient ID plate does not obscure any anatomy of interest.

A right or left marker, identifying the correct wrist, is present on the radiograph and does not superimpose anatomy of interest.
- Place the marker within the collimated light field so it does not superimpose any portion of the affected wrist. When more than one position of the wrist is placed on the same radiograph, only one of the views needs to be marked.

There is no evidence of preventable artifacts, such as bracelets, watches, bandages, and splints.
- Consult with the ordering physician and the patient about whether bandages and splints can be removed.

Contrast and density are adequate to demonstrate the scaphoid fat stripe and the surrounding soft tissue and bony structures of the wrist. Penetration is sufficient to visualize the bony trabecular patterns and the cortical outlines of the carpal bones.
- A high-contrast, low (50 to 60) kVp technique best enhances the soft tissue and bony structures of the wrist.
- The scaphoid fat stripe is one of the soft tissue structures that should be visualized on all oblique wrist

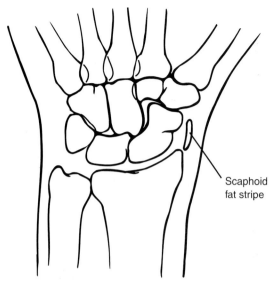

Figure 3-32. Location of scaphoid fat stripe.

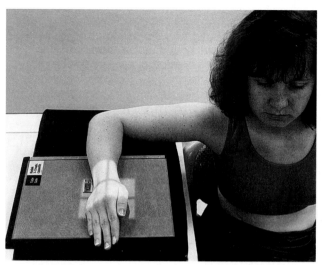

Figure 3-33. Proper patient positioning for oblique wrist radiograph.

radiographs. It is convex and is located just lateral to the scaphoid on a noninjured wrist (Fig. 3–32). A change in the shape of this fat stripe or in its proximity to the scaphoid may indicate joint effusion or a radial side fracture.[2, 3]

The bony trabecular patterns and cortical outlines of the carpal bones are sharply defined.
- Sharply defined radiographic details are obtained when patient motion is controlled, a detail screen and a small focal spot are used, and a short object–image distance (OID) is maintained.

The wrist has been placed in a 45-degree medial oblique position. The trapezoid and trapezium are demonstrated without superimposition, and the trapeziotrapezoidal joint space is open. The scaphoid tuberosity and waist are visualized in profile.[8] There is only a small degree of trapezoid and capitate superimposition.
- To accomplish an oblique wrist radiograph, begin with the wrist in a PA projection with the humerus and the forearm on the same horizontal plane. Externally rotate the hand and wrist until the wrist forms a 45-degree angle with the film (Fig. 3–33). When judging the degree of wrist obliquity, it is best to view the wrist and not the hand. The obliquity of the hand and wrist are not always equal when they are rotated, especially if the humerus and forearm are not positioned on the same horizontal plane for the radiograph.
- ***Determining the Accuracy of Wrist Obliquity:*** On a PA projection radiograph (Rad. 37), the trapezoid and trapezium are superimposed. Placing the wrist in a medial oblique position draws the trapezium from beneath the trapezoid, providing clear visualization of both carpal bones and the joint space (trapeziotrapezoidal) between them. The medial oblique position also rotates the scaphoid tuberosity and waist into profile. The relationships between the trapezoid and trapezium and the trapezoid and capitate

are used to discern an accurate oblique wrist position. If the wrist is not rotated enough, the trapezoid and trapezium are superimposed, and the trapeziotrapezoidal joint space is obscured (see Rad. 38). If wrist obliquity is more than 45 degrees, the trapezium demonstrates minimal trapezoidal superimposition, the capitate is superimposed by the trapezoid, and the trapeziotrapezoidal joint space is obscured (see Rad. 39).

The second carpometacarpal (CM) and the scaphotrapezium joint spaces are demonstrated.
- For the PA projection of the wrist, the CM joints are opened by flexing the hand until the metacarpals are angled at about 10 to 15 degrees with the film. When the hand and wrist are placed in obliquity, the same metacarpal tilt must be maintained to open the second CM and scaphotrapezium joint spaces. If the distal metacarpals are allowed to tilt toward the film, these two joints are obscured (see Rad. 38).

The long axes of the third metacarpal and radius are aligned with the long axis of the collimated field. The scaphoid tuberosity and waist are demonstrated in profile and are not positioned directly next to the radius.
- If the long axes of the third metacarpal and the radius are aligned with the long axis of the collimation field, the patient's wrist is placed in a neutral position. Radial flexion foreshortens the scaphoid, preventing visualization of the scaphoid tuberosity and waist, and positions the scaphoid directly next to the radius (see Rad. 40).

The distal radius is demonstrated without foreshortening. The anterior and posterior carpal-articulating surfaces of the radius are nearly superimposed.
- The distal radial carpal articular surface is concave and slants about 11 degrees from posterior to anterior when the radius and ulna are positioned parallel with

the film.[4] Because the forearm is positioned parallel with the film for an oblique wrist radiograph, the slant of the distal radius causes the posterior margin to be projected slightly (0.25 inch or 0.6 cm) distal to the anterior radial margin, obscuring the radiocarpal joints.

- If a radiograph is obtained that demonstrates an excessive amount of the radial articulating surface, or if open radioscaphoid and radiolunate joint spaces are desired, you should view the distal radioulnar articulation to determine the correcting movement. On the radioulnar articulation, the radial surface that superimposes the ulna is associated with the posterior radial margin.
- If a radiograph is obtained that demonstrates the posterior radial margin too far distal to the anterior margin, the proximal forearm was elevated higher than the distal forearm (see Rad. 41). If the anterior radial margin is demonstrated distal to the posterior margin, the proximal forearm was positioned lower than the distal forearm.
- To demonstrate open radioscaphoid and radiolunate joint spaces (see Rad. 42), position the proximal forearm slightly (5 to 6 degrees) lower than the distal forearm.
- ***Positioning Patient with Thick Proximal Forearm:*** For the patient with a large muscular or thick proximal forearm, allow the proximal forearm to hang off the film or table to position it parallel with the film. If the patient is not positioned in this manner, the radius is foreshortened, demonstrating an excessive amount of radial articular surface, and superimposition of the scaphoid and lunate onto the radius is increased.

The ulnar styloid is in profile at the far medial edge.
- The position of the humerus and elbow determines the placement of the ulnar styloid. The ulnar styloid is demonstrated in profile when the patient's humerus is placed parallel with the film and the elbow is in a lateral position. If the humerus is not abducted, but remains against the patient's side, the ulnar styloid is rotated anteriorly and is no longer demonstrated in profile.

The carpal bones are at the center of the collimated field. The carpal bones, one fourth of the distal ulna and radius, and half of the proximal metacarpals are included within the field.
- The wrist joint is located at a level just distal to the first proximal metacarpal. To obtain an oblique image of the carpal bones with the least amount of distortion, a perpendicular central ray should be placed at this level and centered with the midwrist area. Open longitudinal collimation to include half of the metacarpals. Transverse collimation should be to the wrist skin-line.
- Either half of an 8 × 10 inch (18 × 24 cm) film or one third of a 10 × 12 inch (24 × 30 cm) film placed crosswise should be adequate to include all the required anatomical structures.

Critiquing Radiographs

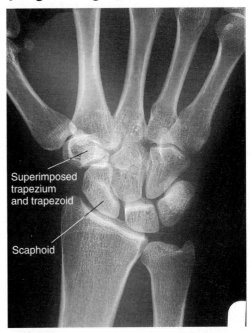

Radiograph 37.

Critique: The trapezoid and trapezium are superimposed, and the scaphoid tuberosity is not demonstrated in profile. This is a PA projection.

Correction: Externally rotate the wrist until it forms a 45-degree angle with the film.

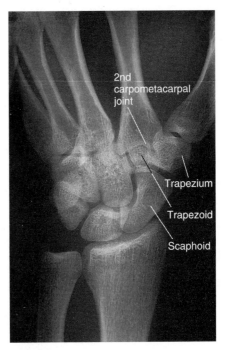

Radiograph 38.

Critique: A portion of the trapezoid and trapezium are superimposed, obscuring the trapeziotrapezoidal joint space. The second CM and scaphotrapezoidal joint spaces are closed. The wrist was rotated less than 45 degrees, and the distal second metacarpal was tilted toward the film.

Correction: Externally rotate the wrist until it forms a 45-degree angle with the film. Elevate the distal metacarpal (10 to 15 degrees from horizontal) higher than the proximal metacarpals.

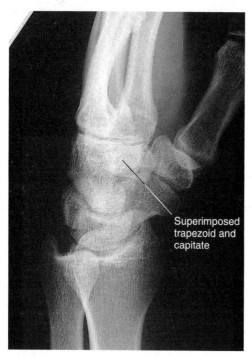

Radiograph 39.

Critique: The trapezoid is superimposing the capitate. The wrist obliquity was more than 45 degrees.

Correction: Internally rotate the wrist until it forms a 45-degree angle with the film.

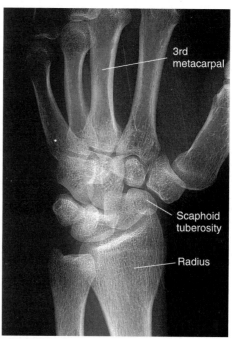

Radiograph 40.

Critique: The scaphoid is foreshortened, and the scaphoid tuberosity is situated next to the radius. The wrist was radially flexed.

Correction: Ulnar-flex the wrist until the long axes of the third metacarpal and the radius are aligned with the long axis of the collimation field.

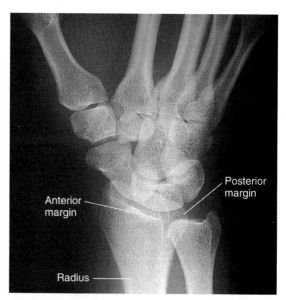

Radiograph 41.

Critique: The posterior margin of the distal radius is quite distal to the anterior margin. The proximal forearm was elevated.

Correction: Lower the proximal forearm until the forearm is parallel with the film. For a patient with a muscular or thick proximal forearm, it may be necessary to allow the proximal forearm to hang off the film or table in order to obtain a parallel forearm.

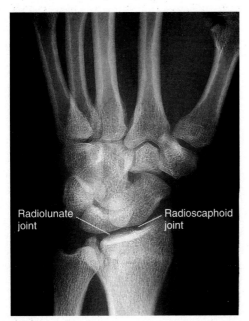

Radiograph 42.

Critique: The anterior and posterior margins of the distal radius are superimposed, demonstrating open radiolunate and radioscaphoid joint spaces. The proximal forearm was positioned slightly (5 to 6 degrees from horizontal) lower than the distal forearm.

Correction: This is an acceptable radiograph. No correction movement is needed.

Wrist: Lateral Position
(Lateromedial Projection)

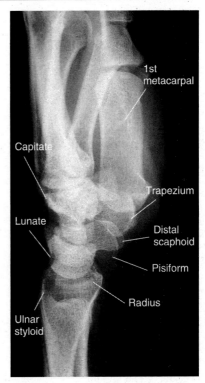

Figure 3-34. Accurately positioned lateral wrist radiograph.

Radiographic Evaluation

Facility's patient identification requirements are visible on radiograph.
- These requirements usually are facility name, patient name, age, and hospital number, and exam time and date.
- The patient ID plate does not obscure any anatomy of interest.

A right or left marker, identifying the correct wrist, is present on the radiograph and does not superimpose anatomy of interest.
- Place the marker within the collimated light field, without superimposing any portion of the affected wrist. When more than one view of the wrist is placed on the same radiograph, only one of the views needs to be marked.

There is no evidence of preventable artifacts, such as bracelets, watches, bandages, and splints.
- Consult with the ordering physician and the patient about whether bandages or splints can be removed.

Contrast and density are adequate to demonstrate the pronator fat stripe, surrounding soft tissue, and bony structures. Penetration is sufficient to visualize the bony trabecular patterns and the cortical outlines of the scaphoid, pisiform, and ulnar styloid.

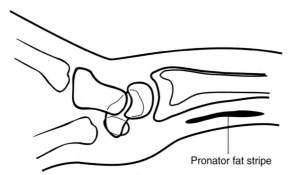

Figure 3–35. Location of pronator fat stripe. (Courtesy Educational Reviews, Inc.) (Reproduced with permission from Martensen K. II. Radiographic Positioning and Evaluation of the Wrist. (In-Service Reviews in Radiologic Technology, vol 16, no 5.) Birmingham, AL: Educational Reviews, Inc., 1992.)

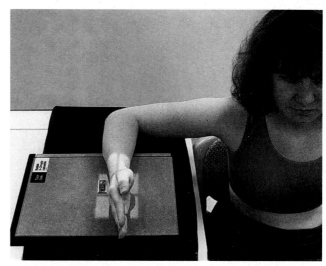

Figure 3–36. Proper patient positioning for lateral wrist radiograph.

- A high-contrast, low (50 to 60) kVp technique best enhances the soft tissue and bony structures of the wrist.
- The pronator fat stripe is one of the soft tissue structures that should be visualized on all lateral wrist radiographs (Fig. 3–35). It is located parallel to the anterior (volar) surface of the distal radius, is normally convex, and lies within 0.25 inch (0.6 cm) of the radial cortex. Bowing or obliteration of this fat stripe may be the only indication of a subtle radial fracture.[9]
- The soft tissue that surrounds the posterior (dorsal) aspect of the wrist should also be visualized. This posterior soft tissue is convex on the noninjured wrist. To the reviewer, a straightening or concave appearance of this surface may indicate swelling and injury.[10]

The bony trabecular patterns and cortical outlines of the carpal bones are sharply defined.
- Sharply defined radiographic details are obtained when patient motion is controlled, a detail screen and a small focal spot are used, and a short object–image distance (OID) is maintained.

The wrist is in a true lateral position. The distal end of the scaphoid and the pisiform, as well as the radius and ulna, are superimposed.
- A lateral position of the wrist is accomplished by flexing the elbow 90 degrees and abducting the humerus until it is parallel with the film, placing the entire arm on the same horizontal plane. Rotate the wrist into a true lateral position with its ulnar (medial) aspect against the cassette (Fig. 3–36).
- To ensure true lateral positioning, place the palmar aspect of your thumb and forefinger against the anterior and posterior aspects, respectively, of the patient's wrist joint, as demonstrated in Figure 3–37. Adjust wrist rotation until your thumb and finger are aligned perpendicular to the film.
- **_Detecting Wrist Rotation:_** The relationship between the pisiform and the distal portion of the scaphoid can best be used to discern whether a true lateral wrist position has been obtained. On a true lateral

radiograph, these two carpals should be superimposed and should be visualized anterior to the capitate and lunate. When the wrist is rotated, the anteroposterior relationship between the distal scaphoid and pisiform changes, and the pronator fat stripe is obscured. If the wrist is rotated externally (hand supinated), the distal scaphoid is visualized posterior to the pisiform (see Rad. 43). If the wrist is rotated internally (hand pronated), the distal scaphoid is visualized anterior to the pisiform[7] (see Rad. 44).

A second method of determining how to reposition a rotated lateral wrist radiograph uses the radius and ulna. Because the exact amount of superimposition of the radius and ulna depends on the position of the humerus, you should always view the pisiform and distal scaphoid relationship when determining whether the wrist is truly lateral. If the distal scaphoid and pisiform are not superimposed and the ulna is posi-

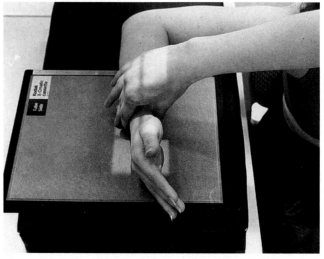

Figure 3–37. Manipulating wrist for true lateral alignment.

tioned anterior to the radius, the patient's wrist was externally rotated (hand supinated) (see Rad. 43). If the distal scaphoid and pisiform are not superimposed and the ulna is positioned posterior to the radius, the patient's wrist was internally rotated (hand pronated) (see Rad. 44).

- ***Mediolateral Wrist Radiograph:*** Routinely, the lateral wrist position is taken with the ulnar side of the wrist against the cassette. If, instead, the radial side of the wrist was placed against the cassette (mediolateral projection), the ulna and pisiform are visualized anterior to the radius and scaphoid, respectively, and the ulnar styloid is demonstrated in profile anteriorly (see Rad. 45).

The carpal bones do not indicate radial or ulnar flexion. The distal scaphoid superimposes the pisiform.

- To obtain a neutral lateral wrist radiograph, align the long axes of the third metacarpal and the midforearm parallel with the film. When the proximal forearm is higher or lower than the distal forearm, the wrist is radial flexed or ulnar flexed, respectively. In radial and ulnar flexion, the distal scaphoid moves but the pisiform's position remains relatively unchanged. Radial flexion of the wrist forces the distal scaphoid anteriorly (Fig. 3–38), resulting in visualization of the pisiform distal to the scaphoid (see Rad. 46). Ulnar flexion shifts the distal scaphoid posteriorly (Fig. 3–38), resulting in visualization of the pisiform proximal to the scaphoid[7] (see Rad. 47). The amount of pisiform and distal scaphoid separation is usually a very small

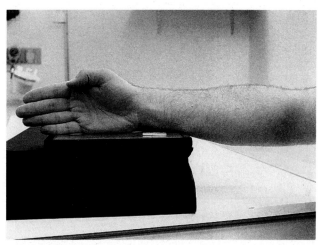

Figure 3-39. Positioning of patient with thick proximal forearm.

degree, because you would be unlikely to position a patient in maximum wrist flexion without being aware of the positioning error. To obtain optimal lateral wrist radiographs, however, we must learn to eliminate even small degrees of flexion.

- ***Positioning Patient with Thick Proximal Forearm:*** For a patient with a large muscular or thick proximal forearm, it may be necessary to allow the proximal forearm to hang off the film or table to maintain a neutral wrist position (Fig. 3–39). If the patient is not positioned in this manner, radial flexion of the wrist will result.

The long axes of the first metacarpal, capitate, and radius are aligned with the long axis of the collimated field.

- If the long axes of the first metacarpal, which is positioned adjacent to the second metacarpal, and the forearm are aligned with the long axis of the collimation field, the patient's wrist is placed in a neutral position.
- When the wrist is flexed or extended, the positions of the scaphoid and lunate are altered. In wrist flexion, the lunate and the distal scaphoid tilt anteriorly (see Rad. 48). In wrist extension, the lunate and distal scaphoid tilt posteriorly (see Rad. 49). Flexion and extension views of the wrist may be specifically requested to demonstrate wrist joint mobility.

The ulnar styloid is demonstrated in profile posteriorly.

- When the humerus and elbow are mispositioned, the placement of the ulna styloid changes. The ulnar styloid is demonstrated posteriorly in profile when the patient's elbow is in a lateral position and the humerus is positioned parallel with the film. If the humerus is not abducted, but remains against the patient's side, the elbow is in or close to an AP projection and the ulnar styloid rotates medially and is no longer demonstrated in profile (see Rad. 50).
- ***Lateral Wrist Position with No Forearm Rotation:*** In contrast to positioning the forearm and

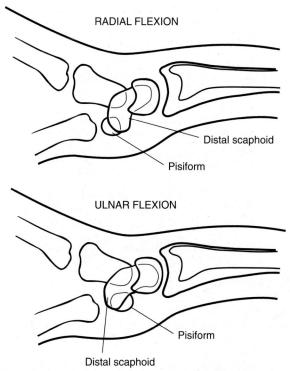

RADIAL FLEXION

Distal scaphoid

Pisiform

ULNAR FLEXION

Pisiform

Distal scaphoid

Figure 3-38. Lateral wrist in radial flexion *(top)* and ulnar flexion *(bottom).*

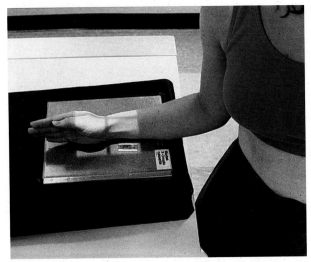

Figure 3-40. Lateral wrist positioning without humeral abduction.

humerus on the same horizontal plane for a lateral wrist radiograph, Dr. Ronald Epner and his colleagues[4] suggest that a lateral wrist radiograph be taken with zero forearm rotation. To accomplish this, the humerus is not abducted but remains positioned against the body with the elbow in an AP projection (Fig. 3–40). Such positioning rotates the ulnar styloid medially, demonstrating it just distal to the midline of the ulnar head (see Rad. 50). Because forearm rotation has been eliminated, the ulnar head also shifts closer to the lunate. Dr. Epner states that this positioning allows for more accurate measuring of the ulnar length. Department policy determines which humerus positioning is performed in your facility.

The trapezium is demonstrated without superimposition of the first proximal metacarpal.

- To obtain optimal visualization of the trapezium, lower the distal first metacarpal until it is at the same level as the second metacarpal. This positioning places the trapezium and metacarpal parallel with the film, demonstrating them without superimposition. If the distal first metacarpal is not lowered, it is foreshortened, and its proximal portion superimposes the trapezium (see Rad. 51).

The carpal bones are at the center of the collimated field. The carpal bones, one fourth of the distal ulna and radius, and half of the proximal metacarpals are included within the field.

- In a lateral position, the wrist joint is located just proximal to the first metacarpal base. To obtain an image of the carpal bones with the least amount of distortion, place a perpendicular central ray at this level and centered to the midwrist area. Open the longitudinal collimation to include half of the metacarpals. Transverse collimation should be to the wrist skin-line.

- Either half of an 8 × 10 inch (18 × 24 cm) film or one third of a 10 × 12 inch (24 × 30 cm) film placed crosswise should be adequate to include all the required anatomical structures.

- ***Wrist Exam Taken to Include More than One Fourth of the Forearm:*** When a wrist exam is requested to include more than one fourth of the distal forearm, the central ray should remain on the wrist joint, and the collimation field should be opened to demonstrate the desired amount of forearm. This method results in an extended, unneeded radiation field distal to the metacarpals. A lead strip placed over this extended radiation field protects the patient's phalanges and prevents any possible backscatter from reaching the film. The advantage of this method over centering the central ray proximal to the wrist joint is an undistorted demonstration of the carpal bones. A lateral wrist radiograph taken with the central ray positioned proximal to the wrist joint demonstrates the distal scaphoid projecting distal to the pisiform (see Rad. 47).

Critiquing Radiographs

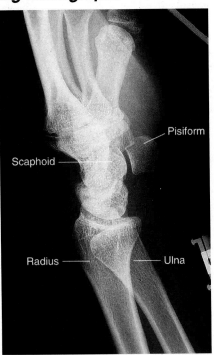

Radiograph 43.

Critique: The wrist is not in a true lateral position. The pisiform is shown anterior to the scaphoid, and the ulna anterior to the radius. The wrist was externally rotated (hand supinated).
Correction: Internally rotate the wrist (pronate the hand) until the wrist is in a true lateral position.

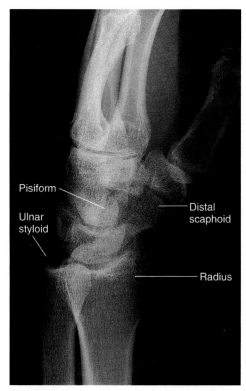

Radiograph 44.

Critique: The wrist is not in a true lateral position. The distal scaphoid is anterior to the pisiform and the radius is anterior to the ulna. The wrist was internally rotated (hand pronated).

Correction: Externally rotate the wrist (supinate the hand) until the wrist is in a true lateral position.

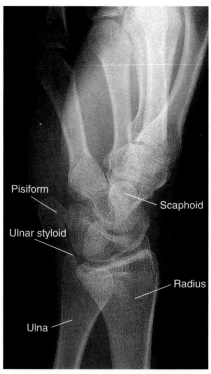

Radiograph 45.

Critique: The ulna and pisiform are demonstrated anterior to the radius and scaphoid, respectively, and the ulnar styloid is visualized in profile anteriorly. The radial side of the wrist was placed against the cassette (mediolateral projection).

Correction: Externally rotate the hand and wrist until the ulnar side of the wrist is placed against the cassette.

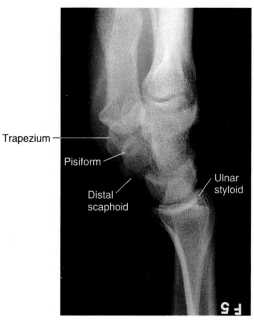

Radiograph 46.

Critique: The pisiform is demonstrated distal to the scaphoid. Two possible positioning errors cause such a radiograph. Either the central ray was not centered with the wrist joint, but was positioned distally, or the wrist was in radial flexion. Note that the ulnar styloid is not in profile but is projecting distal to the midline of the ulnar head. This ulnar positioning indicates that the patient was positioned without humerus abduction as demonstrated in Figure 3–40.

Correction: Center the central ray with the wrist joint, which is located just proximal to the first metacarpal base. Position the wrist in neutral deviation by aligning the long axes of the third metacarpal and the midforearm parallel with the film.

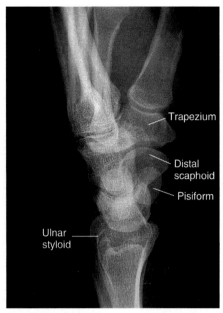

Radiograph 47.

Critique: The distal scaphoid is demonstrated distal to the pisiform. Two possible positioning errors cause such a problem. Either the wrist was in ulnar flexion or the central ray was not centered with the wrist joint but was positioned to the midforearm.

Correction: Position the wrist in neutral deviation by aligning the long axes of the third metacarpal and the midforearm parallel with the film. Center the central ray with the wrist joint, which is located just proximal to the first metacarpal base.

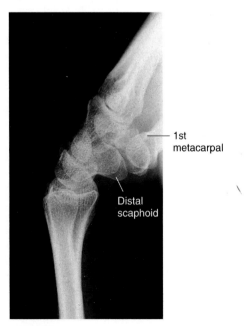

Radiograph 48.

Critique: The first metacarpal is not aligned with the long axis of the collimation field. The wrist was flexed anteriorly.

Correction: If a neutral position is desired, align the long axis of the first metacarpal with the long axis of the collimation field. If a wrist flexion radiograph was taken to evaluate wrist mobility, no correction movement is required.

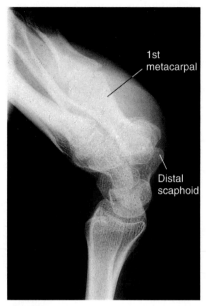

Radiograph 49.

Critique: The first metacarpal is not aligned with the long axis of the collimation field. The wrist is extended posteriorly.

Correction: If a neutral position is desired, align the long axis of the first metacarpal with the long axis of the collimation field. If a wrist extension radiograph was taken to evaluate wrist mobility, no correction movement is required.

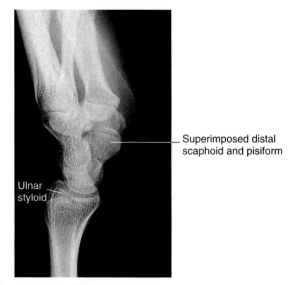

Radiograph 50.

Critique: The pisiform and the distal scaphoid are positioned accurately for a lateral wrist radiograph. The ulnar styloid is not positioned in profile, but is demonstrated projecting distal to the midline of the ulnar head. This ulnar positioning indicates that the humerus was positioned without abduction as demonstrated in Figure 3–40.

Correction: Adjust the patient's humerus to meet your department protocol. If the ulnar styloid is to be demonstrated in profile, abduct the humerus and flex the elbow 90 degrees, placing the forearm and humerus on the same horizontal plane. If department protocol requires that a lateral wrist radiograph be taken without humeral abduction, no correction movement is needed. Consistency in arm position is important to evaluating ulnar length.

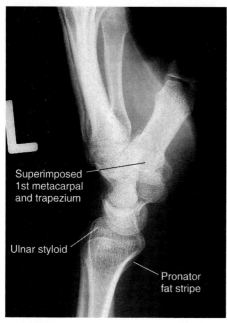

Radiograph 51.

Critique: The first proximal metacarpal is superimposing the trapezium. The thumb was not positioned at the same level as the second metacarpal, but was pointing upward. The ulnar styloid is not in profile.

Correction: Depress the patient's distal thumb until it is at the same level as the second metacarpal. Adjust the patient's humerus to meet your department protocol. If the ulnar styloid is to be demonstrated in profile, abduct the humerus and flex the elbow 90 degrees, placing the forearm and humerus on the same horizontal plane. If department protocol requires that a lateral wrist radiograph be taken without humeral abduction, no correction movement is needed.

Wrist: Ulnar-Flexed, PA Projection
(Scaphoid Position)

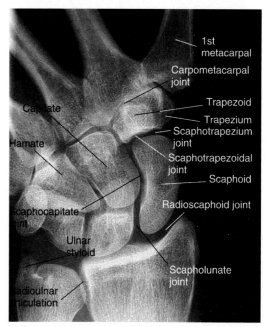

Figure 3–41. Accurately positioned ulnar-flexed PA wrist radiograph.

Radiographic Evaluation

Facility's patient identification requirements are visible on radiograph.

- These requirements usually are facility name, patient name, age, and hospital number, and exam time and date.
- The patient ID plate does not obscure any anatomy of interest.

A right or left marker, identifying the correct wrist, is present on the radiograph and does not superimpose anatomy of interest.

- Place the marker within the collimated light field so it does not superimpose any portion of the affected wrist. It may be necessary to open the light field to include the marker.
- When more than one view of the wrist is placed on the same radiograph, only one of the views needs to be marked.

There is no evidence of preventable artifacts, such as bracelets, watches, bandages, and splints.

- Consult with the ordering physician and the patient about whether bandages or splints can be removed.

Contrast and density are adequate to demonstrate the scaphoid fat stripe and the surrounding soft tissue and bony structures of the wrist. Penetration is sufficient to visualize the bony trabecular patterns and the cortical outlines of the carpal bones.

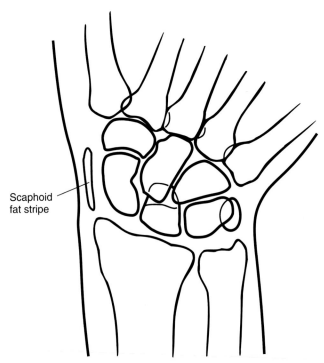

Figure 3-42. Location of scaphoid fat stripe. (Courtesy Educational Review, Inc.) (Reproduced with permission from Martensen K. II. Radiographic Positioning and Evaluation of the Wrist. (In-Service Reviews in Radiologic Technology, vol 16, no 5.) Birmingham, AL: Educational Reviews, Inc., 1992.)

- A high-contrast, low (50 to 60) kVp technique best enhances the soft tissue and bony structures of the wrist.
- The scaphoid fat stripe is one of the soft tissue structures that should be visualized on all scaphoid radiographs (Fig. 3–42). It is convex and is located just lateral to the scaphoid in a noninjured wrist. A change in the convexity of this stripe may signify to the reviewer joint effusion or a scaphoid fracture.[2, 3]

The bony trabecular patterns and cortical outlines of the carpal bones are sharply defined.
- Sharply defined radiographic details are obtained when patient motion is controlled, a detail screen and a small focal spot are used, and a short object–image distance (OID) is maintained.

The wrist is in ulnar flexion, as demonstrated by the alignment of the long axes of the first metacarpal and the radius and by the position of the lunate distal to the radius. The scaphocapitate and scapholunate joints are open, and the distal radius and ulna demonstrate minimal superimposition. The radial and ulnar styloids are at the extreme lateral and medial edges, respectively, of each bone. The scaphotrapezium, scaphotrapezoidal, and second carpometacarpal joint spaces are open.
- To obtain accurate scaphoid positioning, abduct the humerus until it is positioned parallel with the film, and place the elbow in a flexed, lateral position. Then

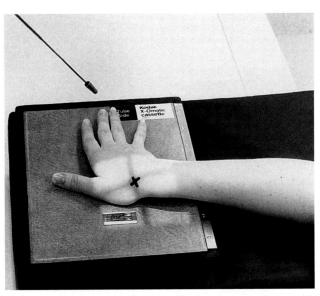

Figure 3-43. Proper patient positioning for ulnar-flexed, PA wrist radiograph. *X* indicates location of scaphoid.

pronate the extended hand and put the wrist in ulnar flexion (Fig. 3–43). Good ulnar flexion has been accomplished when the first metacarpal aligns with the radius.
- ***Advantages of Ulnar Flexion:*** In a neutral, nondeviated PA projection of the wrist, the distal scaphoid tilts anteriorly approximately 20 degrees[11] (Fig. 3–44). Radiographically, the result would be a

NEUTRAL

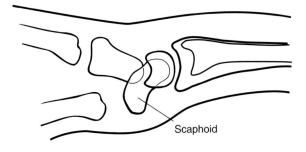

ULNAR FLEXION

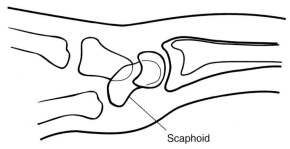

Figure 3-44. Lateral wrist in neutral position *(top)* and in ulnar flexion *(bottom)*.

foreshortened scaphoid. To offset some of this foreshortening and demonstrate all aspects of the scaphoid, place the wrist in ulnar flexion. In ulnar flexion, the distal scaphoid tilts posteriorly, decreasing the degree of foreshortening (Fig. 3–44).

Besides decreasing the degree of scaphoid foreshortening, ulnar flexion positions the wrist in medial obliquity, 10 to 15 degrees with the film. Do not offset this obliquity, because it is needed to demonstrate the open scaphocapitate and scapholunate joint spaces. This small amount of obliquity also closes the radioulnar articulation.

- *Repositioning for Closed Scaphocarpal Joint Spaces:* When closed scaphocarpal joint spaces are obtained, evaluate the surrounding anatomical structure carefully to determine the adjustment required to demonstrate open spaces.

If the scaphocapitate or scapholunate joint spaces are closed, evaluate the amount of radial and ulnar superimposition, as well as of capitate and hamate superimposition, to identify the correct repositioning movement. When these carpal and forearm bones show increased superimposition—compare Figure 3–41 and Radiograph 52 to familiarize yourself with this difference—the wrist was in greater medial obliquity than necessary. Excessive medial obliquity often occurs when the humerus and forearm have not been positioned on the same horizontal plane. Radiographically, one can judge accurate humerus and forearm positioning by evaluating the ulnar styloid. Accurate positioning places the ulnar styloid in profile medially. If the humerus is not positioned parallel with the film and the elbow is not placed in a lateral position, the ulnar styloid is demonstrated distal to the ulnar head (see Rad. 52).

If the scaphocapitate joint is closed but the scapholunate and radioulnar joints are open, the wrist was positioned in a true PA projection without the required 10 to 15 degrees of medial obliquity (see Rad. 53). This mispositioning is a result of inadequate ulnar wrist flexion or hand extension. If the wrist is not ulnar flexed, it is not in 10 to 15 degrees of medial obliquity, and if the hand is flexed, the wrist moves into a true PA projection. Accurate hand positioning also opens the scaphotrapezium, scaphotrapezoidal, and second carpometacarpal joint spaces. If the hand is not extended so that the palm is placed flat against the cassette, but rather is flexed, the second metacarpal base superimposes the trapezoid and trapezium and closes the scaphotrapezium and scaphotrapezoidal joint spaces (see Rad. 54).

The scaphoid is demonstrated without foreshortening, and the long axes of the first metacarpal and radius are aligned with the longitudinally collimated light field. When a scaphoid fracture is indicated, the fracture line is visualized.

- To demonstrate the scaphoid without foreshortening, position the patient's wrist in maximum ulnar flexion; then direct a 15-degree proximal (toward the elbow) central ray angulation to the long axis of the scaphoid.

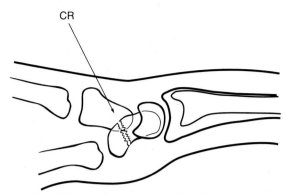

Figure 3–45. Proper alignment of central ray (CR) and fracture.

This ulnar flexion and central ray angulation place the central ray perpendicular with the long axis of the scaphoid waist (Fig. 3–45). Because 70 percent of the fractures occur at the scaphoid waist, most scaphoid fractures should be visualized with this positioning and angulation.

- *Compensating for Inadequate Ulnar Flexion:* One must remember that the position of the distal scaphoid changes with ulnar wrist flexion. Many patients with suspected scaphoid fractures are unable to achieve satisfactory ulnar wrist flexion. Without adequate ulnar flexion, the distal scaphoid is positioned anteriorly. To compensate for this anterior tilt, the central ray angulation should be increased to about 20 degrees to place the central ray and scaphoid waist perpendicular to each other. When the central ray is not aligned parallel with the fracture site, the fracture is obscured (Fig. 3–46).

- *Demonstrating Fractures of Distal and Proximal Scaphoid:* Not all fractures of the scaphoid are at the scaphoid waist; they may be located at the distal or proximal end instead. When a fracture is suspected because of persistent pain and obliteration of the fat stripe but has not been demonstrated on routine views, it may be necessary to use different angles to position the central ray perpendicu-

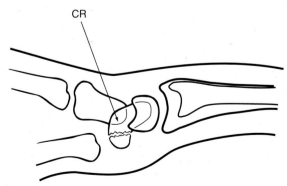

Figure 3–46. Poor alignment of central ray *(CR)* and fracture.

lar with the distal and proximal scaphoid ends. An increase of 5 to 10 degrees in central ray angulation better demonstrates the distal scaphoid, whereas a decrease of 5 to 10 degrees better demonstrates the proximal scaphoid.

Radioscaphoid joint space is open.

- The distal radial carpal articular surface is concave and slants about 11 degrees from posterior to anterior when the radius and ulna are positioned parallel with the film.[6] On a PA projection without a central ray angulation, the posterior radial margin is demonstrated slightly distal to the anterior margin if the radius and ulna are positioned parallel with the film. When a 15-degree proximal central ray angulation is employed for the scaphoid position, the posterior margin is projected slightly proximal to the anterior margin. To demonstrate an open radioscaphoid joint, the anterior and posterior margins of the distal radius should be superimposed. This superimposition is accomplished by elevating the proximal forearm 5 to 6 degrees above the distal forearm.

- ***Repositioning to Demonstrate the Radioscaphoid Joint Space:*** When the radioscaphoid joint space is obscured on a scaphoid radiograph, determine whether the proximal forearm should be elevated or lowered to superimpose the distal radius by viewing the radioulnar articulating surface. On this surface, the edge that superimposes a portion of the ulna is associated with the posterior margin.

The scaphoid is at the center of the collimated field. The carpal bones, the radioulnar articulation, and the proximal first through fourth metacarpals are included within the field.

- To place the scaphoid at the center of the collimated field, center the central ray with the scaphoid. In ulnar flexion, the scaphoid can be palpated halfway between the first metacarpal base and the radial styloid. After the central ray is centered, open the longitudinal collimation to include the first through fourth metacarpal bases and the distal radius. Transverse collimation should be to the medial skin-line.

    Avoid collimating too tightly. It is difficult to determine how to reposition the patient from a poorly positioned radiograph when key anatomical structures are not included.

- Half of an 8 × 10 inch (18 × 24 cm) film placed crosswise should be adequate to include all the required anatomical structures.

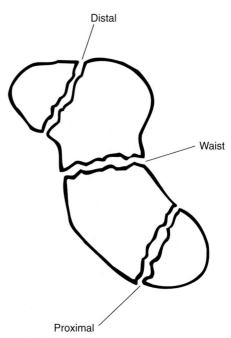

Figure 3–47. Sites of scaphoid fracture.

- ***Mechanics of Scaphoid Fracture:*** The scaphoid is the most commonly fractured carpal bone. One reason for this is its location among the other carpal bones. There are two rows of carpal bones, a distal row and a proximal row, with joint spaces between that allow the wrist to flex. The long scaphoid bone, however, is aligned partially with both of these rows with no joint space separating it from them. When an outstretched hand is dorsiflexed during a fall, the proximal and dorsal carpal rows are flexed at the joints, placing a great deal of stress on the narrow waist of the scaphoid. This stress may result in a fracture.

Three areas of the scaphoid may be fractured: the waist, which sustains about 70 percent of the fractures; the distal end, which sustains 20 percent of the fractures and the proximal end, which sustains 10 percent[12] (Fig. 3–47). Because scaphoid fractures can be at different locations on the scaphoid, precise positioning and central ray angulation are essential to obtain the optimum demonstration of this bone.

Critiquing Radiographs

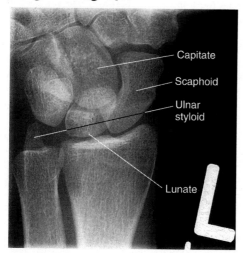

Radiograph 52.

Critique: The scaphocapitate and scapholunate joints are closed, and the lunate superimposes a portion of the scaphoid, indicating that the wrist was placed in greater medial obliquity than necessary. The styloid process is not positioned in profile.

Correction: Decrease the degree of medial wrist obliquity, and position the humerus parallel with the film on the same plane as the forearm.

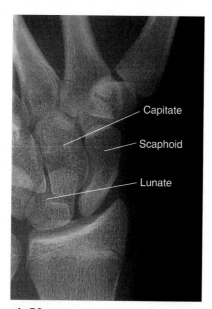

Radiograph 53.

Critique: The scaphocapitate joint space is closed, but the scapholunate, radioulnar, and capitate-hamate joint spaces are open, indicating that the wrist was in a true PA projection. The scaphotrapezium, scaphotrapezoidal, and carpometacarpal joint spaces are closed. The fingers were not positioned flat against the cassette.

Correction: Position the wrist in slight medial obliquity and extend the patient's fingers, placing the hand flat against the cassette.

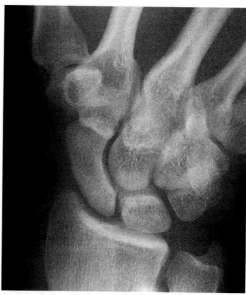

Radiograph 54.

Critique: The scaphotrapezium, scaphotrapezoidal, and carpometacarpal joint spaces are closed. The hand and fingers were not positioned flat against the cassette.

Correction: Extend the patient's fingers, placing the hand flat against the cassette.

FOREARM

Anteroposterior Projection

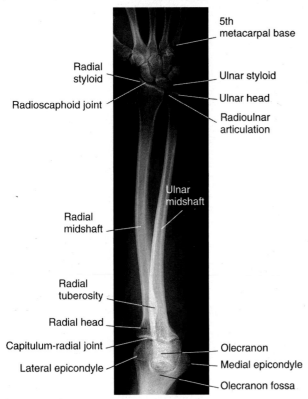

Radial styloid

Radioscaphoid joint

5th metacarpal base

Ulnar styloid

Ulnar head

Radioulnar articulation

Ulnar midshaft

Radial midshaft

Radial tuberosity

Radial head

Capitulum-radial joint

Lateral epicondyle

Olecranon

Medial epicondyle

Olecranon fossa

Figure 3-48. Accurately positioned AP forearm radiograph.

Radiographic Evaluation

Facility's patient identification requirements are visible on radiograph.
- These requirements usually are facility name, patient name, age, and hospital number, and exam time and date.
- The patient ID plate does not obscure any anatomy of interest.

A right or left marker identifying the correct forearm is present on the radiograph and does not superimpose anatomy of interest.
- Place the marker within the collimated light field so it does not superimpose any portion of the forearm.
- When more than one view of the forearm is placed on the same radiograph, only one of the views needs to be marked.

There is no evidence of preventable artifacts, such as bracelets, watches, bandages, and splints.
- Consult with the ordering physician and the patient about whether bandages or splints can be removed.

Contrast and density are adequate to demonstrate the surrounding humeral soft tissue and bony structures. Penetration is sufficient to visualize the bony trabecular patterns and the cortical outlines of the radius and ulna.

- A high-contrast, low (55 to 65) kVp technique enhances the bony and soft tissue structures of the forearm.
- ***Anode-Heel Effect:*** Another exposure factor that should be considered when you are positioning the forearm is the anode-heel effect. Because a long (17-inch [43-cm]) field is used for the length of the adult forearm, there is a difference in the intensity of the beam on the cathode and anode ends of the film. This noticeable intensity variation is a result of greater photon absorption at the thicker "heel" portion of the anode compared with the thinner "toe" portion when a long field is used. Consequently, radiographic density at the anode end of the tube is less than that at the cathode end.[13]

  Using this knowledge to our advantage can help us produce radiographs of the forearm that demonstrate uniform density at both ends. Set an exposure (mAs) that will adequately demonstrate the proximal forearm. Because the anode will absorb some of the photons aimed at the anode end of the film, the distal forearm, which requires less exposure than the proximal forearm, will not be overexposed.

The bony trabecular patterns and cortical outlines of the carpal bones are sharply defined.
- Sharply defined radiographic details are obtained when patient motion is controlled, a detail screen and a small focal spot are used, and a short object–image distance (OID) is maintained.

The long axis of the forearm is aligned with the long axis of the collimated field.
- Aligning the long axis of the forearm with the long axis of the collimated field enables you to collimate tightly without clipping the distal or proximal forearm.

The forearm midshaft is at the center of the collimated field. The wrist radius and ulna, elbow joints, and forearm soft tissue are included within the field.
- A perpendicular central ray is centered to the midshaft of the forearm to place it in the center of the radiograph.
- When the wrist and elbow joints are included on the radiograph, the degree of radiation beam divergence used to radiograph a long body part needs to be considered (Fig. 3–49).
- ***Film Length for the Forearm:*** Choose a film that is long enough to allow at least 1 inch (2.5 cm) of film to extend beyond each joint space; half of a 14 × 17 inch (35 × 43 cm) film placed lengthwise should be adequate.

  To ensure that the film extends beyond the elbow joint, palpate the medial epicondyle, which is located about 0.75 inch (2 cm) proximal to the elbow joint. To ensure that the film extends beyond the wrist joint, palpate the base of the first metacarpal; the wrist joint is located just proximal to this base.
- ***Central Ray Centering and Collimation:*** Once the forearm is accurately positioned in relation to the film, center the central ray with the midshaft of the forearm and open the longitudinal collimation field

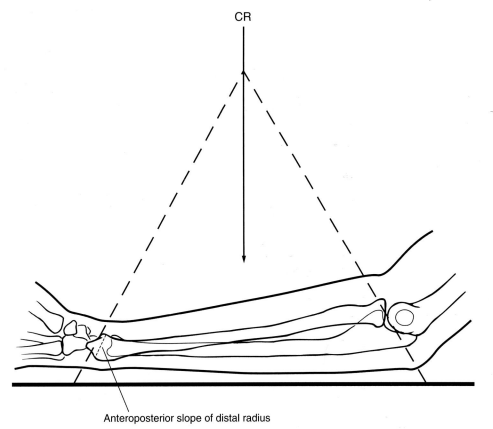

Figure 3-49. Effect of x-ray divergence on elbow and wrist joints. *CR*, central ray.

CR

Anteroposterior slope of distal radius

until it extends just beyond the elbow and the wrist. If the collimation does not extend beyond the joints, adjust the centering point of the central ray until both the elbow and the wrist joint are included within the collimated field without demonstrating an excessive field beyond them. Transverse collimation should be to the forearm skin-line.

DISTAL FOREARM POSITIONING

The distal forearm is positioned in a true AP projection. The radial styloid is demonstrated in profile laterally, and there is minimal superimposition of the metacarpal bases and of the radius and ulna.

- To obtain a true AP projection of the distal forearm, supinate the hand and place the second through fifth metacarpal heads against the cassette (Fig. 3–50).
- ***Detecting Distal Forearm Rotation:*** Rotation of the distal forearm results from inaccurate positioning of the hand and wrist. If the wrist and hand are not positioned in a true AP projection, but are rotated, the radial styloid is no longer in profile, and the distal radius and ulna and the metacarpal bases superimpose. To identify which way the wrist is rotated, evaluate the metacarpal and carpal bones. When the wrist and hand are internally rotated (medial oblique), the laterally located first and second metacarpal bases and carpal bones are superimposed, and the medially located metacarpals, pisiform, and hamate hook are better visualized (see Rad. 55). If the wrist and hand are externally rotated (lateral oblique), the medially

located fourth and fifth metacarpal bases and carpal bones will be superimposed, while the laterally located metacarpals and carpal bones will demonstrate less superimposition.

- ***Distal Forearm Positioning for Fracture:*** Patients with known or suspected fractures may be unable to position both the wrist and elbow joints into a true AP projection simultaneously. In such cases, position the joint closer to the fracture in a true position.

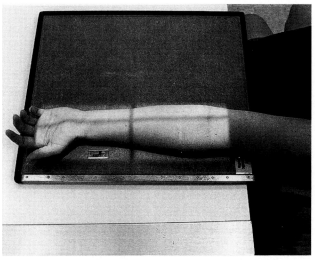

Figure 3-50. Proper AP forearm positioning.

When the fracture is situated closer to the wrist joint, the wrist joint and distal forearm should meet the requirements for a true AP projection, but the elbow and proximal forearm may demonstrate an oblique or lateral position. It may be necessary to position the distal forearm in a PA projection when an AP projection is difficult for the patient. The wrist joint and distal forearm should still be positioned as previously described (see Rad. 56).

The ulnar styloid is projected distally to the midline of the ulnar head.

- The position of the ulnar styloid is determined by the position of the humerus and elbow. When the humerus and elbow position are adjusted but the wrist position is maintained, it is the ulna that rotates and changes position. Positioning the humeral epicondyles parallel with the film for the AP projection of the forearm places the ulnar styloid posterior to the head of the ulna. If the elbow is rotated internally (medially) and the wrist remains in a true AP projection, the ulnar styloid is demonstrated laterally, next to the radius. If the elbow is rotated externally (laterally) and the wrist remains in a true AP projection, the ulnar styloid is demonstrated in profile medially (see Rad. 57).

The anterior and posterior carpal articulating surfaces of the distal radius are superimposed, and the radioscaphoid and radiolunate joint spaces are open.

- The distal radial carpal articular surface is concave and slants at about 11 degrees from posterior to anterior.[6] When the forearm is placed parallel with the film in an AP projection and the central ray is centered to the midforearm, diverged x-rays record the image (Fig. 3–49) much the same as if the central ray were angled toward the wrist joint. If this angle of divergence is parallel with the anteroposterior slant of the distal radius, the resulting radiograph shows superimposed distal radial margins and open radioscaphoid and radiolunate joint spaces.

PROXIMAL FOREARM POSITIONING

The proximal forearm is positioned in a true AP projection. The radial head and tuberosity superimpose the lateral aspect of the proximal ulna by about 0.25 inch (0.6 cm). If included on the film, the medial and lateral humeral epicondyles are demonstrated in profile at the extreme medial and lateral edges of the distal humerus.

- A true AP proximal forearm projection is obtained by palpating the humeral epicondyles and aligning them parallel with the film, placing the proximal radius anterior to the ulna (Fig. 3–50).
- ***Detecting Proximal Forearm Rotation:*** Proximal forearm rotation results when the humeral epicondyles are poorly positioned. Rotation can be identified radiographically when the radial head and tuberosity demonstrate more or less than 0.25 inch (0.6 cm) superimposition on the ulna and when the humeral epicondyles are not visualized in profile. When more than 0.25 inch (0.6 cm) of the radial head

and tuberosity is superimposing the ulna, the elbow has been medially rotated. When less than 0.25 inch (0.6 cm) of radial head and tuberosity is superimposing the ulna, the elbow has been laterally rotated (see Rad. 57).

- ***Proximal Forearm Positioning for Fracture:*** Patients with known or suspected fractures may be unable to position both the wrist and elbow joint into a true AP projection simultaneously. In such cases, position the joint closer to the fracture in the truer position. When the fracture is situated closer to the elbow joint, the elbow joint and proximal forearm should meet the requirements for a true AP projection, whereas the wrist and distal forearm may demonstrate obliquity.

The capitulum-radius joint is either partially or completely closed, and the radial head articulating surface is demonstrated. The olecranon process is situated within the olecranon fossa, and the coronoid is visualized on end.

- The elbow image on an AP forearm radiograph is slightly different from a true AP elbow radiograph, owing to the difference in centering of the central ray. The central ray is placed directly over the elbow joint for an AP elbow radiograph, but it is centered distal to the elbow joint, at the midforearm, for an AP forearm radiograph. With distal centering, diverged rays record the elbow joint image instead of straight central rays, much the same as if the central ray were angled toward the elbow joint (Fig. 3–49). Imaging the elbow with diverged rays projects the radial head into the capitulum-radius joint and causes the anterior margin of the radial head to project beyond the posterior margin, demonstrating its articulating surface.
- ***Effect of Elbow Flexion:*** The positions of the olecranon process and fossa and the coronoid process are determined by the amount of elbow flexion. Accurate forearm positioning requires us to position the elbow in full extension, which places the olecranon process within the olecranon fossa and demonstrates the coronoid process on end. When a forearm radiograph is taken with the elbow flexed and the proximal humerus elevated (Fig. 3–51), the olecranon process moves away from the olecranon fossa and the coronoid shifts proximally. How far the olecranon process is from the fossa depends on the degree of elbow flexion. The greater the elbow flexion, the farther the olecranon process is positioned away from the fossa and the more foreshortened is the distal humerus.

The radial tuberosity is demonstrated in profile medially, and the radius and ulna are visualized parallel with each other.

- When the distal humerus is positioned with the epicondyles parallel with the film, the relationship of the radius and ulna is controlled by wrist positioning. To place the radius and ulna parallel with each other and the radial tuberosity in profile, position the wrist and hand in a true AP projection. When the hand and wrist are pronated, the radius crosses over the ulna, and the

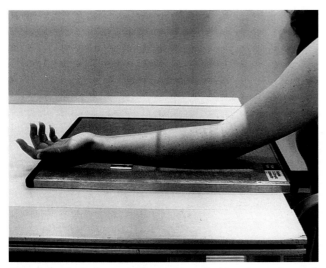

Figure 3-51. Patient positioned for AP forearm radiograph with flexed humerus.

radial tuberosity is rotated posteriorly, out of profile (see Rad. 58).

Critiquing Radiographs

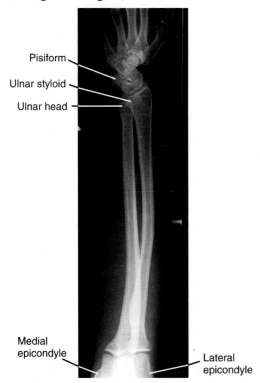

Pisiform

Ulnar styloid

Ulnar head

Medial epicondyle

Lateral epicondyle

Radiograph 55.

Critique: The humeral epicondyles are demonstrated in profile, and the ulnar styloid is demonstrated distal to the midline of the ulnar head. The elbow has been accurately positioned. The first and second metacarpal bases and the laterally located carpal bones are superimposed, and the medially located carpal bones and pisiform are well demonstrated. The radial styloid is not visualized in profile.

Correction: While maintaining the true AP projection of the elbow, rotate the wrist and hand externally until the hand is supinated and the wrist is in an AP projection.

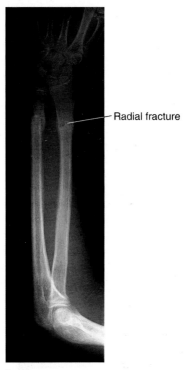

Radial fracture

Radiograph 56.

Critique: There is a fracture located at the distal forearm. The wrist demonstrates a true PA projection, whereas the elbow is in an oblique to lateral position.
Correction: Because the joint closer to the fracture is in the true projection, no repositioning movement is needed.

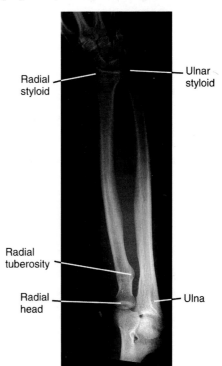

Radial styloid

Ulnar styloid

Radial tuberosity

Radial head

Ulna

Radiograph 57.

Critique: The radial styloid is in profile laterally, and the carpals and metacarpals demonstrate accurate superimposition. The wrist has been accurately positioned. The humeral epicondyles are not in profile, the radial head and tuberosity do not superimpose the ulna, and the ulnar styloid is in profile medially. The elbow has been laterally rotated.

Correction: While maintaining the true AP projection of the wrist and distal forearm, rotate the elbow laterally until the humeral epicondyles are parallel with the film.

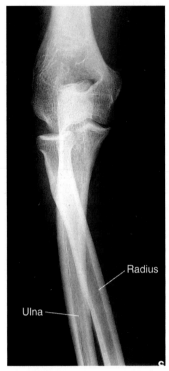

Radiograph 58.

Critique: The radius and ulna are not parallel. The radius is crossed over the ulna, and the radial tuberosity is not demonstrated in profile. For this radiograph, the elbow is in an AP projection, but the wrist and hand are positioned in a PA projection. The distal forearm and wrist joint were not included on the radiograph.

Correction: While maintaining a true AP projection of the elbow, externally rotate the wrist and hand until they are in an AP projection. Center the central ray more distally, and open the longitudinal collimation to include the wrist joint.

Forearm: Lateral Position
(Lateromedial Projection)

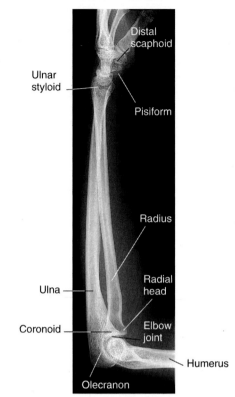

Figure 3-52. Accurately positioned lateral forearm radiograph.

Radiographic Evaluation

Facility's patient identification requirements are visible on radiograph.
- These requirements usually are facility name, patient name, age, and hospital number, and exam time and date.
- The patient ID plate does not obscure any anatomy of interest.

A right or left marker, identifying the correct forearm, is present on the radiograph and does not superimpose anatomy of interest.
- Place the marker within the collimated light field so it does not superimpose any portion of the forearm.

There is no evidence of preventable artifacts, such as bracelets, watches, bandages, and splints.
- Consult with the ordering physician and the patient about whether bandages and splints can be removed.

Contrast and density are adequate to demonstrate the wrist and elbow fat structures, surrounding humeral soft tissue, and bony structures. Penetration is sufficient to visualize the bony trabecular patterns and the cortical outlines of the radius and ulna.

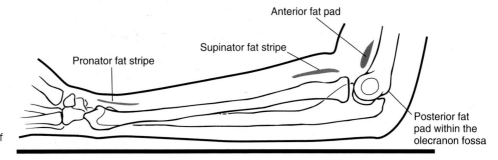

Figure 3–53. Placement of wrist and elbow soft tissue.

- A high-contrast, low (55 to 65) kVp technique enhances the bony and soft tissue structures of the forearm.
- ***Anode-Heel Effect:*** Another exposure factor that should be considered when positioning the forearm is the anode-heel effect. Because a long (17-inch [43-cm]) field is used for the length of the adult forearm, there is a difference in the intensity of the beam that reaches the cathode and anode ends of the film. This noticeable intensity variation is a result of greater photon absorption at the thicker, "heel" portion of the anode compared with the thinner, "toe" portion when a long field is used. Consequently, radiographic density at the anode end of the tube is less than that at the cathode end.[13]

  Using this knowledge to our advantage can help us produce radiographs of the forearm that demonstrate uniform density on both ends. Position the thinner wrist (distal forearm) at the anode end of the tube and the thicker elbow (proximal forearm) at the cathode end. Set an exposure (mAs) that will adequately demonstrate the proximal forearm. Because the anode will absorb some of the photons aimed at the anode end of the film, the distal forearm, which requires less exposure than the proximal forearm, will not be overexposed.
- ***Soft Tissue Structures on Lateral Forearm Radiograph:*** Soft tissue structures of interest located are the anterior and posterior fat pads and the supinator fat stripe at the elbow, and the pronator fat stripe at the wrist (Fig. 3–53). The elbow's anterior fat pad is situated anterior to the distal humerus and the elbow's supinator fat stripe is visualized parallel to the anterior aspect of the proximal radius. A change in the shape or placement of these fat structures indicates joint effusion and elbow injury.[14, 15] The elbow's posterior fat pad is normally obscured on a negative lateral forearm radiograph owing to its location within the olecranon fossa. Upon elbow injury, joint effusion pushes this pad out of the fossa, allowing it to be visualized proximal and posterior to the olecranon process.[14] The wrist's pronator fat stripe is demonstrated parallel to the anterior surface of the distal radius. Bowing or obliteration of this fat stripe may be the only indication of subtle radial fractures.[10]

The bony trabecular patterns and the cortical outlines of the carpal bones are sharply defined.
- Sharply defined details are obtained when patient motion is controlled, a detail screen and a small focal spot are used, and a short object–image distance (OID) is maintained.

The long axis of the forearm is aligned with the long axis of the collimated field.
- Aligning the long axis of the forearm with the long axis of the collimated field enables you to collimate tightly without clipping the distal or proximal forearm.

The forearm midshaft is at the center of the collimated field. The radius and ulna, wrist and elbow joints, and forearm soft tissue are included within the field.
- A perpendicular central ray is centered to the midshaft of the forearm to place the forearm in the center of the radiograph.

  When the wrist and elbow joints are included on the radiograph, the degree of radiation beam divergence used to radiograph a long body part needs to be considered (Fig. 3–54).
- ***Film Length for the Forearm:*** Choose a film that is long enough to allow at least 1 inch (2.5 cm) of film to extend beyond each joint space; half of a 14 × 17 inch (35 × 43 cm) film placed lengthwise should be adequate. To ensure that the film extends beyond the elbow, palpate the medial epicondyle, which is located 0.75 inch (2 cm) proximal to the elbow joint. To ensure that the film extends beyond the wrist joint, palpate the base of the first metacarpal; the wrist joint is located just proximal to this base.
- ***Central Ray Centering and Collimation:*** Once the forearm is accurately positioned with the film, center the central ray to the midshaft of the forearm, and open the longitudinal collimation field until it extends just beyond the elbow and wrist joints. If collimation does not extend beyond the joints, adjust the centering point of the central ray until both the elbow and the wrist joint are included within the collimated field without demonstrating an excessive field beyond them. Transverse collimation should be to the forearm skin-line.

CR

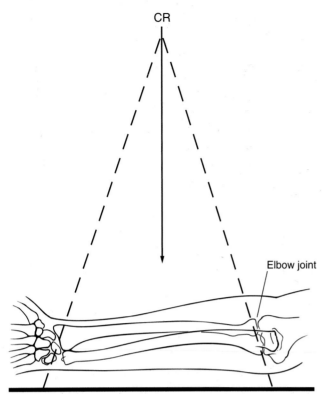

Elbow joint

Figure 3-54. Alignment of x-ray divergence on distal forearm. *CR*, central ray.

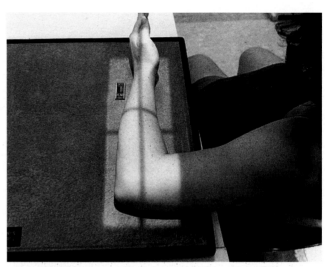

Figure 3-55. Proper patient positioning for lateral forearm radiograph.

Distal Forearm Positioning

The distal forearm is in a true lateral position. The anteroposterior aspect of the distal scaphoid and pisiform are aligned with each other, and a portion of the distal scaphoid is demonstrated slightly distal to the pisiform. The distal radius and ulna are superimposed.

- A true lateral position of the wrist and distal forearm is obtained by rotating the wrist into a lateral position with its ulnar aspect against the cassette (Fig. 3-55). To ensure true lateral positioning, place the palmar aspect of your thumb and forefinger against the anterior and posterior aspects of the patient's wrist joint. Then adjust the rotation until your thumb and finger are aligned perpendicular to the film.
- *Distal Forearm Positioning for Fracture:* Patients with known or suspected fractures may be unable to position both the wrist and elbow joint into a true lateral position simultaneously. In such cases, position the joint closer to the fracture in a true position. When the fracture is situated closer to the wrist joint, the wrist and distal forearm should meet the lateral positioning requirements, indicating a true lateral position, but the elbow and proximal forearm may demonstrate obliquity (see Rad. 59).
- *Verifying a True Lateral Forearm Position:* The pisiform and distal scaphoid relationship can be used to discern whether a true lateral wrist and distal forearm have been obtained. On a accurately positioned lateral forearm, these two bones should be visualized anterior to the capitate and lunate, with

their anterior aspects aligned and a portion of the distal scaphoid projecting distal to the pisiform. It is the diverged x-ray beams used to image the pisiform and scaphoid that cause the distal scaphoid to be projected distal to the pisiform. When the wrist and distal forearm are rotated, the anterior alignment of the scaphoid and pisiform, as well as of the radius and ulna, changes. If the wrist and distal forearm have been externally rotated (supinated), the pisiform is visualized anterior to the distal scaphoid, and the ulna appears anterior to the radius (see Rad. 60). If the wrist and distal forearm have been internally rotated (pronated), the pisiform is visualized posterior to the distal scaphoid, and the radius appears anterior to the ulna (see Rad. 61).

The ulnar styloid is demonstrated in profile posteriorly.

- When the humerus and elbow are mispositioned, the placement of the ulna changes. The ulnar styloid is put in profile by placing the elbow in a lateral position and abducting the humerus until it is parallel with the film, aligning the entire arm on the same horizontal plane. If the humerus is not abducted, nor the elbow positioned laterally, the ulnar styloid is positioned medially, out of profile.

Proximal Forearm and Distal Humerus Positioning

Elbow is flexed 90 degrees.

- When the elbow is flexed 90 degrees, displacement of the anterior or posterior fat pads can be used as a sign to determine diagnosis. Poor elbow positioning, however, also displaces these fat pads and consequently simulates joint pathology. When the elbow is extended, nonpathological displacement of the anterior and posterior fat pads may result from intra-articular pressure and the olecranon's position within the olecranon fossa.

The radial tuberosity is superimposed by the radius and is not demonstrated in profile.

- The extent of radial tuberosity visualization is determined by the position of the wrist and hand. When the wrist and hand are placed in a true lateral position, the radial tuberosity is visualized on the medial aspect of the radius. Because a lateral forearm radiograph is taken in a lateromedial projection, the radius superimposes the radial tuberosity. If the wrist and hand are not positioned in a lateral position, the radial tuberosity placement changes. As the wrist and hand are supinated (externally rotated), the radial tuberosity is visualized in profile anteriorly (see Rad. 60). Pronation (internal rotation) of the wrist and hand visualizes the radial tuberosity in profile posteriorly.

The distal humerus is in a true lateral position. The distal humerus demonstrates three concentric (having the same center) arcs, formed by the trochlear sulcus, capitulum, and medial aspect of the trochlea.[17] The elbow joint space is open, and the radial head superimposes the coronoid.

- A true lateral forearm radiograph is obtained by placing the elbow in a lateral position and abducting the humerus until it is parallel with the film, thereby putting the entire arm on the same horizontal plane. The wrist and hand are then placed in a lateral position, and the medial (ulnar) aspect of the forearm rests against the cassette (see Fig. 3–55). Even though the capitulum is placed anterior to the medial trochlea and the humeral epicondyles are not superimposed for this position, an open joint space may still be obtained. Because the central ray is centered to the midforearm, the diverged x-rays used to image the distal humerus align parallel with the slant of the capitulum and medial trochlea (see Fig. 3–54). The result of this parallelism is an open elbow joint space.
- **Effect of Muscular or Thick Forearm:** Because the patient's forearm rests on its medial (ulnar) surface, the size of the proximal and distal forearm affects the appearance of the elbow joint space. For a patient with a muscular or thick proximal forearm, which is therefore elevated higher than the distal forearm, the capitulum is positioned too far anteriorly and the medial trochlea too posteriorly to align with the x-ray beam divergence. The resulting radiograph demonstrates a closed elbow joint space, and the radial head is positioned distal to the coronoid (see Rad. 61).

  For a patient with a muscular or thick distal forearm, which is elevated higher than the proximal fore-

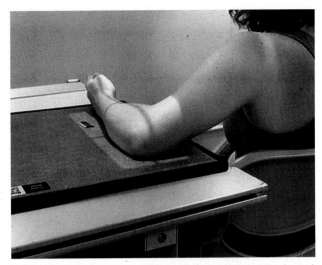

Figure 3-56. Lateral forearm positioning with elevated proximal humerus.

arm, the capitulum is positioned too far posteriorly and the medial trochlea too far anteriorly to align with the x-ray beam divergence. The resulting radiograph demonstrates a closed elbow joint space, and the radial head is positioned proximal to the coronoid (see Rad. 62).

- **Forearm and Humeral Positioning for Fracture:** Patients with known or suspected fractures may be unable to position both the wrist and elbow joint into a true lateral position simultaneously. In such cases, position the joint closer to the fracture in the true position. When the fracture is situated closer to the elbow joint, the elbow joint and proximal forearm should meet the requirements for a true lateral position, whereas the wrist and distal forearm may demonstrate obliquity.
- **Effect of Poor Humeral Positioning:** Misalignment of the capitulum and medial trochlea as well as of the radial head and coronoid is also the result of poor humeral positioning. When the distal surface of the capitulum appears quite distal to the distal surface of the medial trochlea and the radial head is positioned posterior to the coronoid process, the proximal humerus was elevated (see Fig. 3–56 and Rad. 63). When the distal surface of the capitulum appears proximal to the distal surface of the medial trochlea and the radial head is positioned too anteriorly on the coronoid process, the proximal humerus was positioned lower than the distal humerus.

Critiquing Radiographs

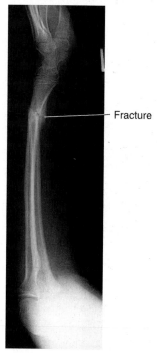

Radiograph 59.

Critique: There is a fracture, located at the distal forearm. The wrist demonstrates a true lateral position, but the elbow is rotated.

Correction: Because the joint closer to the fracture is in the true projection, no repositioning movement is needed.

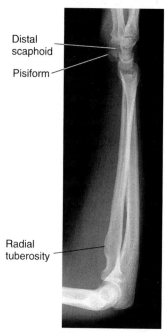

Radiograph 60.

Critique: On this radiograph, the elbow has been accurately positioned. The pisiform is demonstrated anterior to the scaphoid, indicating that the wrist and distal forearm were slightly externally rotated (supinated). The radial tuberosity is visualized in profile anteriorly.

Correction: While maintaining accurate elbow positioning, internally rotate (pronate) the wrist and distal forearm into a true lateral position. This movement will rotate the scaphoid toward the pisiform, aligning their anterior aspects. The radial tuberosity will rotate medially, beneath the radius.

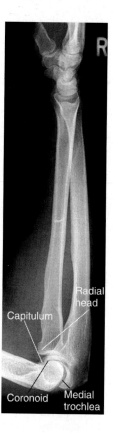

Radiograph 61.

Critique: The distal scaphoid is anterior to the pisiform, indicating that the wrist and hand were internally rotated (pronated). The elbow joint is closed, the capitulum is too far anterior to the medial trochlea, and the radial head is positioned distal to the coronoid process. The proximal forearm was elevated higher than the distal forearm, possibly because the patient has a muscular or thick proximal forearm.

Correction: Raise the distal forearm until the forearm is positioned parallel with the film. Externally rotate (supinate) the wrist and distal forearm until the wrist is in a true lateral position.

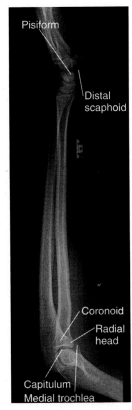

Radiograph 62.

Critique: The capitulum is demonstrated posterior to the medial trochlea, and the radial head is proximal to the coronoid process. The distal forearm was elevated higher than the proximal forearm, possibly because the patient has a muscular or thick distal forearm. The pisiform is demonstrated posterior to the distal scaphoid, indicating that the wrist and hand were internally rotated (pronated).

Correction: Lower the distal forearm until it is positioned parallel with the film. Externally rotate (supinate) the wrist and distal forearm until the wrist is in a true lateral position.

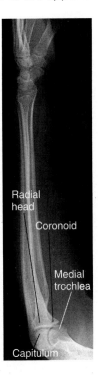

Radiograph 63.

Critique: The wrist is accurately positioned. The distal end of the capitulum is shown distal to the medial trochlea, and the radial head is posterior to the coronoid process. The proximal humerus was elevated as demonstrated in Figure 3–56.

Correction: While maintaining accurate wrist positioning, depress the proximal humerus until the humerus is parallel with the film.

ELBOW

Anteroposterior Projection

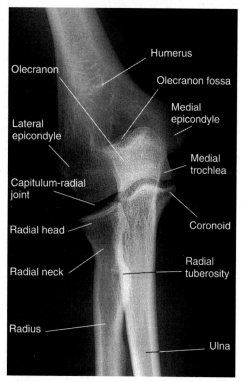

Figure 3-57. Accurately positioned AP elbow radiograph.

Radiographic Evaluation

Facility's patient identification requirements are visible on radiograph.

- These requirements usually are facility name, patient name, age, and hospital number, and exam time and date.
- The patient ID plate does not obscure any anatomy of interest.

A right or left marker, identifying the correct elbow, is present on the radiograph and does not superimpose anatomy of interest.

- Place the marker within the collimated light field so it does not superimpose any portion of the elbow. It may be necessary to open the field to include the marker.
- When more than one view of the elbow is placed on the same radiograph, only one of the views needs to be marked.

There is no evidence of preventable artifacts, such as bandages and splints.

- Consult with the ordering physician and the patient about whether bandages and splints can be removed.

Contrast and density are adequate to demonstrate the surrounding soft tissue and bony structures. Penetration is sufficient to visualize the bony trabecular pat-

terns and the cortical outlines of the distal humerus and proximal forearm.

- A high-contrast, low (55 to 65) kVp technique best enhances the bony and soft tissue structures of the elbow.

The bony trabecular patterns and the cortical outlines of the distal humerus and proximal forearm are sharply defined.

- Sharply defined radiographic details are obtained when patient motion is controlled, a detail screen and a small focal spot are used, and a short object–image distance (OID) is maintained.

The elbow is positioned in a true AP projection. The medial and lateral humeral epicondyles are demonstrated in profile at the extreme medial and lateral edges of the distal humerus, and the radial head and tuberosity superimpose the lateral aspect of the proximal ulna by about 0.25 inch (0.6 cm). The coronoid is demonstrated on end.

- A true AP projection of the elbow is obtained by supinating the patient's hand and externally rotating the forearm and humerus until an imaginary line drawn between the humeral epicondyles is parallel with the film (Fig. 3–58). This positioning places the proximal radius anterior to the ulna.
- ***Detecting Elbow Rotation:*** Rotation of the elbow is a result of poor humeral epicondyle positioning and can be identified radiographically when the (1) epicondyles are not visualized in profile, (2) the radial head and tuberosity are demonstrated with more or less than 0.25 inch (0.6 cm) superimposition of the ulna, and (3) the coronoid is seen in profile. The smaller, lateral humeral epicondyle is more sensitive to rotation, moving out of profile with only a slight degree of elbow rotation.

  If the epicondyles are not demonstrated in profile, evaluate the degree of radial head and tuberosity superimposition of the ulna to determine how to reposition for a true AP projection. If more than 0.25 inch (0.6 cm) of radial head and tuberosity is superimpos-

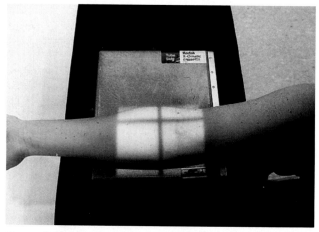

Figure 3-58. Proper patient positioning for AP elbow radiograph.

ing the ulna, the elbow has been medially (internally) rotated (see Rad. 64). If less than 0.25 inch (0.6 cm) of the radial head and tuberosity is superimposing the ulna, the elbow has been laterally (externally) rotated (see Rad. 65).

The radial tuberosity is demonstrated in profile medially, and the radius and ulna are parallel with each other.
- The alignment of the radius and ulna is determined by the position of the humerus and the wrist. When the humerus is positioned with the humeral epicondyles parallel with the film, the radial and ulnar relationship can be adjusted with wrist rotation. For a true AP projection of the elbow, the hand and wrist should also be positioned in an AP projection by supinating the hand. This positioning places the radial tuberosity medially in profile and eliminates crossing of the radius and ulna. As the hand and wrist are pronated, the radius crosses over the ulna, and the radial tuberosity is rotated posteriorly, out of profile (see Rad. 66).

The capitulum–radius joint is open, the radial head articulating surface is not demonstrated, the olecranon process is situated within the olecranon fossa, and the coronoid is demonstrated on end.
- You must use accurate central ray placement and position the elbow in full extension to obtain an open capitulum-radius joint space. When the central ray is centered proximal to the elbow joint space, the capitulum is projected into the joint; when the central ray is centered distal to the elbow joint, the radial head is projected into the joint space (see Rad. 3–67). Poor central ray placement also distorts the radial head, causing its articulating surface to visualize. The degree of joint closure depends on how far the central ray is positioned from the elbow joint. The farther away from the joint the central ray is centered, the more the capitulum-radius joint space is obscured and the more the radial head articulating surface is demonstrated.
- **Effect of Elbow Flexion:** Flexion of the elbow joint also distorts the AP elbow image. With elbow flexion, the capitulum-radial joint closes, the olecranon process moves away from the olecranon fossa, and the coronoid shifts proximally. How a flexed elbow is positioned with respect to the film determines which elbow structures are distorted on the radiograph. If a flexed elbow is resting on the posterior point of the olecranon, with the proximal humerus and the distal forearm elevated as demonstrated in Figure 3–59, both the humerus and the forearm are foreshortened and the capitulum-radial joint is obscured (see Rad. 68). Foreshortening of the proximal humerus is radiographically signified by an oval olecranon fossa that is clearly demonstrated, without the olecranon within it. Foreshortening of the distal forearm occurs radiographically if the radial head articulating surface is visualized partially on end. The severity of the distortion depends on the extent of elbow flexion.

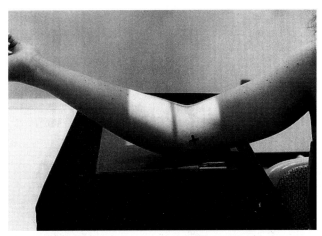

Figure 3-59. Proper elbow positioning for a patient who cannot fully extend the elbow but can extend to at least 30 degrees.

- **Compensating for a Nonextendable Elbow (Partial AP Projections):** An elbow that cannot be extended to at least 30 degrees should be radiographed using separate exposures to image the distal humerus and the proximal forearm—a method referred to as *partial AP projections*.

Figure 3–60 demonstrates how the patient should be positioned to obtain an undistorted AP distal humerus image. Note that the humerus is placed parallel with the film. The resulting radiograph demonstrates an undistorted image of the distal humerus, whereas the proximal forearm is severely distorted and the capitulum-radial joint space is obscured (see Rad. 69).

Figure 3–61 demonstrates how the patient should be positioned to obtain an undistorted AP proximal forearm image. Note that the forearm is placed parallel with the film. The resulting radiograph demonstrates an undistorted image of the proximal forearm and an open capitulum-radial joint, but the distal hu-

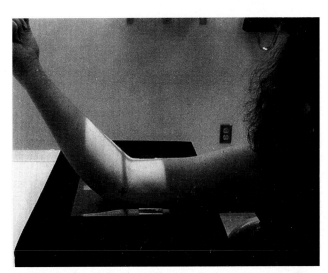

Figure 3-60. Patient positioning for partial AP elbow projection: humerus parallel with film.

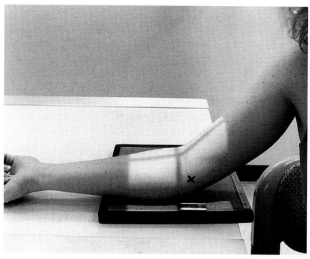

Figure 3-61. Patient positioning for partial AP elbow projection: forearm parallel with film.

merus is severely distorted (see Rad. 70). The capitulum-radial joint space is visualized on the radiograph only if the forearm is positioned parallel with the film.

The elbow joint is at the center of the collimated field. The elbow joint, one fourth of the proximal forearm and distal humerus and the lateral soft tissue are included within the field.

- The elbow joint is located 0.75 inch (2 cm) distal to the easily palpable medial epicondyle. To obtain an image of the elbow joint with the least amount of distortion, place a perpendicular central ray at this level and centered to the mid-elbow. Open longitudinal collimation to include one fourth of the proximal forearm and distal humerus. Transverse collimation should be to the elbow skin-line.
- Half of a 10 × 12 inch (24 × 30 cm) film placed crosswise should be adequate to include all the required anatomical structures.

Critiquing Radiographs

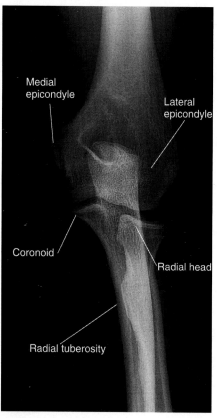

Radiograph 64.

Critique: The humeral epicondyles are not in complete profile, especially the lateral epicondyle. The radial head and tuberosity are superimposing more than 0.25 inch (0.6 cm) of the ulna, and the coronoid is visualized medially. The humerus was medially (internally) rotated.
Correction: Rotate the elbow laterally (externally) until the humeral epicondyles are parallel with the film.

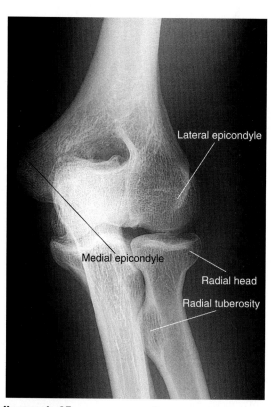

Radiograph 65.

Critique: The humeral epicondyles are not in complete profile, and the radial head and tuberosity are drawn away from the ulna. This radiograph was taken with the humerus in lateral (external) rotation.
Correction: Rotate the elbow medially (internally) until the humeral epicondyles are parallel with the film.

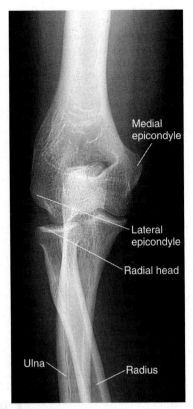

Radiograph 66.

Critique: The radius is crossed over the ulna, and the radial tuberosity is not demonstrated in profile. The hand and wrist were pronated for this radiograph.
Correction: Supinate the hand and wrist into a true AP projection.

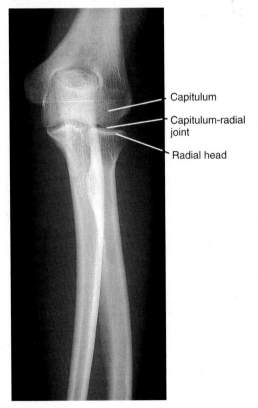

Radiograph 67.

Critique: The capitulum-radial joint space is closed, and the radial head articulating surface is demonstrated. The central ray was centered distal to the joint space.
Correction: Center the central ray to the mid-elbow at a level 0.75 inch (2 cm) distal to the medial epicondyle.

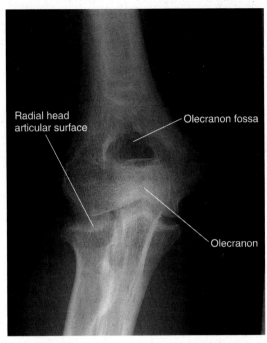

Radiograph 68.

Critique: The capitulum-radial joint space is closed, and the proximal forearm and distal humerus are foreshortened. The elbow was flexed (40 degrees), and the arm was resting on the posterior point of the elbow with the distal forearm and proximal humerus elevated.
Correction: If possible, fully extend the elbow. If the patient is unable to extend the elbow, take two partial AP exposures, one with the forearm and one with the humerus positioned parallel with the film, as demonstrated in Figures 3–60 and 3–61.

139

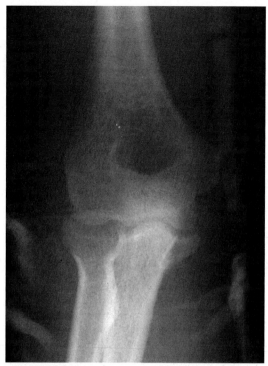

Radiograph 69.

Critique: The distal humerus is demonstrated without foreshortening, but the proximal forearm is severely distorted. The humerus was positioned parallel with the film, but the distal forearm was elevated as demonstrated in Figure 3–60.

Correction: If possible, fully extend the elbow. If the patient is unable to extend the elbow, this is an acceptable view of the distal humerus. A second AP projection of the elbow should be taken with the forearm positioned parallel with the film, as demonstrated in Figure 3–61.

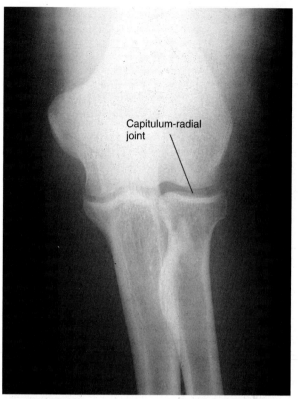

Capitulum-radial joint

Radiograph 70.

Critique: The distal forearm is demonstrated without foreshortening, and the capitulum-radial joint space is open, but the distal humerus is severely distorted. The forearm was positioned parallel with the film, whereas the proximal forearm was elevated as demonstrated in Figure 3–61.

Correction: If possible, fully extend the elbow. If the patient is unable to extend the elbow, this is an acceptable view of the proximal forearm. A second AP projection of the elbow should be taken with the humerus positioned parallel with the film, as demonstrated in Figure 3–60.

Elbow: Medial and Lateral Oblique Positions

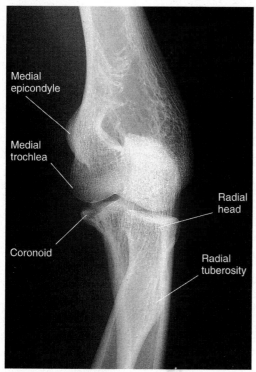

Figure 3-62. Accurately positioned medial oblique elbow radiograph.

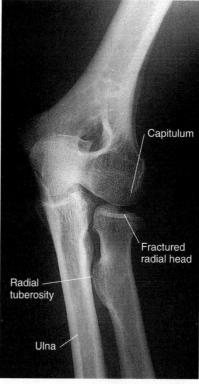

Figure 3-63. Accurately positioned lateral oblique elbow radiograph.

Radiographic Evaluation

Facility's patient identification requirements are visible on radiograph.
- These requirements usually are facility name, patient name, age, and hospital number, and exam time and date.
- The patient ID plate does not obscure any anatomy of interest.

A right or left marker, identifying the correct elbow, is present on the radiograph and does not superimpose anatomy of interest.
- Place the marker laterally within the collimated light field so it does not superimpose any portion of the elbow.

There is no evidence of preventable artifacts, such as bandages and splints.
- Consult with the ordering physician and the patient about whether bandages or splints can be removed.

Contrast and density are adequate to demonstrate the surrounding soft tissue and bony structures. Penetration is sufficient to visualize the bony trabecular patterns and the cortical outlines of the distal humerus and proximal forearm.

- A high-contrast, low (55 to 65) kVp technique best enhances the bony and soft tissue structures of the elbow.

The bony trabecular patterns and cortical outlines of the distal humerus and proximal forearm are sharply defined.
- Sharply defined radiographic details are obtained when patient motion is controlled, a detail screen and a small focal spot are used, and a short object–image distance (OID) is maintained.

The capitulum-radial joint is open, the radial head articulating surface is not demonstrated, and the olecranon process is situated within the olecranon fossa.
- To obtain an open capitulum-radial joint space, you must use accurate central ray placement and position the elbow in full extension. When the central ray is centered proximal to the elbow joint space, the capitulum is projected into the joint; when the central ray is centered distal to the elbow joint, the radial head is projected into the joint space. Poor central ray positioning also distorts the radial head, causing its articulating surface to be visualized. The degree of joint closure and radial head distortion depends on how far the central ray is positioned from the elbow joint. The farther away from the joint the central ray is centered,

the more the capitulum-radial joint space is obscured, and the more the radial head articulation is demonstrated.

- ***Effect of Elbow Flexion:*** Flexion of the elbow joint also distorts the AP elbow image. With elbow flexion, the olecranon process moves away from the olecranon fossa and the coronoid shifts proximally. How the flexed elbow is positioned with respect to the film determines which elbow structures are distorted on the radiograph. If a flexed elbow is resting on the posterior point of the olecranon, with the proximal humerus and the distal forearm elevated, both the humerus and the forearm are foreshortened and the capitulum-radial joint is obscured. Foreshortening of the proximal humerus is radiographically signified by an oval olecranon fossa that is clearly demonstrated but without the olecranon process within it. Foreshortening of the distal forearm occurs radiographically if the radial head articulating surface is visualized partially on end.

  The severity of the distortion depends on the degree of elbow flexion. If the humerus is positioned parallel with the film and the distal forearm is elevated, the radiographic image shows an undistorted distal humerus, but the proximal forearm is severely distorted and the capitulum-radial joint is obscured (see Rad. 71). If the forearm is positioned parallel with the film and the proximal humerus is elevated, the radiographic image shows an undistorted proximal forearm and an open capitulum-radial joint, but the distal humerus is severely distorted.

- ***Oblique Positioning of the Nonextendable Elbow:*** For oblique elbow radiographs, if the patient's condition prevents full elbow extension, the anatomical structure (forearm or humerus) of interest should be positioned parallel with the film. If the radial head or coronoid is of interest, position the forearm parallel with the film (Fig. 3–64). If the capitulum or medial trochlea is of interest, position the humerus parallel with the film. The degree and direction of elbow obliquity are the same as those used for an extended elbow.

The elbow joint is at the center of the collimated field. The elbow joint, one fourth of the proximal forearm and distal humerus, and surrounding soft tissue are included within the field.

- The elbow joint is located 0.75 inch (2 cm) distal to the easily palpable medial humeral epicondyle. To obtain an undistorted image of the elbow joint, place a perpendicular central ray at this level and centered to the mid-elbow. Open longitudinal collimation to include one fourth of the proximal forearm and distal humerus. Transverse collimation should be to the elbow skin-line.
- Half of a 10 × 12 inch (24 × 30 cm) film placed crosswise should be adequate to include all the required anatomical structures.

MEDIAL (INTERNAL) OBLIQUE POSITION

The elbow has been positioned at 45 degrees of medial obliquity. The coronoid process, the trochlear notch, and the medial aspect of the trochlea are demonstrated in profile. The trochlear-coronoid articulation is open, and the radial head and neck superimpose the ulna.

- An accurately positioned medial oblique elbow radiograph is obtained by placing the arm in an AP elbow projection, then internally rotating the hand and humerus until the humeral epicondyles are at a 45-degree angle with the film (Fig. 3–65). When the elbow obliquity is correct, the coronoid process is demonstrated in profile and the radial head and tuberosity superimpose the ulna. If the humeral epicondyles are at less than 45 degrees of obliquity, the radial head is demonstrated posterior to the coronoid process and does not entirely superimpose the ulna (see Rad. 72). If the humeral epicondyles are at more than 45 degrees of obliquity, a portion of the radial head is visualized anterior to the coronoid (see Rad. 73).

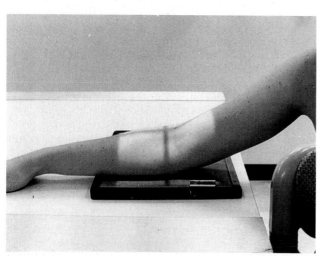

Figure 3–64. Proper patient positioning for oblique elbow radiograph with a flexed elbow.

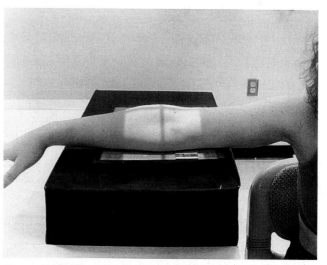

Figure 3–65. Proper patient positioning for medial oblique elbow radiograph.

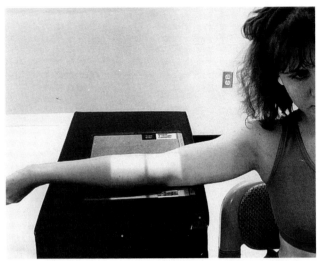

Figure 3-66. Proper patient positioning for lateral oblique elbow radiograph.

LATERAL (EXTERNAL) OBLIQUE POSITION

The elbow has been positioned at 45 degrees of lateral obliquity. The capitulum and radial tuberosity are demonstrated in profile, the radial head, neck, and tuberosity are visualized without superimposing the ulna, and the radioulnar articulation is demonstrated.

- An accurately positioned lateral oblique elbow radiograph is achieved by positioning the arm in an AP projection, then externally rotating the humerus and forearm until the humeral epicondyles form a 45-degree angle with the film (Fig. 3–66). This positioning rotates the radius away from the ulna, demonstrating it without superimposition. If the humeral epicondyles are at less than 45 degrees of obliquity, a portion of the radial head and tuberosity still superimpose the ulna (see Rad. 74). If the humeral epicondyles are at more than 45 degrees of obliquity, the coronoid process superimposes a portion of the radial head, and the radial neck and tuberosity are free of superimposition; the radial tuberosity is no longer in profile (see Rad. 75).

Critiquing Radiographs

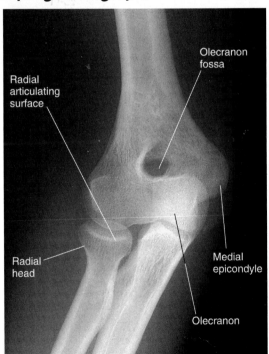

Radiograph 71.

Critique: In this lateral oblique elbow radiograph, the olecranon process is drawn slightly away from the olecranon fossa, the capitulum-radial joint space is closed, and the radial articulating surface is demonstrated. The forearm was not positioned parallel with the film.

Correction: If possible, fully extend the elbow. If the patient is unable to fully extend the elbow and the radial head is of interest, position the forearm parallel with the film, and allow the proximal humerus to be elevated, as demonstrated in Figure 3–64.

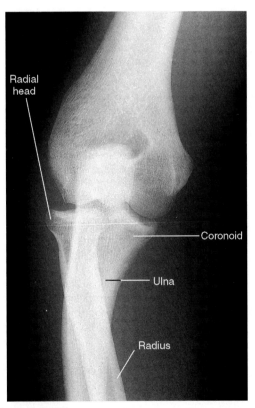

Radiograph 72.

Critique: This is a medial oblique elbow radiograph. The radial head is demonstrated posterior to the coronoid process without complete superimposition of the ulna, and the most proximal aspect of the olecranon is not demonstrated in profile. The degree of elbow obliquity is less than 45 degrees.

Correction: Increase the degree of medial obliquity until the humeral epicondyles are angled at 45 degrees with the film.

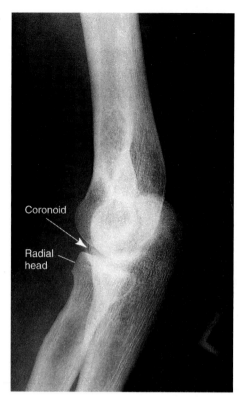

Radiograph 73.

Critique: In this medial oblique elbow radiograph, a portion of the radial head is visualized anterior to the coronoid process, without complete superimposition of the ulna. The degree of elbow obliquity is more than 45 degrees.

Correction: Decrease the degree of medial obliquity until the humeral epicondyles are angled at 45 degrees with the film.

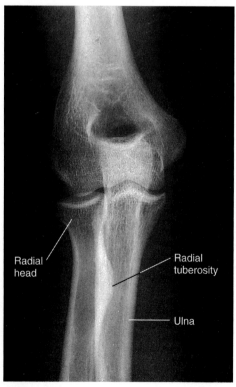

Radiograph 74.

Critique: This is a lateral oblique elbow radiograph. A portion of the radial head and tuberosity is superimposing the ulna, and the radioulnar articulation is obscured. The degree of elbow obliquity is less than 45 degrees. The forearm was not positioned parallel with the film.

Correction: Increase the degree of lateral obliquity until the humeral epicondyles are angled at 45 degrees with the film, and position the forearm parallel with the film.

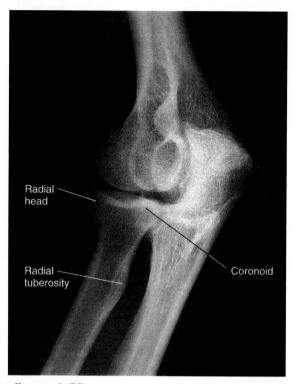

Radiograph 75.

Critique: In this lateral oblique elbow radiograph, the coronoid is superimposing a portion of the radial head, but the radial neck and tuberosity are free of superimposition. The radial tuberosity is not demonstrated in profile. The elbow was angled more than 45 degrees.

Correction: Decrease the degree of lateral obliquity until the humeral epicondyles are angled at 45 degrees with the film.

Elbow: Lateral Position
(Lateromedial Projection)

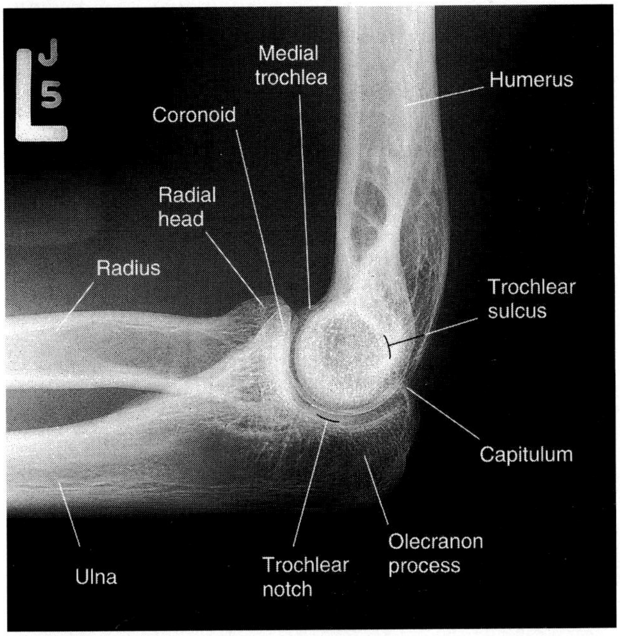

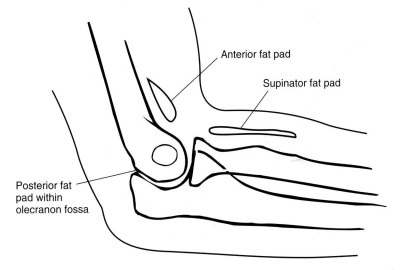

Figure 3-67. Accurately positioned lateral elbow radiograph.

Radiographic Evaluation

Facility's patient identification requirements are visible on radiograph.
- These requirements usually are facility name, patient name, age, and hospital number, and exam time and date.
- The patient ID plate does not obscure any anatomy of interest.

A right or left marker, identifying the correct elbow, is present on the radiograph and does not superimpose anatomy of interest.
- Place the marker within the collimated light field so it does not superimpose any portion of the elbow.
- When more than one view of the elbow is placed on the same radiograph, only one of the views needs to be marked.

There is no evidence of preventable artifacts, such as bandages and splints.
- Consult with the ordering physician and the patient about whether bandages or splints can be removed.

Contrast and density are adequate to demonstrate the anterior, posterior, and supinator fat pads, surrounding soft tissue, and bony structures. Penetration is sufficient to visualize the bony trabecular patterns of the distal humerus and proximal forearm and the cortical outlines of the capitulum, the trochlear sulcus, the medial aspect of the trochlea, and the coronoid process through the radial head.
- A high-contrast, low (55 to 65) kVp technique best enhances the bony and soft tissue structures of the elbow.
- ***Fat Pads on Lateral Elbow Radiograph:*** To evaluate a lateral elbow radiograph, the reviewer not only analyzes the bony structure, but also studies the placement of the soft tissue fat pads. There are three fat pads of interest on a lateral elbow radiograph: the anterior and posterior fat pads and the supinator fat stripe. The *anterior fat pad* should routinely be seen on all lateral elbow radiographs when adequate exposure factors are used. This pad is formed by the superimposed coronoid and radial pads and is situated immediately anterior to the distal humerus (Fig. 3–68). A change in the shape or placement of the anterior fat pad may indicate joint effusion and elbow injury. The *posterior fat pad* is normally obscured on a negative lateral elbow radiograph going to its location within the olecranon fossa (see Fig. 3–68). Upon injury, joint effusion pushes this pad out of the fossa, allowing it to be visualized proximal and posterior to the olecranon fossa.[14] The *supinator fat stripe* is visualized parallel to the anterior aspect of the proximal radius (see Fig. 3–68). Displacement of this fat stripe is useful in diagnosing fractures of the radial head and neck.[15]

Figure 3-68. Locations of fat pads on lateral elbow projection. (Courtesy Educational Reviews, Inc.) (Reproduced with permission from Martensen K. III: The Elbow. (In-Service Reviews in Radiologic Technology, vol 14, no 11.) Birmingham, AL: Educational Reviews, Inc., 1992.)

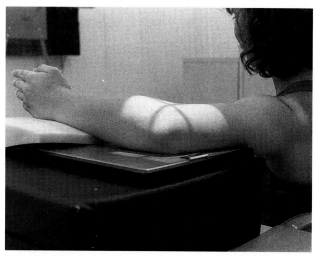

Figure 3-69. Proper patient positioning for lateral elbow radiograph.

The bony trabecular patterns and the cortical outlines of the distal humerus and proximal forearm are sharply defined.

- Sharply defined radiographic details are obtained when patient motion is controlled, a detail screen and a small focal spot are used, and a short object–image distance (OID) is maintained.

The elbow is flexed 90 degrees.

- When the elbow is flexed 90 degrees, the forearm can be elevated to properly align the anatomical structures of the distal humerus, and displacement of the anterior and posterior fat pads can be used as signs to determine diagnosis. If the elbow is not adequately flexed, these fat pads can be displaced by poor positioning instead of joint pathology, interfering with their diagnostic usefulness. When the arm is extended, nonpathological displacement of the anterior fat pad is

due to intra-articular pressure placed on the joint. Nonpathological displacement of the posterior fat pad is a result of positioning of the olecranon within the olecranon fossa, which causes proximal and posterior displacement of the pad[16] (see Rad. 76).

The elbow is in a true lateral position. The distal humerus demonstrates three concentric arcs, which are formed by the trochlear sulcus, capitulum, and medial aspect of the trochlea.[5] The elbow joint space is open, and the radial head superimposes the coronoid process.

- A true lateral elbow radiograph is obtained when the humeral epicondyles are positioned directly on top of one another, placing an imaginary line drawn between them perpendicular to the film. To obtain this humeral epicondyle positioning, place the humerus parallel with the film, and elevate the distal forearm until the palpable medial and lateral epicondyles are superimposed (Fig. 3–69). This positioning aligns the trochlear sulcus, capitulum, and medial trochlea into three concentric (having the same center) arcs (Fig. 3–70). The trochlear sulcus is the small center arc. It moves very little when a positional change is made and works like a pivoting point between the capitulum and the medial aspect of the trochlea. The largest of the arcs is the medial aspect of the trochlea. It is demonstrated very close to and follows the curve of the trochlear notch. The intermediate-sized arc is the capitulum.[15] When these three arcs are in accurate alignment, the elbow joint is visualized as an open space and the radial head superimposes the coronoid process.
- **_Importance of Accurate Positioning:_** The distal humerus, radial head, and coronoid process are misaligned when the proximal humerus and distal forearm are inaccurately positioned. Proximal humerus positioning determines the alignment of the distal surfaces of the capitulum and medial trochlea, whereas distal forearm positioning determines the

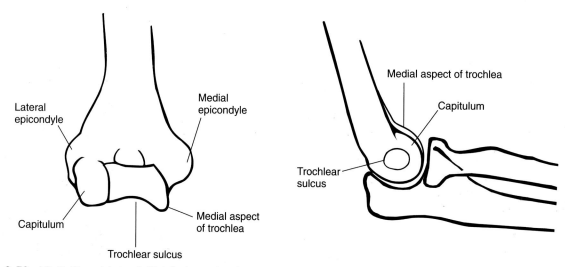

Figure 3-70. AP *(left)* and lateral *(right)* views showing anatomy of the distal humerus. (Reproduced with permission from Martensen K. III: The Elbow. (In-Service Reviews in Radiologic Technology, vol 14, no 11.) Birmingham, AL: Educational Reviews, Inc., 1992.)

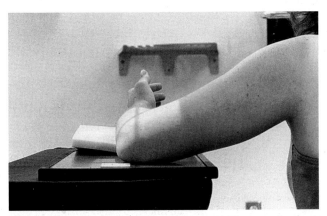

Figure 3-71. Patient positioned for lateral elbow radiograph with elevated proximal humerus.

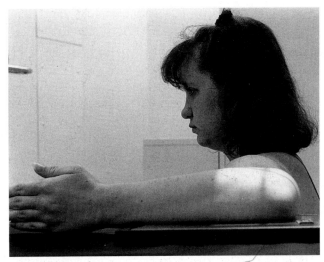

Figure 3-73. Patient positioned for lateral elbow radiograph with depressed distal forearm.

anteroposterior alignment of the capitulum and medial trochlea. Proximal humerus and distal forearm positioning also determines the alignment of the radial head on the coronoid process. Depression or elevation of the proximal humerus moves the radial head anteriorly or posteriorly on the coronoid process, respectively. Depression or elevation of the distal forearm shifts the radial head distally or proximally, respectively, to the coronoid process.

To help understand how the distal humerus and radial head move together, remember that ligaments connect the capitulum and the radial head, so any movement in one causes an equal movement in the other. Precise positioning is a must to obtain a true lateral elbow radiograph. It takes only a small amount of inaccurate positioning to misalign the distal humerus and close the elbow joint space.

- ***Mispositioning of the Proximal Humerus:*** If the proximal humerus is elevated (Fig. 3–71), the radial head is positioned too far posteriorly on the

coronoid process, and the distal capitulum surface is visualized too far distal to the distal surface of the medial trochlea (see Rad. 77). If the proximal humerus is positioned lower than the distal humerus (Fig. 3–72), the radial head is positioned too far anteriorly on the coronoid process, and the distal capitulum surface is visualized too far proximal to the distal medial trochlear surface (see Rad. 78).

- ***Mispositioning of the Distal Forearm:*** When the distal forearm is positioned too low (Fig. 3–73), the radiograph shows the radial head distal to the coronoid process and the capitulum too far anterior to the medial trochlea (see Rad. 79). When the distal forearm is positioned too high (Fig. 3–74), the radiograph shows the radial head proximal to the coronoid process and the capitulum too far posterior to the medial trochlea (see Rad. 80). Carefully evaluate poorly positioned radiographs. Often, both forearm and humeral corrections are needed to obtain accurate positioning.

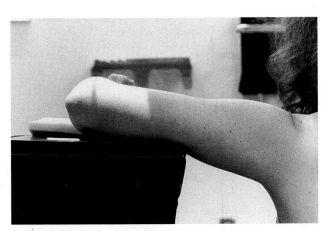

Figure 3-72. Patient positioned for lateral elbow radiograph with depressed proximal humerus.

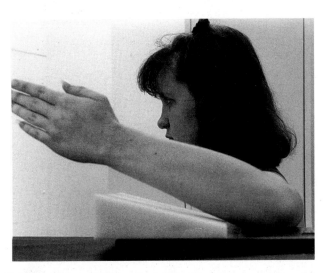

Figure 3-74. Patient positioned for lateral elbow radiograph with elevated distal forearm.

The radial tuberosity is superimposed by the radius and is not demonstrated in profile.

- Visualization of the radial tuberosity is determined by the position of the wrist and hand. When the wrist and hand are placed in a true lateral position, the radial tuberosity is visualized on the medial aspect of the radius. Because a lateral elbow radiograph is taken in a lateromedial projection, the radius superimposes the radial tuberosity. If the wrist and hand are not placed in a lateral position, placement of the radial tuberosity changes. When the wrist and hand are supinated (externally rotated), the radial tuberosity is visualized in profile anteriorly (see Rad. 81). Pronation (internal rotation) of the wrist and hand shows the radial tuberosity in profile posteriorly (see Rad. 82).
- Lateral elbow radiographs using the different hand and wrist positions just described are often taken to study the circumference of the radial head and neck for fractures; they are referred to as *radial head views*.

The elbow joint is at the center of the collimated field. The elbow joint, one fourth of the proximal forearm and distal humerus, and the surrounding soft tissue are included within the field.

- The elbow joint is located 0.75 inch (2 cm) distal to the lateral epicondyle. To obtain an undistorted image of the elbow joint, place a perpendicular central ray at this level and centered to the mid-elbow. Open longitudinal collimation to include one fourth of the proximal forearm and distal humerus. Transverse collimation should be to the elbow skin-line.
- Half of a 10 × 12 inch (24 × 30 cm) film placed crosswise should be adequate to include all the required anatomical structures.

Critiquing Radiographs

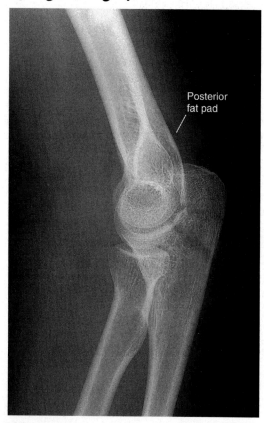

Radiograph 76.

Critique: The elbow is extended. The olecranon is positioned within the olecranon fossa, and the posterior fat pad is demonstrated proximal to the olecranon process. The radial tuberosity is demonstrated in profile posteriorly, indicating that the hand and wrist were pronated.

Correction: If possible, flex the elbow 90 degrees. Position the hand and wrist in a true lateral position.

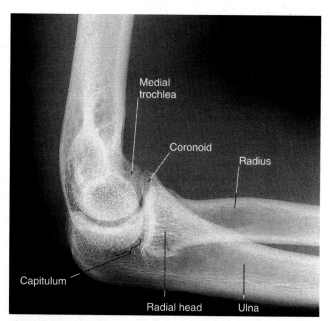

Radiograph 77.

Critique: The radial head is positioned too far posteriorly on the coronoid process, and the distal surface of the capitulum is demonstrated too far distal to the distal surface of the medial trochlea. The patient was positioned with the proximal humerus elevated, as demonstrated in Figure 3–71.

Correction: Lower the proximal humerus until the humeral epicondyles are superimposed and the humerus is positioned parallel with the film. This change will move the capitulum proximally and the medial trochlea distally. Because the capitulum and the trochlea move simultaneously, the amount of adjustment needed is only half of the distance demonstrated between where the two distal surfaces should be on an accurately positioned lateral elbow radiograph and where they are on this radiograph. On this radiograph, this distance is about 0.5 inch (1 cm), so the repositioning adjustment needed is only 0.25 inch (0.6 cm).

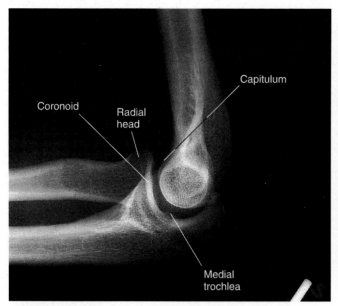

Radiograph 78.

Critique: The radial head is positioned anterior on the coronoid process, and the distal surface of the capitulum is too far proximal to the distal surface of the medial trochlea. The patient was positioned with the proximal humerus depressed, as demonstrated in Figure 3–72.

Correction: Elevate the proximal humerus until the humeral epicondyles are superimposed and the humerus is positioned parallel with the film.

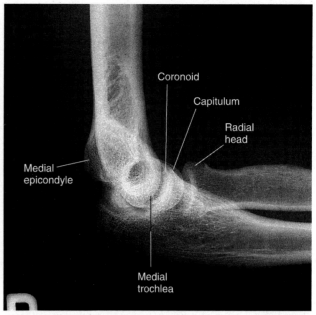

Radiograph 79.

Critique: The radial head is distal to the coronoid process, and the capitulum is visualized too far anterior to the medial trochlea. The patient was placed with the distal forearm positioned too close to the film, as demonstrated in Figure 3–73.

Correction: Elevate the distal forearm until the humeral epicondyles are superimposed. This change will move the capitulum posteriorly and the medial trochlea anteriorly. Because the capitulum and the trochlea move simultaneously, the amount of adjustment required is only half the distance demonstrated between where the two anterior surfaces should be located on an accurately positioned lateral elbow radiograph and where they are on this radiograph.

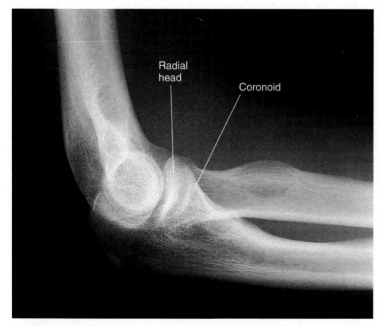

Radiograph 80.

Critique: The radial head is proximal to the coronoid process, and the capitulum is visualized too far posterior to the medial trochlea. The patient was positioned with the distal forearm placed too far away from the film, as demonstrated in Figure 3–74.

Correction: Lower the distal forearm until the humeral epicondyles are superimposed.

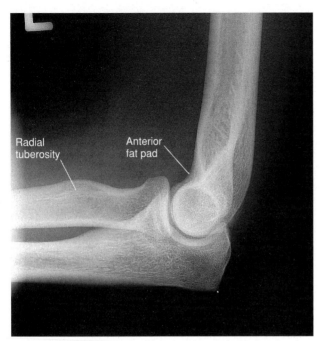

Radiograph 81.

Critique: The elbow joint space is open, and the distal humerus demonstrates accurate alignment. The radial tuberosity is demonstrated in profile anteriorly, indicating that the hand and wrist were supinated.

Correction: If the circumference of the radial head and neck is being evaluated and this is the desired position for the tuberosity, no repositioning movement is needed. If a true lateral elbow image is desired, the hand and wrist should be placed in a true lateral position.

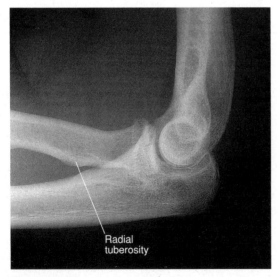

Radiograph 82.

Critique: The elbow joint space is open, and the distal humerus demonstrates accurate alignment. The radial tuberosity is demonstrated in profile posteriorly, indicating that the hand and wrist were pronated (internally rotated).

Correction: If the circumference of the radial head and neck is being evaluated and this is the desired position for the tuberosity, no repositioning movement is needed. If a true lateral elbow image is desired, the hand and wrist should be placed in a true lateral position.

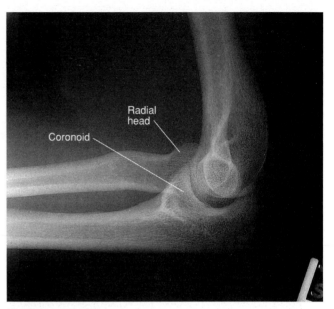

Radiograph 83.

Critique: Two positional problems on this radiograph are preventing the distal humerus from demonstrating accurate alignment. The radial head is positioned anterior and proximal to the coronoid process, and the capitulum is positioned too far proximal and posterior to the medial aspect of the trochlea. The proximal humerus was positioned too low, and the distal forearm was positioned too high, a combination of the errors demonstrated in Figures 3–72 and 3–74.

Correction: Raise the proximal humerus and lower the distal forearm until the humeral epicondyles are superimposed.

Elbow: Radial Head and Capitulum View

The radial head and capitulum view is a special projection taken when a fracture of the radial head or capitulum is suspected.

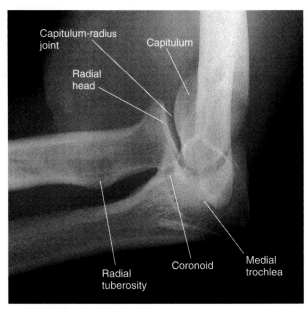

Figure 3-75. Accurately positioned radial head and capitulum radiograph.

Radiographic Evaluation

Facility's patient identification requirements are visible on radiograph.
- These requirements usually are facility name, patient name, age, and hospital number, and exam time and date.
- The patient ID plate does not obscure any anatomy of interest.

A right or left marker, identifying the correct elbow, is present on the radiograph and does not superimpose anatomy of interest.
- Place the marker within the collimated light field so it does not superimpose any portion of the elbow.

There is no evidence of preventable artifacts, such as bandages and splints.
- Consult with the ordering physician and the patient about whether bandages or splints can be removed.

Contrast and density are adequate to demonstrate the surrounding soft tissue and bony structures of the elbow. Penetration is sufficient to visualize the bony trabecular patterns and the cortical outlines of the capitulum, trochlear sulcus, medial aspect of the trochlea, coronoid process, and radial head.
- A high-contrast, low (55 to 65) kVp technique best enhances the bony structures of the elbow.

The bony trabecular patterns and cortical outlines of the radial head and capitulum are sharply defined.
- Sharply defined radiographic details are obtained when patient motion is controlled, a detail screen and a small focal spot are used, and a short object–image distance (OID) is maintained.

The elbow is flexed 90 degrees.
- If the elbow is flexed 90 degrees, the forearm can be elevated to properly align the anatomical structures of the distal humerus.

The anterior aspect of the distal humerus demonstrates three arcs. The largest and most distally located arc is the medial aspect of the trochlea; the smaller center arc is the trochlear sulcus; and the capitulum is the proximal arc. The capitulum-radius joint is open, and the radial head is aligned with the coronoid process.
- An accurately aligned distal humerus, radial head, and coronoid is obtained when the elbow is in a true lateral position. A lateral elbow position is accomplished when the humeral epicondyles are positioned directly on top of one another, placing them perpendicular to the film. To obtain this humeral epicondyle positioning, place the humerus parallel with the film, and elevate the distal forearm until the palpable medial and lateral epicondyles are superimposed (Fig. 3–76). This positioning aligns the capitulum, trochlear sulcus, and medial trochlea into three concentric (having the same center) arcs. The trochlear sulcus is the small center arc; it moves very little when a positional change is made, and works like a pivoting point between the capitulum and the medial aspect of the trochlea. The largest of the arcs is the medial aspect of the trochlea; it is demonstrated very close to and follows the curve of the trochlear notch. The intermediate-sized arc is the capitulum.[5] When these three arcs are in accurate alignment, the capitulum-radius joint is visualized as an open space, and the radial head aligns with the coronoid process.

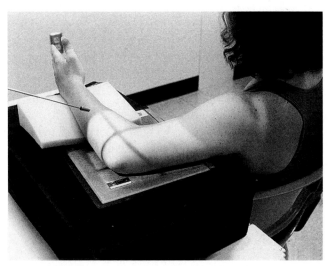

Figure 3-76. Proper patient positioning for radial head and capitulum radiograph.

- **Effect of Distal Forearm Mispositioning:** The alignment of the anterior surfaces of the capitulum, trochlear sulcus, and medial trochlea, as well as the alignment of the radial head and coronoid process, is affected when the distal forearm is positioned. Precise positioning is a must to obtain accurate alignment. It takes only a small amount of inaccurate positioning to close the capitulum-radius joint. If the distal forearm is positioned too low, the radiograph shows a closed capitulum-radius joint space and visualizes the capitulum too far anterior to the medial trochlea and the radial head distal to the coronoid process (see Rad. 84). If the distal forearm is positioned too high, the radiograph shows the capitulum too far posterior to the medial trochlea and the radial head proximal to the coronoid process.

The arcs of the capitulum and medial trochlea are demonstrated without superimposition, and the radial head superimposes only the anterior tip of the coronoid process.

- To accurately separate the arcs of the distal humerus and position the radial head anterior to the coronoid process, position the humerus parallel with the film, and place a 45-degree angulation on the central ray. Then direct the central ray proximally (toward the shoulder). This combination of positioning and angulation projects the anatomical structures (radial head and capitulum) situated farther from the film proximal to those structures (coronoid and medial trochlea) situated closer to the film.

- **Effects of Errors in Positioning or Angulation:** If the central ray is angled accurately but the proximal humerus is depressed lower than the distal humerus, the medial trochlea and capitulum cortices are not clearly defined, the coronoid process is free of radial head superimposition, and the radial neck and tuberosity are superimposed by the ulnar supinator crest (a sharp, prominent ridge running along the lateral margin of the ulna that divides the ulna's anterior and posterior surfaces) (see Rad. 85). The same radiograph could result if the patient was accurately positioned but the central ray was angled more than 45 degrees.

  If the central ray is accurately angled but the proximal humerus is elevated, the medial trochlea demonstrates some capitular superimposition, and the radial head superimposes a greater portion of the coronoid process (see Rad. 86). This same radiograph could result if the patient was accurately positioned but the central ray was angled less than 45 degrees.

The radial head surface of interest is demonstrated in profile.

- The position of the wrist determines which surface of the radial head is placed in profile.
- **Effect of Wrist Position:** When the patient's elbow is placed in a lateral position, wrist rotation causes the radius to rotate around the ulna. This rotation places different radial head surfaces in profile. To determine which surfaces are in profile, one should become familiar with the relationship between the wrist position and visualization of the radial tuberosity. If the patient's wrist is positioned in a PA projection, the radial tuberosity is demonstrated posteriorly, the lateral surface of the radial head appears in profile anteriorly, and the medial surface of the radial head is shown in profile posteriorly (see Fig. 3–75). If the wrist is in a lateral position, the radial tuberosity is not demonstrated in profile, but is superimposed by the radius. In this position, the anterior surface of the radial head appears in profile anteriorly, and the posterior surface is shown in profile posteriorly (see Rad. 84).

The radial head is at the center of the collimated field. The proximal forearm, distal humerus, and the surrounding soft tissue are included within the field.

- To place the radial head in the center of the collimated field, center the central ray 0.75 inch (2 cm) distal (toward the wrist) to the lateral epicondyle. Open the longitudinally and transversely collimated fields to the posterior elbow skin-line.
- An 8 × 10 inch (18 × 24 cm) film placed lengthwise should be adequate to include all the required anatomical structures.

Critiquing Radiographs

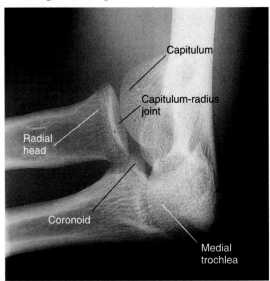

Capitulum

Capitulum-radius joint

Radial head

Coronoid

Medial trochlea

Radiograph 84.

Critique: The capitulum-radius joint space is closed, the radial head is demonstrated distal to the coronoid process, and the capitulum is demonstrated too far anterior to the medial trochlea, indicating that the distal forearm was depressed. The radial tuberosity is not demonstrated in profile, the anterior surface of the radial head is in profile anteriorly, and the posterior surface is in profile posteriorly; the wrist was placed in a lateral position.

Correction: Elevate the distal forearm until the humeral epicondyles are aligned perpendicular to the film. The amount of movement needed is half the distance between how close the anterior surfaces of the capitulum and medial trochlea should be on an accurately positioned radial head and capitulum radiograph and where they are located on this radiograph. If the lateral and medial surfaces of the radial head should be demonstrated in profile, the patient's wrist needs to be placed in a PA projection.

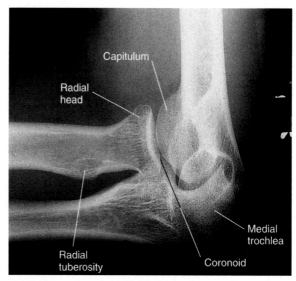

Radiograph 86.

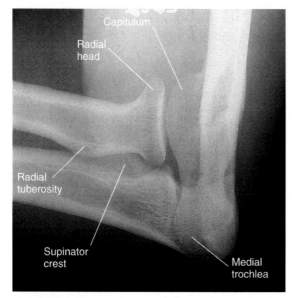

Radiograph 85.

Critique: The distal medial trochlea and capitulum cortices are not clearly defined, the coronoid process is free of radial head superimposition, and the radial neck and tuberosity are superimposed by the ulnar supinator crest. The proximal humerus was depressed lower than the distal humerus.

Correction: Elevate the proximal humerus until the humeral epicondyles are perpendicular to the film.

Critique: The capitulum-radius joint space is closed, the radial head is demonstrated distal to the coronoid process, and the capitulum is demonstrated too far anterior to the medial trochlea, indicating that the distal forearm was depressed. The radial head superimposes more than just the tip of the coronoid, and the medial trochlea and capitulum would demonstrate slight superimposition if the distal forearm had been accurately positioned; the proximal humerus was elevated. The radial tuberosity is demonstrated in profile posteriorly and the lateral surface of the radial head is demonstrated in profile anteriorly, whereas the medial surface is in profile posteriorly; the wrist was placed in a PA projection.

Correction: Elevate the distal forearm and depress the proximal humerus until the humeral epicondyles are aligned perpendicular to the film. If you want the anterior and posterior surfaces of the radial head to be demonstrated in profile, place the wrist in a lateral position.

HUMERUS

Anteroposterior Projection

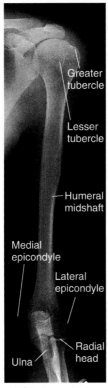

Figure 3-77. Accurately positioned AP humerus radiograph.

Radiographic Evaluation

Facility's patient identification requirements are visible on radiograph.
- These requirements usually are facility name, patient name, age, and hospital number, and exam time and date.
- The patient ID plate does not obscure any anatomy of interest.

A right or left marker identifying the correct humerus is present on the radiograph and does not superimpose anatomy of interest.
- Place marker within the collimated light field, without superimposing any portion of affected humerus or humeral soft tissue.

There is no evidence of preventable artifacts, such as gown snaps, bandages, slings, and splints.
- Consult the ordering physician and the patient about whether bandages, slings, or splints can be removed.

Contrast and density are adequate to demonstrate the surrounding soft tissue and bony structures of the humerus. Penetration is sufficient to visualize the bony trabecular patterns and the cortical outlines of the humerus.

- If the patient's upper arm anteroposterior thickness measures less than 5 inches (13 cm), a grid is not required. For such a patient, a high-contrast, low (60 to 70) kVp technique sufficiently penetrates the bony and soft tissue structures of the humerus without causing excessive scattered radiation to reach the film and hinder radiographic contrast. If the upper arm measures more than 5 inches (13 cm), a grid (device placed between patient and film to absorb scattered radiation) should be used, because this thickness would produce enough scattered radiation to negatively affect the radiographic contrast.[17, 18] When a grid is used, increase the kVp to above 70 to penetrate the thicker humerus and to provide an adequate scale of contrast. Increase the exposure (mAs) by the standard density conversion factor for the grid ratio (number used to express a grid's scatter eliminating ability) being used, to compensate for the scatter and the primary radiation that the grid will absorb.
- ***Anode-Heel Effect:*** Another exposure factor to consider when positioning the humerus is the anode-heel effect. Because a long (17-inch [43-cm]) field is used for the length of the adult humerus, there is a difference in the intensity of the beam that reaches the cathode and anode ends of the film. This noticeable intensity variation is a result of greater photon absorption at the thicker, "heel" portion of the anode compared with the thinner, "toe" portion when a long field is used. Consequently, radiographic density at the anode end of the tube is less than that at the cathode end.

  Using this knowledge to our advantage can help us produce radiographs of the humerus that demonstrate uniform density on both ends. Position the thinner elbow (distal humerus) at the anode end of the tube and the thicker shoulder (proximal humerus) at the cathode end. Set an exposure (mAs) that will adequately demonstrate the proximal humerus. Because the anode will absorb some of the photons aimed at the anode end of the film, the distal humerus, which requires less exposure than the proximal humerus, will not be overexposed.

The bony trabecular patterns and the cortical outlines of the humerus are sharply defined.
- Sharply defined radiographic details are obtained when patient motion and respiration are halted, when a small focal spot is used and a short object–image distance (OID) is maintained.

The humerus is in a true AP projection. The medial and lateral humeral epicondyles are demonstrated in profile, and the radial head and tuberosity are superimposing the lateral aspect of the proximal ulna by about 0.25 inch (0.6 cm). The greater tubercle is demonstrated laterally in profile, the humeral head is demonstrated medially in profile, and the vertical cortical margin of the lesser tubercle is visualized about halfway between the greater tubercle and the humeral head.
- A true AP projection is obtained by placing the patient in either a supine or an upright AP projection, with

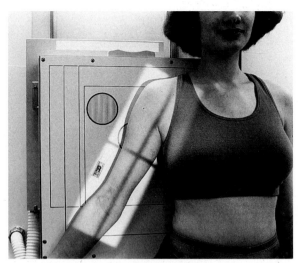

Figure 3-78. Proper patient positioning for AP humerus radiograph: collimator head rotated.

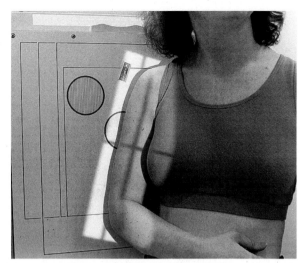

Figure 3-79. Patient positioning for AP humerus radiograph when fracture is located close to shoulder.

the affected arm extended. Supinate the hand and externally rotate the elbow until a line drawn between the palpable humeral epicondyles is aligned parallel with the film (Fig. 3–78). This positioning places the proximal radius anterior to the ulna, causing the radial head and tuberosity to superimpose the lateral ulna by about 0.25 inch (0.6 cm), and the greater tuberosity in profile.

- **Detecting Humeral Rotation:** Rotation of the humerus is a result of poor humeral epicondyle positioning. When the humeral epicondyles and the greater tuberosity are not demonstrated in profile, measure the amount of radial head and tuberosity superimposition of the ulna to determine how the patient should be repositioned. If less than 0.25 inch (0.6 cm) of the radial head and tuberosity are superimposing the ulna, the elbow and humerus have been excessively laterally (externally) rotated (see Rad. 87). If more than 0.25 inch (0.6 cm) of the radial head and tuberosity are superimposing the ulna, the elbow and humerus have been medially (internally) rotated (see Rad. 88).
- **Forearm Positioning for Humeral Fracture:** When a fracture of the humerus is suspected or a followup radiograph is being taken to assess healing of a humeral fracture, the patient's forearm should not be externally rotated to obtain the AP projection, because external rotation of the forearm increases the risk of radial nerve damage.[6] For such an exam, the joint closer to the fracture should be aligned in the true AP projection. If the fracture site is situated closer to the shoulder joint and the arm cannot be externally rotated, the greater tuberosity is placed in profile by rotating the patient's body toward the affected humerus 35 to 40 degrees (Fig. 3–79). Depending on the amount of humeral rotation at the fracture site, the distal humerus may or may not be in a true AP projection (see Rad. 89). If the fracture is situated closer to the elbow joint, extend the arm and rotate the patient's body toward the affected humerus

until the humeral epicondyles are aligned parallel with the film. Depending on the amount of humeral rotation at the fracture site, the greater tuberosity may or may not be in profile.

The long axis of the humerus is aligned with the long axis of the collimated field.

- If the humerus can remain aligned with the long axis of the film while the elbow and shoulder joints are included on the film, align the long axis of the collimated light field with the long axis of the humerus to allow for tight transverse collimation.
- For many adult humeral radiographs, it may be necessary to position the humerus diagonally on the film to include the elbow and shoulder joint. For this positioning, the collimator head or tube column should be turned or rotated to align the long axis of the collimated light field with the long axis of the humerus. (If a grid is used, do not rotate the tube column, or grid cutoff—unwanted absorption of primary radiation—will result.)
- If the collimator head or tube column cannot be adjusted for a diagonal positioning, leave the transversely collimated field open enough to include the shoulder joint and elbow. With this setup, the collimated field includes a large portion of the patient's thorax. Hence, the thorax is exposed to unnecessary radiation, which can be protected by laying a flat contact shield across the patient's thorax. Remember to leave at least 3 inches (7.5 cm) of space between the humeral head and the shield to allow for magnification, so the shoulder joint is not obscured by the shield (Fig. 3–80).

The humeral midshaft is at the center of the collimated field. The shoulder and elbow joints and the lateral humeral soft tissue are included within the field.

- To place the humeral midshaft in the center of the radiograph, palpate the coracoid process and the me-

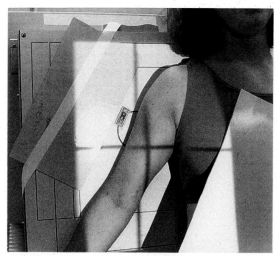

Figure 3-80. Proper patient positioning for AP humerus radiograph using shields when collimator head cannot be rotated.

dial epicondyle, and position the central ray halfway between these two palpable landmarks. When the elbow and shoulder joints are included on the radiograph, the degree of radiation beam divergence that is used for a long body part needs to be considered.

- **Film Length and Positioning:** Choose a film that is long enough to allow at least 1 inch (2.5 cm) of film to extend beyond each joint space; a 14 × 17 inch (35 × 43 cm) film placed lengthwise should be adequate. For a patient with a long humerus, it may be necessary to position the humerus diagonally on the film to obtain the needed film length.

    Palpate the two joints to ensure that the film extends beyond them. The elbow is located about 0.75 inch (2 cm) proximal to the medial epicondyle. The shoulder joint is located at the same level as the palpable coracoid.

- **Central Ray Centering and Collimation:** Once the humerus is accurately positioned with the film and the central ray is centered to the humeral midshaft, open the longitudinal collimated field until it extends 1 inch (2.5 cm) beyond the elbow and shoulder joint. If the collimation does not extend beyond both joints, adjust the centering point of the central ray until both the elbow and the shoulder joint are included within the collimated field without demonstrating an excessive light field beyond them. Transverse collimation should be to the skin-line laterally and to the coracoid medially.

Critiquing Radiographs

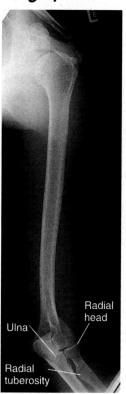

Radial head

Ulna

Radial tuberosity

Radiograph 87.

Critique: The humeral epicondyles are not demonstrated in profile, the radial head and tuberosity do not superimpose the ulna, and the cortical margin of the lesser tuberosity is not shown halfway between the greater tuberosity and the humeral head. The arm was externally rotated more than the required amount.

Correction: Internally rotate the arm until the humeral epicondyles are positioned parallel with the film.

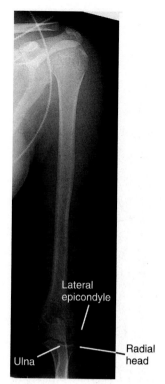

Lateral
epicondyle

Ulna

Radial
head

Radiograph 88.

Critique: Neither the humeral epicondyles nor the greater tuberosity is demonstrated in profile, and the radial head and tuberosity superimpose more than 0.25 inch (0.6 cm) of the ulna. The arm was internally rotated.

Correction: Externally rotate the arm until the humeral epicondyles are positioned parallel with the film.

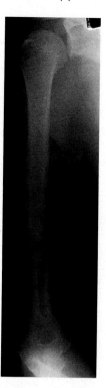

Radiograph 89.

Critique: There is a fracture at the distal humerus. The glenohumeral joint space is demonstrated, indicating that this radiograph was taken with the patient rotated toward the humerus.

Correction: Because the joint closer to the fracture is in a true projection, no repositioning movement is needed.

Humerus: Lateral Position

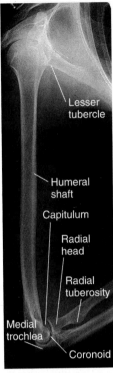

Figure 3–81. Accurately positioned mediolateral humerus radiograph.

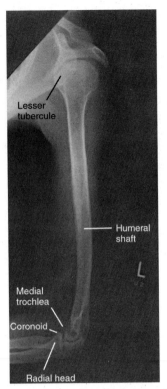

Figure 3–82. Accurately positioned lateromedial humerus radiograph.

Radiographic Evaluation

Facility's patient identification requirements are visible on radiograph.

- These requirements usually are facility name, patient name, age, and hospital number, and exam time and date.
- The patient ID plate does not obscure any anatomy of interest.

A right or left marker identifying the correct humerus, is present on the radiograph and does not superimpose anatomy of interest.

- Place the marker within the collimated light field so it does not superimpose any portion of the affected humerus or humeral soft tissue.

There is no evidence of preventable artifacts, such as gown snaps, bandages, slings, and splints.

- Consult with the ordering physician and the patient about whether bandages, slings, or splints can be removed.

Contrast and density are adequate to demonstrate the surrounding soft tissue and bony structures of the humerus. Penetration is sufficient to visualize the bony trabecular patterns and the cortical outlines of the humerus.

- If the patient's upper arm anteroposterior thickness measures less than 5 inches (13 cm), a grid is not required. For such a patient, a high-contrast, low (60 to 70) kVp technique sufficiently penetrates the bony and soft tissue structures of the humerus without causing excessive scattered radiation to reach the film and hinder contrast. If the patient's upper arm measures more than 5 inches (13 cm), a grid (device placed between patient and film to absorb radiation) should be used, because this thickness would produce enough scattered radiation to negatively affect the radiographic contrast.[19, 20] When a grid is used, increase the penetration to above 70 kVp to penetrate the thicker humerus and to provide an adequate scale of contrast. Increase the exposure (mAs) by the standard density conversion factor for the grid ratio used to compensate for the absorption of the scatter and primary radiation that occurs.

- ***Anode-Heel Effect:*** Another exposure factor to consider when positioning the humerus is the anode-heel effect. Because a long (17-inch [43 cm]) field is used for the length of the adult humerus, there is a difference in the intensity of the beam on the cathode and anode ends of the film. This noticeable intensity variation is a result of increased photon absorption at the thicker, "heel" portion of the anode compared with the thinner, "toe" portion when a large field is

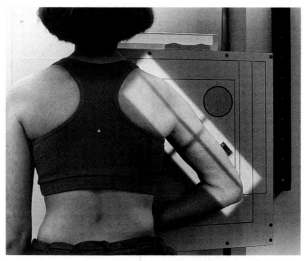

Figure 3–83. Proper patient positioning for mediolateral humerus radiograph.

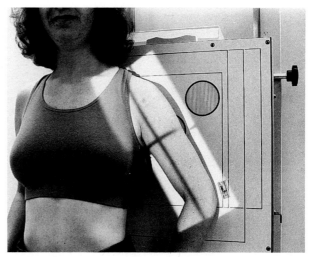

Figure 3–84. Proper patient positioning for lateromedial humerus radiograph.

used. Consequently, radiographic density at the anode end of the tube is less than at the cathode end.[18] Using this knowledge to our advantage can help us produce radiographs of the humerus that demonstrate uniform density at both ends. Position the thinner elbow (distal humerus) at the anode end of the tube and the thicker (proximal humerus) at the cathode end. Set an exposure (mAs) that will adequately demonstrate the proximal humerus. Because the anode will absorb some of the photons aimed at the anode end film, the distal humerus, which requires less exposure than the proximal humerus, will not be overexposed.

The bony trabecular patterns and cortical outlines of the humerus are sharply defined.

- Sharply defined radiographic details are obtained when patient motion and respiration are halted, a small focal spot is used, and a short object–image distance (OID) is maintained. The standing mediolateral projection of the humerus positions the humerus closer to the film, resulting in the less distal humeral magnification.

The humerus is in a true lateral position. The lesser tubercle is demonstrated in profile medially and the humeral head and greater tubercle are superimposed. For a *mediolateral projection*, most of the radial head is demonstrated anterior to the coronoid process, the radial tuberosity is demonstrated in profile, and the capitulum is visualized proximal to the medial trochlea (see Fig. 3–81). For a *lateromedial projection*, the radial head and coronoid process are superimposed, the radial tuberosity is not demonstrated in profile, and the capitulum is visualized distal to the medial trochlea (see Fig. 3–82).

- There are two methods of positioning the patient for a lateral humerus radiograph, mediolateral and lateromedial. The preferred method positions the patient's body in an upright PA projection, with the elbow flexed 90 degrees and the forearm and humerus inter-

nally rotated until an imaginary line connecting the humeral epicondyles is perpendicular to the film: this is a *mediolateral projection* (Fig. 3–83). Have the patient rotate the humerus internally while the body maintains a true PA projection. Do not allow the patient to rotate the body toward the affected humerus instead. Such body obliquity would cause a decrease in density of the proximal humerus compared with the distal humerus (see Rad. 90), because the shoulder tissue would superimpose the proximal humerus. If body rotation cannot be avoided, an increase in exposure (mAs) is required to adequately demonstrate the upper humerus.

- The second method positions the patient's body in an AP projection. The hand is positioned against the patient's side, the elbow is slightly flexed, and the forearm and humerus are internally rotated until an imaginary line connecting the humeral epicondyles is perpendicular to the film; this is a *lateromedial projection* (Fig. 3–84). If the patient's forearm is positioned across the body in an attempt to flex the elbow 90 degrees and the distal humerus is not brought away from the cassette enough to position the humeral epicondyles perpendicular to the film (Fig. 3–85), the radiograph demonstrates the capitulum posterior to the medial trochlea, a distorted proximal forearm, and the lesser tubercle in partial profile (see Rad. 91).

The difference in the anatomical relationship of the distal humerus between the mediolateral and lateromedial projections is a result of x-ray beam divergence. For a lateral humerus radiograph, the central ray is centered to the midhumeral shaft, which is located about 5 inches (13 cm) from the elbow joint. Since the elbow joint is placed so far away from the central ray, diverged x-ray beams are used to image the elbow joint. This causes the anatomical structures positioned farthest from the film to be diverged more distally than the anatomical structures positioned closest to the film. In the mediolateral projection the medial trochlea is placed farther from the film than

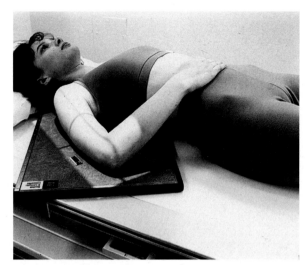

Figure 3-85. Patient positioned for lateromedial humerus radiograph with poor distal humerus alignment.

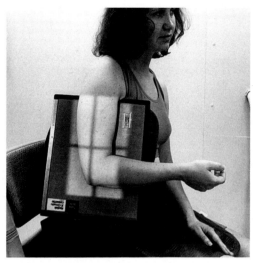

Figure 3-86. Proper patient positioning for distal humerus fracture.

the capitulum. Consequently, x-ray beam divergence will project the medial trochlea distal to the capitulum. In the lateromedial projection the capitulum is situated farther from the film, thus the x-ray beam divergence will project it distal to the medial trochlea.

- **Positioning for a Humeral Fracture:** When a fracture of the humerus is suspected or a follow-up radiograph is being taken to assess healing of a fracture, the patient's forearm or humerus should not be rotated to obtain a lateral position. Rotation of the forearm and humerus would increase the risk of radial nerve damage and displacement of the fracture fragments.[6] Because the forearm should not be rotated for a trauma exam, a lateral radiograph of the proximal and distal humerus must be obtained by positioning the patient differently.
- Distal Humeral Fracture: Obtain a lateral distal humerus radiograph by gently sliding a cassette between the patient and the distal humerus. Adjust the cassette until the epicondyles are positioned perpendicular to the cassette. Place a flat contact protecting shield between the patient and the film to absorb any radiation that would penetrate the cassette and expose the patient. Finally, center the central ray perpendicular to the cassette and distal humerus (Fig. 3–86). Radiographically, this positioning should demonstrate a true lateral position of the distal humerus with superimposition of the epicondyles and of the radial head and coronoid process (see Rad. 92).
- Proximal Humeral Fracture: A lateral radiograph can be achieved by positioning the patient two ways.

  The first method is best done with the patient in an upright position. This position is known as the *trans-scapular Y position*. Begin by placing the patient in a PA upright projection with the humerus positioned as is, and then rotate the patient toward the affected humerus (about 45 degrees) until the scapular body is in a lateral position (see Fig. 3–87 and Rad. 93). Precise positioning and evaluating points for this view

can be studied by referring to the trans-scapular Y position, page 180.

The second method of obtaining a lateral view of the proximal humerus can be accomplished in either an upright or supine position. It is known as the *transthoracic lateral position* (Fig. 3–88). The patient's body is placed in a true lateral position with the affected humerus resting against the grid cassette, and the unaffected arm is raised above the patient's head. To prevent superimposition of the shoulders on the radiograph, either (1) elevate the unaffected shoulder by tilting the midsagittal plane toward the film and using a horizontal central ray or (2) position the shoulders on the same transverse plane and angulate the central ray 10 to 15 degrees cephalically.

For both positions, direct the central ray to the midthorax at the level of the affected shoulder. Use

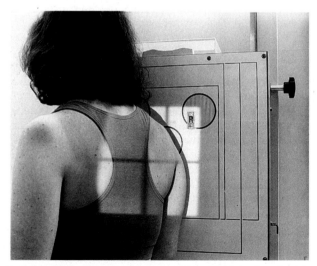

Figure 3-87. Proper trans-scapular Y positioning of patient for proximal humerus fracture.

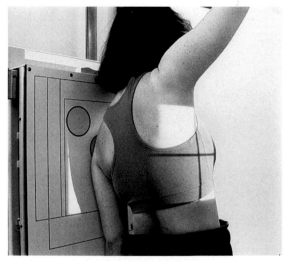

Figure 3–88. Proper transthoracic lateral positioning of patient for proximal humerus fracture.

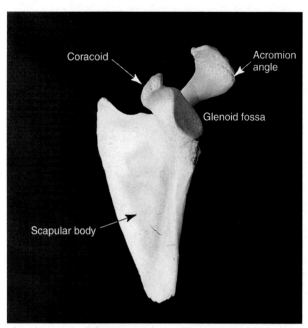

Figure 3–89. Location of acromion angle and coracoid.

breathing technique to blur the vascular lung markings and axillary ribs: A long exposure time (3 seconds) is used while the patient breathes shallowly (costal breathing) during the exposure. An accurately positioned transthoracic radiograph should sharply demonstrate the affected proximal humerus halfway between the sternum and the thoracic vertebrae, without superimposition of the unaffected shoulder (see Rad. 94).

The long axis of the humerus is aligned with the long axis of the collimated field.
- If the patient's humerus can remain aligned with the long axis of the film while the elbow and shoulder joints are included on the film, align the long axis of the collimated light field with the long axis of the humerus to allow for tight transverse collimation. For many adult humeral radiographs, it may be necessary to position the humerus diagonally on the film to include the elbow and shoulder joint. For this positioning, the collimator head or tube column should be turned or rotated to align the long axis of the collimated light field with the long axis of the humerus. (If a grid is used, do not rotate the tube column, or grid cutoff—unwanted absorption of primary radiation—will result.)
- If the collimator head or tube column cannot be adjusted for diagonal positioning, leave the transversely collimated field open enough to include the elbow and shoulder joint. With this setup, the collimated field includes a large portion of the patient's thorax. Hence, the thorax is exposed to unnecessary radiation, which can be protected by laying a flat contact shield across the patient's thorax. Remember to leave at least 3 inches (7.5 cm) of space between the humeral head and the shield to allow for magnifi-

cation, so the shoulder joint is not obscured by the shield.

The humeral midshaft is at the center of the collimated field. The shoulder and elbow joints, the proximal humerus and forearm, and the lateral humeral soft tissue are included within the field.
- To place the humeral midshaft in the center of the radiograph, palpate (1) the acromion angle (Fig. 3–89) for a mediolateral projection or (2) the coracoid for a lateromedial projection as well as the medial epicondyle. Position the central ray with the humeral midshaft at a level halfway between these two palpable landmarks. To include the elbow and shoulder joints on the radiograph, the degree of radiation beam divergence that is used when radiographing a long body part needs to be considered.
- ***Film Length and Positioning:*** Choose a film that is long enough to allow at least 1 inch (2.5 cm) of film to extend beyond each joint space; a 14 × 17 inch (35 × 43 cm) film placed lengthwise should be adequate. On a patient with a long humerus, it may be necessary to position the humerus diagonally on the film to obtain the needed film length. Palpate the joints to ensure that the film extends beyond them. The elbow is located about 0.75 inch (2 cm) proximal to the medial epicondyles. The shoulder joint is located at the same level as the palpable coracoid and acromion angle.
- ***Central Ray Centering and Collimation:*** Once the humerus is accurately positioned with the film and the central ray is centered to the humeral midshaft, open the longitudinal collimated field until it extends 1 inch (2.5 cm) beyond the elbow and shoulder joint. If the collimation does not extend

beyond both joints, adjust the centering point of the central ray until both the elbow and the shoulder joint are included within the collimated field without demonstrating an excessive light field beyond them. Transverse collimation should be to the skin-line laterally and to (1) the lateral scapular border for the mediolateral projection or (2) the coracoid for the lateromedial projection.

Critiquing Radiographs

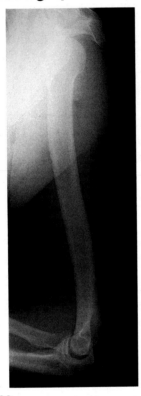

Radiograph 90.

Critique: This is a mediolateral projection. The density is lighter at the proximal humerus than at the distal humerus. The torso was not in a true PA projection but was rotated toward the humerus, increasing the tissue thickness at the proximal humerus.

Correction: Rotate the torso away from the proximal humerus into a true PA projection.

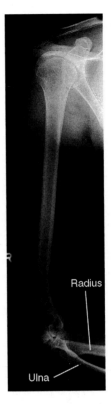

Radiograph 91.

Critique: This is a lateromedial projection. The humerus is not in a lateral position. The epicondyles are not superimposed, the capitulum is posterior to the medial trochlea, and the proximal forearm is distorted. The forearm was positioned across the patient's body and the distal humerus was not drawn away from the table to place the epicondyles perpendicular to the film, as demonstrated in Figure 3–85.

Correction: Position the patient as demonstrated in Figure 3–84, with the distal humerus positioned adjacent to the film, aligning the humeral epicondyles perpendicular to the film.

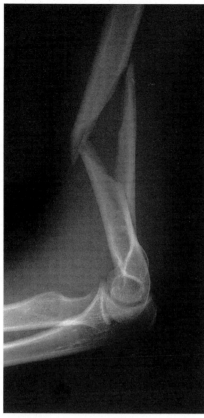

Radiograph 92.

Critique: This is a fractured lateral distal humeral radiograph. The patient was accurately positioned.
Correction: No correction movement is required.

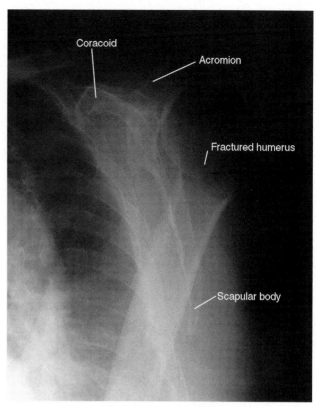

Coracoid

Acromion

Fractured humerus

Scapular body

Radiograph 93.

Critique: This is a trans-scapular Y view of a fractured proximal humerus. The radiograph demonstrates accurate positioning. The scapular body is in a true lateral position. The scapular body, acromion, and coracoid form a Y, with the scapular body as the leg and the acromion and coracoid as the arms.
Correction: No correction movement is required.

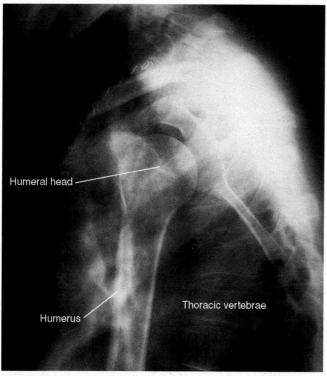

Humeral head

Humerus

Thoracic vertebrae

Radiograph 94.

Critique: This is a transthoracic view of the proximal humerus. This radiograph demonstrates accurate positioning. The unaffected shoulder is superior to the affected shoulder, and the humerus is clearly demonstrated halfway between the thoracic vertebrae and the sternum.
Correction: No correction movement is required.

References

1. Bontrager KL, Anthony BT. Textbook of Radiographic Positioning and Related Anatomy, ed 2. St Louis: CV Mosby, 1987, p 97.
2. Andersen JL, Gron P, Longhoff O. The scaphoid fat stripe in the diagnosis of carpal trauma. Acta Radiologica 29:97–99, 1988.
3. Ramin JE, Terry DW. The navicular fat stripe: A useful roentgen feature for evaluating wrist trauma. AJR 124:25–28, 1975.
4. Epner RA, Bowers WH, Guilford WB. Ulnar variance—the effect of wrist positioning and roentgen filming techniques. J Hand Surg 7:298–305, 1982.
5. Berquist TH. Imaging of Orthopedic Trauma and Surgery. Philadelphia: WB Saunders, 1986, p 643.
6. Farrar EL, Kilcoyne RF. Handbook of Orthopedic Terminology. Boca Raton, FL: CRC Press, 1991.
7. Gilula LA. Carpal injuries: Analytic approach and case exercises. AJR 133:503–517, 1977.
8. Gilula LA. The Traumatized Hand and Wrist. Philadelphia: WB Saunders, 1992, pp 222–226.
9. MacEwan DW. Changes due to trauma in the fat plane overlying the pronator quadratus muscle: A radiologic sign. Radiology 82:879–886, 1964.
10. Gilula LA, Destouet JM, Weeks PM, et al. Roentgenographic diagnosis of the painful wrist. Clin Orthop 187:52–64, 1984.
11. Stecher WR. Roentgenography of the carpal navicular bone. AJR 37:704–705, 1937.
12. Rogers LF. Radiology of Skeletal Trauma. New York: Churchill Livingstone, 1982, pp 532–533.
13. Bushong SC. Radiologic Science for Technologists, ed 4. St. Louis: CV Mosby, 1988, pp 118–119.
14. Griswold R. Elbow fat pads: A radiography perspective. Radiol Technol 53:303–307, 1982.
15. Rogers SL, MacEwan DW. Changes due to trauma in the fat plane overlying the supinator muscle: A radiographic sign. Radiology 92:954–958, 1969.
16. Murry WA, Seigel MJ. Elbow fat pads with signs and extended differential diagnosis. Radiology 124:659–665, 1977.
17. Carroll QB. Fuch's Principles of Radiographic Exposure, Processing and Quality Control, ed 4. Springfield, IL: Charles C Thomas, 1990, p 154.
18. Bushong SC. Radiologic Science for Technologists, ed 5. St. Louis: CV Mosby, 1993.

CHAPTER **4**

Radiographic Critique of the Shoulder

SHOULDER

Anteroposterior Projection

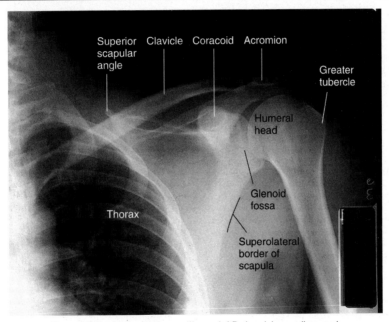

Figure 4-1. Accurately positioned AP shoulder radiograph.

Radiographic Evaluation

Facility's patient identification requirements are visible on radiograph.
- These requirements usually are facility name, patient name, age, and hospital number, and exam time and date.
- The patient ID plate is positioned inferiorly so as not to obscure anatomy of interest.

A right or left marker, identifying correct shoulder, is present on the radiograph and does not superimpose anatomy of interest.
- Place the marker laterally within the collimated light field so it does not superimpose any portion of the shoulder.
- An arrow or word marker should also be used to indicate internal or external humeral rotation.

There is no evidence of preventable artifacts, such as gown snaps, undergarments, slings, and splints.
- Consult with the ordering physician and the patient about whether slings or splints can be removed.

Contrast and density are adequate to demonstrate the surrounding soft tissue and bony structures of the shoulder. Penetration is sufficient to visualize the bony trabecular patterns and cortical outlines of the clavicle, glenoid fossa, coracoid, acromion, and lesser and greater tubercles.
- An optimal 73 to 80 kVp technique with a grid sufficiently penetrates the shoulder girdle and provides contrast that enhances the bony and soft tissue structures of the shoulder. A grid should be used to absorb the scattered radiation produced by the shoulder, reducing fog and providing a higher-contrast radiograph.

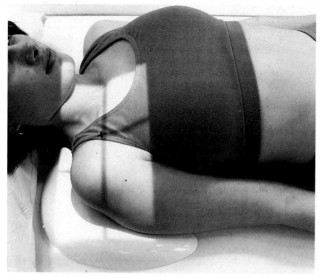

Figure 4-2. Proper neutral AP shoulder positioning with compensating filter.

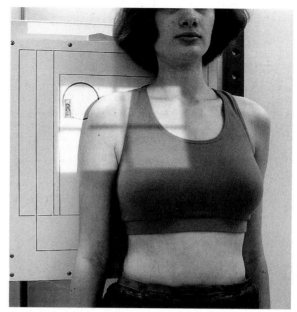

Figure 4-3. Proper neutral AP shoulder positioning.

- When an exposure (mAs) is set that adequately demonstrates the glenohumeral joint, the laterally located acromion and clavicular end are overexposed, because of the difference in AP body thickness between these two regions. A compensating filter placed over or under the lateral clavicle region can be used to obtain uniform density across the entire shoulder (Fig. 4–2).

The bony trabecular patterns and cortical outlines of the proximal humerus and shoulder girdle are sharply defined.

- Sharply defined radiographic details are obtained when patient motion and respiration are halted, when a small focal spot is used, and when a short object–image distance (OID) is maintained.

The shoulder girdle is demonstrated in an AP projection. The scapula is rotated, visualizing the glenoid fossa, the superolateral border of the scapula is seen without thorax superimposition, and the clavicle is demonstrated horizontally, with the medial end of the clavicle positioned next to the lateral vertebral column. When the humeral head is not dislocated, the posterior portion of the glenoid fossa and the medial margin of the humeral head are superimposed.

- A true AP shoulder projection is achieved by placing the patient in either a supine or an upright AP projection, with the shoulders positioned at equal distances from the table or upright grid holder (Fig. 4–3). When the patient is positioned in a true AP projection, the scapular body is at 35 to 45 degrees of obliquity, with the lateral scapula situated more anteriorly than the medial scapula, and the glenoid fossa articulating surface is visualized.

   The amount of scapular obliquity and glenoid fossa visualization depends on the degree of shoulder retraction. Retraction or backward movement of the shoulder is a result of the gravitational pull placed on the shoulder when the patient is in a supine position. It causes the scapular body to be positioned more nearly

parallel with the film. On an AP shoulder projection, the clavicle should be demonstrated horizontally, with the medial end positioned next to the lateral vertebral column without excessive curvature or transverse foreshortening.

- **Upright Positioning for Kyphosis:** For the kyphotic patient there is less patient discomfort if the radiograph is taken in an upright position. If it is not possible to place the kyphotic patient in an upright position, use angled sponges under the shoulders and thorax to place the shoulders at equal distances from the table. A table sponge also helps ease patient discomfort.
- **Detecting Rotation:** Rotation on an AP shoulder radiograph is detected by evaluating the images of the scapular body, glenoid fossa, and clavicle. When the patient is rotated toward the affected shoulder (places affected shoulder closer to film than unaffected shoulder), the scapular body is positioned parallel with the film and appears wider on the radiograph. The thorax superimposes the superolateral scapular region, the glenoid fossa and scapular neck are positioned more in profile, and the clavicle is transversely foreshortened, with the medial clavicular end shifted away from the vertebral column (see Rad. 1). When the patient is rotated away from the affected shoulder, the scapular body demonstrates increased transverse foreshortening, the thorax superimposes a smaller amount of the scapula, the glenoid fossa demonstrates increased visualization, and the medial clavicular end superimposes the vertebral column (see Rad. 2).
- **Effect of Shoulder Dislocation:** The AP shoulder projection is taken to detect shoulder fractures, as well as humeral head dislocations. When the shoulder is not dislocated, the humeral head is centered to and slightly superimposed over the glenoid fossa. Shoulder dislocation can result in positioning of the humeral

head either anterior or posterior and inferior to the glenoid fossa. Anterior dislocation, which is more common (95%), results in the humeral head's being demonstrated anteriorly, beneath the coracoid[2] (see Rad. 3). Posterior dislocations, which are uncommon (2–4%), result in the humeral head's being demonstrated posteriorly, beneath the acromion or spine of the scapula.[2, 3]

The scapular body is demonstrated without longitudinal foreshortening. The coracoid and acromion are at the same level, the superior scapular angle is superimposed by the midclavicle, and the acromion and humeral head demonstrate slight superimposition.

- Foreshortening of the scapula is a result of positioning of the patient's upper midcoronal plane with a forward arch or curve. This foreshortening can be avoided by instructing the patient to arch the upper vertebral column and shoulders posteriorly, until a straight vertebral column is obtained.
- ***Compensating for Kyphosis:*** For the kyphotic patient, little can be done to improve patient positioning, but a cephalic central ray angulation can be used to offset the forward angle of the scapula. The central ray should be angled perpendicular to the scapular body.
- ***Detecting Scapular Foreshortening:*** Radiographically, a foreshortened scapula is demonstrated when the coracoid is visualized inferior to the acromion, the superior scapular angle is projected superior to the clavicle, and the acromion and humeral head are no longer superimposed (see Rad. 4). The severity of foreshortening depends on the degree of forward thoracic curvature.

The humerus is aligned parallel with the body, and the glenoid fossa faces laterally.

- Proper AP shoulder positioning is accomplished with zero humeral abduction. When the humerus is abducted, it is demonstrated away from the body, the glenoid fossa shifts superiorly, and the scapular body glides around the thorax, moving anteriorly (see Rad. 5). The amount of scapular movement demonstrated depends on the degree of humeral abduction.

The glenohumeral joint space and the coracoid are at the center of the collimated field. The glenohumeral joint, the lateral two thirds of the clavicle, the proximal third of the humerus, and the superior scapula are included within the field.

- When the central ray is centered to the palpable coracoid process, the glenohumeral joint is centered within the collimated field. The coracoid can be palpated 0.75 inch (2 cm) inferior to the midpoint of the lateral half of the clavicle and medial to the humeral head (Fig. 4–4). Even on very muscular patients, the concave pocket formed inferior to the lateral half of the clavicle and medial to the humeral head can be used to center the central ray. Beware of using positioning instructions to center the central ray a certain number of

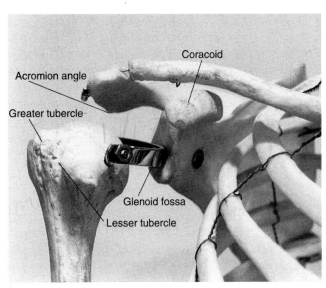

Figure 4-4. Location of coracoid.

inches or centimeters from the top of the shoulder; these methods do not take into account the variance in muscle and fat thickness at the shoulder top of different patients.

- Open the longitudinal collimation enough to include the top of the shoulder. Transverse collimation should be to the lateral humeral skin-line.
- A 10 × 12 inch (24 × 30 cm) film placed crosswise should be adequate to include all the required anatomical structures. The film may be placed lengthwise to visualize more of the humerus.

HUMERAL HEAD POSITIONING

The position of the humeral epicondyles with respect to the film determines which anatomical aspect of the humeral head is demonstrated in profile.

- ***Positioning for Suspected Fracture or Dislocation:*** On a patient with suspected shoulder dislocations or humeral fractures, the humerus should not be rotated. Take the exposure with the humerus positioned as it is.

In *neutral rotation*, the greater tubercle is partially demonstrated in profile laterally, and the humeral head is partially demonstrated in profile medially (see Fig. 4–1).

- Accurate neutral humeral head rotation is accomplished by placing the patient's palm against the thigh and aligning the humeral epicondyles at a 45-degree angle with the film (see Fig. 4–3).

In *external rotation*, the greater tubercle is demonstrated in profile laterally, the humeral head is demonstrated in profile medially, and the vertical cortical outline of the lesser tubercle is visualized about halfway between the greater tubercle and the medial aspect of the humeral head (see Rad. 6).

- Accurate external humeral head rotation is obtained by externally rotating the patient's arm until the humeral epicondyles are aligned parallel with the film (Fig. 4–5).

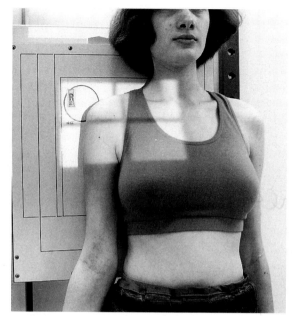

Figure 4–5. Proper external AP shoulder positioning.

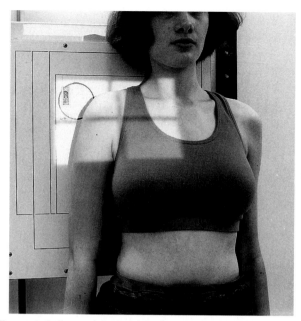

Figure 4–6. Proper internal AP shoulder positioning.

In *internal rotation*, **the lesser tubercle is demonstrated in profile medially, and the humeral head is superimposed by the greater tubercle (see Rad. 7).**
- Accurate internal humeral head rotation is obtained by internally rotating the patient's arm until the humeral epicondyles are aligned parallel with the film (Fig. 4–6).

- Internal humeral rotation may also cause the scapula to move anteriorly, transversely foreshortening the scapular body, and cause the humeral head to demonstrate increased glenoid fossa superimposition.

Critiquing Radiographs

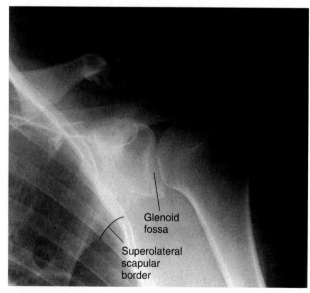

Glenoid
fossa

Superolateral
scapular
border

Radiograph 1.

Critique: The glenoid fossa is nearly in profile, with only a small amount of the articulating surface demonstrated, the superolateral border of the scapula is superimposed by the thorax, and the medial clavicular end has been rolled away from the vertebral column. The patient was rotated toward the affected shoulder.

Correction: Rotate the patient away from the affected shoulder into a true AP projection, with the shoulders positioned at equal distances from the table.

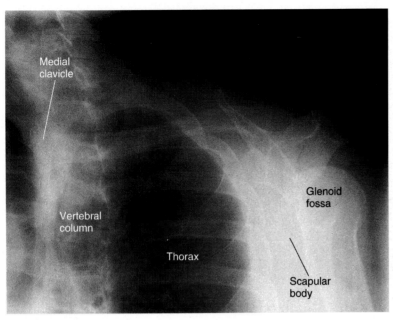

Radiograph 2.

Critique: The scapular body is drawn from beneath the thorax and is foreshortened, the glenoid fossa's articulating surface is demonstrated on end, and the medial clavicular end is superimposing the vertebral column. The patient was rotated toward the unaffected shoulder.

Correction: Rotate the patient toward the affected shoulder into a true AP projection, with the shoulders positioned at equal distances from the table.

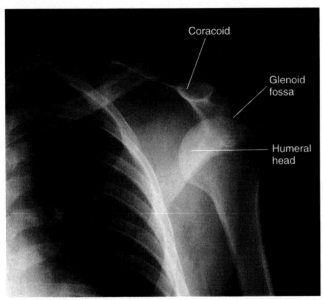

Radiograph 3.

Critique: The humeral head is demonstrated below the coracoid. The patient's shoulder is dislocated.

Correction: No correction movement is needed.

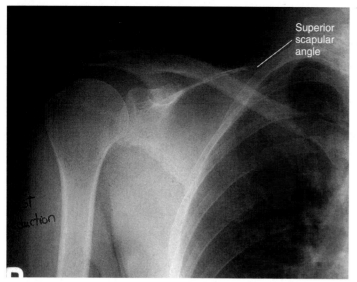

Radiograph 4.

Critique: The coracoid is visualized slightly inferior to the acromion, the superior scapular angle is demonstrated superior to the clavicle, and the acromion and humeral head demonstrate no superimposition. The patient's upper thoracic vertebrae are arched forward.
Correction: Instruct the patient to arch the upper thorax and shoulders posteriorly until a straight vertebral column is obtained. For a kyphotic patient whose vertebral column cannot be straightened, bring the central ray perpendicular to the scapular body by angling it cephalically.

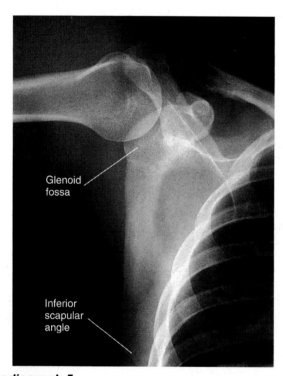

Radiograph 5.

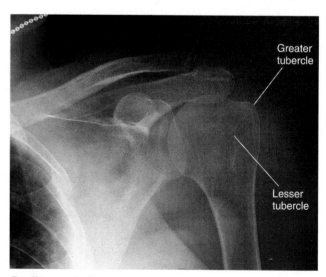

Radiograph 6.

Critique: The humerus is visualized at a 90-degree angle with the body, the glenoid fossa faces superiorly, and the lateral scapular body is drawn away from the thorax. The humerus was abducted.
Correction: Position the humerus next to the patient's body.

Critique: The greater tubercle is demonstrated in profile laterally, and the cortical margin of the lesser tubercle is visualized about halfway between the greater tubercle and the humeral head. The patient's humerus was externally rotated.
Correction: No correction movement is needed if the greater tubercle is wanted in profile. If a neutral position is desired, position the humeral epicondyles at a 45-degree angle with the film (see Fig. 4–3). To demonstrate the lesser tubercle in profile, internally rotate the arm until the humeral epicondyles are perpendicular to the film (see Fig. 4–6).

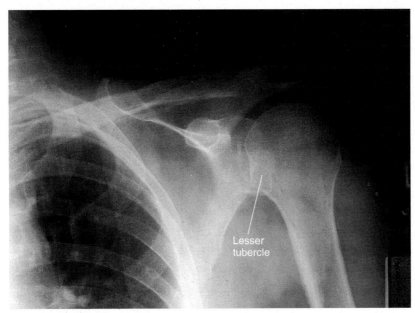

Critique: The lesser tubercle is demonstrated in profile medially, and the greater tubercle and humeral head are superimposed. The patient's humerus was internally rotated.

Correction: No correction movement is needed if the lesser tubercle is wanted in profile. If a neutral position is desired, position the humeral epicondyles at a 45-degree angle with the film (see Fig. 4–3). To demonstrate the greater tubercle in profile, externally rotate the arm until the humeral epicondyles are parallel with the film (see Fig. 4–4).

Radiograph 7.

Shoulder: Axial Position (Inferosuperior Projection)

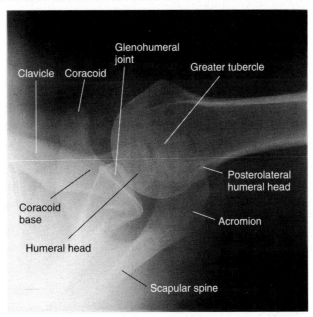

Figure 4–7. Accurately positioned axillary shoulder radiograph.

Radiographic Evaluation

Facility's patient identification requirements are visible on radiograph.

- These requirements usually are facility name, patient name, age, and hospital number, and exam time and date.
- Position the patient ID plate toward the distal humerus so it does not obscure anatomy of interest.

A right or left marker, identifying the correct shoulder, is present on the radiograph and does not superimpose anatomy of interest.

- Place the marker anteriorly within the collimated light field, so it does not superimpose any portion of the shoulder.

There is no evidence of preventable artifacts, such as gown snaps or grid lines.

- If a grid is used for the inferosuperior shoulder projection, the central ray must remain perpendicular to the grid to prevent grid cutoff and grid line artifacts.

Contrast and density are adequate to demonstrate the surrounding soft tissue and bony structures of the shoulder girdle and proximal humerus. Penetration is sufficient to visualize the bony trabecular patterns and cortical outlines of the humeral head, glenoid fossa, coracoid, acromion, and lateral clavicle.

- If the patient's inferosuperior shoulder thickness measurement is under 5 inches (13 cm), a grid is not required. For such a patient, a high-contrast, low (65) kVp technique sufficiently penetrates the bony and soft tissue structures of the shoulder and proximal humerus without causing excessive scattered radiation to reach the film and hinder contrast. If the patient's inferosuperior measurement is over 5 inches (13 cm), a grid should be employed, because this thickness would produce enough scattered radiation to negatively affect radiographic contrast.[1, 4]
- When a grid is used, increase the kVp above 70 to penetrate the thicker shoulder and to provide an adequate scale of contrast. Increase the exposure (mAs) by the standard density conversion factor for the grid ratio being used, to compensate for the scatter and for the primary radiation that the grid will absorb.

The bony trabecular patterns and cortical outlines of the shoulder girdle and proximal humerus are sharply defined.

- Sharply defined recorded details are obtained when patient motion is controlled and a short object–image distance (OID) is maintained.

The inferior and superior margins of the glenoid fossa are nearly superimposed, with only a small amount of humeral head superimposition. The lateral edge of the coracoid base is aligned with the glenoid fossa.

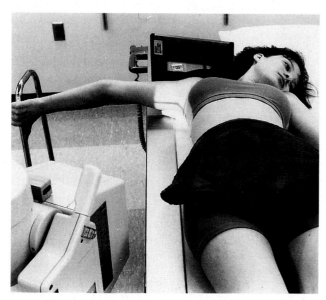

Figure 4-8. Proper axillary shoulder positioning.

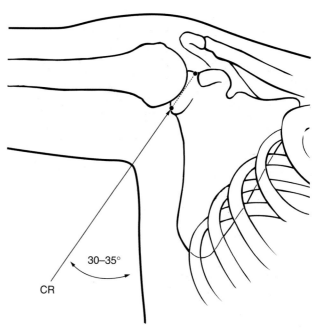

Figure 4-9. Placement of glenoid fossa with arm abducted 90 degrees. *CR*, central ray.

- The axial position of the shoulder is obtained by placing the patient supine on the radiographic table in a true AP projection with the affected shoulder next to the lateral edge of the table. The patient's arm is then abducted 90 degrees from the body, and a horizontal beam is directed to the axilla, parallel with the glenohumeral joint space (Fig. 4–8).
- ***Effect of Humeral Abduction on Central Ray Alignment:*** Because there are no palpable structures to help align the central ray with the glenohumeral joint, we must rely on our knowledge of scapular movement upon humeral abduction to align it. Abduction of the arm is accomplished by combined movements of the glenohumeral joint and the scapula as they glide around the thoracic cavity. The ratio of movement in these two articulations is two parts glenohumeral to one part scapulothoracic, with the initial movement being primarily glenohumeral.[3] If the patient's arm is not abducted, the glenoid fossa is angled about 20 degrees with the lateral body surface.

On a patient who is not experiencing severe pain with the 90-degree humeral abduction, the scapular movement angles the glenoid fossa to about 30 to 35 degrees with the lateral body surface (Fig. 4–9). Consequently, to align the central ray parallel with the glenohumeral joint on such a patient, the angle between the lateral body surface and central ray should be 30 to 35 degrees.

Because the glenoid fossa faces superiorly when the arm is abducted, if a patient is unable to fully abduct the arm, the angle between the lateral body surface and central ray needs to be decreased to align it parallel with the glenohumeral joint (Fig. 4–10). Because the first 60 degrees of humeral abduction involves primarily movement of the glenohumeral joint without accompanying scapular movement, the angle between the central ray and lateral body surface

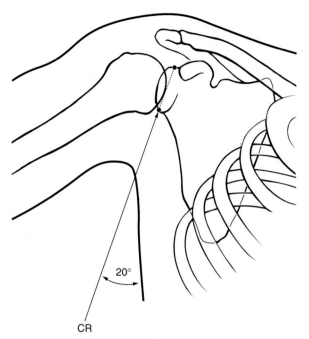

Figure 4-10. Placement of glenoid fossa with arm abducted less than 90 degrees. *CR,* central ray.

should be about 20 degrees when the humerus is abducted up to 60 degrees.

- *Detecting Inaccurate Central Ray Alignment:* Inaccurate alignment of the central ray with the glenohumeral joint space can be signified on a radiograph by the increased demonstration of the glenoid fossa and the greater humeral head superimposition on the glenoid fossa. Whether the angle between the central ray and the lateral body surface should be increased or decreased can be determined by viewing the relationship of the coracoid base to the glenoid fossa. If the glenoid fossa has been projected lateral to the coracoid base, the angle was too small and needs to be increased. (Closely compare the coracoid base and glenoid fossa relationships in Fig. 4–7 and Rad. 8.) If the glenoid fossa has been projected medial to the lateral edge of the coracoid base, the angle was too large and needs to be decreased (see Rad. 9).

Angulation of the cassette with the central ray can cause a small degree of glenohumeral joint distortion. To eliminate this possible distortion, align the central ray with the patient, then position the cassette vertically at the top of the affected shoulder so it is perpendicular to the central ray.

The long axis of the humeral shaft is demonstrated without foreshortening. The proximal humerus is demonstrated without distortion, as indicated by visualization of a portion of the humeral head proximal to the greater tubercle.

- Distortion of the humeral shaft and head can be prevented when the patient's humerus is placed in 90-degree abduction. If the patient is unable to abduct the arm to 90 degrees, the humeral shaft and head demonstrate foreshortening (see Rad. 10). The severity of the distortion present depends on how close to 90

degrees the patient was able to abduct the humerus. The more the humerus is abducted, the less distortion is demonstrated.

The lesser tuberosity is demonstrated in profile anteriorly, and the posterolateral aspect of the humeral head is in profile posteriorly.

- The lesser tubercle and the posterolateral aspect of the humeral head are positioned in profile when the arm is extended, then externally rotated until an imaginary line connecting the humeral epicondyles is as nearly perpendicular to the table as the patient can achieve, and the thumb is pointing toward the floor. This position is often difficult for the patient to hold. It is best to center the central ray and set up the film position before asking the patient to externally rotate the arm. It is also easier for the patient to hold this position if he or she is allowed to grasp an IV pole or foot stand.
- This exaggerated external rotation is especially helpful in identifying a compression fracture of the posterolateral aspect of the humeral head. This compression fracture, a result of an anterior shoulder dislocation, is known as the Hill-Sachs defect.[5] If the arm is extended without exaggerated external rotation, an imaginary line connecting the humeral epicondyles is placed somewhat parallel with the tabletop, the humeral head and neck are in profile posteriorly, and the lesser tubercle is partially in profile anteriorly, but the posterolateral aspect of the humeral head is not visualized (see Rad. 9). If the patient's elbow is flexed so the hand can be used to hold the film in place, the humerus is capable of greater external rotation, and the resulting radiograph demonstrates the greater tubercle in profile posteriorly (see Rad. 8).

The humeral head is centered within the collimated field. The glenoid fossa, coracoid, scapular spine, acromion, and a third of the proximal humerus are included within the field.

- To ensure that the scapular spine is included within the radiograph, elevate the patient's shoulder about 2 inches (5 cm) from the tabletop with a sponge or folded washcloth. If the shoulder is not elevated, the posterior portion of the humerus and shoulder may not be included on the radiograph (see Rad. 11).
- To include the coracoid on the radiograph, instruct the patient to turn the face away from the affected shoulder, then laterally flex the neck and tilt the head toward the unaffected shoulder. Place a cassette at the patient's superior shoulder top, perpendicular to the tabletop and resting snugly against the patient's neck. If the cassette is not positioned snugly against the patient's neck, the coracoid and possibly the glenoid fossa and proximal humerus may not be included on the radiograph (see Rad. 12).
- To align the central ray with the glenohumeral joint, center the central ray horizontally to the midaxillary region at the same level as the coracoid. (Palpate, to locate the coracoid prior to humeral abduction.) This centering does not position the glenohumeral joint in the center of the radiograph, because the film cannot be positioned medially enough to center the joint in the film.

- Open the longitudinal collimation slightly beyond the coracoid, and transversely collimate to the proximal humeral skin-line.
- An 8 × 10 inch (18 × 24 cm) film placed crosswise should be adequate to include all the required anatomical structures.

Critiquing Radiographs

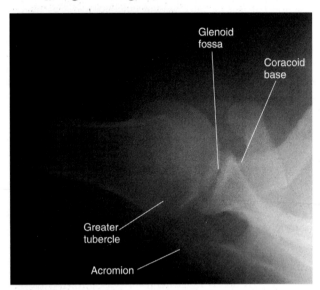

Radiograph 8.

Critique: The glenohumeral joint is obscured, the glenoid fossa is demonstrated lateral to the lateral edge of the coracoid base, and the greater tubercle is in profile posteriorly. The angle formed between the lateral body surface and the central ray was less than required to align the central ray parallel with the glenohumeral joint space. The arm was flexed so the patient's hand could support the film's position.

Correction: Increase the angle between the lateral body surface and the central ray, extend the patient's arm, and use a sandbag to hold the film in the correct position.

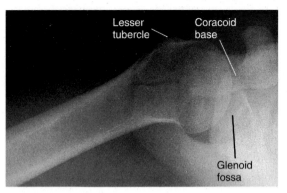

Radiograph 9.

Critique: The glenohumeral joint is obscured, the glenoid fossa is demonstrated medial to the lateral edge of the coracoid base, the humeral neck and head are demonstrated in profile posteriorly, and a portion of the lesser tuberosity is in profile anteriorly. The angle formed between the lateral body surface and the central ray was larger than needed to align the central ray parallel with the glenohumeral joint space, and the arm was extended without exaggerated external rotation.

Correction: Decrease the angle between the lateral body surface and central ray. If the posterolateral aspect of the humeral head is of interest, increase the external rotation of the arm until the thumb is pointing toward the floor.

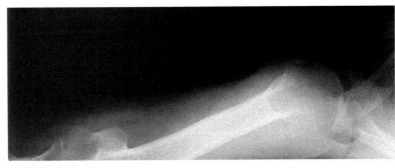

Radiograph 10.

Critique: The glenoid fossa and coracoid are accurately demonstrated, but the humerus has been severely foreshortened. The arm was not abducted 90 degrees from the body.
Correction: If possible, have the patient abduct the humerus 90 degrees from the body. If patient cannot abduct the humerus, no correction movement is needed.

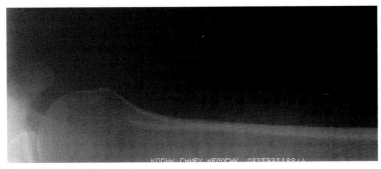

Radiograph 11.

Critique: The acromion, scapular spine, and posterior aspect of the proximal humerus are not included on the radiograph. The patient's shoulder was not adequately elevated off the tabletop.
Correction: Elevate the shoulder at least 2 inches (5 cm) off the tabletop with a sponge or folded washcloth.

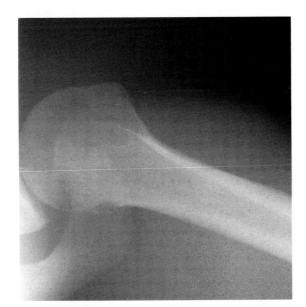

Radiograph 12.

Critique: The coracoid and a portion of the glenoid fossa are not included on the radiograph. The patient's head was not turned or tilted enough toward the unaffected shoulder to adequately position the film medially.
Correction: Turn the patient's face, and tilt the head toward the unaffected shoulder. Then snugly position the edge of the cassette against the patient's neck.

Shoulder: Glenoid Cavity (Fossa) Position (Grashey Method)

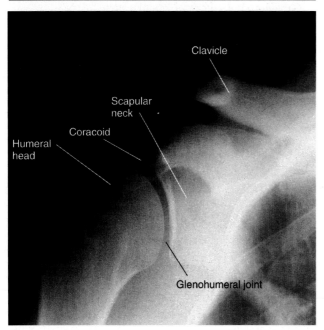

Figure 4–11. Accurately positioned Grashey shoulder radiograph.

Radiographic Evaluation

Facility's patient identification requirements are visible on radiograph.

- These requirements usually are facility name, patient name, age, hospital number, and exam time and date.
- The patient ID plate does not obscure anatomy of interest.

A right or left marker, identifying the correct shoulder, is present on the radiograph and does not superimpose anatomy of interest.

- Place the marker laterally within the collimated light field so it does not superimpose any portion of the shoulder or humerus.

There is no evidence of preventable artifacts, such as gown snaps, undergarments, and slings.

- Consult with the ordering physician and the patient about whether a shoulder sling can be removed.

Contrast and density are adequate to demonstrate the surrounding soft tissue and bony structures of the shoulder. Penetration is sufficient to visualize the bony trabecular patterns and the cortical outlines of the scapular neck, glenoid fossa, humeral head, and coracoid.

- An optimal 73 to 80 kVp technique sufficiently penetrates the shoulder and provides radiographic contrast that will enhance the shoulder's bony and soft tissue structures. A grid should be used to absorb the scattered radiation produced by the shoulder, reducing fog and further improving radiographic contrast.

The bony trabecular patterns and cortical outlines of the scapular neck, glenoid fossa, and humeral head are sharply defined.

- Sharply defined radiographic details are obtained when patient motion and respiration are halted, a small focal spot is used, and a short object–image distance (OID) is maintained.

The glenoid fossa is demonstrated in profile, the glenohumeral joint space is open, and the lateral coracoid demonstrates about 0.25 inch (0.6 cm) of superimposition of the humeral head. The clavicle is transversely foreshortened.

- To obtain a radiograph that demonstrates the glenoid fossa in profile and an open glenohumeral joint space, the patient's scapular body must be positioned parallel with the film. This is accomplished by placing the patient in an upright AP projection, then rotating the patient's body about 45 degrees toward the affected shoulder (Fig. 4–12). A 45-degree posterior oblique position routinely opens the glenohumeral joint space as long as the patient is upright and the affected shoulder is in a neutral position without protraction.
- **Effect of Shoulder Protraction on the Required Degree of Patient Obliquity:** Protraction or forward movement of the shoulder occurs as a result of pressure that is placed on the affected shoulder when the patient leans against the upright grid holder. The sternoclavicular and acromioclavicular joints function cooperatively to allow the shoulder to be drawn forward. When the shoulder is drawn forward, the scapula glides around the thorax, moving the lateral portion of the scapula anteriorly.[3] This increase in forward shoulder positioning places the scapular body at a larger angle with the film, thus

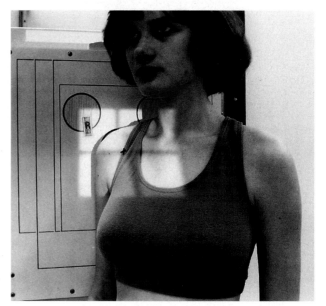

Figure 4–12. Proper positioning for Grashey shoulder radiograph.

requiring an increase in patient obliquity to bring the scapular body parallel with the film for the Grashey method.

An increase in patient obliquity is also necessary when the exam is performed on a kyphotic or supine patient. Because of the vertebral column curvature, the kyphotic patient's shoulders are situated anteriorly, aligning them similarly to protracted shoulders. In the supine position, the shoulder of interest is forced forward by the pressure of the body on the shoulder when the patient is rotated. In both of these situations, a radiograph can be obtained that demonstrates the glenoid fossa in profile and an open glenohumeral joint space, although they are often superimposed by the thoracic cavity. On such a radiograph the anatomical relationships of the bony structures can still be seen, but the soft tissue structures are difficult to evaluate (see Rad. 13).

- ***Recommended Method of Determining Degree of Body Obliquity:*** The most accurate method of determining the amount of patient obliquity needed for all Grashey shoulder radiographs is to palpate the patient's coracoid and acromion angle, then rotate the patient toward the affected shoulder until the coracoid superimposes the acromion angle, aligning an imaginary line connecting them perpendicular to the film (Fig. 4–13).
- ***Detecting Incorrect Obliquity:*** Inadequate body obliquity can be identified on a radiograph as a closed glenohumeral joint space.

Whether the body has been rotated too much or too little can be determined by viewing the relationship of the coracoid with the humeral head and by observing the degree of transverse clavicle foreshortening. If obliquity was excessive, the glenohumeral joint space is closed, more than just the lateral tip of the coracoid superimposes the humeral head, and the clavicle demonstrates excessive transverse foreshortening (see Rad. 14). If obliquity was insufficient, the glenohumeral joint space is closed, the lateral tip of the coracoid demonstrates very little if any superimposition of the humeral head, and the clavicle demonstrates little foreshortening (see Rad. 15).

- ***Evaluating the Supine or Kyphotic Patient's Radiograph:*** When evaluating a Grashey radiograph on a supine or kyphotic patient, you cannot use the clavicle as a guide to determine repositioning because the clavicle always demonstrates excessive foreshortening (see Rad. 16). For these radiographs, use only the coracoid position as the repositioning guide.
- ***Repositioning for Grashey View:*** When repositioning for an excessive or insufficient obliquity on a Grashey view, remember that the glenohumeral joint space is narrow, and the needed repositioning movement is only half of the distance demonstrated between the anterior and posterior margins of the glenoid fossa. In most cases, you need to move the patient only a few degrees to obtain an open joint space, so it is important to carefully evaluate and make mental notes on how the patient was positioned for the initial exam. If a repeat is needed, start with the patient position used for the initial exam; then adjust the position from this starting point.

The glenoid fossa is facing laterally and the clavicle is horizontal.

- When the shoulders are positioned on the same transverse plane, the glenoid fossa faces laterally and the clavicle is positioned horizontally. If the affected shoulder is elevated, the glenoid fossa faces upward, and the clavicle is aligned somewhat vertically (see Rad. 17).

The glenohumeral joint is at the center of the collimated field. The glenoid fossa, humeral head, coracoid, acromion, and distal clavicle are included within the field.

- Center a perpendicular central ray with the palpable coracoid process to place the glenohumeral joint at the center of the collimated field. The coracoid can be palpated 0.75 inch (2 cm) inferior to the midpoint of the lateral half of the clavicle and medial to the humeral head. Even on very muscular patients, the concave pocket formed inferior to the lateral half of the clavicle and medial to the humeral head can be used to center the central ray.
- Open the longitudinal collimated field enough to include the shoulder top and transversely collimate to the lateral humeral skin-line.
- An 8 × 10 inch (18 × 24 cm) film placed lengthwise or crosswise should be adequate to include all the required anatomical structures.

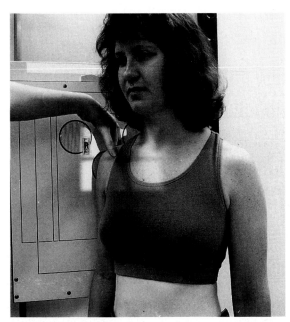

Figure 4–13. Alignment of coracoid and acromion for Grashey shoulder radiograph.

Critiquing Radiographs

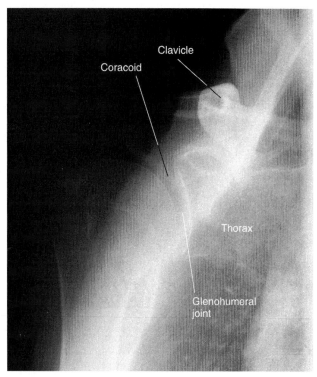

Radiograph 13.

Critique: The glenohumeral joint space is open, and the lateral tip of the coracoid is superimposing the humeral head. The clavicle demonstrates excessive foreshortening, and the thorax is superimposing the glenohumeral joint space. Either the patient was kyphotic or the radiograph was taken with the patient leaning against the upright grid holder or in a supine position. The shoulder and scapula were protracted, and the patient was rotated more than the 45 degrees to obtain an open glenohumeral joint space.

Correction: If the patient is kyphotic or the exam had to be performed with the patient in a recumbent position, no repositioning movement is required. If the patient was leaning against the upright grid holder, position the patient's upper midcoronal plane in a vertical position, and place the affected shoulder in a neutral position. Less patient obliquity will be required with this new positioning.

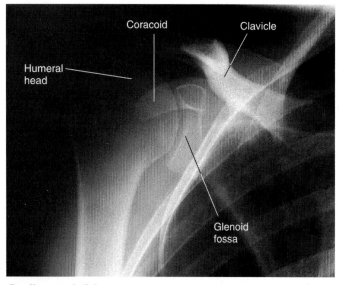

Radiograph 14.

Critique: The glenohumeral joint space is closed, more than 0.25 inch (0.6 cm) of the lateral tip of the coracoid is superimposing the humeral head, and the clavicle demonstrates excessive transverse foreshortening. Patient obliquity was excessive.

Correction: Decrease the degree of patient obliquity. The amount of decrease required is only half of the distance between the anterior and posterior margins of the glenoid fossa.

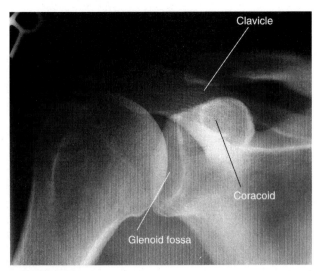

Radiograph 15.

Critique: The glenohumeral joint space is closed, the lateral tip of the coracoid does not superimpose the humeral head, and the clavicle demonstrates little foreshortening. Patient obliquity was insufficient.

Correction: Increase the degree of patient obliquity, thus moving the coracoid toward the humeral head and shifting the anterior and posterior margins of the glenoid fossa toward each other.

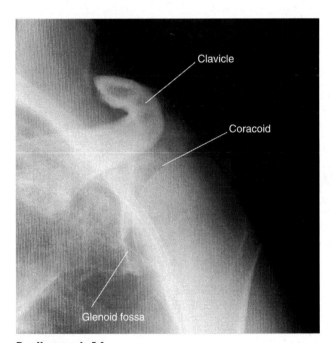

Radiograph 16.

Critique: The clavicle demonstrates excessive foreshortening, and the thorax is superimposing the glenohumeral joint space. The glenohumeral joint space is closed, and more than the lateral coracoid tip superimposes the humeral head. The affected shoulder was protracted and patient obliquity was excessive.

Correction: If possible, position the patient's upper midcoronal plane vertically, and place the shoulders in a neutral position. Decrease the degree of patient obliquity.

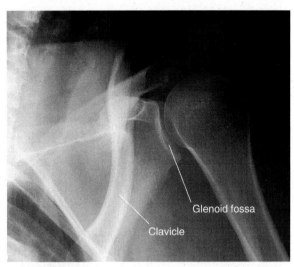

Radiograph 17.

Critique: The glenoid fossa is facing upward, and the clavicle is vertical. The affected shoulder was elevated above the unaffected shoulder.

Correction: Position the shoulders on the same transverse plane.

Shoulder: Anterior Oblique Position
(Trans-scapular Y Position)

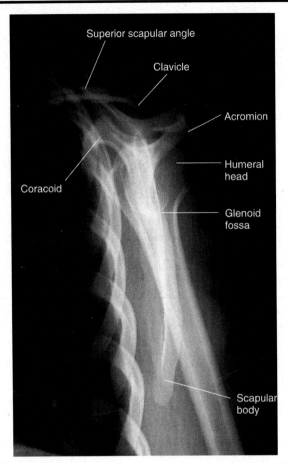

Figure 4–14. Accurately positioned trans-scapular Y shoulder radiograph.

Radiographic Evaluation

Facility's patient identification requirements are visible on radiograph.

- These requirements usually are facility name, patient name, age, and hospital number, and exam time and date.
- The patient ID plate does not obscure anatomy of interest.

A right or left marker, identifying the correct shoulder, is present on the radiograph and does not superimpose anatomy of interest.

- Place the marker laterally within the collimated light field so it does not superimpose any portion of the scapula or humerus.

There is no evidence of preventable artifacts, such as gown snaps, undergarments, and slings.

- Consult with the ordering physician and the patient about whether the shoulder sling can be removed.

Contrast and density are adequate to demonstrate the surrounding soft tissue and bony structures of the

shoulder. **Penetration is sufficient to visualize the bony trabecular patterns and the cortical outlines of the glenoid fossa, humeral head, acromion, and coracoid.**

- An optimal 75 to 80 kVp technique sufficiently penetrates the scapular body and demonstrates the outline of the glenoid fossa while still providing contrast that will enhance other bony and soft tissue shoulder structures.
- A grid should be used to absorb the scattered radiation produced by the shoulder, reducing fog and further improving radiographic contrast.

The bony trabecular patterns and cortical outlines of the glenoid fossa and humeral head are sharply defined.

- Sharply defined radiographic details are obtained when patient motion and respiration are halted, a small focal spot is used, and a short object–image distance (OID) is maintained.
- The standing anterior oblique patient position places the scapula closest to the film, resulting in the least amount of scapular magnification and the greatest scapular detail.

The scapular body is in a true lateral position. The lateral and vertebral (medial) scapular borders are superimposed, and the scapular body does not superimpose the thoracic cavity. The scapular body, acromion, and coracoid form a Y, with the scapular body as the leg and the acromion and coracoid as the arms. The glenoid fossa is demonstrated on end at the converging point of the arms and leg of the Y.

- To place the scapular body in a lateral position, begin by placing the patient in an upright PA projection, with the affected arm dangling freely. This nonelevated arm position aligns the vertebral border of the scapula parallel with the film, allowing the coracoid and the acromion to be demonstrated in profile. From this PA projection, rotate the patient's body toward the affected scapula until the lateral and vertebral scapular borders are superimposed (Fig. 4–15).
- ***Amount of Body Obliquity Required:*** The degree of body obliquity required to superimpose the scapular borders for the trans-scapular Y position has been questioned. Some radiographic positioning textbooks state that the midcoronal plane should form a 60-degree angle with the film.[6, 7] This degree of obliquity originated from the observations made by Rubin and colleagues[8] of the Y shoulder formation while they were evaluating 60-degree oblique chest radiographs. A later study of the trans-scapular Y position presented by De Smet[9] in 1979 found that a 45-degree anterior oblique was the optimal obliquity for this view.

   The controversy between these two observations may lie in the position of the humerus. For a 60-degree anterior oblique chest radiograph, the patient's humerus is abducted and the hand is placed on the patient's crest. When the patient is rotated, the shoulder is retracted (drawn backward). This humerus and shoulder positioning causes the scapula to glide around the thoracic cavity, moving toward the spinal column. When the scapula is in this posterior position,

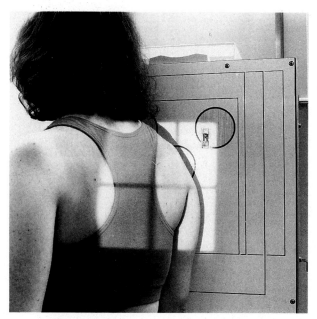

Figure 4–15. Proper trans-scapular Y positioning.

the patient's body needs to be rotated more to bring the scapular body lateral. The 1979 report by De Smet[9] states that the humerus is to hang freely. Because the humerus and shoulder are not forced backward when the arm dangles freely, the scapula is positioned slightly more anteriorly, thus needing less obliquity to bring it into a lateral position.

- ***Recommended Method of Determining Degree of Body Obliquity:*** I have found that the best method of determining the correct degree of patient obliquity is to palpate the scapular anatomy. First, palpate the coracoid and the acromion angle, and locate the midpoint of an imaginary line drawn between them. Next, locate the medial border of the scapula. Rotate the patient toward the affected shoulder until the medial scapular border is aligned with a point midway between the acromion and coracoid. This positioning sets up the Y formation with the scapular body positioned between the acromion and coracoid. Once the correct obliquity is determined, have the patient step toward the film until the patient's shoulder just touches the upright grid and film holder. The exact degree of obliquity varies from patient to patient, depending on shoulder roundness, arm position, and pressure placed on the shoulder when patient touches the film holder.
- ***Posterior Oblique Positioning:*** For a patient who is supine, the trans-scapular Y position can be obtained by performing a posterior oblique radiograph. Palpate the acromion, coracoid, and vertebral scapular borders in the same way as described for the standing anterior oblique position, and rotate the patient toward the unaffected shoulder until the vertebral scapular border lies midway between the acromion and coracoid. The anatomical relationship of the bony structures of the scapula should be aligned identically on anterior and posterior oblique Y view radiographs. The posterior oblique radiograph, however, demon-

strates increased magnification of the scapula and humerus (see Rad. 18).
- ***Detecting Mispositioning:*** If the patient obliquity is not accurate for the trans-scapular Y position, the Y formation of the scapula is not formed, the medial and lateral borders of the scapular body are not superimposed but are visualized next to each other, and the glenoid fossa is not demonstrated on end.

  To determine whether patient obliquity needs to be increased or decreased to superimpose the scapular body and position the glenoid fossa on end, identify the borders of the scapula. The lateral border is thick, with a rough appearance, whereas the cortical outline of the vertebral border demonstrates a single thin line. If the lateral border is demonstrated next to the ribs, and the vertebral border is visualized laterally, patient obliquity was excessive (see Rad. 19). If the vertebral border is demonstrated next to the ribs and the lateral border is visualized laterally, patient obliquity was insufficient to superimpose the borders (see Rad. 20).

If the shoulder is *not* dislocated, the humeral head superimposes directly over the glenoid fossa. When the shoulder has been dislocated, the scapular Y formation should be demonstrated as described previously, although the humeral head is seen either anterior or posterior to the glenoid fossa.
- One indication for the trans-scapular Y position is to determine whether a shoulder dislocation exists and, if so, whether it is dislocated anteriorly or posteriorly. When the shoulder is being radiographed to rule out a dislocation or a scapular or humeral head fracture, the patient's humerus should not be moved but should be allowed to dangle freely. The position of the humeral head in relation to the glenoid fossa should not be a positioning concern to the radiographer. As long as the scapula is positioned in a Y formation, proper positioning has been obtained.
- ***Detecting Shoulder Dislocation:*** The cortical outline of the glenoid fossa is visualized as a circular density at the junction of the coracoid, acromion, and scapular body. Normally, the humeral head is superimposed over this junction. When the humeral head is not positioned over the glenoid fossa, a shoulder dislocation exists and will result in positioning of the humeral head either anterior or posterior and inferior to the glenoid fossa. An anterior dislocation, which is more common (95%), results in the humeral head's being demonstrated anteriorly, beneath the coracoid[2] (see Rad. 21). A posterior dislocation, which is uncommon (2–4%), results in the humeral head's being demonstrated posteriorly, beneath the acromion[2, 3] (Fig. 4–16).

The scapula is demonstrated without longitudinal foreshortening and the superior scapular angle is superimposing the clavicle.
- Longitudinal foreshortening of the scapula is prevented when the patient's shoulders remain on the same transverse plane and the midcoronal plane remains vertical. The most common way to cause fore-

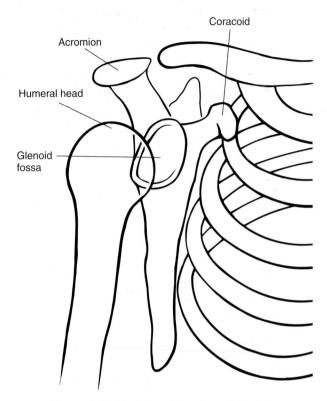

Figure 4-16. Posterior dislocation of shoulder.

shortening of the scapula is to lean the patient's upper midcoronal plane and shoulder toward the film. This forward position causes the glenoid fossa, acromion, and coracoid to project inferiorly and the superior scapular angle and spine to project superiorly. Radiographically, a longitudinally foreshortened scapula demonstrates the superior scapular angle above the clavicle and the scapular spine above the acromion (see Rad. 22).

- **Positioning for Kyphosis:** On a patient with spinal kyphosis, the scapula is longitudinally foreshortened because of the forward curvature of the vertebral column. To offset this curvature and obtain a scapula without foreshortening, the central ray may be angled perpendicular to the vertebral scapular border. This angulation can be obtained by palpating the vertebral scapular border and aligning the central ray perpendicular to it. For anterior oblique views, the angulation would be caudal, and for posterior oblique views, the angulation would be cephalic.

The midscapular body is at the center of the collimated field. The entire scapula, which includes the inferior angle, coracoid, and acromion, and the proximal humerus are included within the field.

- To place the midscapular body in the center of the collimated field, center a perpendicular central ray to the vertebral border of the scapula halfway between the inferior scapular angle and the acromial angle. Each of these anatomical structures is palpable and should be used to ensure accurate positioning.

- Open the longitudinal collimation enough to include the acromion and inferior scapular angles. Transverse collimation should be to the lateral humeral skin-line.
- A 10 × 12 inch (24 × 30 cm) film placed lengthwise should be adequate to include all the required anatomical structures.

Critiquing Radiographs

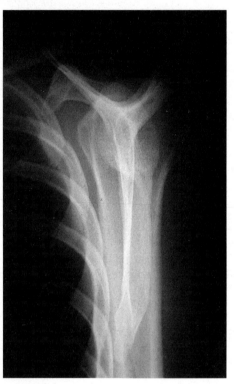

Radiograph 18.

Critique: The vertebral and lateral borders of the scapular body are superimposed, the coracoid and acromion form the upper arms of a Y, and the cortical outline of the glenoid fossa is visualized at the Y's arm and leg junction. The patient was accurately positioned. Note the increased amount of magnification of the scapula and humerus compared with the radiograph shown in Figure 4–14. This radiograph was taken with the patient in a posterior oblique position.

Correction: No correction movement is needed. If the patient can stand, the anterior oblique position would demonstrate less magnification.

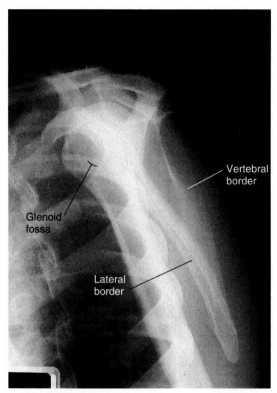

Radiograph 19.

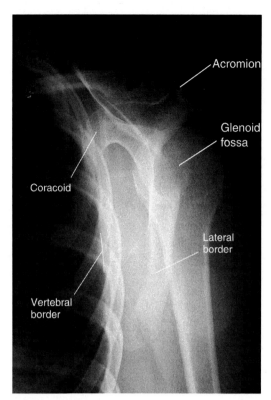

Radiograph 20.

Critique: The lateral and vertebral borders of the scapula are demonstrated without superimposition, and the glenoid fossa is not demonstrated on end, but is seen medially. The lateral scapular border is demonstrated next to the ribs, and the vertebral border is visualized laterally. The patient was rotated more than needed to superimpose the scapular body.
Correction: Decrease the patient obliquity. The amount of decrease is half the distance demonstrated between the vertebral and lateral scapular borders.

Critique: The lateral and vertebral borders of the scapula are demonstrated without superimposition, and the glenoid fossa is not demonstrated on end, but is seen laterally. The vertebral scapular border is demonstrated next to the ribs, whereas the lateral border is visualized laterally. The patient was not rotated enough to superimpose the scapular body.
Correction: Increase the patient obliquity.

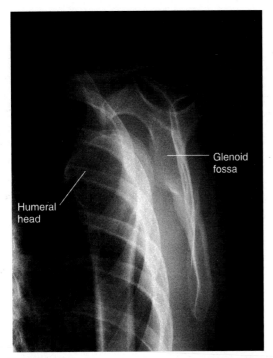

Radiograph 21.

Critique: The scapular body, acromion, and coracoid are accurately positioned into a Y formation, and the cortical outline of the glenoid fossa is demonstrated at the junction of the arms and leg of the Y. The humeral head is demonstrated anterior to the glenoid fossa, directly inferior to the coracoid. The shoulder is anteriorly dislocated.

Correction: No correction movement is required.

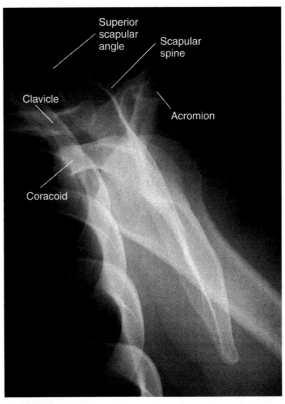

Radiograph 22.

Critique: The scapular body, acromion, and coracoid are accurately aligned, but the superior scapular angle is demonstrated superior to the coracoid, and the spine is demonstrated superior to the acromion. The scapula is foreshortened. The patient's upper midcoronal plane and shoulder were leaning forward.

Correction: Position the patient with the shoulders on the same transverse plane and the midcoronal plane vertical.

CLAVICLE

Anteroposterior Projection

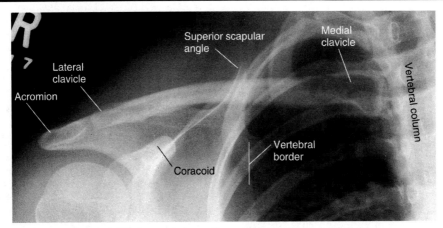

Figure 4-17. Accurately positioned AP clavicular radiograph.

Radiographic Evaluation

Facility's patient identification requirements are visible on radiograph.
- These requirements usually are facility name, patient name, age, hospital number, and exam time and date.
- The patient ID plate does not obscure anatomy of interest.

A right or left marker, identifying the correct clavicle, is present on the radiograph and does not superimpose anatomy of interest.
- Place the marker laterally within the collimated light field so it does not superimpose any portion of the clavicle.

There is no evidence of preventable artifacts, such as gown snaps, undergarments, and slings.
- Consult with the ordering physician and the patient about whether a sling can be removed.

Contrast and density are adequate to demonstrate the surrounding soft tissue and bony structures of the clavicle. Penetration is sufficient to visualize the bony trabecular patterns and cortical outlines of the clavicle.
- An optimal 73 to 80 kVp technique sufficiently penetrates the clavicle and provides contrast that will enhance the bony and soft tissue structures of the shoulder. A grid should be used to absorb the scattered radiation produced by the shoulder, reducing fog and providing a higher contrast radiograph.
- Because the anteroposterior shoulder thickness varies at either end of the clavicle, it is difficult to set an exposure (mAs) that adequately demonstrates the entire clavicle on the same radiograph. An exposure set to visualize the medial (sternal) end overexposes the lateral end, and an exposure set to visualize the lateral end underexposes the medial end. To even out this density difference and demonstrate both ends of the clavicle adequately on the same radiograph, position a compensating filter over or under the lateral end of the clavicle. With the exposure set to adequately demonstrate the medial end, the compensating filter absorbs some of the x-ray photons that would normally overexpose the lateral end, resulting in uniform clavicular density.

The bony trabecular patterns and cortical outlines of the clavicle are sharply defined.
- Sharply defined radiographic details are obtained when patient motion and respiration are halted, when a small focal spot is used, and a short object–image distance (OID) is maintained.
- Although a PA projection would position the clavicle closer to the film, resulting in less magnification and greater radiographic detail, the AP projection is the more commonly performed because it causes less patient discomfort during positioning and allows the clavicle to be easily palpated.

The clavicle is demonstrated in a true AP projection. The medial end lies next to the lateral edge of the vertebral column, and the thoracic cavity superimposes

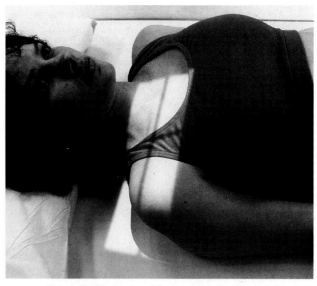

Figure 4-18. Proper AP clavicular positioning.

the vertebral scapular border and a small amount of the scapular body.
- A true AP projection of the clavicle is obtained by placing the patient in either a supine or upright position with the shoulders at equal distances from the table or upright film holder (see Fig. 4–18).
- ***Positioning for Kyphosis:*** For the kyphotic patient, there is less patient discomfort if the radiograph is taken with the patient in an upright position. If it is not possible to place the kyphotic patient in an upright position, use angled sponges under the shoulders and thorax to place the shoulders at equal distances from the table. A table sponge also helps with patient comfort.
- ***Detecting Clavicular Rotation:*** Rotation on an AP clavicle radiograph is detected by evaluating the relationships of the medial clavicle with the vertebral column and of the scapular body with the thoracic cavity. If the patient is rotated away from the affected clavicle, the medial end of the clavicle superimposes the vertebral column and the scapular body moves away from the thoracic cavity (see Rad. 23). If the patient is rotated toward the affected clavicle, the medial end of the clavicle draws away from the vertebral column, the thoracic cavity demonstrates increased superimposition of the scapular body, and the clavicle is transversely foreshortened (see Rad. 24).

The clavicle and scapula are demonstrated without inferosuperior foreshortening. The lateral clavicular end aligns with the most superior portion of the acromion, and the midclavicle superimposes the superior scapular angle.
- Inferosuperior foreshortening of the clavicle and scapula results when the patient's upper midcoronal plane was allowed to arch forward. This forward positioning can often be avoided by instructing the patient to arch the upper thorax and shoulders backwards, straightening the vertebral column.

- *Angulation for Kyphosis:* For the kyphotic patient, little can be done to improve positioning, but a cephalic central ray angulation can be used to offset the forward angle of the scapula. The central ray should be angled enough to align it perpendicular to the scapular body.
- *Detecting Inferosuperior Foreshortening:* Radiographically, inferosuperior foreshortening of the clavicle and scapula is demonstrated when the entire lateral end of the clavicle superimposes the scapular spine and when the superior scapular angle is projected superior to the midclavicle (see Rad. 25).

The midclavicle is at the center of the collimated field. The lateral, middle, and medial thirds of the clavicle and the acromion are included within the field.

- The midclavicle is located by palpating the medial and lateral ends of the clavicle and centering the central ray halfway between them.
- Open the longitudinal and transverse collimation enough to include all aspects of the medial and lateral clavicular ends.
- A 10 × 12 inch (24 × 30 cm) film placed crosswise should be adequate to include all the required anatomical structures.

Critiquing Radiographs

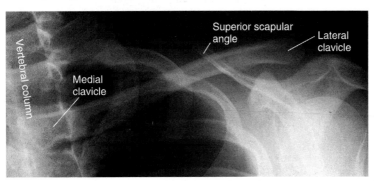

Radiograph 23.

Critique: The medial end of the clavicle is superimposing the vertebral column, and the vertebral border of the scapula is positioned away from the thoracic cavity. The patient was rotated away from the affected clavicle for this radiograph.

Correction: Place the patient in a true AP projection by rotating the patient toward the affected clavicle. The shoulders should be placed at equal distances from the film.

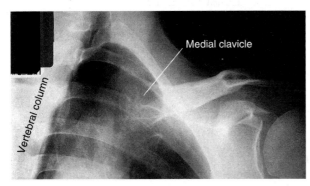

Radiograph 24.

Critique: The medial end of the clavicle is drawn away from the vertebral column, the vertebral and lateral borders of the scapula are superimposed by the thoracic cavity, and the clavicle is transversely foreshortened. The patient was rotated toward the affected shoulder for this radiograph.

Correction: Place the patient in a true AP projection by rotating the patient away from the affected clavicle. The shoulders should be placed at equal distances from the film.

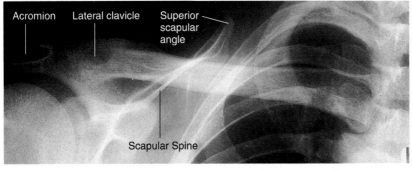

Radiograph 25.

Critique: The lateral end of the clavicle superimposes the scapular spine, and the superior scapular angle is projected above the midclavicle. The clavicle and scapula have been inferosuperiorly foreshortened.

Correction: Instruct the patient to arch the upper thorax and shoulders backwards, straightening the upper vertebral column and midcoronal plane.

Clavicle: Anteroposterior Axial Position

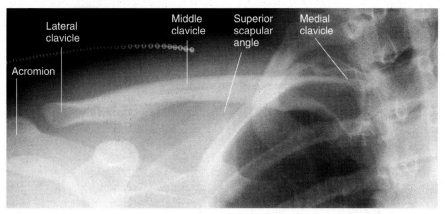

Figure 4–19. Accurately positioned AP axial clavicular radiograph.

Radiographic Evaluation

Facility's patient identification requirements are visible on radiograph.

- These requirements usually are facility name, patient name, age, and hospital number, and exam time and date.
- The patient ID plate does not obsure anatomy of interest.

A right or left marker, identifying the correct clavicle, is present on the radiograph and does not superimpose anatomy of interest.

- Place the marker laterally within the collimated light field, so it does not superimpose any portion of the clavicle.
- An arrow marker pointing cephalad should be used to indicate that a cephalic central ray angulation was used.

There is no evidence of preventable artifacts, such as gown snaps, undergarments, and slings.

- Consult with the ordering physician and the patient about whether a sling can be removed.

Contrast and density are adequate to demonstrate the surrounding soft tissue and bony structures of the clavicle. Penetration is sufficient to visualize the bony trabecular patterns and the cortical outlines of the clavicle.

- An optimal 73 to 80 kVp technique sufficiently penetrates the clavicle and provides contrast that enhances the bony and soft tissue structures of the shoulder. A grid should be used to absorb the scattered radiation produced by the shoulder, reducing fog and providing a higher contrast radiograph.
- Because the anteroposterior shoulder thickness varies at either end of the clavicle, it is difficult to set an exposure (mAs) that adequately demonstrates the entire clavicle on the same radiograph. To even out this density difference and adequately demonstrate both ends of the clavicle on the same radiograph, position

a compensating filter over or under the lateral clavicle. With an exposure set to adequately demonstrate the medial (sternal) end of the clavicle, the compensating filter absorbs some of the x-ray photons that would normally overexpose the lateral end, resulting in uniform clavicular density.

The bony trabecular patterns and cortical outlines of the clavicle are sharply defined.

- Sharply defined radiographic details are obtained when patient motion and respiration are halted, a small focal spot is used, and a short object–image distance (OID) is maintained.
- Although a PA projection would position the clavicle closer to the film, resulting in less magnification and greater radiographic detail, the AP projection is more commonly performed, because it produces less patient discomfort during positioning and allows the clavicle to be easily palpated.

The clavicle is demonstrated in an AP axial projection without body rotation. The medial end of the clavicle lies next to the lateral edge of the vertebral column, and the thoracic cavity superimposes the vertebral scapular border and a small amount of the scapular body.

- An AP axial projection of the clavicle is accomplished by placing the patient in either a supine or upright position with shoulders positioned at equal distances from the table or upright film holder (see Fig. 4–20).
- **Detecting Clavicular Rotation:** Rotation on an AP axial clavicle radiograph is detected by evaluating the relationships of the medial clavicle with the vertebral column and of the scapular body with the thoracic cavity. If the patient is rotated away from the affected clavicle, the medial end of the clavicle superimposes the vertebral column, and the scapular body moves away from the thoracic cavity. If the patient is rotated toward the affected clavicle, the medial end of the clavicle is drawn away from the vertebral column, the thoracic cavity demonstrates

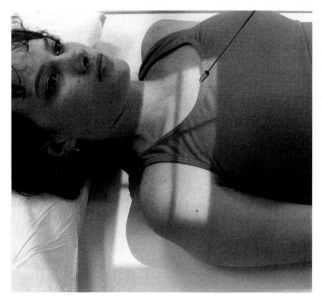

Figure 4-20. Proper AP axial clavicular positioning.

imposes the scapula and ribs. This is why the routine views for a clavicle include an axial projection. An axial projection is accomplished by angulating the central ray 15 to 30 degrees cephalically when it is taken in an AP projection. Even though the amount of angulation used may vary with the radiography department, all radiographs result in superior projection of the clavicle. The larger the angle, the farther superior the clavicle is projected. Ideally, because 80 percent of clavicle fractures occur at the middle third and 15 percent at the lateral third, the central ray should be angled enough to project the lateral and middle thirds of the clavicle superior to the thorax and scapula.[2]

Compare Radiographs 26 and 27, and note how an increase in cephalic angulation has projected the lateral and middle thirds of the clavicle above the scapula. The clavicle fracture demonstrated on these radiographs is quite obvious, but one can see that a subtle nondisplaced fracture could be obscured by the scapular structures if an AP axial projection were not included in the exam.

increased superimposition of the scapular body, and the clavicle is transversely foreshortened (see Rads. 23 and 24; rotation results on the AP and AP axial are the same, but the clavicle on the AP axial projection would be situated more superiorly).

The medial end of the clavicle superimposes the first and second ribs, the middle and lateral thirds of the clavicle are demonstrated superior to the acromion, and the clavicle bows slightly upward.

- It is difficult to demonstrate a nondisplaced fracture of the clavicle on the AP projection, because it super-

The midclavicle is at the center of the collimated field. The lateral, middle, and medial thirds of the clavicle and the acromion are included within the field.

- The midclavicle is located by palpating the lateral and medial ends of the clavicle and centering the central ray just inferior to the clavicle, halfway between the ends.
- Open the longitudinal and transverse collimation enough to include all aspects of the lateral and medial clavicular ends.
- A 10 × 12 inch (24 × 30 cm) film placed crosswise should be adequate to include all the required anatomical structures.

Critiquing Radiographs

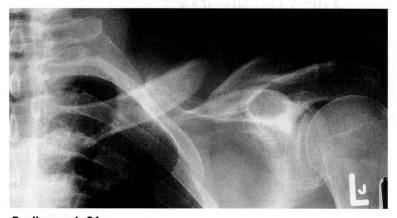

Radiograph 26.

Critique: The lateral and middle thirds of the clavicle are superimposed by the scapula. The cephalic central ray angulation was not adequate to project the lateral and middle thirds of the clavicle superior to the scapula.

Correction: Increase the cephalic central ray angulation. A starting guideline would be to increase the angle 5 degrees for every 0.25 inch (0.6 cm) you want the clavicle to move. For this radiograph, the central ray angle should be increased about 20 degrees.

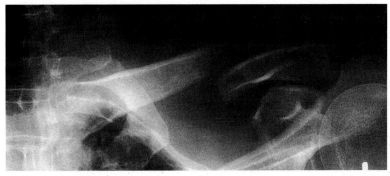

Radiograph 27.

Critique: The lateral and middle thirds of the clavicle are projected above the scapula. A displaced fracture of the middle third of the clavicle is evident.

Correction: No correction movement is needed.

ACROMIOCLAVICULAR (AC) JOINT

Anteroposterior Projection

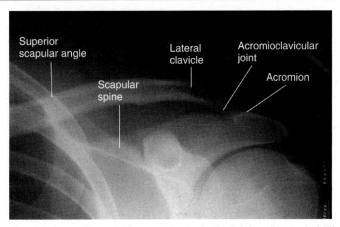

Figure 4-21. Accurately positioned AP acromioclavicular joint radiograph (without weights).

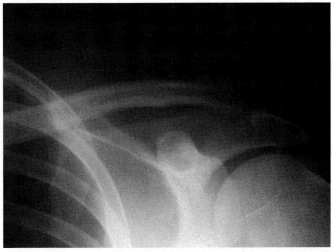

Figure 4-22. Accurately positioned AP acromioclavicular joint radiograph (with weights).

Radiographic Evaluation

Facility's patient identification requirements are visible on radiograph.

- These requirements usually are facility name, patient name, age, and hospital number, and exam time and date.
- The patient ID plate does not obscure anatomy of interest.

A right or left marker, identifying the correct acromioclavicular (AC) joint, is present on the radiograph. The weight-bearing radiograph displays an arrow marker pointing downward. Markers do not superimpose anatomy of interest.

- Place the marker(s) laterally within the collimated light field, without superimposing any portion of the clavicle.
- Two AP radiographs are taken of the AC joint, one with the patient holding weights and one without weights. To discern one from the other, an arrow marker should be placed, pointing downward, on the weight-bearing radiograph.

There is no evidence of preventable artifacts, such as gown snaps, undergarments, and slings.

- Consult with the ordering physician and the patient about whether a sling can be removed.

Contrast and density are adequate to demonstrate the surrounding soft tissue and bony structures of the lateral clavicle and acromion. Penetration is sufficient to visualize the bony trabecular patterns and the cortical outlines of the lateral clavicle and acromion.

- If the patient's anteroposterior AC joint area measurement is under 5 inches (13 cm), a grid is not required. For such a patient, an optimal 50 to 60 kVp technique sufficiently penetrates the bony and soft tissue structures of the AC joint without causing excessive scattered radiation to reach the film and hinder contrast. If the patient's anteroposterior AC joint area measurement is over 5 inches (13 cm), a grid should be employed, because this thickness would produce enough scattered radiation to negatively affect radiographic contrast.[1, 4]
- When a grid is used, increase the kVp above 70 to penetrate the thicker shoulder and to provide an adequate scale of contrast, and increase the exposure (mAs) by the standard density conversion factor for the grid ratio being used, to compensate for the scatter and for the primary radiation that the grid will absorb.

The bony trabecular patterns and cortical outlines of the lateral clavicle and acromion are sharply defined.

- Sharply defined radiographic details are obtained when patient motion and respiration are halted, a small focal spot is used, and a short object–image (OID) is maintained.

The lateral clavicle and acromion are demonstrated in a true AP projection. The lateral clavicle is nearly horizontal and there is approximately 0.125 inch (0.3 cm) of space between the lateral clavicle and the acromial apex.

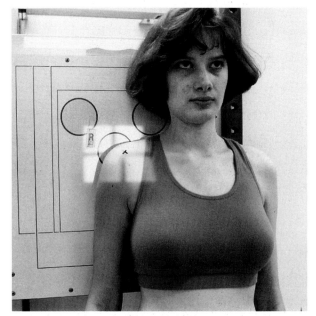

Figure 4–23. Proper AP acromioclavicular joint positioning (without weights).

- An AP projection of the AC joint is obtained by placing the patient in an upright position with both shoulders positioned at equal distances from the upright film holder (Fig. 4–23).
- **_Weight-Bearing AC Joint Radiographs:_** To evaluate the AC joint for possible injury to the acromioclavicular ligament—which extends between the lateral clavicular end and the acromion—the AP projection should be taken first without weights. Then a second AP projection should be taken with the patient holding 10 to 15 lb (4.5 to 7 kg) weights (Fig. 4–24). If there is injury to the acromioclavicular

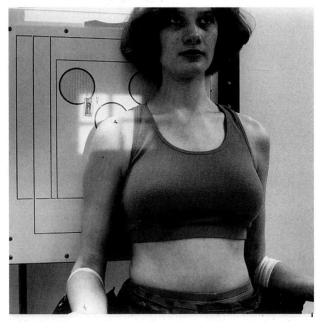

Figure 4–24. Proper AP acromioclavicular joint positioning (with weights).

ligament, the AC joint space is wider on the weight-bearing radiograph than on the radiograph taken without weights.

For the weight-bearing radiograph, equal weights should be attached to the arms regardless of whether the exam is unilateral (one side) or bilateral (both sides), keeping the shoulders on the same transverse plane. Attach the weights to the patient's wrists or slide them onto the patient's forearms after the elbows are flexed to 90 degrees, and instruct the patient to allow the weights to depress the shoulders.

- ***Detecting Rotation:*** Rotation on an anteroposterior AC joint radiograph is detected by evaluating the relationships of the lateral clavicle with the acromion apex and of the scapular body with the thoracic cavity. If the patient was rotated toward the affected AC joint, the lateral end of the clavicle and the acromion apex are rotated out of profile, resulting in a narrowed or closed AC joint. The thoracic cavity also moves toward the scapular body, increasing the amount of scapular body superimposition (see Rad. 28, right shoulder). If the patient is rotated away from the affected AC joint, the lateral end of the clavicle and the acromion apex demonstrate a slightly greater AC joint space with only a small amount of rotation and may be closed with a greater degree of rotation. The scapular body demonstrates decreased thoracic cavity superimposition (see Rad. 28, left shoulder).

The lateral clavicle and acromion are demonstrated without inferosuperior foreshortening. The lateral clavicle is demonstrated without superimposing the acromion or scapular spine.

- Inferosuperior foreshortening of the clavicle and acromion results when the patient's upper midcoronal plane is allowed to arch forward. This forward positioning can often be avoided by instructing the patient to arch the upper thorax and shoulders backwards, straightening the vertebral column.
- ***Positioning for Kyphosis:*** For the kyphotic patient little can be done to improve patient positioning, but a cephalic central ray angulation can be used to offset the forward angle of the scapula. The central ray should be angled enough to align it perpendicular to the scapular body.
- ***Detecting Inferosuperior Foreshortening:*** Radiographically, inferosuperior foreshortening of the clavicle and acromion is demonstrated when the lateral clavicle superimposes the acromion and scapular spine (see Rad. 29).

The AC joint of interest is at the center of the collimated field on a unilateral AC joint radiograph; the lateral clavicle and the acromion are included within the field. The vertebral column is at the center of the collimated field on a bilateral AC joint radiograph; the clavicles and AC joints are included within the field.

- ***Unilateral AC Joint Radiograph:*** Center a perpendicular central ray to the AC joint of interest. The AC joint is located by palpating along the clavicle until the most lateral tip is reached, then moving about 0.5 inch (1 cm) inferiorly. Open the longitudinally

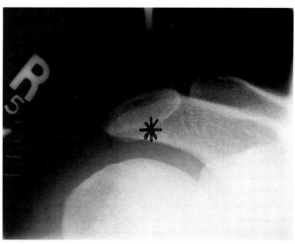

Figure 4-25. Acromioclavicular joint radiograph taken without weights and showing good centering. Star indicates location of central ray.

and transversely collimated field to about a 4-inch (10-cm) field size. An 8 × 10 inch (18 × 24 cm) film placed crosswise should be adequate to include all the anatomical structures.

- ***Bilateral AC Joint Radiograph:*** Center a perpendicular central ray to the midsagittal plane at a level 1.5 inch (4 cm) superior to the jugular notch. Open the longitudinally collimated field to about a 4-inch (10-cm) field size; the transversely collimated field should be left open the full length of the film size used. A 14 × 17 inch (35 × 43 cm) film placed crosswise should be adequate to include all the anatomical structures. For patients who have broad shoulders and do not fit both on a film this size, it may be necessary to take each AC joint separately, as described previously. This method is not recommended, since it unnecessarily exposes the thyroid and uses diverged x-rays to record the AC joints.
- ***Ensuring Identical Central Ray Alignment:*** Repalpate for the AC joint or mark on the patient

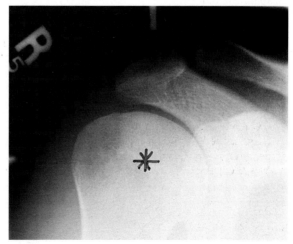

Figure 4-26. Acromioclavicular joint radiograph taken with weights and showing poor centering. Star indicates location of central ray.

where the central ray was positioned for the first radiograph taken, to ensure that the same centering is obtained when the patient is given weights. Because the shoulders are depressed when weights are used, the AC joint moves inferiorly. If the central ray is not centered the same for both radiographs, x-ray beam divergence may result in a false reading. Compare Figures 4–25 and 4–26, radiographs of the same patient, taken without weights and with weights, respectively. One must wonder whether the separation demonstrated on the weight-bearing radiograph is due to ligament injury or poor central ray centering.

Critiquing Radiographs

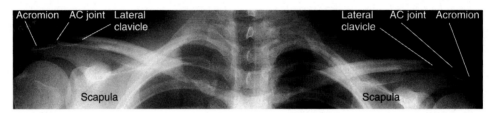

Radiograph 28.

Critique: The right AC joint is closed, and the right scapular body demonstrates greater thoracic superimposition than the left; the left AC joint is open. The patient was rotated onto the right shoulder.

Correction: Rotate the patient toward the left shoulder until the shoulders are at equal distances from the film.

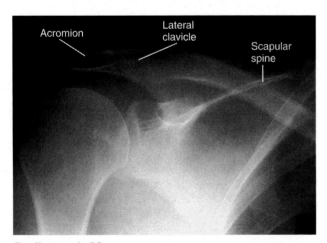

Radiograph 29.

Critique: The lateral end of the clavicle superimposes on the acromion and the scapular spine. The clavicle and acromion have been inferosuperiorly foreshortened.

Correction: Instruct the patient to arch the upper thorax and shoulders backwards, straightening the upper vertebral column and midcoronal plane.

SCAPULA

Anteroposterior Projection

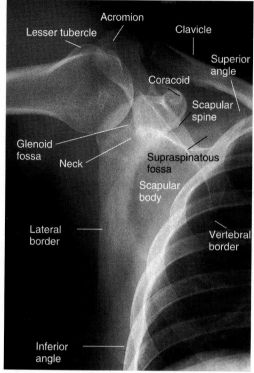

Figure 4-27. Accurately positioned AP scapular radiograph.

Radiographic Evaluation

Facility's patient identification requirements are visible on radiograph.

- These requirements usually are facility name, patient name, age, and hospital number, and exam time and date.
- The patient ID plate does not obscure anatomy of interest.

A right or left marker, identifying the correct scapula is present on the radiograph and does not superimpose anatomy of interest.

- Place the marker laterally within the collimated light field, so it does not superimpose any portion of the scapula.

There is no evidence of preventable artifacts, such as gown snaps, undergarments, and slings.

- Consult with the ordering physician and the patient about whether a sling can be removed.

Contrast and density are adequate to demonstrate the surrounding soft tissue and bony structures of the scapula. Penetration is sufficient to visualize the bony trabecular patterns and the cortical outlines of the scapular neck and body, acromion, coracoid, and glenoid fossa.

- An optimal 70 to 75 kVp technique sufficiently penetrates the scapular, shoulder, and thoracic structures and provides contrast that will enhance the bony and soft tissue structures of the scapula. A grid should be used to absorb the scattered radiation that is produced by the shoulder and thoracic cavity, reducing fog and further improving radiographic contrast.
- ***Radiographic Density of Shoulder Girdle and Thoracic Cavity:*** Although the anteroposterior thickness is about the same across the entire scapula, the overall radiographic density is not uniform. Radiographically, the medial portion of the scapula, which is superimposed by the thoracic cavity, demonstrates darker density than the lateral scapula, which is superimposed by the soft tissue of the shoulder girdle. This radiographic density difference is a result of the difference in density (number of atoms per given area) that exists between the thoracic cavity and the shoulder soft tissue.

  The thoracic cavity is largely composed of air, which contains very few atoms in a given area, whereas the same area of soft tissue contains many compacted atoms. As the radiation goes through the patient's body, fewer photons are absorbed in the thoracic cavity than in the shoulder girdle, because there are fewer atoms in the thoracic cavity for the photons to interact with. Consequently, more photons penetrate the thoracic cavity to expose the film than penetrate the shoulder girdle.

  Taking the exposure on expiration can help to decrease the radiographic density of the portion of the scapula that is superimposed by the thoracic cavity, by reducing the air and slightly compressing the tissue in this area. If the AP scapular radiograph is taken on inspiration, the medial scapular body demonstrates increased density (see Rad. 30).

The bony trabecular patterns and cortical outlines of the scapula are sharply defined.

- Sharply defined radiographic details are obtained when patient motion is controlled, a small focal spot is used, and a short object–image distance (OID) is maintained.
- Patient respiration also determines how well the scapular details are demonstrated. Some positioning textbooks suggest that a breathing technique be used to better visualize the vertebral border and medial scapular body through the air-filled lungs.[6, 7] Although visualization of this anatomy would be improved with such a technique, it is difficult to obtain a long enough exposure time (3 seconds) to adequately blur the ribs and vascular lung markings when the overall exposure (mAs) needed for an AP scapula radiograph is so small. If an adequate exposure time cannot be set to use breathing technique, the exposure should be taken on expiration.

The scapula is demonstrated in an AP projection without transverse or longitudinal foreshortening. The anterior and posterior margins of the glenoid fossa are nearly superimposed.

- When the patient's body is positioned in a true AP projection with the arms against the sides, the scapular body is placed at a 35 to 45 degree angle with the film, with the lateral scapula situated more anteriorly than the medial scapula. This positioning results in transverse foreshortening of the scapular body.

- **Methods of Positioning for an AP Scapular Projection:** There are two ways in which the patient can be positioned to obtain a true AP projection of the scapular body. The first method, referred to as the Grashey method, is accomplished by rotating the patient toward the affected scapula. Precise positioning and evaluating points on this view can be further studied by referring to the Grashey method discussion of this book (page 176). The second method, which is the preferred method because it draws the lateral aspect of the scapula from beneath the thoracic cavity, leaves the patient's body in an AP projection. An AP scapular radiograph is obtained by abducting the humerus, then supinating the hand and flexing the elbow to externally rotate the arm (Fig. 4–28). Each of these arm movements, with the sternoclavicular and acromioclavicular joints, works to retract (force backward) the shoulder. When the humerus is abducted and the shoulder retracted, the scapula glides around the thoracic surface, moving the scapula laterally and posteriorly.[3] This movement of the scapula places it in an AP projection. To take advantage of gravity and obtain maximum shoulder retraction, take the radiograph with the patient in a supine position.

- **Detecting Poor Shoulder Retraction:** Mispositioning of the scapula can be identified by evaluating the image of the scapular body and glenoid fossa. If the patient's arm is not sufficiently externally rotated and abducted, and the shoulder sufficiently retracted, the transverse scapular body is foreshortened and the glenoid fossa is demonstrated somewhat on end (see Rad. 31).

- **Detecting Longitudinal Foreshortening:**

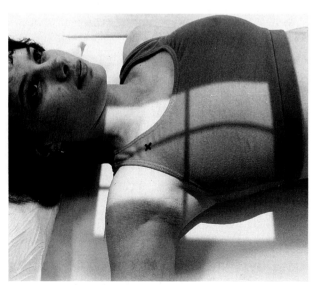

Figure 4-28. Proper AP scapular positioning.

Longitudinal foreshortening of the scapular body is caused by poor midcoronal plane positioning and most often results when the AP scapular radiograph is taken in the upright position or on a kyphotic patient. To prevent such foreshortening, position the patient's midcoronal plane vertically when the patient is upright. Radiographically, a foreshortened scapula is demonstrated when the coracoid is visualized inferior to the clavicle, and the acromion and humeral head are no longer superimposed (see Rad. 4).

- **Angulation for Kyphosis:** Longitudinal foreshortening of the scapular body on the kyphotic patient cannot be improved with patient positioning, but a cephalic central ray angulation can be used to offset the forward angle of the scapula. Angle the central ray to align it perpendicular to the scapular body.

The lateral border of the scapula is demonstrated without thoracic cavity superimposition, and the supraspinatous fossa and the superior border of the scapula are demonstrated without superimposition of the clavicle. The thoracic cavity superimposes the vertebral (medial) border of the scapula. The humeral shaft demonstrates at least 90 degrees of abduction.

- Visualizing the lateral portion of the scapula with adequate density often causes the medial scapula, which is superimposed by the thoracic cavity, to demonstrate excessive density. To increase the proportion of scapular body located "outside" the thoracic cavity, the humerus should be abducted.

- **Effect of Humeral Abduction:** Abduction of the humerus is accomplished by combined movements of the shoulder joint and rotation of the scapula around the thoracic cage. The ratio of movement in these two articulations is two parts glenohumeral to one part scapulothoracic.[3] When the arm is abducted, the lateral scapula is drawn from beneath the thoracic cavity, and the glenoid fossa is elevated. It takes at least 90 degrees of humeral abduction to demonstrate the lateral border without thoracic cavity superimposition, and the supraspinatous fossa and superior angle without clavicle superimposition. The farther the arm is abducted, the more of the lateral scapular body is demonstrated without thoracic cavity superimposition. If the arm is not abducted, the inferolateral border of the scapula is superimposed by the thoracic cavity and the clavicle superimposes the supraspinatous fossa and superior scapular angle (see Rad. 32).

- **Positioning for Trauma:** Trauma patients often experience great pain with arm abduction. Because of this pain, the abduction movement takes place almost entirely at the glenohumeral articulation, instead of using the combined movements of the glenohumeral and scapulothoracic articulations. When the scapulothoracic articulation is not involved with the movement of humeral abduction, the inferolateral border and inferior angle of the scapula remain superimposed by the thoracic cavity, and the supraspinatous fossa and superior border remain superimposed by the clavicle (see Rad. 30). In this situation, little can be done to draw the scapula away from the thoracic cavity, although one can take the exposure on expiration and use a technique that better demonstrates the parts of the scapula superimposed by the thorax.

The midscapular body is at the center of the collimated field. The entire scapula, consisting of the inferior and superior angles, the coracoid, acromion, and glenoid fossa, is included within the field.

- To ensure that the entire scapula, from the coracoid to the inferior angle, is included on the radiograph, center a perpendicular central ray about 3 inches (7.5 cm) inferior to the palpable coracoid. The coracoid can be palpated 0.75 inch (2 cm) inferior to the midpoint of the lateral half of the clavicle and medial to the humeral head. Even on very muscular patients, the concave pocket formed inferior to the lateral half of the clavicle and the medial humeral head can be used to center the central ray. The coracoid should be palpated prior to abducting the arm. This positioning accurately aligns the horizontal and transverse aspects of the scapula. If the arm can not be adequately abducted, the transverse centering should be 0.50 inch (1 cm) more medial.
- Once the central ray has been centered, open the longitudinal collimation to the top shoulder skin-line. Transverse collimation should be to the lateral body skin-line.
- A 10 × 12 inch (24 × 30 cm) film placed lengthwise should be adequate to include all the required anatomical structures.

Critiquing Radiographs

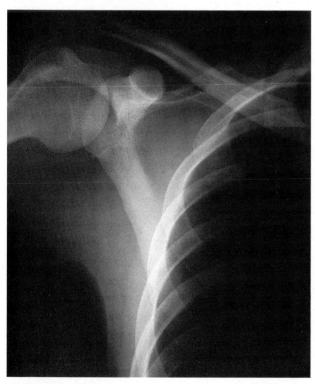

Radiograph 30.

Critique: The portion of the scapula superimposed by the thoracic cavity demonstrates excessive density. The exam was taken on inspiration. Although the humerus demonstrates nearly 90 degrees of abduction, the inferolateral border is superimposed by the thorax, because of the pain the patient experienced when the arm was abducted.

Correction: Take the exposure on expiration or use a breathing technique.

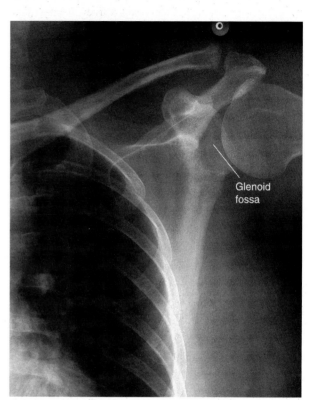

Radiograph 31.

Critique: The transverse axis of the scapular body is foreshortened, and the glenoid fossa is demonstrated. This AP scapular radiograph was taken with the patient in an upright position, resulting in insufficient shoulder retraction.

Correction: Place the patient supine to maximize shoulder retraction, or instruct the patient to retract the shoulder toward the film.

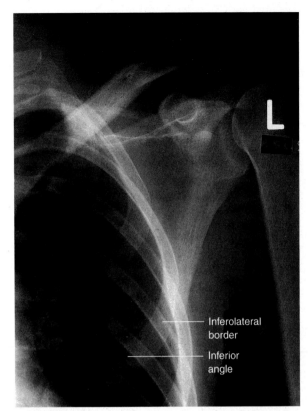

Radiograph 32.

Critique: The inferolateral border of the scapula is superimposed by the thoracic cavity, and the superior angle is superimposed by the clavicle. The humeral shaft is not abducted 90 degrees with the body.

Correction: Abduct the humerus 90 degrees from the body. This adjustment will draw the inferolateral border of the scapula away from the thoracic cavity and shift the superior angle away from the clavicle.

Scapula: Lateral Position
(Lateromedial or Mediolateral Projection)

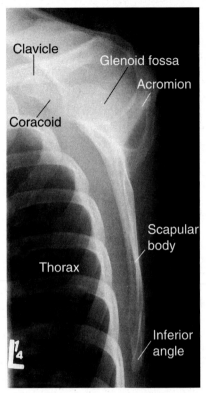

Figure 4-29. Accurately positioned lateral scapular radiograph.

Radiographic Evaluation

Facility's patient identification requirements are visible on radiograph.

- These requirements usually are facility name, patient name, age, and hospital number, and exam time and date.
- The patient ID plate does not obscure anatomy of interest.

A right or left marker, identifying the correct scapula, is present on the radiograph and does not superimpose anatomy of interest.

- Place the marker laterally and within the collimated light field so it does not superimpose any portion of the scapula.

There is no evidence of removable artifacts such as gown snaps, undergarments, and slings.

- Consult with the ordering physician and the patient about whether a sling can be removed.

Contrast and density are adequate to demonstrate the surrounding scapular soft tissue and bony structures of the scapula. Penetration is sufficient to visualize the bony trabecular patterns and the cortical outlines of

the scapular body, acromion, coracoid, and superior angle of the scapula.

- An optimal 75 to 80 kVp technique sufficiently penetrates the scapular body and provides the contrast needed to enhance the bony and soft tissue scapular structures.
- A grid should be used to absorb the scattered radiation produced by the shoulder, reducing fog and improving radiographic contrast.

The bony trabecular patterns and cortical outlines of the scapula are sharply defined.

- Sharply defined radiographic details are obtained when patient motion is controlled, a small focal spot is used, and a short object–image distance (OID) is maintained.
- The standing anterior oblique position places the scapula closer to the film, resulting in less scapular magnification and greater scapular detail.

The scapular body is in a true lateral position. The lateral and vertebral (medial) scapular borders are superimposed, and the scapular body is demonstrated without superimposing the thoracic cavity.

- The scapular body is placed in a lateral position by first placing the patient in an upright PA projection with the affected arm drawn across the chest so the hand can grasp the unaffected shoulder. From this position, rotate the patient's body toward the affected scapula until the lateral and vertebral scapular borders are superimposed (Fig. 4–30).
- The degree of body obliquity required to superimpose the scapular borders depends on the degree of humeral elevation. As the humerus is elevated, the inferior angle of the scapula glides around the thoracic cage, moving the scapula more anteriorly.[3] The more the

scapula glides around the thorax, the less body obliquity is required to superimpose the vertebral and lateral scapular borders.

- To position the scapular body perpendicular to the film and demonstrate it with the least amount of foreshortening, elevate the arm to a 90-degree angle with the body.
- The proper degree of body rotation for any arm position is determined by palpating the lateral and vertebral scapular borders. Because the superior portions of the lateral and vertebral borders are heavily covered with muscles, it is best to palpate them just superior to the inferior scapular angle.[10] Adjusting the arm position slightly while palpating can also help in locating the scapular borders and inferior angle. Once these anatomical structures are located, rotate the patient's body until the vertebral border of the scapula superimposes the lateral border and the inferior scapular angle is positioned in profile.
- ***Positioning the Supine Patient:*** For the supine patient, a lateral scapula radiograph is accomplished by placing the patient in a posterior oblique position. The lateral and vertebral scapular borders and the inferior scapular angle should be palpated using the same method as described for the standing patient; however, the patient is rotated toward the unaffected shoulder to superimpose the vertebral and lateral scapular borders and place the inferior angle in profile (Fig. 4–31).
- ***Detecting Inaccurate Rotation:*** If the body was not accurately rotated for a lateral scapular radiograph, the borders of the scapula are not superimposed, but are visualized next to each other. When such a radiograph has been produced, one can determine whether patient obliquity was excessive or insufficient by identifying the scapular borders. The lateral

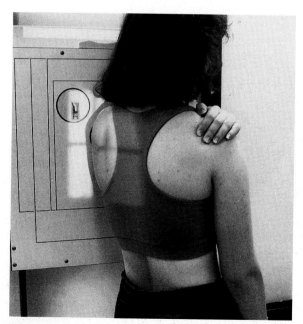

Figure 4–30. Proper standing lateral scapular positioning.

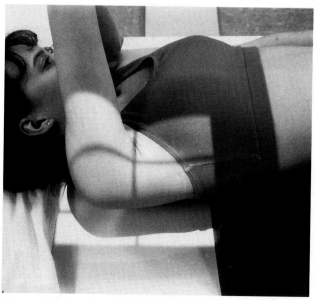

Figure 4–31. Proper recumbent lateral scapular positioning.

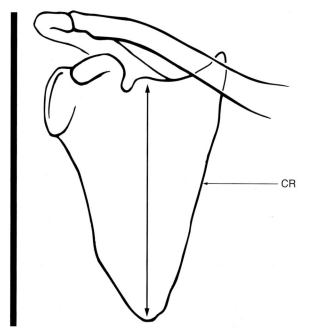

Figure 4–32. Long axis of scapular body parallel with film. *CR*, central ray.

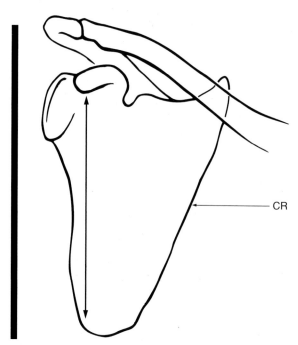

Figure 4–34. Lateral border of scapula parallel with film. *CR*, central ray.

border is thick, with a rough appearance, but the cortical outline of the vertebral border demonstrates a single thin line. If the lateral border is demonstrated next to the ribs and the vertebral border is visualized laterally, the patient has been rotated too much (see Rad. 33). If the vertebral border is demonstrated next to the ribs and the lateral border is visualized laterally, the patient was not rotated enough to superimpose the borders (see Rad. 34).

The humerus is drawn away from the superior scapular body, and the superior angle superimposes the coracoid base.

- Eighty percent of scapular fractures involve the body or neck of the scapula. The neck of the scapula is best visualized on the AP projection, because it is demonstrated on end in the lateral position. If a fracture of the scapular body is present or suspected, the lateral position should be taken to demonstrate the anteroposterior alignment of the fracture.
- ***Effect of Humeral Elevation on Scapular Visualization:*** To best demonstrate the scapular body, position its long axis parallel with the long axis of the film by elevating the humerus to a 90-degree angle with the patient's body (Figs. 4–32 and 4–33). This positioning causes the scapula to glide anteriorly

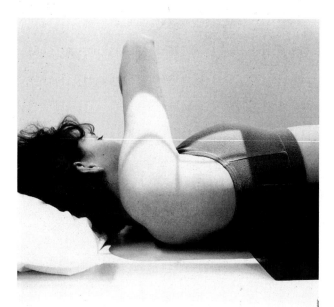

Figure 4–33. Proper arm positioning for lateral scapula.

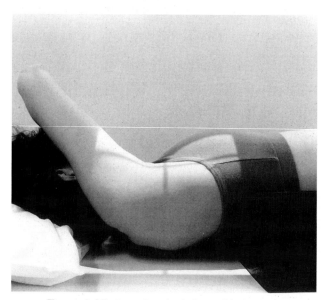

Figure 4–35. Arm elevated above 90 degrees.

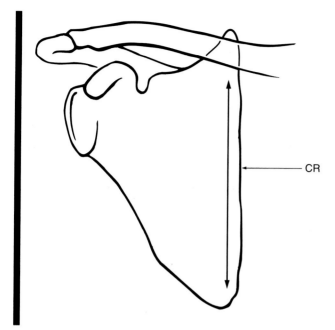

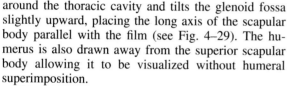

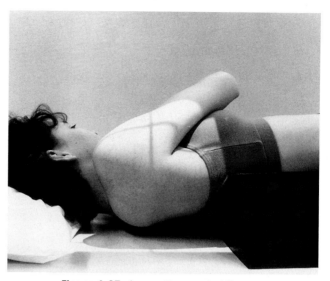

Figure 4-37. Arm resting against thorax.

Figure 4-36. Vertebral border of scapula parallel with film. *CR,* central ray.

around the thoracic cavity and tilts the glenoid fossa slightly upward, placing the long axis of the scapular body parallel with the film (see Fig. 4–29). The humerus is also drawn away from the superior scapular body allowing it to be visualized without humeral superimposition.

If humeral elevation is increased above 90 degrees with the patient still grasping the opposite shoulder, the lateral border of the scapula is placed parallel with the film (Figs. 4–34 and 4–35). This positioning distorts the superior scapular body and demonstrates the superior scapular angle and scapular spine below the coracoid and acromion, respectively (see Rad. 4–35).

If the humerus is not elevated, but rests on the patient's chest with the patient still grasping the opposite shoulder, the vertebral border of the scapula is positioned parallel with the film (Figs. 4–36 and 4–37). This arm positioning produces a shoulder image that is similar to that obtained for the trans-scapular Y-position: The superior scapular body superimposes the glenoid fossa and the proximal humerus (see Rad. 36), the coracoid and acromion are visualized in profile, and the anteroposterior relationship of the humeral head and glenoid fossa is demonstrated.

For each of these arm positions, the degree of patient obliquity needed to place the scapular body in a lateral position varies. The more the humerus is elevated, the less the patient needs to be rotated.

The midscapular body is at the center of the collimated field. The entire scapula, consisting of the inferior angle, coracoid, and acromion is included within the field.

- To place the midscapular body in the center of the collimated field and still include the coracoid, center a perpendicular central ray 1 inch (2.5 cm) anterior to the vertebral border of the scapula, halfway between the inferior scapular angle and the acromion angle. Each of these anatomical structures is palpable and should be used to ensure accurate positioning.

- Open the longitudinal collimation enough to include both the acromion and inferior scapular angles. Transverse collimation should be to the closest lateral skin-line.

- A 10 × 12 inch (24 × 30 cm) film placed lengthwise should be adequate to include all the required anatomical structures.

Critiquing Radiographs

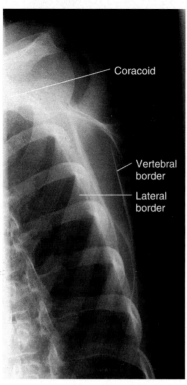

Radiograph 33.

Critique: The lateral and vertebral borders of the scapula are demonstrated without superimposition. The lateral border is next to the ribs, and the vertebral border is demonstrated laterally. The patient was rotated more than required for this radiograph.

Correction: Decrease the patient obliquity. The amount of change required is half of the distance demonstrated between the lateral and vertebral borders. When patient obliquity is decreased, the lateral border moves away from the thoracic cavity, and the vertebral border moves closer to the thoracic cavity.

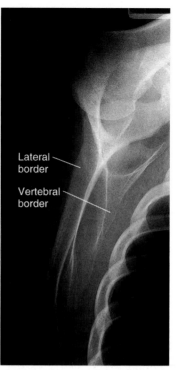

Radiograph 34.

Critique: The lateral and vertebral borders of the scapula are demonstrated without superimposition. The thick lateral border is demonstrated laterally, and the vertebral border is visualized next to the ribs. The patient was not rotated enough for this radiograph.

Correction: Increase the patient obliquity. The amount of change necessary is half of the distance demonstrated between the lateral and vertebral borders.

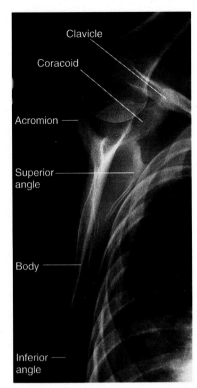

Radiograph 35.

Critique: The lateral and vertebral borders of the scapula are superimposed, indicating that patient obliquity was adequate. Note that the superior angle is visualized next to the thoracic cavity, inferior to the coracoid. The patient's arm was elevated more than 90 degrees, positioning the lateral border of the scapula parallel with the film (see Fig. 4–34 and 4–35).

Correction: Depress the arm, positioning it at a 90-degree angle with the body. This depression causes the inferior angle to draw posteriorly around the thoracic cavity. Because of this posterior scapular movement, it is necessary to increase patient obliquity slightly to obtain a lateral scapula. It is suggested that the scapular borders and inferior angle be repalpated to obtain accurate patient obliquity.

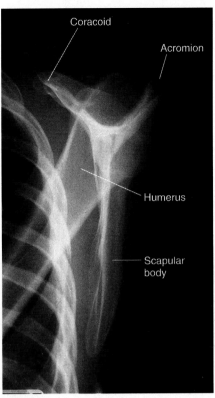

Radiograph 36.

Critique: The superior scapular body is superimposed by the glenoid fossa and the proximal humeral head, the coracoid and acromion are clearly demonstrated and the glenoid fossa is demonstrated "on end." The patient's arm was not elevated but was rested on the patient's chest, positioning the vertebral border of the scapula parallel with the film (Figs. 4–36 and 4–37).

Correction: To best demonstrate the scapular body, the arm should be elevated to approximately 90 degrees with the body. If the coracoid and acromion or the anteroposterior relationship between the glenoid fossa and humeral head are of interest, no correction movement is needed.

References

1. Carrol QB. Fuch's Principles of Radiographic Exposure, Processing and Quality Control, ed 4. Springfield, IL: Charles C Thomas, 1990, p 154.
2. Rogers LF. Radiology of Skeletal Trauma. New York: Churchill Livingstone, 1982.
3. Clemente CD. Gray's Anatomy, ed 30. Philadelphia: Lea & Febiger, 1985.
4. Bushong SC. Radiologic Science for Technologists, ed 5. St Louis: CV Mosby, 1993, p 238.
5. Rafert JA, Long BW, Hernandez EM, Kreipke DL: Axillary shoulder with exaggerated rotation: The Hill-Sachs defect. Radiol Technol 62:18–21, 1990.
6. Bontrager KL. Radiographic Positioning and Related Anatomy, ed 3. St. Louis: Mosby Year Book, 1993, p 161.
7. Ballinger PW. Radiographic Positioning and Radiologic Procedures, ed 7. St. Louis: Mosby Year Book, 1991, pp 128–129.
8. Rubin SA, Gray RL, Green WR. The scapular "Y": A diagnostic aid in shoulder trauma. Radiology 110:725–726, 1974.
9. De Smet AA. Anterior oblique projection in radiography of the traumatized shoulder. AJR 134:515–518, 1980.
10. Warwick R, Williams PL. Gray's Anatomy, ed 36. Philadelphia: WB Saunders, 1980, pp 353–357.

CHAPTER 5

Radiographic Critique of the Lower Extremity

TOE

Anteroposterior Projection

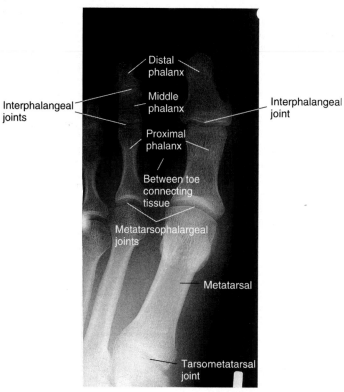

Figure 5-1. Accurately positioned AP toe radiograph.

Radiographic Evaluation

Facility's patient identification requirements are visible on radiograph.
- These requirements usually are facility name, patient name, age, and hospital number, and exam time and date.
- The patient ID plate is positioned toward the heel so as not to obscure any anatomy of interest.

A right or left marker, identifying the correct foot, is present on the radiograph and does not superimpose anatomy of interest.

- Place the marker within the collimated light field so it does not superimpose any portion of the affected toe.
- When more than one view of the toe is placed on the same film, only one of the views needs to be marked.

There is no evidence of preventable artifacts, such as bandages and splints.
- Consult with the ordering physician and the patient about whether bandages or splints can be removed.

Contrast and density are adequate to demonstrate the surrounding soft tissue and bony structures of the affected digit. Penetration is sufficient to visualize the

bony trabecular patterns and cortical outlines of the phalanges and metatarsal head.

- An optimal 50 to 60 kVp technique sufficiently penetrates the bony and soft tissue structures of the affected toe and provides high radiographic contrast.

The bony trabecular patterns and cortical outlines of the phalanges are sharply defined.

- Sharply defined recorded details are obtained when patient motion is controlled, a detail screen and a small focal spot are used, and a short object–image distance (OID) is maintained.

The digit demonstrates no rotation. Soft tissue width and midshaft concavity are equal on either side of the phalanges.

- A true AP projection of the toe is obtained by flexing the supine patient's knee until the plantar foot surface rests flat against the cassette. The lower leg, ankle, and foot should remain aligned, and equal pressure should be applied across the plantar surface (Fig. 5–2).

- ***Detecting Toe Rotation:*** Toe rotation is controlled by the position of the foot. Take a few minutes to study a toe skeleton and note that in an AP projection concavity of the midshaft of the proximal phalanx is equal on either side. As the toe skeleton is rotated medially or laterally, the concavity increases on the side rolled away from the film and decreases on the side positioned toward the film. The same results can be seen in the soft tissue that surrounds the phalanges. More soft tissue width is evident on the surface rolled away from the film than on the surface rolled toward the film.

    Look for this midshaft concavity and soft tissue width variation to indicate rotation on a toe radiograph. With lateral toe rotation phalangeal soft tissue width and midshaft concavity are greater on the side

positioned away from the lateral foot surface (see Rad. 1). With medial toe rotation, phalangeal soft tissue width and midshaft concavity are greater on the side positioned away from the medial foot surface (see Rad. 2). If the patient's toenail is visualized, which is often the case on the first toe, it can also be used to determine the direction of toe rotation. The nail rotates in the same direction the foot was rotated.

The interphalangeal (IP) and metatarsophalangeal (MP) joints appear as open spaces, and the phalanges are demonstrated without foreshortening.

- The IP and MP joint spaces are open and the phalanges are demonstrated without foreshortening when the toe was fully extended and a perpendicular central ray was centered to the MP joint. This toe positioning and central ray placement align the joint spaces perpendicular to the film and parallel with the central ray. They also prevent foreshortening of the phalanges, because the long axes of the phalanges are aligned parallel with the film and perpendicular to the central ray. If the toe is not extended, the resulting radiograph demonstrates closed joint spaces and foreshortened phalanges (see Rad. 3).

- ***Central Ray Angulation for Nonextendable Toes:*** On patients who are unable to extend their toes, the central ray should be angled proximally (toward the heel). The degree of angulation depends on the amount of toe flexion. Angle the central ray until it is perpendicular to the phalanx of interest or parallel with the joint space of interest.

The long axis of the affected digit is aligned with the long axis of the collimated field.

- Aligning the long axis of the toe with the long axis of the collimated field enables you to collimate tightly without clipping the distal phalanx or distal metatarsal.

There is no soft tissue overlap from adjacent digits.

- Spreading the toes slightly prevents soft tissue overlapping from adjacent toes. It is difficult to evaluate the soft tissue of an affected toe when it is superimposed by other soft tissue.

The MP joint is at the center of the collimated field. The distal and proximal phalanges and half of the metatarsal are included within the field.

- Centering a perpendicular central ray to the MP joint places the joint in the center of the radiograph.
- Open the longitudinal collimated field to include the distal phalanx and the distal half of the metatarsal. You can ensure that half of the metatarsal is included on the radiograph by extending the light field 2 inches (5 cm) proximal to the between-toe interconnecting tissue. Transverse collimation should be to the toe skin-line.
- One third of an 8 × 10 inch (18 × 24 cm) film placed crosswise should be adequate to include all the required anatomical structures.

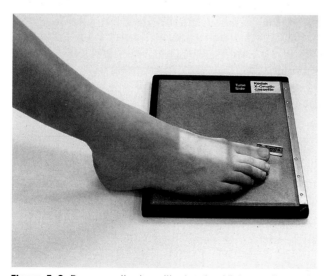

Figure 5-2. Proper patient positioning for AP toe radiograph.

Critiquing Radiographs

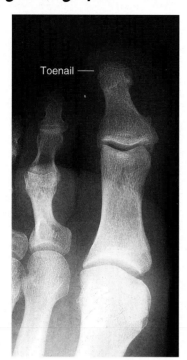

Radiograph 1.

Critique: The phalanges demonstrate greater soft tissue width and midshaft concavity on the medial surface. The outline of the toenail is visualized on the opposite (lateral) side. The foot was laterally rotated.

Correction: Medially rotate the foot and toe until they are flat against the cassette.

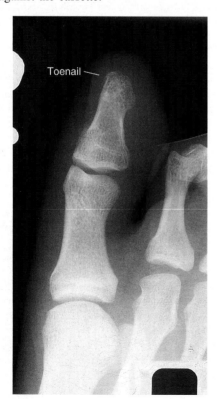

Radiograph 2.

Critique: The phalanges demonstrate greater soft tissue width and midshaft concavity on the lateral surface. The outline of the toenail is visualized on the medial surface. The foot was medially rotated.

Correction: Laterally rotate the foot and toe until they are flat against the cassette.

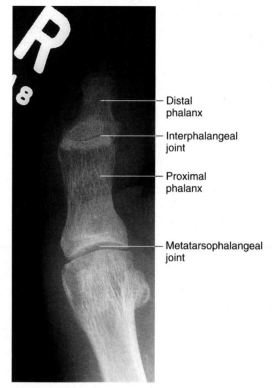

Radiograph 3.

Critique: The IP and MP joint spaces are closed, and the phalanges are foreshortened. The patient's toe was flexed and the central ray was not adequately angled to open these joints or to demonstrate the phalanges without foreshortening.

Correction: If the patient's condition allows, extend the toe, placing it flat against the cassette. If the patient is unable to extend the toe, angle the central ray proximally until it is aligned perpendicular to the phalanx of interest or parallel with the joint space of interest.

Toe: Oblique Position

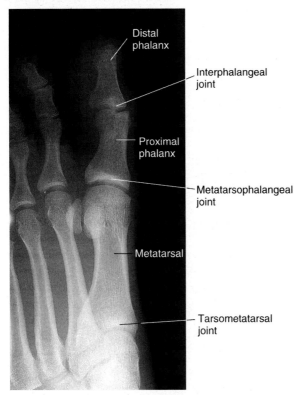

Figure 5-3. Accurately positioned oblique toe radiograph.

Radiographic Evaluation

Facility's patient identification requirements are visible on radiograph.

- These requirements usually are facility name, patient name, age, and hospital number, and exam time and date.
- The patient ID plate is positioned toward the heel so as not to obscure anatomy of interest.

A right or left marker, identifying the correct foot, is present on the radiograph and does not superimpose anatomy of interest.

- Place the marker within the collimated light field so it does not superimpose upon any anatomy of interest.

There is no evidence of preventable artifacts, such as bandages and splints.

- Consult with the ordering physician and the patient about whether bandages or splints can be removed.

Contrast and density are adequate to demonstrate the surrounding soft tissue and bony structures of the affected digit. Penetration is sufficient to visualize the bony trabecular patterns and cortical outlines of the phalanges and metatarsal head.

- An optimal 50 to 60 kVp technique sufficiently penetrates the bony and soft tissue structures of the toe and provides high radiographic contrast.

The bony trabecular patterns and cortical outlines of the phalanges are sharply defined.

- Sharply defined recorded details are obtained when patient motion is controlled, a detail screen and a small focal spot are used, and a short object–image distance (OID) is maintained.

The digit is rotated 45 degrees. There is twice as much soft tissue width and more phalangeal and metatarsal concavity on the side of the digit rotated away from the film.

- An oblique toe radiograph is accomplished by placing the affected foot on the cassette and then rotating the foot until the affected toe is rotated 45 degrees from the AP projection (Fig. 5–4).
- When the first through third toes are of interest, the foot should be rotated medially. When the fourth and fifth toes are of interest, the foot should be rotated laterally. The variation in rotation for the different toes is to obtain an oblique position with the least amount of OID.
- **Toe Midshaft Concavity with Various Positions and Projections:** Examine a toe skeleton in an AP projection and in an oblique and a lateral position. Note how the midshaft concavity of the proximal phalanx varies as the digit is rotated. In an AP projection, the midshaft concavity is equal on the two sides. In an oblique position, the midshaft concavity is greater on the side rolled away from the film than on the side positioned closer to the film. In a lateral position, the posterior aspect of the digit demonstrates more concavity than the anterior aspect. Results are similar in the soft tissue that surrounds the digit. More soft tissue width is evident on the surface that demonstrates greater midshaft concavity and is rotated away from the film.
- **Verifying Toe Rotation on Oblique Radiograph:** To verify the accuracy of rotation on an oblique toe radiograph and to determine the proper way to reposition the patient when digit obliquity was insufficient or excessive, study the midshaft concavity of the proximal phalanx and compare the soft tissue width on either side of the digit. Radiographically, a toe at 45 degrees of obliquity demonstrates more phalangeal midshaft concavity and twice as much soft

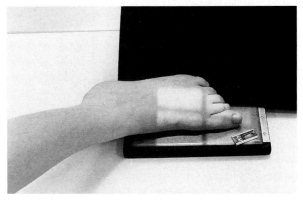

Figure 5-4. Proper patient positioning for oblique toe radiograph.

tissue width on the side positioned farther from the film. When the midshaft concavity of the proximal phalanx and soft tissue width are closer to equal on either side of the digit, the toe was not adequately rotated (see Rad. 4). When the soft tissue width differences between the sides of the digit are more than twice as much and when the posterior aspect of the proximal phalanx's midshaft demonstrates more concavity than the anterior aspect, the toe was rotated more than 45 degrees for the radiograph (see Rad. 5).

The interphalangeal (IP) and metatarsophalangeal (MP) joints are visualized as open spaces, and the phalanges are demonstrated without foreshortening.

- The IP and MP joint spaces are open and the phalanges are demonstrated without foreshortening when the toe was fully extended and a perpendicular central ray was centered to the MP joint. This toe positioning and central ray placement align the joint spaces perpendicular to the film and parallel with the central ray. They also prevent foreshortening of the phalanges, because the long axes of the phalanges are aligned parallel with the film and perpendicular to the central ray. If the toe was not extended, the resulting radiograph demonstrates closed joint spaces and foreshortened phalanges (see Rad. 6).
- ***Central Ray Angulation for Nonextendable Toes:*** On patients who are unable to extend their toes, the central ray should be angled proximally. The degree of angulation depends on the amount of toe flexion. Angle the central ray until it is perpendicular to the phalanx of interest or parallel with the joint space of interest.

The long axis of the affected digit is aligned with the long axis of the collimated field.

- Aligning the long axis of the toe with the long axis of the collimated field enables you to collimate tightly without clipping the distal phalanx or distal metatarsal.

There is no soft tissue or bony overlap from adjacent digits.

- The adjacent toes should be drawn away from the affected toe to prevent overlapping. It may be necessary to use tape or another immobilization device to maintain the unaffected toe's position. If the unaffected toes are not drawn away, they may superimpose the affected toe (see Rad. 7). It is difficult to evaluate the affected digit when it is superimposed by other digits.

The MP joint is at the center of the collimated field. The distal and proximal phalanges and half of the metatarsal are included within the field.

- Centering a perpendicular central ray to the MP joint places the joint in the center of the radiograph.
- Open the longitudinal collimation to include the distal phalanx and the distal half of the metatarsal. You can ensure that half of the metatarsal is included on the radiograph by extending the light field 2 inches (5 cm) proximal to the between-toe interconnecting tissue. Transverse collimation should be to the toe skin-line.

- One third of an 8 × 10 inch (18 × 24 cm) film placed crosswise should be adequate to include all the required anatomical structures.

Critiquing Radiographs

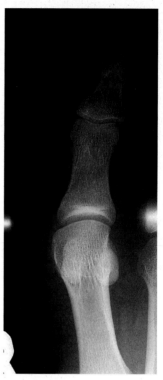

Radiograph 4.

Critique: Soft tissue width and midshaft concavity on either side of the phalanges are nearly equal. The toe was rotated less than 45 degrees.

Correction: Increase toe and foot obliquity until the affected toe is at a 45-degree angle with the film.

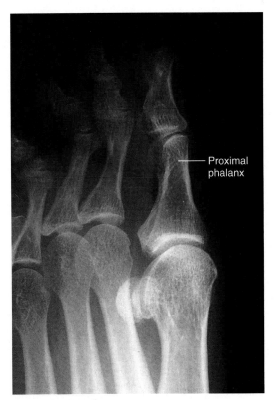

Radiograph 5.

Critique: The proximal phalanx demonstrates more concavity on the posterior aspect of the foot than the anterior aspect. The toe has been rotated close to a lateral position.
Correction: Decrease toe and foot obliquity until the affected toe is at a 45-degree angle with the film.

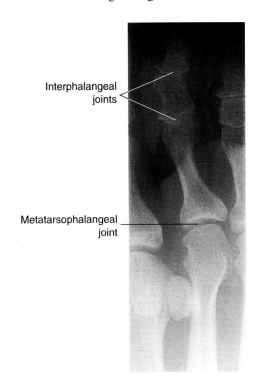

Radiograph 6.

Critique: The IP and MP joint spaces are obscured, and the phalanges are foreshortened. The patient's toe was flexed, and the central ray was not angled to open these joints or to demonstrate the phalanges without foreshortening.
Correction: If the patient's condition allows, extend the toe, placing it flat against the cassette. If the patient's toe cannot be extended, angle the central ray posteriorly until it is aligned perpendicular to the phalanx of interest or parallel with the joint space of interest.

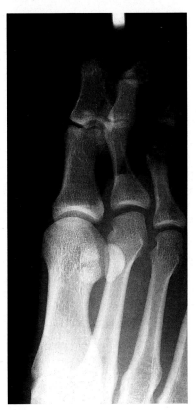

Radiograph 7.

Critique: There is soft tissue and bony overlap of the adjacent digit onto the affected digit. The toes were not spread apart.
Correction: Draw the unaffected toes away from the affected toe. It may be necessary to use tape or another immobilization device if the patient is unable to maintain the position.

Toe: Lateral Position

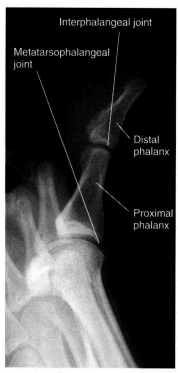

Interphalangeal joint

Metatarsophalangeal joint

Distal phalanx

Proximal phalanx

Figure 5-5. Accurately positioned lateral toe radiograph.

Radiographic Evaluation

Facility's patient identification requirements are visible on radiograph.

- These requirements usually are facility name, patient name, age, and hospital number, and exam time and date.
- Patient ID plate is positioned so as not to obscure anatomy of interest.

A right or left marker, identifying the correct foot, is present on the radiograph and does not superimpose anatomy of interest.

- Place the marker within the collimated light field so it does not superimpose any portion of the affected toe.

There is no evidence of preventable artifacts, such as bandages and splints.

- Consult with the ordering physician and the patient about whether bandages or splints can be removed.

Contrast and density are adequate to demonstrate the surrounding soft tissue and bony structures of the affected digit. Penetration is sufficient to visualize the bony trabecular patterns and cortical outlines of the phalanges and metatarsal head.

- An optimal 50 to 60 kVp technique sufficiently penetrates the bony and soft tissue structures of the affected toe and provides high radiographic contrast.

The bony trabecular patterns and the cortical outlines of the phalanges are sharply defined.

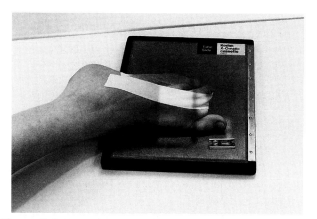

Figure 5-6. Proper patient positioning for lateral radiograph of the first toe.

- Sharply defined recorded details are obtained when patient motion is controlled, a detail screen and a small focal spot are used, and a short object–image distance (OID) is maintained.

The digit is demonstrated in a true lateral position: The posterior surface of the proximal phalanx demonstrates more concavity than the anterior surface, whereas the anterior surface of the distal phalanx demonstrates more concavity than the posterior surface. The soft tissue outline of the nail, when seen, is demonstrated in profile anteriorly.

- A lateral toe radiograph is accomplished by rotating the foot and toe until the affected toe is placed in a lateral position.
- Whether the foot is medially or laterally rotated to obtain this goal depends on which toe is being radiographed. When the first, second, and third toes are radiographed, rotate the foot medially (Fig. 5–6). When the fourth and fifth toes are radiographed, rotate the foot laterally (Fig. 5–7).
- ***Toe Midshaft Concavity with Various Positions and Projections:*** To understand the difference between a true lateral digit and one that is rotated, study a toe skeleton in a lateral and an oblique

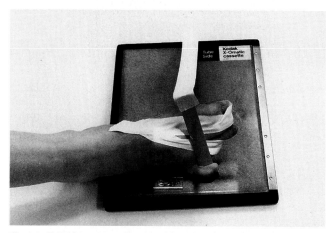

Figure 5-7. Proper patient positioning for lateral radiograph of the fourth toe.

position. Note how the midshaft concavity of the proximal phalanx varies as the digit is rotated. In a lateral position, the posterior surface of the proximal phalanx demonstrates more concavity than the anterior surface. In an oblique position, concavity is about equal on either side of the midshafts of the proximal and distal phalanges. The soft tissue widths on either side of the phalanges also change in the lateral and oblique positions. More soft tissue is present on the side of the digit that demonstrates the greater midshaft concavity (see Rad. 8).

The long axis of the digit is aligned with the long axis of the collimated field.

- Placing the long axis of the toe in alignment with the long axis of the collimated field allows you to collimate tightly without clipping the distal phalanx and metatarsophalangeal (MP) joint space.

There is no soft tissue or bony overlap from adjacent toes.

- The adjacent toes should be drawn away from the affected toe to prevent overlapping. It may be necessary to use tape or another immobilization device to maintain the unaffected toe's position. If the unaffected toes are not drawn away, they may superimpose the affected toe (see Rad. 9).

The interphalangeal (IP) joint is at the center of the collimated field. The distal and proximal phalanges and the MP joint space are included within the field.

- Centering a perpendicular central ray to the IP joint places the joint in the center of the radiograph.
- Open the longitudinal collimation to include the distal phalanx and MP joint space. The MP joint space is located about 1 inch (2.5 cm) proximal to the between-toe interconnecting tissue. Transverse collimation should be to the toe skin-line.
- One third of an 8 × 10 inch (18 × 24 cm) film placed crosswise should be adequate to include all the required anatomical structures.

Critiquing Radiographs

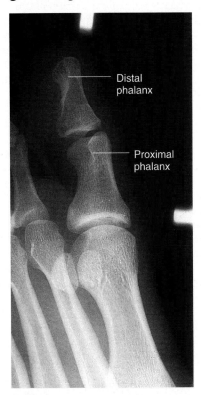

Radiograph 8.

Critique: The proximal and distal phalanges demonstrate nearly equal midshaft concavity, and there is approximately twice as much soft tissue on one side of the phalanges as on the other side. The foot was not rotated enough to place the toe in a true lateral position.

Correction: Increase the patient's toe and foot obliquity until the affected toe is in a true lateral position. For this patient, it may also be necessary to draw the unaffected toes away from the affected toe to prevent superimposition.

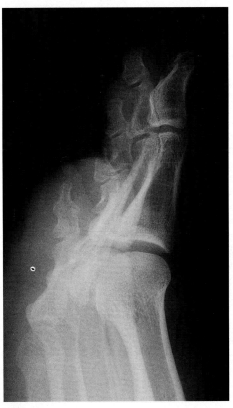

Radiograph 9.

Critique: There is soft tissue and bony overlap of digits. The adjacent unaffected digits were not drawn away from the affected digit.

Correction: The patient's unaffected toes should be drawn away from the affected toe. It may be necessary to use tape or another immobilization device to help the patient maintain this position.

FOOT

AP (Dorsoplantar) Projection

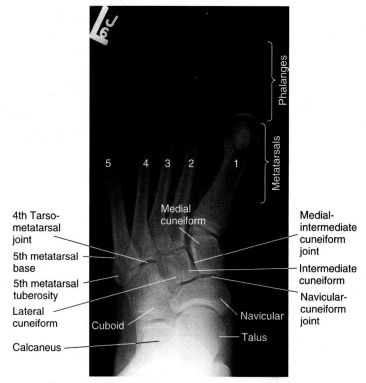

Figure 5-8. Accurately positioned AP foot radiograph.

Radiographic Evaluation

Facility's patient identification requirements are visible on radiograph.

- These requirements usually are facility name, patient name, age, and hospital number, and exam time and date.
- Patient ID plate is positioned toward the heel so as not to obscure anatomy of interest.

A right or left marker, identifying the correct foot, is present on the radiograph and does not superimpose anatomy of interest.

- Place the marker within the collimated light field so it does not superimpose any portion of the foot.
- When more than one view of the foot is placed on a film, only one of the views needs to be marked.

There is no evidence of preventable artifacts, such as bandages and splints.

- Consult with the ordering physician and the patient about whether bandages and splints can be removed.

Contrast and density are adequate to demonstrate the surrounding soft tissue and bony structures of the foot. Penetration is sufficient to visualize the bony trabecular patterns and cortical outlines of the phalanges, metatarsals, and tarsals.

- An optimal 55 to 65 kVp technique sufficiently penetrates the bony and soft tissue structures of the foot and provides high radiographic contrast.
- When an exposure (mAs) is set that will adequately demonstrate the proximal metatarsals and tarsals, the distal metatarsals and phalanges are often overexposed because of the difference in AP foot thickness in these two regions. A compensating filter placed over the phalanges and metatarsophalangeal (MP) joints can be used to absorb some of the photons that reach these areas, thus obtaining uniform foot density (Fig. 5–9). The filter should be positioned so it extends 1 inch (2.5 cm) proximal to the between-toe interconnecting tissue in order to cover the MP joints.

The bony trabecular patterns and the cortical outlines of the phalanges, metatarsals, and tarsals are sharply defined.

- Sharply defined recorded details are obtained when patient motion is controlled, a detail screen and a small focal spot are used, and a short object–image distance (OID) is maintained.

The foot demonstrates a true AP projection: The joint space between the medial (first) and intermediate (second) cuneiforms is open, about 0.75 inch (2 cm) of the calcaneus is demonstrated without talar superimposi-

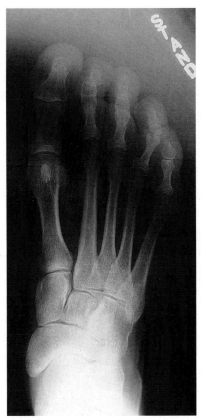

Figure 5-9. AP foot radiograph with compensating filter used on the toes.

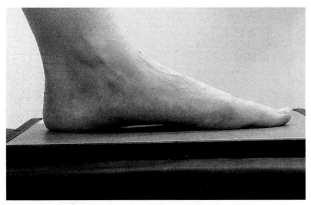

Figure 5-11. Low longitudinal foot arch.

tion, and there is equal concavity on either side of the first metatarsal midshaft.

- A true AP projection of the foot is obtained by flexing the supine patient's knee and placing the plantar foot surface against the cassette (Fig. 5–10). The lower leg, ankle, and foot should remain aligned, and equal pressure should be applied across the plantar surface.
- ***Effect of Foot Rotation:*** If the lower leg, ankle, and foot are not aligned or if more pressure is placed on the medial or lateral plantar surface, foot rotation will result, and the medial and intermediate cuneiform

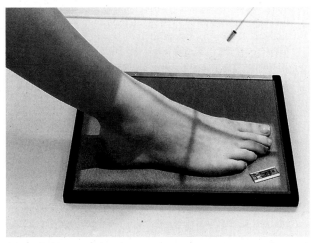

Figure 5-10. Proper patient positioning for AP foot radiograph.

joint space will be closed. When the foot is rotated laterally, the navicular tuberosity, which superimposes itself on an AP projection, is rolled into profile, and the talus moves over the calcaneus, resulting in less than 0.75 inch (2 cm) of calcaneal visualization without talar superimposition. There is also an increase in metatarsal base superimposition (see Rad. 10).

When the foot is rotated medially, the talus moves away from the calcaneus, resulting in greater than 0.75 inch (2 cm) calcaneal visualization without talar superimposition. There is also a decrease in superimposition of the metatarsal bases (see Rad. 11).

- ***Standing AP Projection of the Foot:*** This view may also be obtained with the patient in a standing position. An AP standing foot radiograph should meet the same evaluating criteria used for a nonstanding AP foot radiograph.

The tarsometatarsal and navicular-cuneiform joint spaces are open.

- The bones of the foot with their ligament and muscular structures are arranged in a longitudinal arch that is visible on the medial foot surface. This arch places the tarsometatarsal and navicular-cuneiform joint spaces at a set angle with the film.
- To demonstrate these joints as open spaces, angle the central ray until it is aligned parallel with them. This is accomplished on most patients by using a 10- to 15-degree proximal (toward the heel) angle. The exact degree of angulation depends on the height of the longitudinal arch. A 10-degree angle should be used when the patient's longitudinal arch is low, as demonstrated in Figure 5–11. A 15-degree angle is needed on a patient with a high arch, as demonstrated in Figure 5–12. Omitting the central ray angulation or employing an inaccurate one results in obstructed tarsometatarsal and navicular-cuneiform joint spaces (see Rad. 12).

The long axis of the foot is aligned with the long axis of the collimated field.

- Aligning the midfoot (third metatarsal) with the longitudinally collimated field allows you to tightly collimate without clipping the distal or proximal foot.

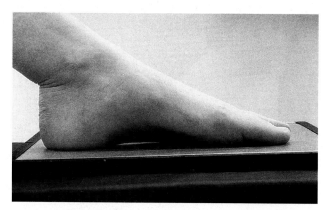

Figure 5-12. High longitudinal foot arch.

The proximal second and third metatarsal bases are at the center of the collimated field. The proximal calcaneus, talar neck, tarsals, metatarsals, phalanges, and surrounding foot soft tissue are included within the field.

- To place the second and third metatarsal bases in the center of the radiograph, center the central ray to the midline of the foot at a level 0.50 inch (1 cm) distal to the fifth metatarsal tuberosity. The fifth metatarsal tuberosity can be palpated along the lateral foot surface, about halfway between the ball of the foot and the heel.
- Open the longitudinal collimation enough to include the phalanges. Transverse collimation should be to the foot skin-line.
- Half of a 10 × 12 inch (24 × 30 cm) film placed lengthwise should be adequate to include all the required anatomical structures.

Critiquing Radiographs

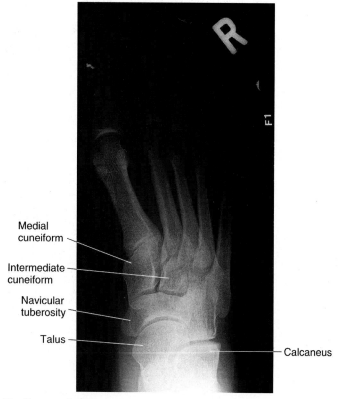

Medial cuneiform

Intermediate cuneiform

Navicular tuberosity

Talus

Calcaneus

Radiograph 10.

Critique: The joint space between the medial and intermediate cuneiforms is closed, the navicular tuberosity is demonstrated in profile, and less than 0.75 inch (2 cm) of the calcaneus is demonstrated without talar superimposition. More pressure was placed on the patient's lateral plantar surface than on the medial surface, resulting in lateral foot rotation.

Correction: Rotate the foot medially until there is equal pressure over the entire plantar surface. The lower leg, ankle, and foot should be aligned.

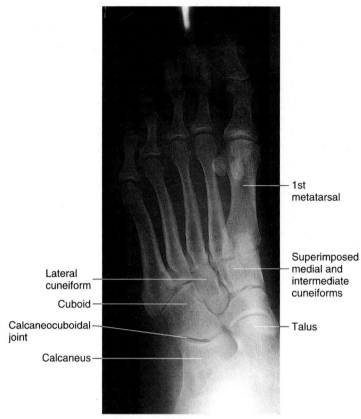

Lateral
cuneiform

Cuboid

Calcaneocuboidal
joint

Calcaneus

1st
metatarsal

Superimposed
medial and
intermediate
cuneiforms

Talus

Radiograph 11.

Critique: The joint space between the medial and intermediate cuneiforms is closed, the calcaneus demonstrates no talar superimposition, and the metatarsal bases demonstrate decreased superimposition. More pressure was placed on the patient's medial plantar surface than on the lateral surface, resulting in medial foot rotation.

Correction: Rotate the foot laterally until there is equal pressure over the entire plantar surface. The lower leg, ankle, and foot should be aligned.

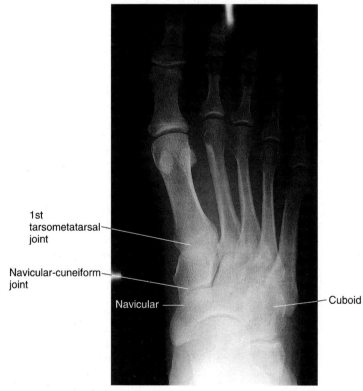

1st
tarsometatarsal
joint

Navicular-cuneiform
joint

Navicular

Cuboid

Radiograph 12.

Critique: The tarsometatarsal and navicular-cuneiform joint spaces are obscured. The central ray was not aligned parallel with these joint spaces.

Correction: Direct the central ray 10 to 15 degrees proximally. Less angulation is needed on patients with low longitudinal arches, whereas more angulation is required on patients with high arches.

Foot: Medial (Internal) Oblique Position

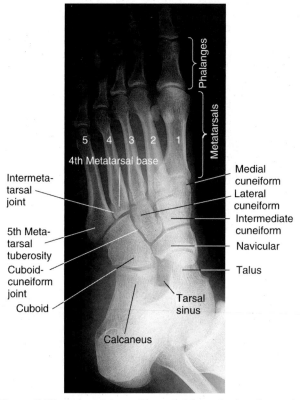

Figure 5-13. Accurately positioned oblique foot radiograph.

Radiographic Evaluation

Facility's patient identification requirements are visible on radiograph.
- These requirements usually are facility name, patient name, age, and hospital number, and exam time and date.
- Patient ID plate is positioned toward the heel so as not to obscure anatomy of interest.

A right or left marker, identifying the correct foot, is present on the radiograph and does not superimpose anatomy of interest.
- Place the marker within the collimated light field so it does not superimpose any portion of the foot.

There is no evidence of preventable artifacts, such as bandages and splints.
- Consult with the ordering physician and the patient about whether bandages and splints can be removed.

Contrast and density are adequate to demonstrate the surrounding soft tissue and bony structures of the foot. Penetration is sufficient to visualize the bony trabecular patterns and cortical outlines of the phalanges, metatarsals, and tarsals.
- An optimal 55 to 65 kVp technique sufficiently penetrates the bony and soft tissue structures of the foot and provides high radiographic contrast.

- When an exposure (mAs) is set that will adequately demonstrate the proximal metatarsals and tarsals, the distal metatarsals and phalanges are often overexposed because of the difference in AP foot thickness in these two regions. A compensating filter placed over the patient's phalanges and distal metatarsals can be used to obtain uniform foot density. The filter should be positioned so it extends about 1 inch (2.5 cm) proximal to the between-toe interconnecting tissue in order to cover the metatarsal heads.

The bony trabecular patterns and the cortical outlines of the phalanges, metatarsals, and tarsals are sharply defined.
- Sharply defined recorded details are obtained when patient motion is controlled, a detail screen and a small focal spot are used, and a short object–image distance (OID) is maintained.

The foot demonstrates adequate obliquity: The joint spaces surrounding the cuboid are demonstrated as open spaces, the first and second intermetatarsal joints are closed but the second through fifth intermetatarsal joint spaces are open, and the tarsi sinus and fifth metatarsal tuberosity are well visualized.
- To accomplish an oblique foot radiograph, begin with the patient in a supine position with the knee flexed until the plantar foot surface rests against the cassette.

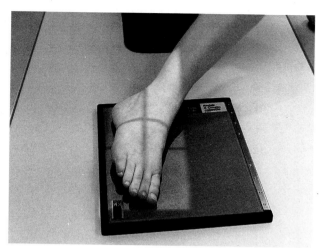

Figure 5-14. Proper patient positioning for oblique foot radiograph.

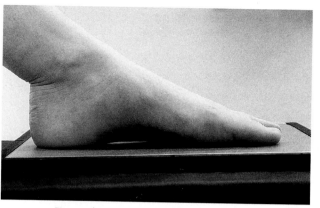

Figure 5-16. High longitudinal foot arch.

Medially (internally) rotate the patient's leg and foot until the foot forms a 30- to 45-degree angle with the film (Fig. 5-14).

- **Determining Required Obliquity:** To determine whether a 30- or 45-degree rotation is needed, view the medial aspect of the patient's foot in an AP projection to judge the height of the patient's longitudinal arch. I have found that less obliquity is required on a patient with a low longitudinal arch than on a patient with a high arch. If the patient has a low arch, such as that demonstrated in Figure 5-15, rotate the patient's foot about 30 degrees; if the patient's arch is high, as demonstrated in Figure 5-16, rotate the foot about 45 degrees. The degree of foot obliquity is easier to judge when the lower leg, ankle, and foot remain aligned as the foot is rotated.

The cuneiform-cuboid joint space is the most sensitive of the joint spaces that surround the cuboid and closes if foot obliquity is only slightly inadequate. The degree of foot obliquity that is required to open this joint as well as the other joint spaces depends on the height of the patient's longitudinal arch. Figures 5-17 and 5-18 demonstrate oblique and lateral foot radiographs taken on a patient with a high longitudinal arch. The oblique radiograph was taken with the

patient's foot rotated 45 degrees medially. In comparison, Figures 5-19 and 5-20 demonstrate oblique and lateral foot radiographs taken on a patient with a low longitudinal arch. For this oblique radiograph, the patient's foot was rotated 30 degrees medially.

On the lateral foot radiographs, the height of the longitudinal arches can be compared by evaluating the amount of cuboid demonstrated distal to the navicular. Note that more of the cuboid is visualized distal to the navicular on the lateral foot radiograph in Figure 5-18 than in Figure 5-20.

Even though the cuboid and intermetatarsal joint spaces are open on both oblique radiographs, they were taken with different degrees of obliquity. This

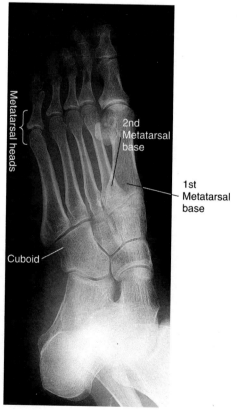

Figure 5-17. Oblique foot radiograph of a patient with a high longitudinal arch.

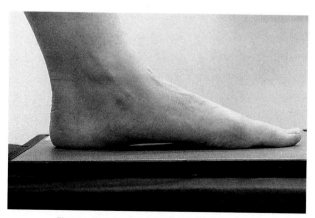

Figure 5-15. Low longitudinal foot arch.

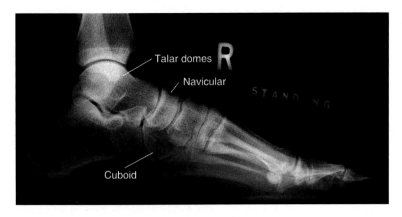

Figure 5-18. Lateral foot radiograph of a patient with a high longitudinal arch.

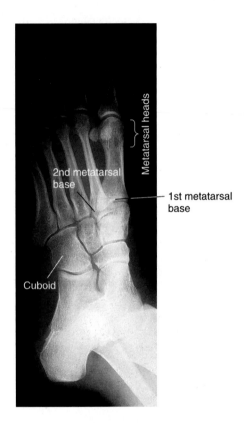

Figure 5-19. Oblique foot radiograph of a patient with a low longitudinal arch.

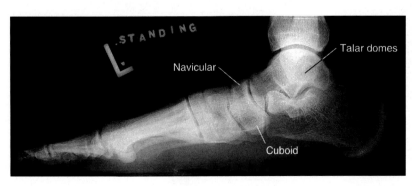

Figure 5-20. Lateral foot radiograph of a patient with a low longitudinal arch.

can be confirmed by studying the amount of first and second metatarsal base superimposition and the amount of space demonstrated between the metatarsal heads. When the foot is rotated medially, the first metatarsal base rotates beneath the second metatarsal base, and the second through third metatarsal heads move closer together. The greater the foot obliquity, the greater the superimposition of the metatarsal heads. Carefully evaluate the first and second metatarsal bases and the metatarsal heads on Figures 5–17 and 5–19 to familiarize yourself with the difference.

- ***Under-Rotation versus Over-Rotation:*** If the degree of foot obliquity is inadequate for an oblique foot radiograph, the lateral cuneiform-cuboid, navicular-cuboid, and second through fifth intermetatarsal joint spaces are closed. To determine whether the patient has been over- or under-rotated, evaluate the fourth and fifth intermetatarsal joint spaces. If these joint spaces are closed and the fourth metatarsal base is superimposing the fifth metatarsal base, the foot was not rotated enough (see Rad. 13). If the fourth and fifth intermetatarsal joint space is closed and the fifth proximal metatarsal is superimposing the fourth metatarsal tubercle, the foot was over-rotated (see Rad. 14). The fourth metatarsal tubercle is a rounded, protruding surface located just distal to the fourth metatarsal base.

The long axis of the foot is aligned with the long axis of the collimated field.

- Aligning the midfoot (third metatarsal) with the longitudinally collimated centering line aligns the foot's long axis with the collimated field. This alignment allows you to collimate tightly without clipping the distal or proximal foot.

The third metatarsal base is at the center of the collimated field. The phalanges, metatarsals, tarsals, calcaneus, and surrounding foot soft tissue are included within the field.

- Centering a perpendicular central ray to the midline of the foot at the level of the fifth metatarsal tuberosity places the base of the proximal third metatarsal in the center of the radiograph. The fifth tuberosity can be palpated about halfway between the ball of the foot and the heel.
- Open the longitudinal collimation enough to include the phalanges and calcaneus. Transverse collimation should be to the foot skin-line.
- Half of a 10 × 12 inch (24 × 30 cm) film placed lengthwise should be adequate to include all the required anatomical structures.

Critiquing Radiographs

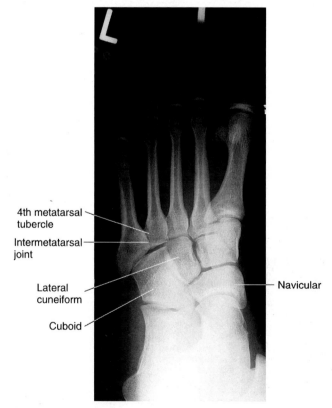

4th metatarsal tubercle

Intermetatarsal joint

Lateral cuneiform

Cuboid

Navicular

Radiograph 13.

Critique: The lateral cuneiform-cuboid, navicular-cuboid, and third through fifth intermetatarsal joint spaces are closed. The fourth metatarsal tubercle is demonstrated without superimposition of the fifth metatarsal. The foot was not medially rotated enough.

Correction: Increase the medial foot obliquity. The amount of increase needed is half the amount of fourth and fifth metatarsal base superimposition demonstrated on the radiograph.

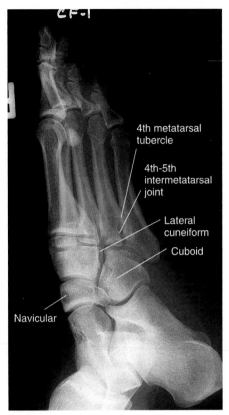

4th metatarsal
tubercle

4th-5th
intermetatarsal
joint

Lateral
cuneiform

Cuboid

Navicular

Radiograph 14.

Critique: The lateral cuneiform-cuboid, navicular-cuboid, and intermetatarsal joint spaces are closed, and the fifth proximal metatarsal is superimposing the fourth metatarsal tubercle. The patient's foot was over-rotated.
Correction: Decrease the medial foot obliquity.

Foot: Lateral Position (Mediolateral Projection)

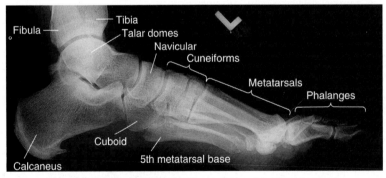

Figure 5-21. Accurately positioned lateral foot radiograph.

Radiographic Evaluation

Facility's patient identification requirements are visible on radiograph.
- These requirements usually are facility name, patient name, age, and hospital number, and exam time and date.
- Patient ID plate is positioned so as not to obscure anatomy of interest.

A right or left marker, identifying the correct foot, is present on the radiograph and does not superimpose anatomy of interest.
- Place the marker within the collimated light field so it does not superimpose any portion of the foot.

There is no evidence of preventable artifacts, such as bandages and splints.

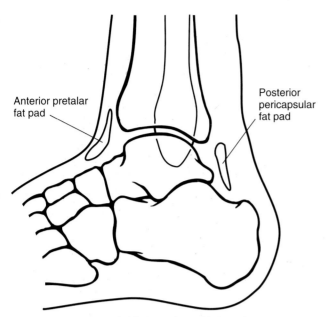

Figure 5-22. Location of fat pads.

- Consult with the ordering physician and the patient about whether bandages and splints can be removed.

Contrast and density are adequate to demonstrate the surrounding soft tissue and bony structures of the foot. Penetration is sufficient to visualize the bony trabecular patterns and cortical outlines of the phalanges, metatarsals, tarsals, calcaneus, and talus.

- An optimal 55 to 65 kVp technique sufficiently penetrates the bony and soft tissue structures of the foot and provides high radiographic contrast.
- **_Fat Pads on the Foot and Ankle:_** Two soft tissue structures located around the foot and ankle may indicate joint effusion and injury: the anterior pretalar fat pad and the posterior pericapsular fat pad. The anterior pretalar fat pad is visualized anterior to the ankle joint and rests next to the neck of the talus (Fig. 5–22). Surrounding the ankle joint is a fibrous, synovium-lined capsule that is attached to the borders of the tibia, fibula, and talus. Upon injury or disease invasion, the synovium membrane secretes synovial fluid, resulting in distention of the fibrous capsule.[1, 2] Anterior fibrous capsule distention results in displacement of the anterior pretalar fat pad. Because neither the fibrous capsule nor the ankle ligaments can be detected on plain radiography, displacement of this fat pad indicates joint effusion and the possibility of underlying injuries.[1, 3]

  The posterior fat pad is positioned within the indentation formed by the articulation of the posterior tibia and talar bones (see Fig. 5–22). This fat pad is displaced in the same manner as the anterior pretalar fat pad, although it is less sensitive and requires more fluid evasion to be displaced.[2]

The bony trabecular patterns and cortical outlines of the metatarsals, tarsals, calcaneus, and talus are sharply defined.

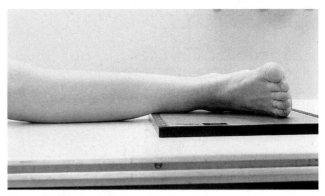

Figure 5-23. Accurate positioning of lower leg for a lateral foot radiograph.

- Sharply defined recorded details are obtained when patient motion is controlled, a detail screen and a small focal spot are used, and a short object–image distance (OID) is maintained.

The foot is in a true lateral position: The domes of the talus are superimposed, the tibiotalar joint is open, and the distal fibula is superimposed by the posterior half of the distal tibia.

- To obtain a true lateral foot radiograph, begin with the patient in a supine position with the leg extended (Fig. 5–23) and the foot dorsiflexed until its long axis forms a 90-degree angle with the lower leg. Rotate the patient and affected leg until the lateral foot surface is against the cassette; then adjust the degree of rotation until the surface is aligned parallel with the film (Fig. 5–24). For most patients, this positioning places the lower leg parallel with the radiographic tabletop. If this is not the case, as for a patient with a large upper thigh, the foot and film should be elevated until the lower leg is brought parallel with the tabletop.
- **_Importance of Proper Positioning:_** Do not try to adjust the leg in an attempt to position the plantar foot surface perpendicular to the film or directly superimpose the metatarsals. The true relationship of this surface to the film and the metatarsals to one another depends on the height of the patient's longitudinal arch and the incline of the calcaneus. Adjusting

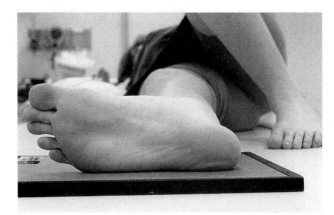

Figure 5-24. Accurate positioning of the lateral foot surface.

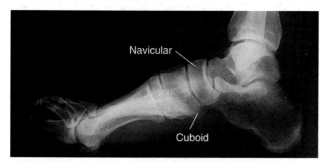

Figure 5-25. Accurate positioning of the lateral foot of a patient with a low arch.

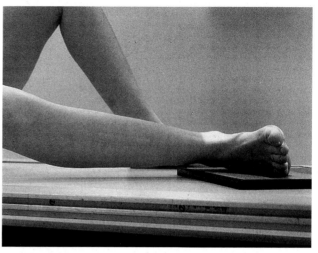

Figure 5-26. Poor positioning of the knee and lower leg for a lateral foot radiograph.

the patient's plantar surface may result in poor talar dome positioning and an erroneous longitudinal arch height.

The height of the longitudinal arch can be determined by measuring the amount of cuboid demonstrated distal to the navicular. The average foot radiograph demonstrates about 0.50 inch (1 cm) of the cuboid, as shown in Figure 5–21. Because the bones that form the foot arch are held in position by ligaments and tendons, weakening of these tissues may result in a decreased or low arch.[4] Radiographically, this decrease in arch height is demonstrated as a decrease in the amount of cuboid visualized distal to the navicular. Figure 5–25 shows a lateral foot radiograph of a patient with a low longitudinal arch. Note that only a small amount of cuboid is demonstrated without navicular superimposition. When such a radiograph is obtained, evaluate the talar domes to ensure that this cuboid-navicular relationship is a result of a low arch and not poor positioning. The talar domes should be superimposed.

- **Talar Domes:** The domes of the talus are formed by the most medial and lateral aspects of the talar's trochlear surface. Radiographically, they are visualized as domed structures that articulate with the tibia. On a true lateral foot radiograph, the talar domes should be superimposed and appear as one and the tibiotalar joint is open. When the lateral foot is mispositioned, the domes are individually demonstrated, and they obscure the tibiotalar joint. Misalignment of the domes results from poor knee or foot positioning.

- **Effect of Lower Leg Positioning on Talar Dome Superimposition:** Often, if the knee is not fully extended (Fig. 5–26) or if the distal tibia is not elevated to place the lower leg parallel with the film (on patients with large upper thighs), the proximal tibia is positioned farther from the table than the distal tibia. The resulting radiograph demonstrates the lateral talar dome proximal to the medial talar dome, and the height of the longitudinal arch appears less than it actually is, because the cuboid shifts proximally and the navicular moves distally in this position (see Rad. 15). If the distal tibia is positioned farther from the table than the proximal tibia, the medial talar dome is demonstrated proximal to the lateral dome, and the height of the longitudinal arch appears higher

than it actually is because the cuboid shifts distally and the navicular moves proximally in this position (see Rad. 16).

When viewing a lateral foot radiograph that demonstrates one of the talar domes proximal to the other, evaluate the height of the longitudinal arch to determine which dome is the proximal dome. If the navicular superimposes most of the cuboid, the lateral dome is the proximal dome; if the navicular superimposes very little of the cuboid, the medial dome is the proximal dome.

- **Effect of Foot Positioning on Talar Dome Superimposition:** To demonstrate accurate anterior and posterior alignment of the talar domes, position the lateral surface of the foot parallel with the film. If this surface is not parallel with the film, the talar domes are demonstrated one anterior to the other. When the leg is rotated more than needed to place the

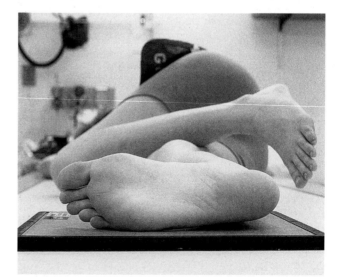

Figure 5-27. Poor lateral foot positioning with the calcaneus elevated.

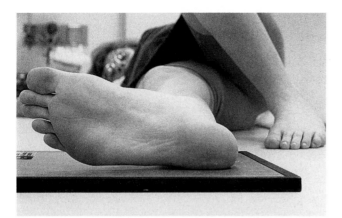

Figure 5-28. Poor lateral foot positioning with the calcaneus depressed.

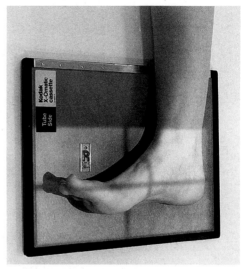

Figure 5-29. Lateral foot radiograph with accurate central ray *(CR)* centering and collimation.

lateral foot surface parallel with the film, as demonstrated in Figure 5–27, the medial talar dome is demonstrated anterior to the lateral talar dome (see Rad. 17). If the leg is not rotated enough to place the lateral foot surface parallel with the film, as demonstrated in Figure 5–28, the medial talar dome is demonstrated posterior to the lateral talar dome (see Rad. 18).

When viewing a lateral foot radiograph that demonstrates one of the talar domes anterior to the other, view the position of the fibula in relationship to the tibia to determine how to reposition the patient. On most accurately positioned lateral foot radiographs, the fibula is positioned in the posterior half of the tibia. If the fibula is demonstrated more posteriorly in this relationship on a poorly positioned foot radiograph, the medial talar dome is anterior, and the patient was positioned with the forefoot depressed and the heel elevated, as demonstrated in Figure 5–27. If the fibula is demonstrated more anteriorly in this relationship, the medial talar dome is posterior, and the patient was positioned with the forefoot elevated and the heel depressed, as demonstrated in Figure 5–28.

Carefully evaluate poorly positioned lateral foot radiographs. Often, both knee and foot corrections are needed simultaneously to obtain accurate positioning.

The long axis of the foot is positioned at a 90-degree angle with the lower leg and is aligned with the long axis of the collimated field.

- In most cases, when a patient is relaxed, the foot rests in plantar flexion. Plantar flexion results in a forced flattening of the anterior pretalar fat pad, reducing its usefulness in the detection of joint effusion[2] (see Rad. 19). Consequently, it is best to dorsiflex the foot, placing its long axis at a 90-degree angle with the lower leg. This positioning also places the tibiotalar joint in a neutral position and helps keep the leg and foot from rolling too far anteriorly. Anterior foot rotation elevates the heel and rotates the foot.
- Aligning the long axis of the foot with the long axis of the collimated field allows tight collimation without clipping the proximal or distal foot.

The proximal metatarsals are at the center of the collimated field. The phalanges, metatarsals, tarsals, talus, calcaneus, 1 inch (2.5 cm) of the distal lower leg, and the surrounding foot soft tissue are included within the field.

- Centering a perpendicular central ray halfway between the distal toes and heel and the anteroposterior aspect of the foot places the metatarsals at the center of the collimated field.
- Open the longitudinal collimation enough to include the patient's toes and heel. Transverse collimation should be to a point 1 inch (2.5 cm) proximal to the medial malleolus (Fig. 5–29).
- An 8 × 10 inch (18 × 24 cm) film placed diagonally or a 10 × 12 inch (24 × 30 cm) film placed crosswise should be adequate to include all the required anatomical structures.

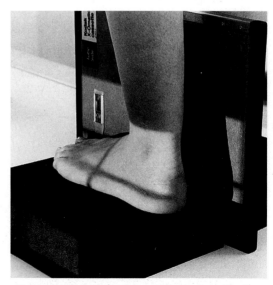

Figure 5-30. Proper lateromedial foot positioning.

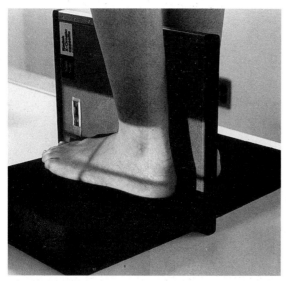

Figure 5–31. Poor lateromedial foot positioning.

STANDING LATEROMEDIAL PROJECTION

A standing lateromedial foot projection is accomplished by placing the film against the medial aspect of the foot and aligning the lateral foot surface parallel with the film, as demonstrated in Figure 5–30. Notice that the patient's heel is situated slightly away from the film when the lateral foot surface is parallel with the film. The resulting radiograph should meet all the evaluation requirements listed for the mediolateral projection.

The most common misposition for the standing lateromedial projection of the foot shows the medial talar dome positioned anterior to the lateral talar dome and the distal fibula positioned too posteriorly on the tibia (see Rad. 17). This misposition is a result of aligning the medial foot surface parallel with the film, as demonstrated in Figure 5–31, rather than the lateral surface.

Critiquing Radiographs

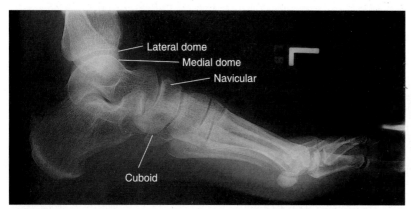

Radiograph 15.

Critique: The tibiotalar joint space is obscured, and one talar dome is demonstrated proximal to the other dome. Because the navicular superimposes most of the cuboid, the lateral dome is the proximal dome. The proximal tibia was elevated, as demonstrated in Figure 5–26.

Correction: Extend the knee, positioning the lower leg parallel with the film, as demonstrated in Figure 5–23. If the knee was extended for this radiograph, elevate the lower leg until it is positioned parallel with the film.

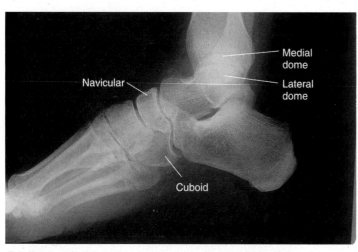

Radiograph 16.

Critique: The tibiotalar joint space is obscured, and one talar dome is demonstrated proximal to the other dome. Because more than 0.50 inch (1 cm) of cuboid is visualized distal to the navicular, the medial dome is the proximal dome. The distal tibia was elevated. The phalanges are not demonstrated.

Correction: Position the lower leg parallel with the film, and shift the central ray and film 1 inch (2.5 cm) distally.

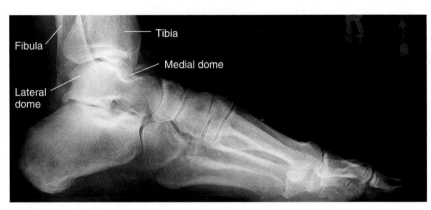

Radiograph 17.

Critique: The medial talar dome is positioned anterior to the lateral dome, as indicated by the posterior position of the fibula on the tibia. The lateral foot surface was not positioned parallel with the film. If this is a mediolateral projection, the forefoot was depressed and heel was elevated, as demonstrated in Figure 5–27. If this is a standing lateromedial projection, the medial surface of the patient's heel was placed next to the cassette, as demonstrated in Figure 5–31.

Correction: For a mediolateral projection, elevate the patient's forefoot and depress the patient's heel until the lateral foot surface is positioned parallel with the film, as demonstrated in Figure 5–24. For a standing lateromedial projection, draw the patient's heel away from the film until the lateral foot surface is positioned parallel with the film, as demonstrated in Figure 5–30.

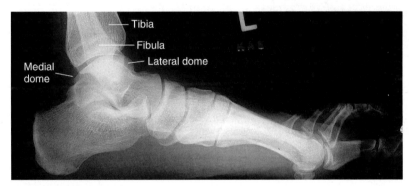

Radiograph 18.

Critique: The medial talar dome is positioned posterior to the lateral dome, as indicated by the anterior position of the distal fibula on the tibia. The lateral foot surface was not positioned parallel with the film, but was positioned with the forefoot elevated and heel depressed, as demonstrated in Figure 5–28.

Correction: Depress the patient's forefoot and elevate the heel until the lateral foot surface is positioned parallel with the film, as demonstrated in Figure 5–24.

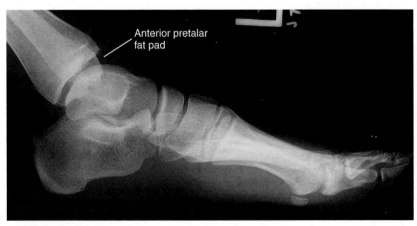

Radiograph 19.

Critique: The lower leg and long axis of the foot do not form a 90-degree angle. The patient's foot was in plantar flexion. There is also a small amount of foot rotation.

Correction: Dorsiflex the foot until the lower leg and long axis of the foot form a 90-degree angle.

CALCANEUS

Axial (Plantodorsal) Projection

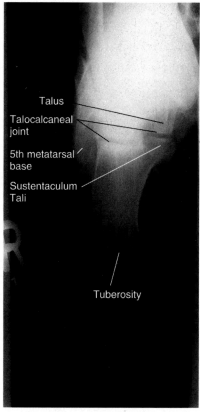

Talus

Talocalcaneal joint

5th metatarsal base

Sustentaculum Tali

Tuberosity

Figure 5-32. Accurately positioned axial calcaneal radiograph.

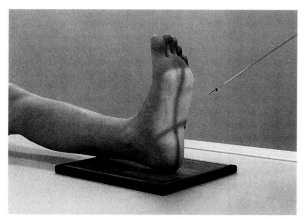

Figure 5-33. Proper axial calcaneal radiograph positioning.

Radiographic Evaluation

Facility's patient identification requirements are visible on radiograph.
- These requirements usually are facility name, patient name, age, and hospital number, and exam time and date.
- Patient ID plate is positioned so as not to obscure anatomy of interest.

A right or left marker, identifying the correct calcaneus, is present on the radiograph and does not superimpose anatomy of interest.
- Place the marker within the collimated light field so it does not superimpose any portion of the calcaneus.

There is no evidence of preventable artifacts, such as bandages and splints.
- Consult with the ordering physician and the patient about whether bandages and splints can be removed.

Contrast and density are adequate to demonstrate the surrounding soft tissue and bony structures of the calcaneus. Penetration is sufficient to visualize the bony trabecular patterns and cortical outlines of the calcaneal tuberosity and the talocalcaneal joint space.

- An optimal 60 to 70 kVp technique sufficiently penetrates the bony and soft tissue structures of the calcaneus and provides high radiographic contrast.

The bony trabecular patterns and cortical outlines of the calcaneal tuberosity and the talocalcaneal joint space are sharply defined.
- Sharply defined recorded details are obtained when patient motion is controlled, a detail screen and a small focal spot are used, and a short object–image distance (OID) is maintained.

The talocalcaneal joint is demonstrated as an open space, and the calcaneal tuberosity is visualized without distortion.
- The talocalcaneal joint space is demonstrated as an open space, and the calcaneal tuberosity is visualized without distortion, when the correct central ray angulation and foot position are used. For a patient who has foot mobility, place the foot in a neutral, vertical position, and direct a 40-degree central ray angulation toward the plantar foot surface (Fig. 5–33). This positioning places the central ray parallel with the talocalcaneal joint space and perpendicular to the calcaneal tuberosity (Fig. 5–34).
- ***Compensating for Plantar-Flexed or Dorsiflexed Foot:*** When the patient's foot is dorsiflexed beyond a 90-degree position with the lower leg or is plantar flexed, the central ray needs to be adjusted to maintain its accurate position with the calcaneal joint space and tuberosity. If the patient's foot is dorsiflexed beyond the vertical position and a 40-degree angulation were used, the calcaneal joint spaces would be obscured and the tuberosity elongated (Fig. 5–35 and Rad. 20). For this situation, the central ray angulation should be decreased to maintain accurate central ray alignment. If the patient's foot is plantar flexed and a 40-degree central ray angulation were used, the calcaneal joint spaces would be obscured and the tuberosity foreshortened (Rad. 21 and Fig. 5–36). For this situation, the central ray angulation should be increased to maintain accurate central ray alignment.

The angulation that is required for each of these situations can be estimated by locating the base of the

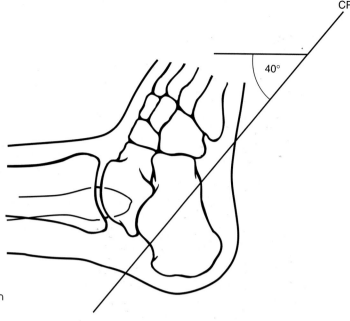

Figure 5-34. Central ray angled 40 degrees with foot in 90-degree position. *CR*, central ray.

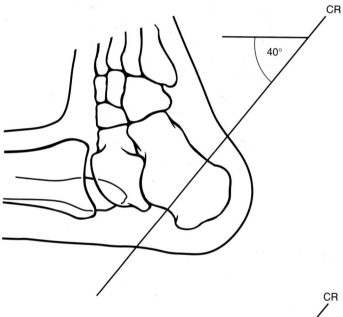

Figure 5-35. Central ray angled 40 degrees with foot in dorsiflexion. *CR*, central ray.

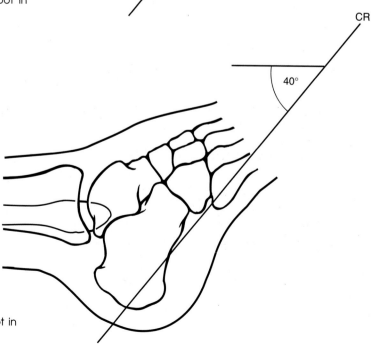

Figure 5-36. Central ray angled 40 degrees with foot in plantar flexion. *CR*, central ray.

fifth metatarsal and the distal portion of the lateral malleolus. The fifth metatarsal base is palpable on the lateral foot surface about halfway between the ball of the foot and the heel. Once these structures are located, angle the central ray parallel with an imaginary line drawn between them. When the axial calcaneal radiograph is taken with the foot in plantar flexion and the central ray is angled to demonstrate the joint space, the tuberosity is elongated (see Rad. 22).

Neither the first nor the fourth and fifth distal metatarsals are visualized on the medial or lateral aspect of the foot, respectively.

- To prevent calcaneal tilting, place the ankle in a true AP projection without medial or lateral rotation. If the ankle is rotated medially, the first metatarsal is demonstrated medially (see Rad. 23). If the ankle is laterally rotated, the fourth and fifth metatarsals are demonstrated laterally (see Rad. 24).

The proximal calcaneal tuberosity is at the center of the collimated field. The calcaneal tuberosity and the talocalcaneal joint space are included within the field.

- Centering the central ray to the midline of the foot at the level of the fifth metatarsal base places the proximal tuberosity in the center of the collimated field.
- Open the longitudinal collimation enough to include the patient's entire heel. Transverse collimation should be to the heel skin-line.
- Half of an 8 × 10 inch (18 × 24 cm) film placed crosswise should be adequate to include all the required anatomical structures.

Critiquing Radiographs

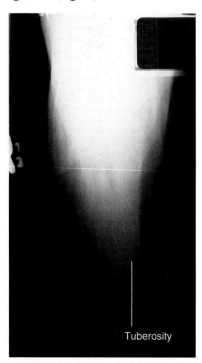

Radiograph 20.

Critique: The talocalcaneal joint space is obscured, and the calcaneal tuberosity is elongated. The foot was dorsiflexed beyond the vertical position, and a 40-degree central ray angulation was used.

Correction: Plantar-flex the foot to a vertical position and use a 40-degree angulation. If the patient cannot plantar-flex the foot, decrease the degree of central ray angulation, aligning the central ray with the fifth metatarsal base and the distal aspect of the lateral malleolus.

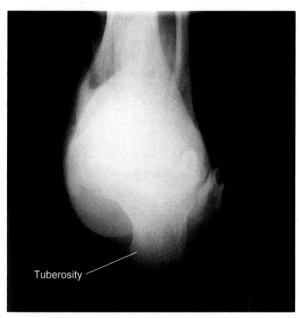

Radiograph 21.

Critique: The talocalcaneal joint space is obscured, and the calcaneal tuberosity is foreshortened. The foot was in plantar flexion and the standard 40-degree central ray angulation was used.

Correction: If patient condition allows, dorsiflex the foot to a vertical, neutral position. If the patient cannot dorsiflex the foot, increase the central ray angulation, aligning the central ray with the fifth metatarsal base and the distal aspect of the lateral malleolus.

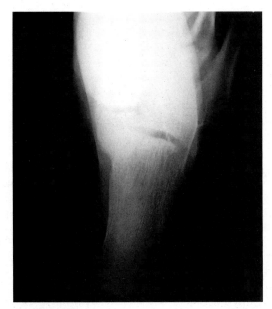

Radiograph 22.

Critique: The talocalcaneal joint space is demonstrated, and the calcaneal tuberosity is greatly elongated. The foot was in plantar flexion, and the central ray was angled so it was aligned with an imaginary line that connects the fifth metatarsal tuberosity and the tip of the lateral malleolus.

Correction: No correction movement is needed. Elongation is not preventable if the patient's foot cannot be dorsiflexed.

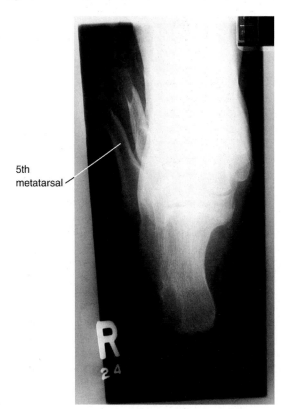

Radiograph 24.

Critique: The fourth and fifth metatarsals are demonstrated laterally. The ankle was laterally rotated.

Correction: Internally rotate the leg until the ankle is in an AP projection.

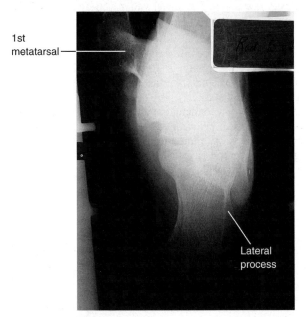

Radiograph 23.

Critique: The first metatarsal is demonstrated medially. The ankle was medially rotated.

Correction: Position the ankle in an AP projection.

Calcaneus: Lateral Position
(Mediolateral Projection)

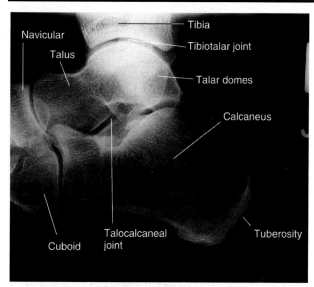

Figure 5–37. Accurately positioned lateral calcaneal radiograph.

Radiographic Evaluation

Facility's patient identification requirements are visible on radiograph.
- These requirements usually are facility name, patient name, age, and hospital number, and exam time and date.
- Patient ID plate is positioned so as not to obscure anatomy of interest.

A right or left marker, identifying the correct calcaneus, is present on radiograph and does not superimpose anatomy of interest.
- Place the marker within the collimated light field so it does not superimpose any portion of the calcaneus.

There is no evidence of preventable artifacts, such as bandages and splints.
- Consult with the ordering physician and the patient about whether bandages and splints can be removed.

Contrast and density are adequate to demonstrate the surrounding soft tissue and bony structures of the calcaneus. Penetration is sufficient to visualize the bony trabecular patterns and cortical outlines of the calcaneus, sinus tarsi, and talus, and all calcaneus-articulating tarsal bones.
- An optimal 55 to 65 kVp technique sufficiently penetrates the bony and soft tissue structures of the calcaneus and provides high radiographic contrast.

The bony trabecular patterns and cortical outlines of the calcaneus, talus, and calcaneus-articulating tarsal bones are sharply defined.
- Sharply defined recorded details are obtained when patient motion is controlled, a detail screen and a small focal spot are used, and a short object–image distance (OID) is maintained.

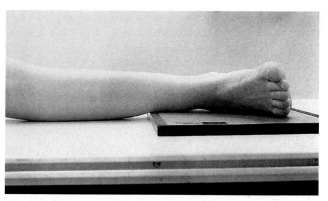

Figure 5–38. Proper lower leg positioning for lateral calcaneal radiograph.

The calcaneus and distal tibia and fibula are in a true lateral position: The domes of the talus are superimposed, the tibiotalar joint space is open, and the distal fibula is superimposed by the posterior half of the distal tibia.
- To obtain a true lateral calcaneal radiograph, begin with the patient in a supine position, with the leg extended (Fig. 5–38) and the foot dorsiflexed until its long axis forms a 90-degree angle with the lower leg. Rotate the patient and the affected leg until the lateral foot surface is against the cassette; then adjust the degree of rotation until the surface is aligned parallel with the film (Fig. 5–39). For most patients, this positioning places the lower leg parallel with the radiographic tabletop. If this is not the case, as for a patient with a large upper thigh, the foot and film should be elevated to place the lower leg parallel with the tabletop.
- ***Importance of Proper Positioning:*** Do not try to adjust the leg in an attempt to position the plantar foot surface perpendicular to the film or directly superimpose the metatarsals. The true relationship of this surface to the film and the metatarsals to one another depends on the height of the patient's longitudinal arch and incline of the calcaneus. Radiographically, the average foot arch demonstrates about 0.50 inch (1 cm) of the cuboid distal to the navicular.

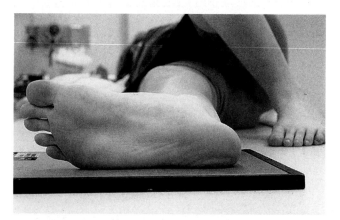

Figure 5–39. Proper lateral foot surface positioning for lateral calcaneal radiograph.

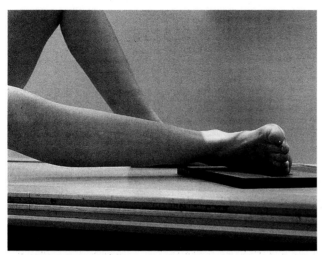

Figure 5-40. Poor knee and lower leg positioning for lateral calcaneal radiograph.

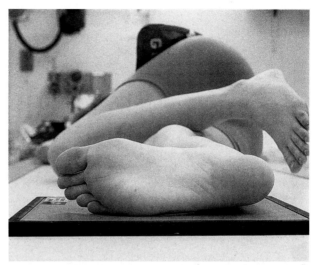

Figure 5-41. Poor lateral foot positioning with the calcaneus elevated.

- *Talar Domes:* The domes of the talus are formed by the most medial and lateral aspects of the talar's trochlear surface. They are visualized on a lateral calcaneal radiograph as domed structures that articulate with the tibia. When a true lateral calcaneus view has been obtained, the talar domes should be superimposed and appear as one, and the tibiotalar joint should be open. If the lateral calcaneus is mispositioned, the domes are individually demonstrated and they obscure the tibiotalar joint. Misalignment of the domes will result from poor knee and/or foot positioning.

- *Effect of Lower Leg Positioning on Talar Dome Superimposition:* Often, if the knee is not fully extended (Fig. 5–40) or if the distal tibia is not elevated to place the lower leg parallel with the film (on a patient with a large upper thigh), the proximal tibia is positioned farther from the table than the distal tibia. The resulting radiograph demonstrates the lateral talar dome proximal to the medial talar dome, and the height of the longitudinal arch appears less than it actually is, because the cuboid shifts proximally and the navicular moves distally in this position (see Rad. 25). If the distal tibia is positioned farther from the table than the proximal tibia, the medial talar dome is demonstrated proximal to the lateral dome, and the height of the longitudinal arch appears higher than it actually is, because the cuboid shifts distally and the navicular moves proximally (see Rad. 26).

  When viewing a lateral calcaneal radiograph that demonstrates one of the talar domes proximal to the other, evaluate the height of the longitudinal arch to determine which dome is the proximal dome. If the navicular superimposes most of the cuboid, the lateral dome is the proximal dome; if the navicular superimposes very little of the cuboid, the medial dome is the proximal dome.

- *Effect of Foot Positioning on Talar Dome Superimposition:* To demonstrate accurate anterior and posterior alignment of the talar domes, the lateral surface of the foot should be positioned parallel

with the film. If this surface is not parallel with the film, the talar domes are demonstrated one anterior to the other. When the leg is rotated more than needed to place the lateral foot surface parallel with the film, as demonstrated in Figure 5–41, the medial talar dome is demonstrated anterior to the lateral talar dome (see Rad. 27). If the leg is not rotated enough to place the lateral foot surface parallel with the film, as demonstrated in Figure 5–42, the medial talar dome is demonstrated posterior to the lateral talar dome (see Rad. 28).

When viewing a lateral calcaneus radiograph that demonstrates one of the talar domes anterior to the other, view the position of the fibula in relationship to the tibia to determine how the patient should be repositioned. On most accurately positioned lateral calcaneus radiographs, the fibula is positioned in the posterior half of the tibia. On a poorly positioned calcaneus radiograph, if the fibula is demonstrated more posteriorly, the medial talar dome is anterior, and the patient was positioned with the forefoot depressed and the heel elevated, as demonstrated in

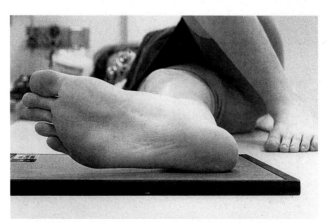

Figure 5-42. Poor lateral foot positioning with the calcaneus depressed.

Figure 5–41. If the fibula is demonstrated more anteriorly, the medial domes are posterior, and the patient was positioned with the forefoot elevated and the heel depressed, as demonstrated in Figure 5–42.

Carefully evaluate poorly positioned lateral calcaneal radiographs. Often, both knee and foot corrections are needed simultaneously to obtain accurate positioning.

The long axis of the foot is positioned at a 90-degree angle with the lower leg.

- In most cases, when a patient is relaxed, the foot rests in plantar flexion, making it difficult for the patient to maintain a true lateral position. Often the patient rotates the foot too far anteriorly, elevating the heel and rotating the foot (see Rad. 29). Consequently, it is best to dorsiflex the patient's foot, placing its long axis at a 90-degree angle with the lower leg.

The midcalcaneus is at the center of the collimated field. The tibiotalar joint, talus, calcaneus, and calcaneus-articulating tarsal bones are included within the field.

- Center a perpendicular central ray to the midcalcaneus to place the calcaneus in the center of the collimated field. Centering to the midcalcaneus better demonstrates the calcaneus and the surrounding calcaneotarsal and talocalcaneal articulations, allowing for accurate calcaneal inclination measurements and for visualization of calcaneal tuberosity displacement.[3]
- Open the longitudinal collimation enough to include the calcaneus and tibiotalar joint, which is located at the level of the palpable medial malleolus. Including the tibiotalar joint on all lateral calcaneal radiographs

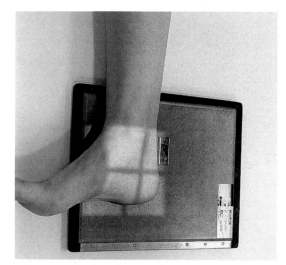

Figure 5–43. Accurate lateral calcaneal radiograph with central ray *(CR)* centering and collimation.

provides a method of judging rotation and determining how to reposition when a rotated lateral calcaneal radiograph has been obtained. Transverse collimation should be to the calcaneal tuberosity and the calcaneotarsal joint spaces. You can ensure that the calcaneotarsal joint spaces are included by extending the transverse collimation at least 2 inches (5 cm) anterior to the medial malleolus (Fig. 5–43).

- Half of an 8 × 10 inch (18 × 24 cm) film placed crosswise should be adequate to include all the required anatomical structures.

Critiquing Radiographs

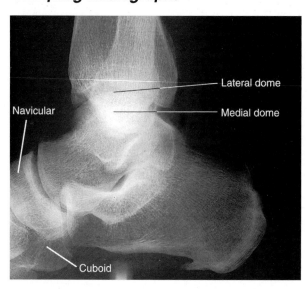

Radiograph 25.

Critique: The tibiotalar joint space is obscured, and one talar dome is demonstrated proximal to the other dome. Because the navicular superimposes most of the cuboid, the lateral dome is the proximal dome. The proximal tibia was elevated, as demonstrated in Figure 5–40.

Correction: Extend the knee to position the lower leg parallel with the film, as demonstrated in Figure 5–38. If the knee was extended for this radiograph, elevate the lower leg until it is positioned parallel with the film.

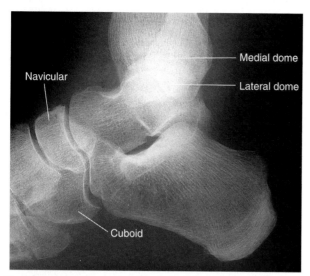

Radiograph 26.

Critique: The tibiotalar joint space is obscured, and one talar dome is demonstrated proximal to the other dome. Because more than 0.50 inch (1 cm) of cuboid is visualized distal to the navicular, the medial dome is the proximal dome. The distal tibia was elevated.

Correction: Position the lower leg parallel with the film.

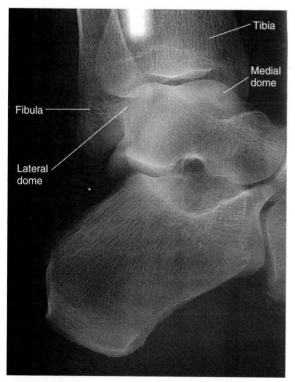

Radiograph 27.

Critique: The medial talar dome is positioned anterior to the lateral talar dome, as indicated by the posterior position of the fibula on the tibia. The lateral foot surface was not positioned parallel with the film. The patient's forefoot was depressed and the heel was elevated, as demonstrated in Figure 5–41.

Correction: Elevate the patient's forefoot and depress the heel until the lateral foot surface is parallel with the film, as demonstrated in Figure 5–39.

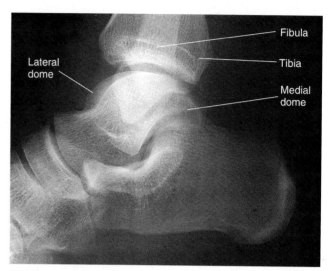

Radiograph 28.

Critique: The medial talar dome is positioned posterior to the lateral dome, as indicated by the anterior position of the distal fibula on the tibia. The lateral foot surface was positioned not parallel with the film but with the forefoot elevated and the heel depressed, as demonstrated in Figure 5–42.

Correction: Depress the patient's forefoot and elevate the heel until the lateral foot surface is positioned parallel with the film, as demonstrated in Figure 5–39.

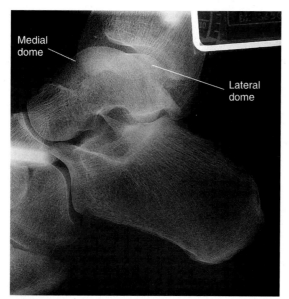

Medial dome

Lateral dome

Radiograph 29.

Critique: The lower leg and the long axis of the foot do not form a 90-degree angle, and the medial talar dome is positioned anterior to the lateral dome. The patient's foot was in plantar flexion, allowing the leg to roll too far anteriorly and resulting in an elevated heel.

Correction: Dorsiflex the foot until the lower leg and the long axis of the foot form a 90-degree angle. Adjust patient rotation until the lateral foot surface is positioned parallel with the film, as demonstrated in Figure 5–39.

ANKLE

Anteroposterior Projection

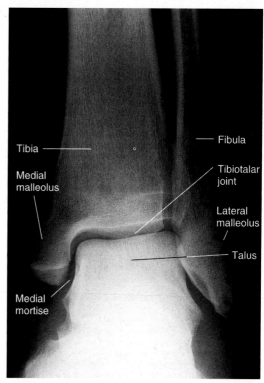

Tibia

Medial malleolus

Medial mortise

Fibula

Tibiotalar joint

Lateral malleolus

Talus

Figure 5–44. Accurately positioned AP ankle radiograph.

Radiographic Evaluation

Facility's patient identification requirements are visible on radiograph.
- These requirements usually are facility name, patient name, age, and hospital number, and exam time and date.
- Patient ID plate is positioned toward the proximal tibia so as not to obscure anatomy of interest.

A right or left marker, identifying the correct ankle, is present on the radiograph and does not superimpose anatomy of interest.
- Place the marker within the collimated light field so it does not superimpose any portion of the ankle.
- When more than one view of the ankle is placed on a film, only one of the views needs to be marked.

There is no evidence of preventable artifacts, such as bandages and splints.
- Consult with the ordering physician and the patient about whether bandages and splints can be removed.

Contrast and density are adequate to demonstrate the surrounding soft tissue and bony structures of the ankle. Penetration is sufficient to visualize the bony trabecular patterns and cortical outlines of the talus and distal tibia and fibula.

- An optimal 55 to 65 kVp technique sufficiently penetrates the bony and soft tissue structures of the ankle and provides high radiographic contrast.

The bony trabecular patterns and cortical outlines of the talus and distal tibia and fibula are sharply defined.

- Sharply defined recorded details are obtained when patient motion is controlled, a detail screen and a small focal spot are used, and a short object–image distance (OID) is maintained.

The ankle is demonstrated in a true AP projection: The medial mortise (tibiotalar articulation) is open, and the distal tibia and talus partially superimpose the distal fibula, closing the lateral mortise (fibulotalar articulation).

- An AP projection of the ankle is obtained by positioning the patient supine on the radiographic table, with the leg fully extended and the foot dorsiflexed until its long axis is placed in a vertical position (Fig. 5–45). In this position, the intermalleolar line (imaginary line drawn between the medial and lateral malleoli) is at a 15- to 20-degree angle with the film. The medial malleolus is positioned farther from the film than the lateral malleolus.
- ***Detecting Direction of Ankle Rotation:*** If the ankle was not positioned in a true AP projection but is rotated laterally or medially, the medial mortise is obscured. When an AP ankle radiograph demonstrates a closed medial mortise, one can determine which way the patient's leg was rotated by evaluating the amount of tibia and talar superimposition of the fibula. In lateral rotation, the tibia and talus demonstrate greater superimposition of the fibula, and the posterior aspect of the medial malleolus (Fig. 5–46) is situated lateral to the anterior aspect (see Rad. 30). In medial rotation, the fibula is demonstrated with little if any talar superimposition (see Rad. 31).

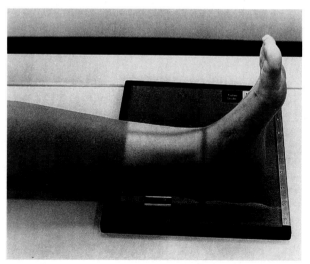

Figure 5–45. Proper patient positioning for AP ankle radiograph.

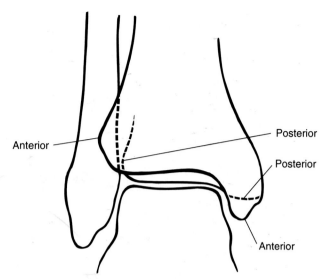

Figure 5–46. Anatomy of anterior and posterior ankle.

The tibiotalar joint space is open, and the tibia is demonstrated without foreshortening.

- The tibiotalar joint is open and the tibia is demonstrated without foreshortening if the patient's lower leg was positioned parallel with the film and the central ray was centered at the level of the tibiotalar joint.
- ***Evaluating the Openness of the Tibiotalar Joint:*** Radiographically, you can determine whether an open joint was obtained and whether the tibia is demonstrated without foreshortening by evaluating the anterior and posterior margins of the distal tibia. On an accurately positioned AP ankle radiograph, the anterior margin is visualized about 0.125 inch (3 mm) proximal to the posterior margin (Fig. 5–46). If the proximal lower leg was elevated or the central ray was centered proximal to the tibiotalar joint, the anterior tibial margin is projected distally, resulting in a narrowed or obscured tibiotalar joint space (see Rad. 32). If the distal lower leg was elevated or the central ray was centered distal to the tibiotalar joint, the anterior tibial margin is projected more proximal to the posterior margin than on a true AP ankle radiograph, expanding the tibiotalar joint space and demonstrating the tibial articulating surface (see Rad. 33).
- ***Effect of Foot Positioning on Tibiotalar Joint Visualization:*** The position of the foot also determines how well the tibiotalar joint space is demonstrated. The patient's foot should be placed vertically, with its long axis positioned at a 90-degree angle with the lower leg. When the ankle radiograph is taken with the foot dorsiflexed, the trochlear surface of the talus is wedged into the anterior tibial region,[5] resulting in a narrower-appearing joint space. If the foot is plantar flexed, the calcaneus is moved proximally, beneath the body of the talus, resulting in talocalcaneal superimposition and possibly hindering visualization of the talar trochlear surface.

The long axis of the tibia is aligned with the long axis of the collimated field.

- This alignment, which allows tight collimation without clipping the distal tibia or fibula, is accomplished by aligning the collimator's longitudinal light line with the middle of the lower leg.

The tibiotalar joint space is at the center of the collimated field. The distal fourth of the tibia and fibula, the talus, and the surrounding ankle soft tissue are included within the field.

- To place the tibiotalar joint in the center of the radiograph, center a perpendicular central ray to the ankle midline at the level of the palpable medial malleolus. The medial malleolus is located at the same level as the tibiotalar joint space. Open the longitudinal collimation to include the calcaneus and one fourth of distal lower leg. Transverse collimation should be to the ankle skin-line.

- Half of a 10 × 12 inch (24 × 30 cm) film placed crosswise should be adequate to include all the required anatomical structures.
- ***Ankle Exam to Include More Than One Fourth of the Lower Leg:*** If an ankle exam order requests that more than one fourth of the distal lower leg be included, the central ray should remain on the ankle joint, and the collimated field should be opened to demonstrate the desired amount of lower leg. This method will result in an unneeded radiation field extending beyond the foot and ankle, but it should not cause an increase in patient dosage because no additional patient tissue is exposed. A flat contact shield placed over this extended radiation field prevents backscattered radiation from reaching the film. The advantage of this method over centering the central ray proximal to the ankle joint is an undistorted view of the ankle joint.

Critiquing Radiographs

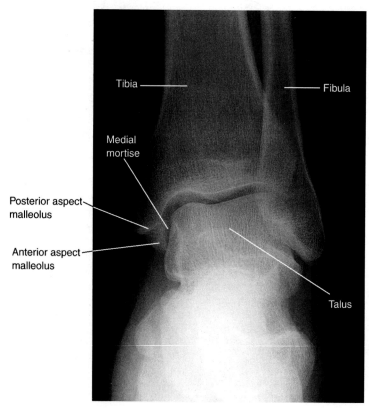

Radiograph 30.

Critique: The ankle was not placed in a true AP projection. The medial mortise is obscured, the tibia and talus demonstrate increased superimposition of the fibula, and the posterior aspect of the medial malleolus is situated lateral to the anterior aspect. The ankle was laterally rotated.

Correction: Rotate the leg medially, placing the long axis of the foot in a vertical position.

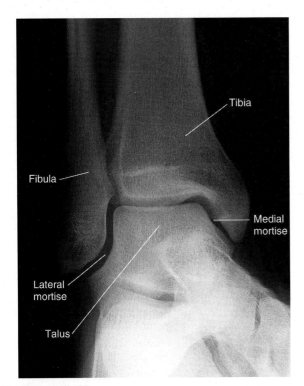

Radiograph 31.

Critique: The ankle was not placed in a true AP projection. The medial mortise is obscured, and the fibula demonstrates no talar superimposition. The ankle was medially rotated.

Correction: Rotate the leg laterally, placing the long axis of the foot in a vertical position.

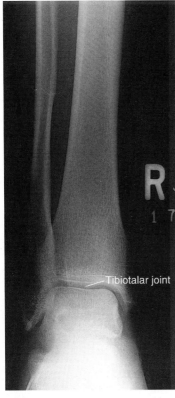

Radiograph 32.

Critique: The tibiotalar joint is closed. The anterior tibial margin has been projected into the joint space. Either the proximal tibia was elevated owing to knee flexion, or the central ray was centered superior to the tibiotalar joint.

Correction: Extend the knee, lowering the proximal tibia until the lower leg is parallel with the film, or center the central ray to the tibiotalar joint (located at the level of the medial malleolus).

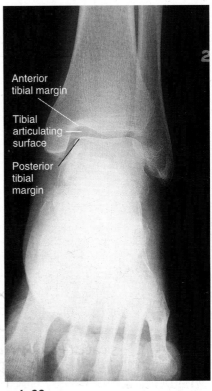

Radiograph 33.

Critique: The tibiotalar joint is distorted. The anterior tibial margin is projected superior to the posterior margin, and the tibial articulating surface is demonstrated. Either the distal tibia was elevated or the central ray was centered inferior to the tibiotalar joint.

Correction: Depress the distal tibia or elevate the proximal tibia until the lower leg is placed parallel with the film, or center the central ray to the tibiotalar joint at the level of the medial malleolus.

235

Ankle: Medial (Internal) Oblique Position

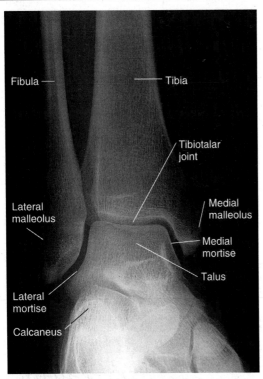

Figure 5-47. Accurately positioned oblique ankle radiograph.

Radiographic Evaluation

Facility's patient identification requirements are visible on radiograph.
- These requirements usually are facility name, patient name, age, and hospital number, and exam time and date.
- Patient ID plate is positioned so as not to obscure anatomy of interest.

A right or left marker, identifying the correct ankle, is present on the radiograph and does not superimpose anatomy of interest.
- Place the marker within the collimated light field so it does not superimpose any portion of the ankle. When more than one view of the ankle is placed on a film, it is necessary to mark only one of the views.

There is no evidence of preventable artifacts, such as bandages and splints.
- Consult with the ordering physician and the patient about whether bandages and splints can be removed.

Contrast and density are adequate to demonstrate the surrounding soft tissue and bony structures of the ankle. Penetration is sufficient to visualize the bony trabecular patterns and cortical outlines of the talus and distal tibia and fibula.
- An optimal 55 to 60 kVp technique sufficiently penetrates the bony and soft tissue structures of the ankle and provides high radiographic contrast.

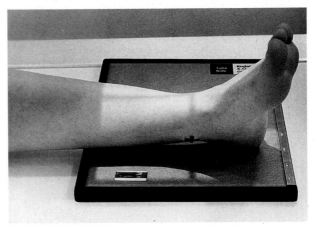

Figure 5-48. Proper patient positioning for oblique ankle radiograph.

The bony trabecular patterns and cortical outlines of the talus and distal tibia and fibula are sharply defined.
- Sharply defined recorded details are obtained when patient motion is controlled, a detail screen and a small focal spot are used, and a short object–image distance (OID) is maintained.

The ankle demonstrates adequate obliquity: The distal fibula is demonstrated without talar superimposition, visualizing an open lateral mortise (talofibular joint), and the lateral and medial malleoli are demonstrated in profile.
- To obtain an accurately positioned oblique ankle radiograph, place the patient in a supine AP projection with the leg extended and the foot positioned vertically (Fig. 5–48). While viewing the plantar surface of the foot, place your index fingers on the most prominent aspects of the lateral and the medial malleoli. Rotate the patient's entire leg medially (15 to 20 degrees) until your index fingers and the malleoli are positioned at equal distances from the film (Fig. 5–49). An imaginary line drawn between the malleoli (intermalleolar line) is then aligned parallel with the film. This rota-

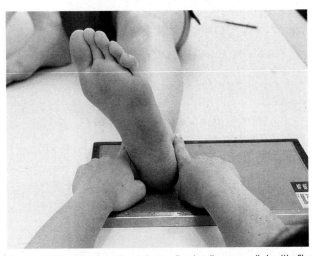

Figure 5-49. Aligning the intermalleolar line parallel with film for the oblique ankle radiograph.

tion moves the fibula away from the talus to demonstrate an open lateral mortise.

- **Detecting Ankle Rotation:** When the ankle are inadequately rotated, the distal fibula and talus are partially superimposed and the lateral mortise will be closed. To determine whether the ankle has been over- or under-rotated, evaluate the visualization of the medial mortise (tibiotalar joint) and the tarsi sinus (opening between the calcaneus and talus). If the medial mortise is demonstrated as an open space and the tarsi sinus has not been visualized, the patient's leg and ankle were not rotated enough (see Rad. 34). If the medial mortise is closed and the tarsi sinus has been visualized, the patient's leg and ankle were over-rotated (see Rad. 35).

The tibiotalar joint space is open, and the tibia is demonstrated without foreshortening.

- The tibiotalar joint space is open and the tibia is demonstrated without foreshortening when the patient's lower leg was positioned parallel with the film and the central ray was centered at the level of the tibiotalar joint (see Fig. 5–48).
- **Evaluating the Openness of the Tibiotalar Joint:** Radiographically, you can determine whether the positioning and alignment goals have been met by evaluating the anterior and posterior margins of the distal tibia. On an accurately positioned oblique ankle radiograph, the anterior margin should be visualized about 0.125 inch (3 mm) proximal to the posterior margin. If the proximal lower leg was elevated or the central ray was centered proximal to the tibiotalar joint, the anterior tibial margin is projected distally, resulting in a narrowed or obscured tibiotalar joint. If the patient's distal lower leg was elevated or the central ray was centered distal to the tibiotalar joint, the anterior tibial margin is projected too far superior to the posterior margin, expanding the tibiotalar joint space and demonstrating the tibial articulating surface (see Rad. 36).

The calcaneus is demonstrated distal to the lateral mortise and fibula.

- To position the calcaneus distal to the lateral mortise and fibula, place the foot in a neutral position by positioning its long axis at a 90-degree angle with the lower leg. If the foot was plantar flexed for an oblique radiograph, the calcaneus obscures the distal aspect of the lateral mortise and the distal fibula (see Rad. 37).

The long axis of the tibia is aligned with the long axis of the collimated field.

- This alignment, which allows tight collimation without clipping the distal tibia or fibula, is accomplished by aligning the collimator's longitudinal light line with the middle of the lower leg.

The tibiotalar joint space is at the center of the collimated field. The distal fourth of the fibula and tibia, the talus, and the surrounding ankle soft tissue are included within the field.

- To place the tibiotalar joint in the center of the radiograph, center a perpendicular central ray to the ankle

midline at the level of the palpable medial malleolus. The medial malleolus is located at the same level as the tibiotalar joint space. Open the longitudinal collimation to include the calcaneus and one fourth of the distal lower leg. Transverse collimation should be to the ankle skin-line.

- Half of a 10 × 12 inch (24 × 30 cm) film placed crosswise should be adequate to include all the required anatomical structures.
- **Ankle Exam to Include More Than One Fourth of the Lower Leg:** If an ankle exam order requests that more than one fourth of the distal lower leg be included, the central ray should remain on the ankle joint, and the collimated field should be opened to demonstrate the desired amount of lower leg. This method results in an unneeded radiation field extending beyond the ankle and foot but should not cause an increase in patient dosage because no additional patient tissue is exposed. A flat lead contact strip placed over this extended radiation field prevents backscattered radiation from reaching the film. The advantage of this method over centering the central ray proximal to the ankle joint is an undistorted view of the ankle joint.

Critiquing Radiographs

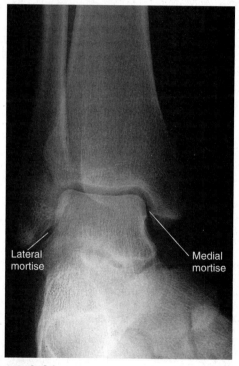

Radiograph 34.

Critique: The lateral mortise (talofibular joint) is closed, and the medial mortise is demonstrated as an open space. The tarsi sinus is not visualized. The patient's leg and ankle were not rotated medially enough.

Correction: Rotate the entire leg medially until the most prominent aspects of the lateral and medial malleoli are positioned at equal distances from the film, as demonstrated in Figure 5–49.

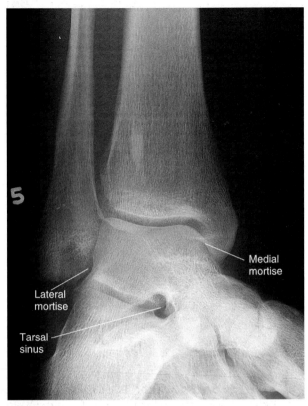

Radiograph 35.

Critique: The lateral and medial mortises are closed, and the tarsi sinus is demonstrated. The patient's leg and ankle were rotated too far medially.

Correction: Rotate the entire leg laterally until the most prominent aspects of the lateral and medial malleoli are positioned at equal distances from the film, as demonstrated in Figure 5–49.

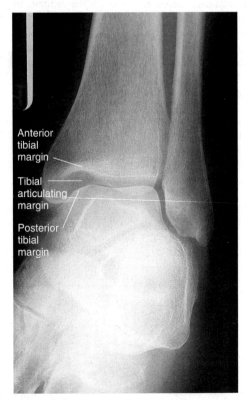

Radiograph 36.

Critique: The tibiotalar joint space is expanded. The anterior tibial margin has been projected superior to the posterior margin, and the tibial articulating surface is demonstrated. Either the distal tibia was elevated or the central ray was centered distal to the tibiotalar joint.

Correction: Depress the distal tibia or elevate the proximal tibia until the lower leg is placed parallel with the film, or center the central ray to the tibiotalar joint at the level of the medial malleolus.

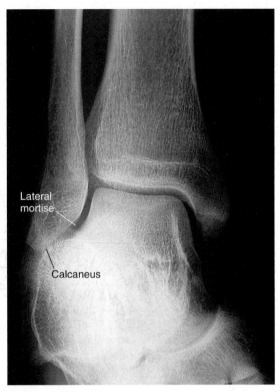

Radiograph 37.

Critique: The calcaneus is obscuring the distal aspect of the lateral mortise and distal fibula. The foot was in plantar flexion for the radiograph.

Correction: Dorsiflex the foot until its long axis forms a 90-degree angle with the lower leg.

Ankle: Lateral Position (Mediolateral Projection)

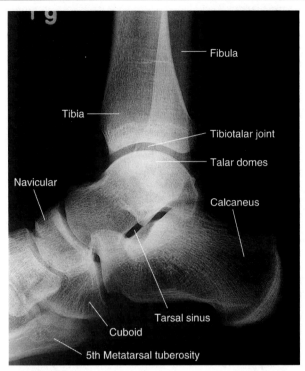

Figure 5-50. Accurately positioned lateral ankle radiograph.

Radiographic Evaluation

Facility's patient identification requirements are visible on radiograph.
- These requirements usually are facility name, patient name, age, and hospital number, and exam time and date.
- Patient ID plate is positioned so as not to obscure anatomy of interest.

A right or left marker, identifying the correct ankle, is present on the radiograph and does not superimpose anatomy of interest.
- Place the marker within the collimated light field so it does not superimpose any portion of the ankle.

There is no evidence of preventable artifacts, such as bandages and splints.
- Consult with the ordering physician and the patient about whether bandages and splints can be removed.

Contrast and density are adequate to demonstrate the surrounding soft tissue and bony structures of the ankle. Penetration is sufficient to visualize the bony trabecular patterns and cortical outlines of the distal tibia and fibula, tarsals, talus, calcaneus, and proximal fifth metatarsal.
- An optimal 55 to 65 kVp technique sufficiently penetrates the bony and soft tissue structures of the ankle and provides high radiographic contrast.

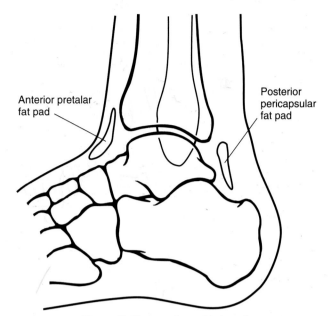

Figure 5-51. Location of fat pads.

- **Fat Pads on the Ankle:** Two soft tissue structures located around the ankle may indicate joint effusion and injury: the anterior pretalar fat pad and the posterior pericapsular fat pad. The anterior pretalar fat pad is visualized anterior to the ankle joint and rests next to the neck of the talus (Fig. 5–51). Surrounding the ankle joint is a fibrous, synovium-lined capsule attached to the borders of the tibia, fibula, and talus. Upon injury or disease invasion, the synovium membrane secretes synovial fluid, resulting in distention of the fibrous capsule.[1, 2] Distention of the anterior fibrous capsule results in displacement of the anterior pretalar fat pad. Because neither the fibrous capsule nor the ankle ligaments can be demonstrated on plain radiography, displacement of this fat pad indicates joint effusion and the possibility of underlying injuries.[1, 3]

  The posterior fat pad, positioned within the indentation formed by the articulation of the posterior tibia and talar bones (Fig. 5–51), is displaced in the same manner as the anterior pretalar fat pad, although it is less sensitive and requires more fluid evasion to be displaced.[2]

The bony trabecular patterns and cortical outlines of the distal fibula and tibia, talus, and fifth metatarsal base are sharply defined.
- Sharply defined recorded details are obtained when patient motion is controlled, a detail screen and a small focal spot are used, and a short object–image distance (OID) is maintained.

The ankle is in a true lateral position: The domes of the talus are superimposed, the tibiotalar joint is open, and the distal fibula is superimposed by the posterior half of the distal tibia.
- To obtain a true lateral ankle radiograph, begin with the patient in a supine position, with the leg extended

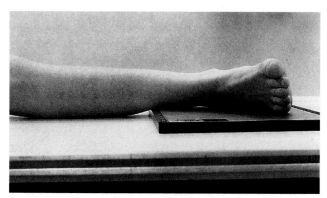

Figure 5–52. Proper knee and lower leg positioning for lateral ankle radiograph.

(Fig. 5–52) and the foot dorsiflexed until its long axis forms a 90-degree angle with the lower leg. Rotate the patient and affected leg until the lateral foot surface is against the cassette; then adjust the degree of rotation until the surface is aligned parallel with the film (Fig. 5–53). For most patients, this positioning places the lower leg parallel with the radiographic tabletop. If this is not the case, as with a patient with a large upper thigh, the foot and film should be elevated until the lower leg is parallel with the tabletop.

- **Importance of Proper Positioning:** Do not try to adjust the leg in an attempt to position the plantar foot surface perpendicular to the film or to directly superimpose the metatarsals. The true relationship of this surface to the film and the metatarsals to one another depends on the height of the patient's longitudinal arch and the incline of the calcaneus. Adjusting the patient's plantar surface may result in poor talar dome positioning and an erroneous longitudinal arch height.

The height of the longitudinal arch can be determined by measuring the amount of cuboid distal to the navicular. The average foot arch demonstrates approximately 0.50 inch (1 cm) of the cuboid, as shown in Figure 5–50. Because the bones that form the foot arch are held in position by ligaments and tendons, weakening of these tissues may result in a decreased or low arch. Radiographically, this decrease in arch height is demonstrated as a decrease in the amount of cuboid visualized distal to the navicular; this appearance can result from poor positioning as well as a low arch. Evaluate the talar domes to determine the cause, because on an accurately positioned lateral ankle radiograph, the talar domes should be superimposed.

- **Talar Domes:** The domes of the talus are formed by the most medial and lateral aspects of the talar's trochlear surface. Radiographically, they are visualized as domed structures that articulate with the tibia. On a true lateral ankle radiograph, the talar domes appear as one and the tibiotalar joint is open. Misalignment of the domes results from poor knee or foot positioning.

- **Effect of Lower Leg Positioning on Talar Dome Superimposition:** Often, if the knee is not fully extended (Fig. 5–54) or if the distal tibia is not elevated to place the lower leg parallel with the film (on a patient with a large upper thigh), the proximal tibia is positioned farther from the table than the distal tibia. The resulting radiograph demonstrates the lateral talar dome proximal to the medial talar dome, and the height of the longitudinal arch appears less than it actually is, because the cuboid shifts proximally and the navicular moves distally in this position (see Rad. 38). If the distal tibia is positioned farther from the table than the proximal tibia, the medial talar dome is demonstrated proximal to the lateral dome, and the height of the longitudinal arch appears greater than it actually is, because the cuboid shifts distally and the navicular moves proximally (see Rad. 39).

When viewing a lateral ankle radiograph that demonstrates one of the talar domes proximally to the other, evaluate the height of the longitudinal arch to determine which dome is the proximal dome. If the navicular superimposes most of the cuboid, the lateral dome is the proximal dome. If the navicular superimposes very little of the cuboid, the medial dome is the proximal dome.

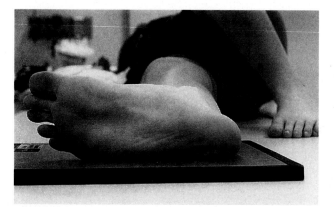

Figure 5–53. Proper lateral foot surface positioning for lateral ankle radiograph.

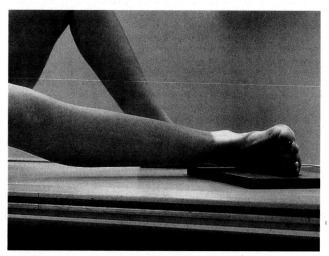

Figure 5–54. Poor knee and lower leg positioning for lateral ankle radiograph.

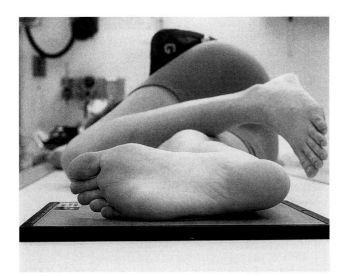

Figure 5–55. Poor foot positioning with the calcaneus elevated.

- **Effect of Foot Positioning on Talar Dome Superimposition:** To demonstrate accurate anterior and posterior alignment of the talar domes, position the lateral surface of the foot parallel with the film. If this surface is not parallel with the film, the talar domes are demonstrated one anterior to the other. When the leg is rotated more than needed to place the lateral foot surface parallel with the film, as demonstrated in Figure 5–55, the medial talar dome is demonstrated anterior to the lateral talar dome (see Rad. 40). If the leg is not rotated enough to place the lateral foot surface parallel with the film, as demonstrated in Figure 5–56, the medial talar dome is demonstrated posterior to the lateral talar dome (see Rad. 41).

When viewing a lateral ankle radiograph that demonstrates one of the talar domes anterior to the other, observe the position of the fibula in relationship to the tibia to determine how the patient should be repositioned. On most accurately positioned lateral ankle radiographs, the fibula is positioned in the posterior half of the tibia. On a poorly positioned radiograph,

if the fibula is demonstrated more posteriorly, the medial dome is anterior, and the patient was positioned with the forefoot depressed and the heel elevated, as demonstrated in Figure 5–55. If the fibula is demonstrated more anteriorly, the medial domes are posterior, and the patient was positioned with the forefoot elevated and the heel depressed, as demonstrated in Figure 5–56.

Carefully evaluate poorly positioned lateral ankle radiographs. Often, both knee and foot corrections are needed simultaneously to obtain accurate positioning.

The long axis of the foot is positioned at a 90-degree angle with the lower leg.

- In most cases, when the patient is relaxed, the foot rests in plantar flexion. Plantar flexion results in a forced flattening of the anterior pretalar fat pad, reducing its usefulness in the detection of joint effusion[2] (see Rad. 42). Consequently, it is best to dorsiflex the patient's foot, placing its long axis at a 90-degree angle with the lower leg. This positioning also places the tibiotalar joint in a neutral position and helps prevent the leg from rolling too far anteriorly. Anterior foot rotation elevates the heel and rotates the foot.

The long axis of the tibia is aligned with the long axis of the collimated field.

- Aligning the middle of the lower leg with the longitudinal collimator centering line aligns the tibial long axis with the long axis of the collimated field, allowing tight collimation without clipping the distal tibia or fibula.

The tibiotalar joint is at the center of the collimated field. The talus, 1 inch (2.5 cm) of the fifth metatarsal base, the surrounding ankle soft tissue, and the distal fourth of the fibula and tibia are included within the field.

- Centering a perpendicular central ray to the ankle midline at the level of the palpable medial malleolus places the tibiotalar joint in the center of the collimated field (Fig. 5–57).

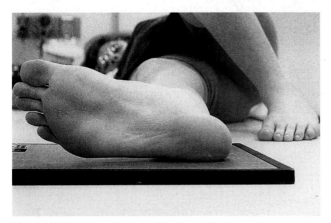

Figure 5–56. Poor foot positioning with the calcaneus depressed.

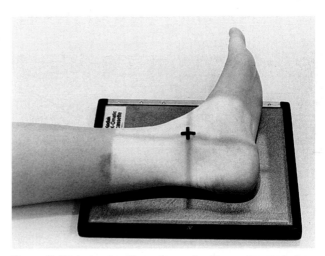

Figure 5–57. Lateral ankle radiograph with proper central ray (CR) centering and collimation.

- Open the longitudinal collimation enough to include the calcaneus and one fourth of the distal tibia and fibula. Transversely collimate to include 3 inches (7.5 cm) of the proximal forefoot, ensuring that approximately 1 inch (2.5 cm) of the fifth metatarsal base is included on the radiograph. An inversion injury of the foot and ankle may result in a fracture of the fifth metatarsal base, known as a Jones fracture (see Rad. 43). Including the fifth metatarsal base on the lateral ankle radiograph allows it to be evaluated for a Jones fracture.

- An 8 × 10 inch (18 × 24 cm) film placed lengthwise should be adequate to include all the required anatomical structures.

- **Ankle Exam to Include More Than One Fourth of the Lower Leg:** If an ankle exam order requests that more than one fourth of the distal lower leg be included, the central ray should remain on the ankle joint, and the collimated field should be opened to demonstrate the desired amount of lower leg. This method results in an unneeded radiation field beyond the heel but should not cause an increase in patient dosage because no additional patient tissue is exposed. A flat lead contact strip placed over this extended radiation field prevents backscattered radiation from reaching the film. The advantage of this method over centering the central ray proximal to the ankle joint is an undistorted view of the ankle joint.

Critiquing Radiographs

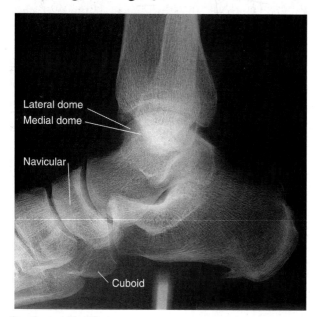

Radiograph 38.

Critique: The tibiotalar joint space is obscured, and one talar dome is demonstrated proximal to the other dome. Because the navicular superimposes most of the cuboid, the lateral dome is the proximal dome. The proximal tibia was elevated, as demonstrated in Figure 5–54.

Correction: Extend the knee to position the lower leg parallel with the film, as demonstrated in Figure 5–52. If the knee was extended for this radiograph, elevate the lower leg until it is positioned parallel with the film.

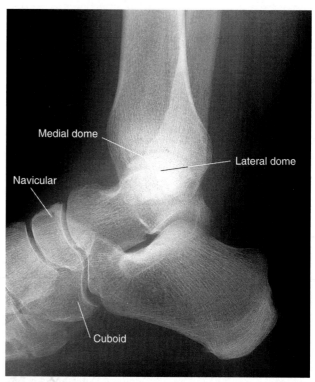

Radiograph 39.

Critique: The tibiotalar joint space is obscured, and one talar dome is demonstrated proximal to the other dome. Because more than 0.50 inch (1 cm) of cuboid is visualized distal to the navicular, the medial dome is the proximal dome. The distal tibia was elevated.

Correction: Position the lower leg parallel with the film.

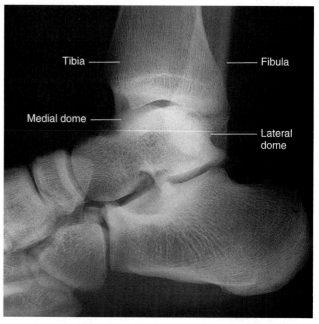

Radiograph 40.

Critique: The medial talar dome is positioned anterior to the lateral talar dome, as indicated by the posterior position of the fibula on the tibia. The lateral foot surface was not positioned parallel with the film. The patient's forefoot was depressed and the heel elevated, as demonstrated in Figure 5–55.

Correction: Elevate the patient's forefoot, and depress the heel until the lateral foot surface is parallel with the film, as demonstrated in Figure 5–53.

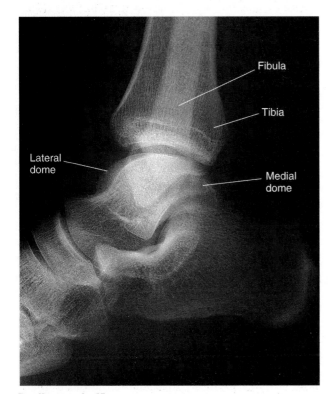

Radiograph 41.

Critique: The medial talar dome is positioned posterior to the lateral dome, as indicated by the anterior position of the distal fibula on the tibia. The lateral foot surface was positioned not parallel with the film, but with the forefoot elevated and the heel depressed, as demonstrated in Figure 5–56.

Correction: Depress the forefoot and elevate the heel until the lateral foot surface is positioned parallel with the film, as demonstrated in Figure 5–53.

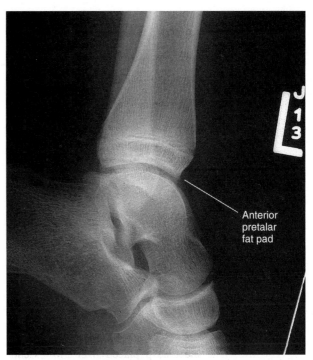

Radiograph 42.

Critique: The lower leg and long axis of the foot do not form a 90-degree angle. The patient's foot was in plantar flexion.

Correction: Dorsiflex the foot until the lower leg and long axis of the foot form a 90-degree angle.

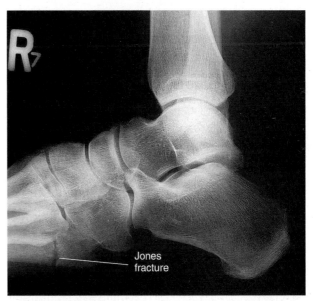

Radiograph 43.

Critique: The domes of the talus are superimposed, and the lower leg and long axis of the foot form a 90-degree angle. The ankle was accurately positioned. There is a Jones fracture of the fifth metatarsal base.

Correction: No repositioning movement is needed.

LOWER LEG

Anteroposterior Projection

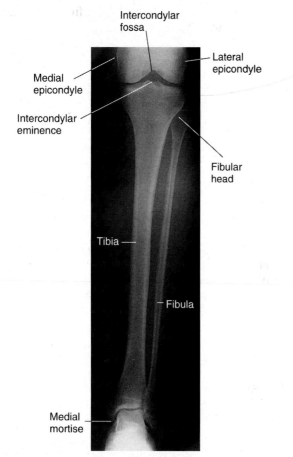

Figure 5-58. Accurately positioned AP lower leg radiograph.

Radiographic Evaluation

Facility's patient identification requirements are visible on radiograph.

- These requirements usually are facility name, patient name, age, and hospital number, and exam time and date.
- Patient ID plate is positioned so as not to obscure anatomy of interest.

A right or left marker, identifying the correct leg, is present on the radiograph and does not superimpose anatomy of interest.

- Place the marker within the collimated light field so it does not superimpose any portion of the affected leg.

There is no evidence of preventable artifacts, such as bandages and splints.

- Consult the ordering physician and the patient about whether bandages or splints can be removed.

Adequate contrast and density exist to demonstrate the surrounding soft tissue and bony structures of the lower leg. There is sufficient penetration to visualize the bony

trabecular patterns and cortical outlines of the tibia and fibula.

- An optimal 60 to 65 kVp technique sufficiently penetrates the bony and soft tissue structures of the lower leg and provides a high radiographic contrast.
- **Anode-Heel Effect:** Another exposure factor that should be considered when positioning the lower leg is the anode-heel effect. Because a long (17-inch [43-cm]) field is used for the length of the adult lower leg, there is a difference in intensity of the beam on the cathode and anode ends of the film. This noticeable intensity variation is a result of increased photon absorption at the thicker, "heel" portion of the anode compared with the thinner, "toe" portion when a long field is used. Consequently, radiographic density at the anode end of the tube is less than that at the cathode end.[6]

  Using this knowledge to our advantage can help us produce radiographs of the lower leg that demonstrate uniform density at both ends. Position the thicker proximal lower leg at the cathode end of the tube and the thinner distal lower leg at the anode end. Then set an exposure (mAs) that adequately demonstrates the proximal lower leg. Because the anode will absorb some of the photons aimed at the anode end of the film, the distal lower leg, which requires less exposure than the proximal lower leg, will not be overexposed.

The bony trabecular patterns and cortical outlines of the tibia and fibula are sharply defined.

- Sharply defined radiographic details are obtained when patient motion is controlled, a detail screen and a small focal spot are used, and a short object–image distance (OID) is maintained.

The lower leg demonstrates a true AP projection. The medial mortise (tibiotalar joint) is open, and the distal tibia and talus partially superimpose the distal fibula, closing the lateral mortise (talofibular joint). The fibular midshaft is free of tibial superimposition. The medial and lateral femoral epicondyles are demonstrated in profile, the intercondylar eminence is centered within the intercondylar fossa, and the head of the fibula is slightly superimposed by the tibia.

- To obtain an AP projection of the lower leg, place the patient in a supine position with the knee fully extended. Internally rotate the leg until the medial and lateral femoral epicondyles are positioned at equal distances from the film and an imaginary line drawn between the epicondyles is positioned parallel with the film. Dorsiflex the foot until its long axis is placed vertically (Fig. 5–59).
- **Detecting Lower Leg Rotation:** Rotation of the lower leg is a result of poor femoral epicondyle positioning and can be identified radiographically in the relationship of the fibula to the tibia and talus. When the patient's leg is laterally (externally) rotated, the fibula shifts toward and eventually beneath the tibia, obscuring the medial mortise (see Rad. 44). If only a small degree of rotation is present, it may be evident at the distal lower leg and undetectable at the proximal lower leg. When the patient's leg is medially (internally) rotated, the head of the fibula draws away

Labels on figure:
Intercondylar fossa
Lateral epicondyle
Medial epicondyle
Intercondylar eminence
Fibular head
Tibia
Fibula
Medial mortise

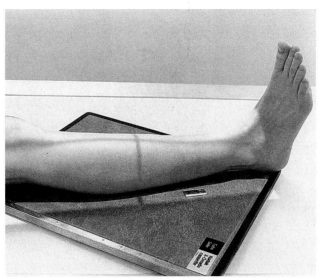

Figure 5-59. Proper patient positioning for AP lower leg radiograph.

from the tibia and the base of the fibula draws away from the talus. The tibia and talus demonstrate a gradual decrease in fibular superimposition with increased rotation (see Rad. 45).

- ***Positioning for Fracture:*** For a patient with a known or suspected fracture who is unable to position both the ankle and knee into a true AP projection simultaneously, position the joint closer to the fracture in the truer position. When the fracture is situated closer to the ankle, the ankle should meet the preceding requirements for a true distal lower leg AP projection (see Rad. 46). When the fracture is situated closer to the knee, the knee should meet the requirements for a true proximal lower leg AP projection. Depending on the degree of tibial and fibular rotation

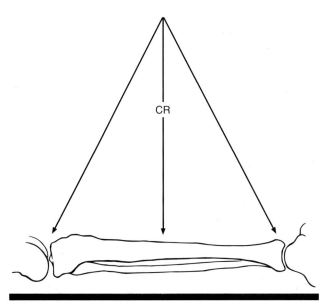

Figure 5-60. Effect of x-ray divergence on AP lower leg radiograph. *CR*, central ray.

at the fracture site, the other joint may or may not be in a true AP projection.

The femorotibial and tibiotalar joint spaces are closed.

- The proximal tibia slopes distally from the anterior condylar margin to the posterior condylar margin by about 5 degrees.[6] When the lower leg is placed parallel with the film and the central ray is centered to the midshaft of the lower leg, x-rays that diverge in the opposite direction are used to record the image of the proximal tibia (Fig. 5–60). The distal lower leg also slopes distally from the anterior tibial margin to the posterior margin, by about 3 degrees. Although the x-rays diverge in the same direction as the slope of the distal tibia, they diverge at a greater angle. Because the angle of x-ray divergence is not aligned parallel with either the proximal or distal tibia, the knee and ankle joints are demonstrated as closed spaces on an AP lower leg radiograph.

The long axis of the lower leg is aligned with the long axis of the collimation field.

- Aligning the long axis of the lower leg with the long axis of the collimated field enables you to collimate tightly without clipping the distal or proximal lower leg.

The tibial midshaft is at the center of the collimated field. The tibia, fibula, ankle, knee, and surrounding lower leg soft tissue are included within the field.

- A perpendicular central ray is centered to the midshaft of the lower leg to place it in the center of the radiograph.
- To include the ankle and knee joints on the radiograph, you must consider the degree of x-ray beam divergence that occurs during radiography of a long body part (Fig. 5–60). A 14 × 17 inch (35 × 43 cm), diagonally placed film should be adequate to include both the ankle and the knee. To ensure that both joints are included, the film should extend 1 inch (2.5 cm) beyond each joint space. The ankle is located at the level of the medial malleolus, and the knee is located 0.75 inch (2 cm) distal to the palpable medial epicondyle.
- Once the lower leg is accurately positioned with the film, center the central ray to the midshaft of the tibia, and open the longitudinal collimation field until it extends just beyond both the knee and the ankle. If the collimation does not extend beyond the joints, adjust the centering point of the central ray until both the knee and ankle are included within the collimated field, without demonstrating an excessive field beyond either joint.
- On patients with long lower legs that need to be placed diagonally on the film, it may be necessary to raise the source–image distance (SID) above the standard 40 inches (102 cm) to obtain a longitudinally collimated field long enough to include both joints on the same film.
- Transverse collimation should be to the lower leg skin-line.

Critiquing Radiographs

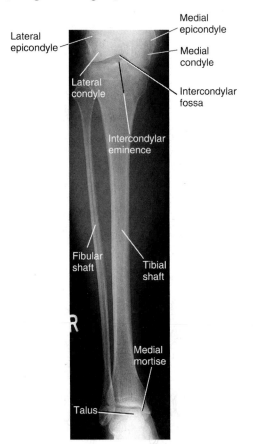

Radiograph 44.

Critique: The talotibial articulation (medial mortise) is closed, and the tibia and talus demonstrate increased fibular superimposition. The lower leg was laterally rotated. The amount of rotation demonstrated on this radiograph is minimal, because rotation is detectable at the ankle joint but not at the knee joint.

Correction: If an open talotibial articulation is important, medially (internally) rotate the leg. Otherwise, no correction movement is needed.

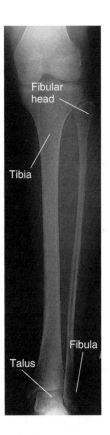

Radiograph 45.

Critique: The distal fibula is free of talar superimposition, and the proximal fibula is free of tibial superimposition. The leg was medially rotated.

Correction: Laterally (externally) rotate the leg until the femoral epicondyles are positioned at equal distances from the film.

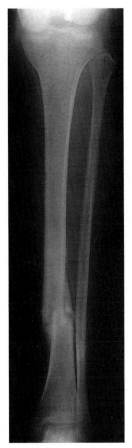

Radiograph 46.

Critique: There is a distal tibial and fibular fracture. The ankle joint is positioned in a true AP projection, but the knee joint demonstrates medial rotation. This rotation is caused by rotation at the fracture site.
Correction: No correction movement is required.

Lower Leg: Lateral Position
(Mediolateral Projection)

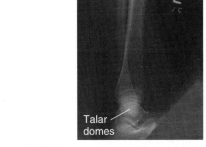

Figure 5-61. Accurately positioned lateral lower leg radiograph.

Radiographic Evaluation

Facility's patient identification requirements are visible on radiograph.
- These requirements usually are facility name, patient name, age, and hospital number, and exam time and date.
- Patient ID plate is positioned so as not to obscure anatomy of interest.

A right or left marker, identifying the correct leg, is present on the radiograph and does not superimpose anatomy of interest.
- Place the marker within the collimated light field so it does not superimpose any portion of the affected leg.

There is no evidence of preventable artifacts, such as bandages and splints.
- Consult the ordering physician and the patient about whether bandages and splints can be removed.

Contrast and density are adequate to demonstrate the surrounding soft tissue and bony structures of the lower leg. Penetration is sufficient to visualize the bony trabecular patterns and cortical outlines of the tibia and fibula.

- An optimal 60 to 65 kVp technique sufficiently penetrates the bony and soft tissue structures of the lower leg and provides a high radiographic contrast.
- **Anode-Heel Effect:** Another exposure factor that should be considered in positioning of the lower leg is the anode-heel effect. Because a long (17- inch [43-cm]) field is used for the length of the adult lower leg, there is a difference in the intensity of the beam on the cathode and anode ends of the film. This noticeable intensity variation results from increased photon absorption at the thicker, "heel" portion of the anode compared with the thinner, "toe" portion when a long field is used. Consequently, radiographic density at the anode end of the tube is less than that at the cathode end.[6]

   Using this knowledge to our advantage can help us produce radiographs of the lower leg that demonstrate uniform density at both ends. Position the thicker proximal lower leg at the cathode end of the tube, and the thinner distal lower leg at the anode end. Then set an exposure (mAs) that will adequately demonstrate the proximal lower leg. Because the anode absorbs some of the photons aimed at the anode end of the film, the distal lower leg, which requires less exposure than the proximal lower leg, will not be overexposed.

The bony trabecular patterns and cortical outlines of the tibia and fibula are sharply defined.

- Sharply defined radiographic details are obtained when patient motion is controlled, a detail screen and a small focal spot are used and a short OID is maintained.

The lower leg demonstrates a true lateral position. The anterior and the posterior aspects of the talar domes are aligned, and the distal fibula is superimposed by the posterior half of the distal tibia. The fibular midshaft is free of tibial superimposition. The tibia partially superimposes the fibular head and the medial femoral condyle is demonstrated posterior to the lateral condyle if the leg is extended; the condyles are superimposed if the knee is flexed at least 30 degrees (compare Fig. 5–61 and Rad. 47).

- To obtain a true lateral lower leg radiograph, begin by placing the patient in a supine position, with the leg extended and the foot dorsiflexed until it forms a 90-degree angle with the lower leg. Next, rotate the leg, positioning the lateral foot surface against the cassette and the femoral epicondyles perpendicular to the cassette (Fig. 5–62).
- **Detecting Leg Rotation:** If the distal lower leg was not placed in a true lateral position, the tibiofibular relationship is altered. If the patient's leg was rotated anteriorly (patella positioned too close to film and heel elevated off film), the distal fibula is situated too far posterior on the tibia, the medial talar dome is demonstrated anterior to the lateral dome (the medial dome is also demonstrated distal to the lateral dome, owing to the diverged x-rays used to record the ankle joint), and the fibular head is demonstrated free of tibial superimposition (see Rad. 48). If the patient's leg was rotated posteriorly (patella positioned too far away from film and forefoot elevated off film), the distal fibula is situated too far anterior on the tibia, the medial talar dome is demonstrated posterior to the lateral dome, and the fibular head and neck and possibly the midshaft are superimposed by the tibia (see Rad. 49).

   Superimposition of the femoral condyles is not a good indication of rotation on a lateral lower leg radiograph. The amount of their superimposition depends on the degree of knee flexion and the way in which the diverged x-ray beams are aligned with the medial condyle. See page 262 on the lateral knee for a discussion of central ray alignment and the superimposition of the femoral condyles.
- **Positioning for Fracture:** For a patient with a known or suspected fracture who is unable to position both the ankle and knee into a true lateral position simultaneously, position the joint closer to the fracture in the truer position. If the fracture is situated closer to the distal lower leg, the distal lower leg should meet the preceding requirements for a true lateral position. If the fracture is situated closer to the proximal lower leg, the proximal lower leg should meet

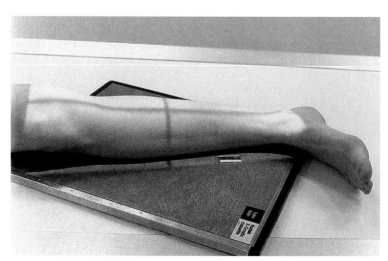

Figure 5–62. Proper patient positioning for lateral lower leg radiograph.

the preceding requirements for a true lateral position. Depending on the degree of tibial and fibular rotation at the fracture site, the other end of the lower leg may or may not be in a true lateral position.

The long axis of the lower leg is aligned with the long axis of the collimated field.

- Aligning the long axis of the lower leg with the long axis of the collimated field enables you to collimate tightly without clipping the distal or proximal lower leg.

The tibial midshaft is at the center of the collimated field. The tibia, fibula, ankle, knee, and surrounding lower leg soft tissue are included within the field.

- A perpendicular central ray is centered to the midshaft of the lower leg to place the midshaft in the center of the radiograph.
- To include the ankle and knee joints on the radiograph, you must consider the degree of x-ray beam divergence that occurs in radiography of a long body part. A 14 × 17 inch (35 × 43 cm) film placed diagonally should be adequate to include both the ankle and the knee. To ensure that both joints are included, the film should extend 1 inch (2.5 cm) beyond each joint space. The ankle is located at the level of the medial malleolus, and the knee is located 0.75 inch (2 cm) distal to the palpable medial epicondyle.
- Once the lower leg is accurately positioned with the film, center the central ray to the midshaft of the tibia, and open the longitudinal collimation until it extends just beyond both the knee and the ankle. If the collimation does not extend beyond the joints, adjust the centering point of the central ray until both the knee and ankle are included within the collimated field, without demonstrating an excessive field beyond either joint.
- On patients with long lower legs that have to be placed diagonally on the film, it may be necessary to raise the source–image distance (SID) above the standard 40 inches (102 cm) to obtain a longitudinally collimated field long enough to include both joints on the same radiograph.
- Transverse collimation should be to the lower leg skin-line.

Critiquing Radiographs

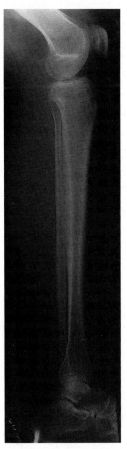

Radiograph 47.

Critique: The distal and proximal ends of the fibula are superimposed by the tibia, whereas the fibular midshaft is free of superimposition. The knee is flexed about 45 degrees, and the femoral condyles are superimposed.

Correction: No correction movement is required, although knee flexion may result in elevation of the proximal lower leg and foreshortening of the tibia and fibula.

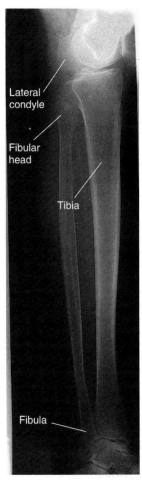

Radiograph 48.

Critique: The distal fibula is situated too far posterior on the tibia, the medial talar dome is anterior to the lateral dome, and the fibular head is free of tibial superimposition. The leg was rotated anteriorly.

Correction: Posteriorly rotate the leg until the lateral foot surface is positioned parallel with the film and the femoral epicondyles are perpendicular to the film.

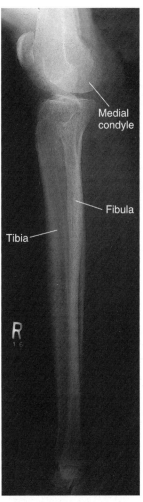

Radiograph 49.

Critique: The distal fibula is situated too far anterior on the tibia, the medial talar dome is posterior to the lateral dome, and the fibular head and midshaft are superimposed by the tibia. The leg was rotated posteriorly.

Correction: Anteriorly rotate the leg until the lateral foot surface is positioned parallel with the film and the femoral epicondyles are perpendicular to the film.

KNEE

Anteroposterior Projection

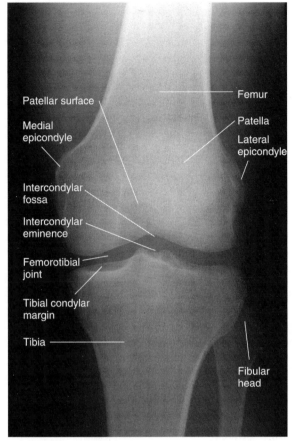

Figure 5-63. Accurately positioned AP knee radiograph.

Radiographic Evaluation

Facility's patient identification requirements are visible on radiograph.

- These requirements usually are facility name, patient name, age, and hospital number, and exam time and date.
- Patient ID plate is positioned so as not to obscure anatomy of interest.

A right or left marker, identifying the correct knee, is present on the radiograph and does not superimpose anatomy of interest.

- Place the marker within the collimated light field so it does not superimpose any portion of the knee.

There is no evidence of preventable artifacts, such as bandages and splints.

- Consult with the ordering physician and the patient about whether bandages and splints can be removed.

Contrast and density are adequate to demonstrate the surrounding soft tissue and bony structures of the knee. Penetration is sufficient to visualize the bony trabecular

patterns and cortical outlines of the patella, intercondylar eminence, fibular head, proximal tibia, and distal femur.

- If the patient's AP knee thickness measures under 5 inches (13 cm), a grid is not required. For such a patient, a high-contrast, low (60 to 70) kVp technique sufficiently penetrates the bony and soft tissue structures of the knee without causing excessive scattered radiation to reach the film and hinder contrast. If the patient's AP knee thickness measures over 5 inches (13 cm), a grid should be used, because this thickness would produce enough scattered radiation to negatively affect radiographic contrast.[6, 8] When a grid is used, increase the kVp above 70 to penetrate the thicker knee and to provide an adequate scale of contrast. Increase the exposure (mAs) by the standard density conversion factor for the grid ratio being used, to compensate for the scatter and the primary radiation the grid will absorb.

The bony trabecular patterns and cortical outlines of the distal femur, proximal tibia and fibula, and patella are sharply defined.

- Sharply defined recorded details are obtained when patient motion is controlled, a small focal spot is used, and a short object–image distance (OID) is maintained.

The knee demonstrates a true AP projection. The medial and lateral femoral epicondyles are demonstrated in profile, the femoral condyles are symmetrical, the intercondylar eminence is centered within the intercondylar fossa, and the fibular head is slightly superimposed by the tibia.

- To obtain an AP knee radiograph, place the patient in a supine position with the knee fully extended. Internally rotate the leg until an imaginary line drawn between the medial and lateral femoral epicondyles is positioned parallel with the film (Fig. 5–64). This positioning places the medial and lateral femoral epicondyles at equal distances from the film as well as

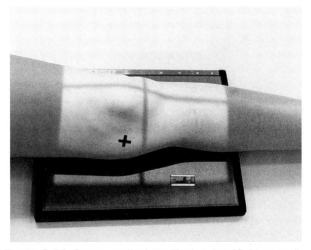

Figure 5-64. Proper patient positioning for AP knee radiograph.

medially and laterally in profile, respectively. It also centers the intercondylar eminence within the intercondylar fossa and draws the fibular neck and a portion of the fibular head from beneath the tibia.

- **Effect of Rotation:** If the femoral epicondyles are not positioned parallel with the film, a true AP projection has not been obtained. If the patient's leg was not internally rotated enough to place the epicondyles at equal distances from the film, they are not in profile, the medial femoral condyle appears larger than the lateral condyle, and the fibular head, neck, and possibly shaft are superimposed by the tibia (see Rad. 50). If the patient's leg was internally rotated more than needed to place the femoral epicondyles at equal distances from the film, the epicondyles are not demonstrated in profile, the lateral femoral condyle appears larger than the medial condyle, and the head of the fibula demonstrates very little if any superimposition by the tibia (see Rad. 51).

The femorotibial (knee) joint space is open, the anterior and posterior condylar margins of the tibia are superimposed, the intercondylar eminence and tubercles are demonstrated in profile, and the fibular head is demonstrated about 0.50 inch (1 cm) distal to the tibial plateau.

- The anterior and posterior condylar margins of the tibia are superimposed if the correct central ray angulation, as determined by the patient's upper thigh and buttocks thickness, is used. By studying the tibial plateau region, you will see that the tibial plateau

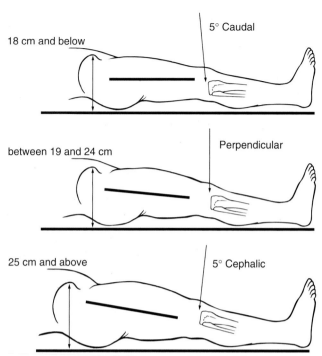

Figure 5-66. Determining central ray (CR) angle from the patient's thigh thickness. (Reproduced with permission from Martensen K: Alternative AP knee method assures open joint space. Radiol Technol 64:19–23, 1992. Courtesy *Radiologic Technology*, published by the American Society of Radiologic Technologists.)

slopes distally about 5 degrees from the anterior condylar margin to the posterior condylar margin on both the medial and lateral aspects[9] (Fig. 5–65). Only if the central ray is aligned parallel with the tibial plateau slope is an open femorotibial joint space obtained.

- **Determining the Central Ray Angulation:** When a patient is placed in a supine position, the degree and direction of the central ray angulation required depends on the thickness of the patient's upper thigh and buttocks. This thickness determines how the lower leg and the tibial plateau align with the film.

Figure 5–66 shows a guideline that can be used to determine the central ray angulation for different body sizes; it illustrates the relationship of the tibial plateau to the tabletop as the patient's upper thigh thickness increases. Note that there is a decrease in femoral decline and a shift in the direction of the tibial plateau slope as the thickness of the thigh decreases. Because of this plateau shift, the central ray angulation must also be adjusted to keep it parallel with the plateau and to obtain an open femorotibial joint.

For optimal AP knee radiographs, measure each patient from ASIS (anterior superior iliac spine) to the tabletop on either side to determine the central ray angulation to use for each knee exam. When measuring this distance, do not include the patient's abdominal tissue. Keep the calipers situated laterally next to the ASIS. If the measurement is 18 cm or below, a 5-degree caudal angle should be used. If the measure-

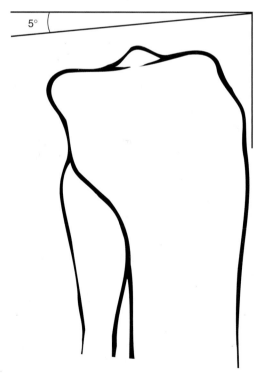

Figure 5-65. Slope of the proximal tibia. (Reproduced with permission from Martensen K: Alternative AP knee method assures open joint space. Radiol Technol 64:19–23, 1992. Courtesy *Radiologic Technology*, published by the American Society of Radiologic Technologists.)

ment is 19 to 24 cm, a perpendicular beam should be used. If the measurement is above 24 cm, a 5-degree cephalad angle should be used.[9]

Using the correct central ray angulation not only results in an open femorotibial joint space but also provides optimal visualization of the intercondylar eminence and tubercles without foreshortening.

- **Evaluation of Joint Space Narrowing:** From an adequately positioned AP knee radiograph, joint space narrowing is evaluated by measuring the medial and the lateral aspects of the femorotibial joint, which are also referred to as *compartments*. The measurement of each of these compartments is obtained by determining the distance between the most distal femoral condylar surface and the posterior condylar margin of the tibia on each side.[10] Comparison of these measurements with each other, with measurements from previous radiographs, or with the other knee determines joint space narrowing or a valgus or varus deformity. In *valgus deformity*, the lateral compartment is narrower than the medial compartment; in *varus deformity*, the medial compartment is narrower (see Rads. 52 and 53).

  Precise measurements of the compartments are necessary to ensure early detection of joint space narrowing and are best obtained when the femorotibial joint space is completely open.[11] If an inaccurate central ray angulation was used for an AP knee radiograph, the femorotibial joint is narrowed or obscured, the intercondylar eminence and tubercles are foreshortened, and the tibial plateau is demonstrated.

- **Effect of Poor Central Ray Angulation:** When viewing an AP knee radiograph for which an inaccurate central ray angulation was used, you can determine how to adjust the angulation by judging the contour of the proximal ridges of the femoral condyles and by evaluating the shape of the fibular head and its proximity to the tibial plateau. If the proximal ridges of the femoral condyles are concave and the fibular head is foreshortened and is demonstrated more than 0.50 inch (1 cm) distal to the tibial plateau, the angle was too cephalic (see Rad. 54). If the proximal ridges of the femoral condyles are convex and the fibular head is elongated and demonstrated less than 0.50 inch (1 cm) distal to the tibial plateau, the central ray was angled too caudally (see Rad. 55).

- **Compensating for the Nonextendable Knee:** If the patient is unable to fully extend the knee, an open femorotibial joint can be obtained by (1) aligning the central ray perpendicular with the anterior lower leg surface, (2) decreasing the angulation about 5 degrees, and (3) placing the central ray parallel with the tibial plateau. For example, if the central ray is perpendicular to the anterior lower leg surface when a 15-degree cephalic angulation is used, the angle should be decreased to 10 degrees if the knee cannot be extended (see Rad. 56).

The patella lies just superior to the patellar surface of the femur and is situated slightly lateral to the knee midline.[12] The intercondylar fossa is partially demonstrated.

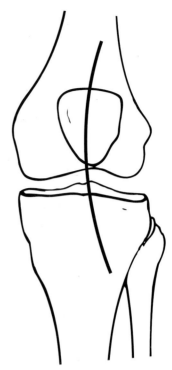

Figure 5–67. Movement of patella upon knee flexion.

- The position of the patella and the degree of intercondylar fossa demonstration are determined by the amount of knee flexion. To visualize the patella and fossa as required, the leg must be in full extension. As the knee is flexed, the patella shifts distally and medially onto the patellar surface of the femur and then laterally into the intercondylar fossa, duplicating a C-shaped path that is open laterally (Fig. 5–67). Thus, the patella is demonstrated at different locations depending on the degree of knee flexion. Generally, when the knee is flexed 20 degrees, the patella is demonstrated on the patellar surface. Between 30 and 70 degrees of knee flexion, the patella is demonstrated between the patellar surface and the intercondylar fossa. At 90 degrees to full knee flexion, the patella is demonstrated within the intercondylar fossa.[3, 12]

- The extent of intercondylar fossa visualization also changes with knee flexion. In full extension, only a slight indentation between the distal medial and lateral femoral condyles indicates the location of the intercondylar fossa. As the knee is flexed, the amount of intercondylar fossa that is demonstrated increases. When the knee is flexed to between 50 and 60 degrees, the intercondylar fossa is seen in profile (see Rad. 56). When the knee is flexed less than 50 degrees or more than 60 degrees, visualization of the fossa will decrease.

- **Patellar Subluxation:** With patellar subluxation, the patella may be situated more laterally on an AP knee radiograph than normal[13] (see Rad. 57). When a radiograph is produced that demonstrates a laterally situated patella, evaluate the symmetry of the femoral condyles and the relationship of the tibia and fibular head to rule out external rotation before assuming that the patella is subluxed. External rotation also results in a laterally located patella.

The femorotibial joint is at the center of the collimated field. One fourth of the distal femur and proximal lower leg and the surrounding soft tissue are included within the field.

- Center the central ray to the midline of the knee at a level 0.75 inch (2 cm) distal to the palpable medial epicondyle to place the femorotibial joint in the center of the collimated field. Open the longitudinal collimation enough to include one fourth of the distal femur and proximal lower leg. Transverse collimation should be to the knee skin-line.
- An 8 × 10 inch (18 × 24 cm) film placed lengthwise should be adequate to include all the required anatomical structures.

Critiquing Radiographs

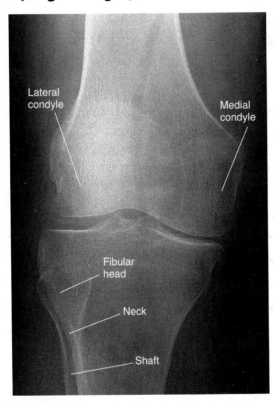

Radiograph 50.

Critique: The femoral epicondyles are not in profile, the medial femoral condyle appears larger than the lateral condyle, and the fibular head, neck, and shaft are almost entirely superimposed by the tibia. The leg was externally rotated.
Correction: Internally rotate the leg until the femoral epicondyles are at equal distances from the film.

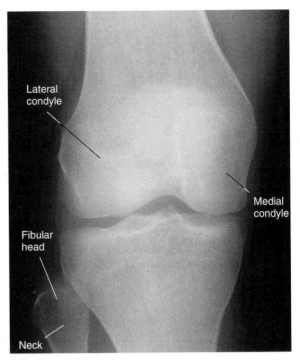

Radiograph 51.

Critique: The femoral epicondyles are not in profile, the lateral femoral condyle appears larger than the medial condyle, and the tibia demonstrates very little superimposition of the fibular head. The leg was internally rotated.
Correction: Externally rotate the leg until the femoral epicondyles are at equal distances from the film.

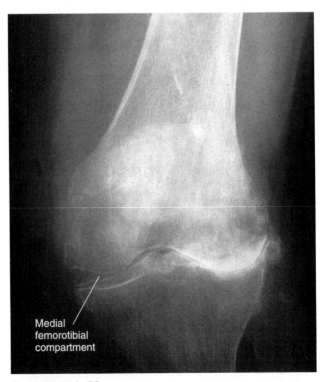

Radiograph 52.

Critique: The lateral femorotibial compartment is narrower than the medial femorotibial compartment. The patient's knee demonstrates a valgus deformity.
Correction: No correction movement is required.

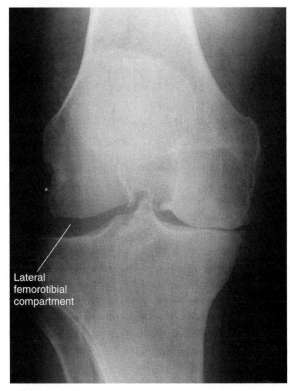

Radiograph 53.

Critique: The medial femorotibial compartment is narrower than the lateral femorotibial compartment. The patient's knee demonstrates a varus deformity.
Correction: No correction movement is required.

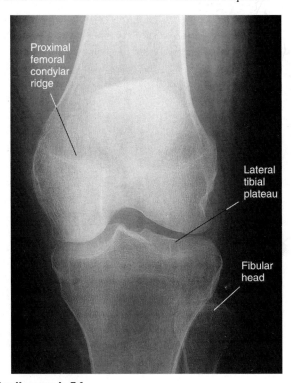

Radiograph 54.

Critique: The femorotibial joint space is obscured, the medial and lateral tibial plateau is demonstrated, the proximal ridges of the femoral condyles are concave, and the fibular head is foreshortened and demonstrated more than 0.50 inch (1 cm) distal to the tibial plateau. Excessive cephalad angulation is indicated.
Correction: Angle the central ray caudally about 5 degrees for every 0.25 inch (0.6 cm) of tibial plateau demonstrated. For this radiograph, about 0.50 inch of the tibial plateau is demonstrated between the anterior and posterior tibial margins. The central ray should be adjusted about 10 degrees, because a 5-degree cephalad angle was used. When the radiograph is repeated, a 5-degree caudal angle should be used.

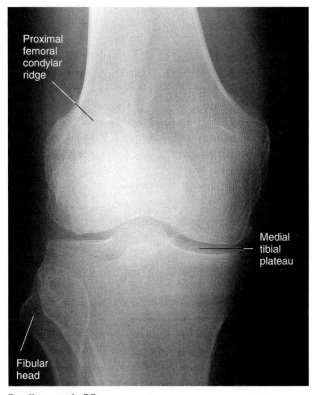

Radiograph 55.

Critique: The medial femorotibial joint space is closed, the proximal ridges of the femoral condyles are convex, and the fibular head is elongated and demonstrated less than 0.50 inch (1 cm) distal to the tibial plateau. Excessive caudal angulation is indicated.
Correction: If an open medial femorotibial joint space is desired, the central ray should be adjusted cephalically.

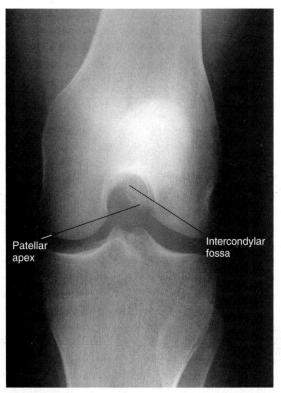

Radiograph 56.

Critique: This is an AP knee radiograph taken with the knee flexed about 50 to 60 degrees and the central ray aligned parallel with the tibial plateau. The femorotibial joint space is open, the intercondylar fossa is demonstrated in profile, and the patellar apex superimposes the intercondylar fossa.

Correction: If the patient's condition allows, fully extend the knee. If the patient is unable to extend the knee, no correction movement is required.

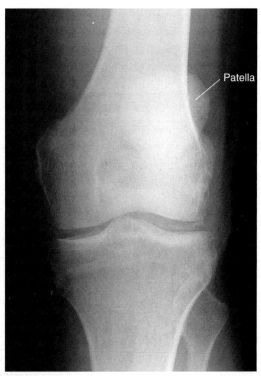

Radiograph 57.

Critique: The knee demonstrates no signs of rotation even though the patella is superimposed over the lateral aspect of the knee. The patient has a subluxed patella.

Correction: No correction movement is required.

Knee: Medial and Lateral Oblique Positions

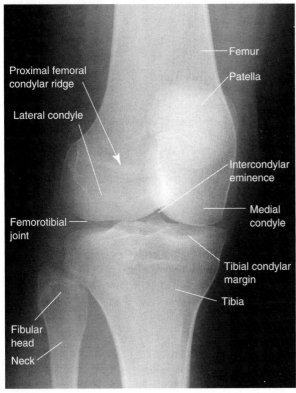

Figure 5–68. Accurately positioned medially oblique knee radiograph.

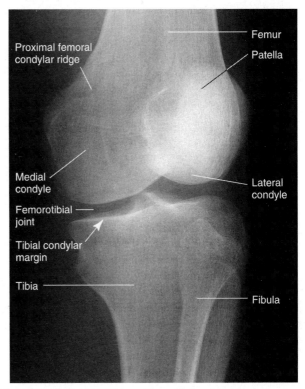

Figure 5–69. Accurately positioned laterally oblique knee radiograph.

Radiographic Evaluation

Facility's patient identification requirements are visible on radiograph.

- These requirements usually are facility name, patient name, age, and hospital number, and exam time and date.
- Patient ID plate is positioned so as not to obscure anatomy of interest.

A right or left marker, identifying the correct knee, is present on the radiograph and does not superimpose anatomy of interest.

- Place the marker within the collimated light field so it does not superimpose any portion of the knee.

There is no evidence of preventable artifacts, such as bandages and splints.

- Consult with the ordering physician and the patient about whether bandages and splints can be removed.

Contrast and density are adequate to demonstrate the surrounding soft tissue and bony structures of the knee. Penetration is sufficient to visualize the bony trabecular patterns and cortical outlines of the patella, tibial eminence, fibular head, proximal tibia, and distal femur.

- If the patient's AP knee thickness measures under 5 inches (13 cm), a grid is not required. For such a patient, a high-contrast, low (60 to 70) kVp technique

sufficiently penetrates the bony and soft tissue structures of the knee without causing excessive scattered radiation to reach the film and hinder contrast. If the patient's AP knee thickness measures over 5 inches (13 cm), a grid should be used, because this thickness would produce enough scattered radiation to negatively affect radiographic contrast.[6, 8]

- When a grid is used, increase the kVp above 70 to penetrate the thicker knee and to provide an adequate scale of contrast. Increase the exposure (mAs) by the standard density conversion factor for the grid ratio being used, to compensate for the scatter and primary radiation the grid will absorb.

The bony trabecular patterns and cortical outlines of the distal femur, proximal tibia and fibula and patella are sharply defined.

- Sharply defined recorded details are obtained when patient motion is controlled, a small focal spot is used, and a short object–image distance (OID) is maintained.

The femorotibial joint space is open. The anterior and posterior condylar margins of the tibia are superimposed, and the fibular head is about 0.50 inch (1 cm) distal to the tibial plateau.

- The anterior and posterior condylar margins of the tibia are superimposed by the use of the correct central

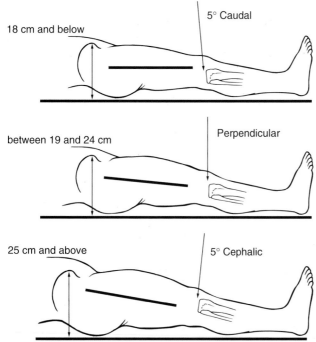

Figure 5–70. Determining central ray *(CR)* angle from the patient's thigh thickness. (Reproduced with permission from Martensen K: Alternative AP knee method assures open joint space. Radiol Technol 64:19–23, 1992. Courtesy *Radiologic Technology*, published by the American Society of Radiologic Technologists.)

ray angulation as determined by the patient's upper thigh and buttocks thickness. By studying the tibial plateau region, you will see that the tibial plateau slopes distally about 5 degrees from the anterior condylar margin to the posterior condylar margin on both the medial and lateral aspects.[7] Only if the central ray is aligned parallel with this slope is a truly open joint space obtained.

- **Determining the Central Ray Angulation:** When a patient is placed in a supine position, the degree and direction of the central ray angulation required depends on the thickness of the patient's upper thigh and buttocks, because it is this thickness that will determine the central ray angulation that should be used for different body sizes. Figure 5–70 demonstrates how the relationship of the tibial plateau varies as the patient's upper thigh thickness changes.

For optimal oblique knee radiographs, measure each patient from the anterior superior iliac spine (ASIS) to the tabletop after the patient has been accurately positioned, to determine the correct central ray angulation to use for each exam. When measuring this distance, do not include the patient's abdominal tissue in the measurement. Keep the calipers situated laterally, next to the ASIS. If the measurement is 18 cm or below, a 5-degree caudal angle should be used. If the measurement is 19 to 24 cm, a perpendicular beam should be used. If the measurement is above 24 cm, a 5-degree cephalad angle should be used.[9]

If an inaccurate central ray angulation was used for an oblique knee radiograph, the femorotibial joint space is narrowed or obscured, and the anterior and posterior margins of the tibial plateau are not superimposed.

- **Effect of Poor Central Ray Angulation:** When looking at an oblique knee radiograph for which an inaccurate central ray angulation was used, you can determine how to adjust the angulation by judging the contour of the proximal ridges of the femoral condyles and by evaluating the shape of the fibular head and its proximity to the tibial plateau. If the proximal ridges of the femoral condyles are concave and the fibular head is foreshortened and demonstrated more than 0.50 inch (1 cm) distal to the tibial plateau, the cephalad angle was too great (see Rad. 62). If the proximal ridges of the femoral condyles are convex and the fibular head is elongated and demonstrated less than 0.50 inch (1 cm) distal to the tibial plateau, the caudad angle was too great.

The femorotibial joint is at the center of the collimated field. One fourth of the distal femur and the proximal lower leg are included within the field.

- The central ray should be centered to the midline of the knee at the level of the femorotibial joint, which is located 0.75 inch (2 cm) distal to the palpable medial femoral epicondyle, to place the femorotibial joint in the center of the collimated field. Open the longitudinal collimation to include one fourth of the distal femur and the proximal lower leg. Transverse collimation should be to the knee skin-line.
- An 8 × 10 inch (18 × 24 cm) film placed lengthwise should be adequate to include all the required anatomical structures.

MEDIAL (INTERNAL) OBLIQUE POSITION

The knee has been rotated 45 degrees medially. The fibular head is demonstrated free of tibial superimposition, and the lateral femoral condyle is visualized in profile without medial condyle superimposition.

- An accurately positioned medial oblique knee radio-

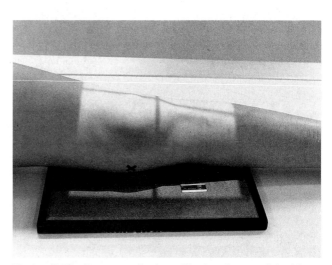

Figure 5–71. Proper patient positioning for medial oblique knee radiograph.

film, the tibia partially superimposes the fibular head (see Rad. 58). If the femoral epicondyles are rotated more than 45 degrees with the film, the femoral condyles are nearly superimposed (see Rad. 59).

LATERAL (EXTERNAL) OBLIQUE POSITION

The knee has been rotated 45 degrees laterally. The fibular head, neck, and shaft are superimposed by the tibia, and the fibular head is aligned with the anterior edge of the tibia. The medial femoral condyle is demonstrated in profile without lateral condyle superimposition.

- An accurately positioned lateral oblique knee radiograph is obtained by placing the patient in an AP knee projection, then externally rotating the leg until an imaginary line drawn between the medial and lateral femoral epicondyles is positioned at a 45-degree angle with the film (Fig. 5–72). This position places the medial condyle in profile and rotates the tibia onto the fibula. If the femoral epicondyles are rotated less than 45 degrees with the film, the fibular head is demonstrated in the center of the tibia (see Rad. 60). If the femoral epicondyles are rotated more than 45 degrees with the film, the fibular head is aligned with the posterior edge of the tibia and the femoral condyles are nearly superimposed (see Rad. 61).

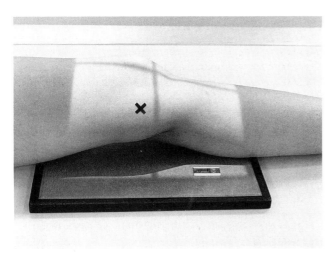

Figure 5–72. Proper patient positioning for lateral oblique knee radiograph. *X* indicates medial femoral epicondyle.

graph is obtained by placing the patient in an AP knee projection, then internally rotating the leg until an imaginary line drawn between the medial and lateral femoral epicondyles is positioned at a 45-degree angle with the film (Fig. 5–71). This position places the lateral condyle in profile and rotates the fibular head from beneath the tibia. If the femoral epicondyles are rotated less than 45 degrees with the

Critiquing Radiographs

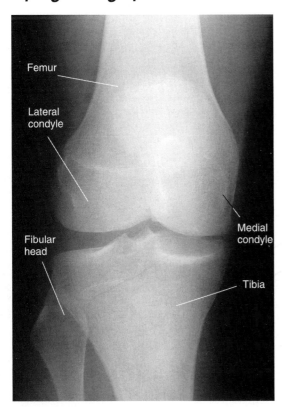

Radiograph 58.

Critique: This is a medial oblique knee radiograph. The tibia partially superimposes the fibular head. The patient's knee was rotated less than 45 degrees.

Correction: Increase the medial knee obliquity until the femoral epicondyles are aligned at a 45-degree angle with the film.

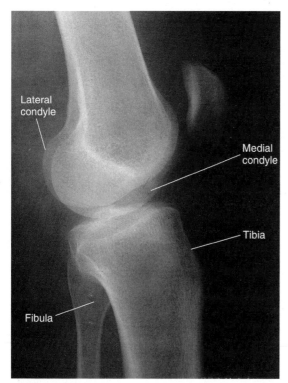

Radiograph 59.

Critique: This is a medial oblique knee radiograph. The medial femoral condyle superimposes the lateral condyle. The patient's knee was rotated more than 45 degrees.

Correction: Decrease the medial knee obliquity until the femoral epicondyles are aligned at a 45-degree angle with the film.

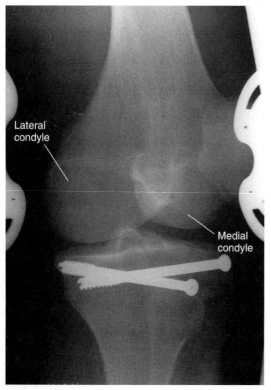

Radiograph 60.

Critique: This is a lateral oblique knee radiograph. The fibula is aligned with the center of the tibia. The patient's knee was rotated less than 45 degrees.

Correction: Increase the lateral knee obliquity until the femoral epicondyles are aligned at a 45-degree angle with the film.

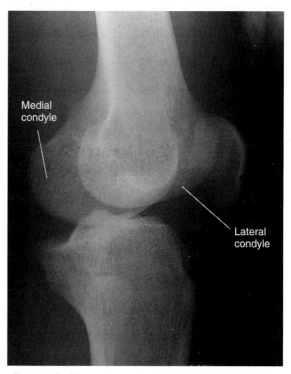

Radiograph 61.

Critique: This is a lateral oblique knee radiograph. The fibula is aligned with the posterior edge of the tibia, and the femoral condyles are nearly superimposed. The patient's knee was rotated more than 45 degrees.

Correction: Decrease the lateral knee obliquity until the femoral epicondyles are aligned at a 45-degree angle with the film.

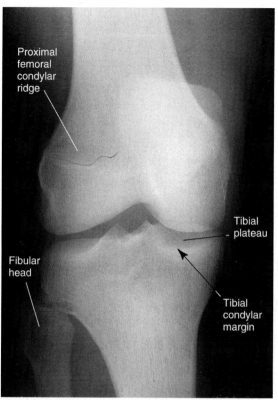

Proximal
femoral
condylar
ridge

Fibular
head

Tibial
- plateau

Tibial
condylar
margin

Radiograph 62.

Critique: This is a medial oblique knee radiograph. The fibular head is demonstrated without tibial superimposition, and the lateral femoral condyle is demonstrated in profile, indicating accurate obliquity. The femorotibial joint space is obscured, the proximal ridges of the femoral condyles are concave, and the fibular head is foreshortened and demonstrated more than 0.50 inch (1 cm) distal to the tibial plateau. The cephalad angle was too great.

Correction: Decrease the degree of central ray angulation about 5 degrees for every 0.25 inch (0.6 cm) of tibial plateau demonstrated. For this radiograph, approximately 0.25 inch of the tibial plateau is demonstrated between the anterior and posterior tibial margins; thus, the central ray should be adjusted about 5 degrees.

Knee: Lateral Position (Mediolateral Projection)

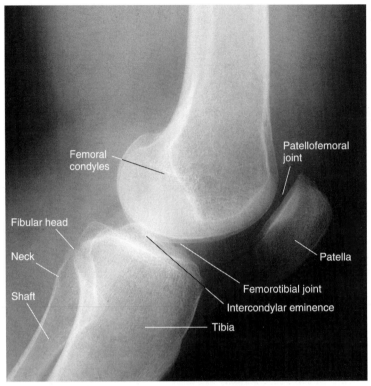

Femoral condyles

Patellofemoral joint

Fibular head

Neck

Shaft

Patella

Femorotibial joint

Intercondylar eminence

Tibia

Figure 5-73. Accurately positioned lateral knee radiograph.

Radiographic Evaluation

Facility's patient identification requirements are visible on radiograph.
- These requirements usually are facility name, patient name, age, and hospital number, and exam time and date.
- Patient ID plate is positioned so as not to obscure anatomy of interest.

A right or left marker, identifying the correct knee, is present on the radiograph and does not superimpose anatomy of interest.
- Place the marker within the collimated light field so it does not superimpose any portion of the knee.

There is no evidence of preventable artifacts, such as bandages and splints.
- Consult with the ordering physician and the patient about whether bandages and splints can be removed.

Contrast and density are adequate to demonstrate the surrounding soft tissue and bony structures of the knee. Penetration is sufficient to visualize the bony trabecular patterns and cortical outlines of the patella, femoral condyles, proximal tibia and distal femur.

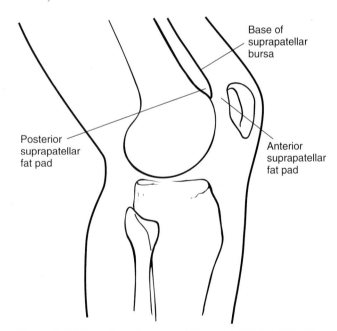

Base of suprapatellar bursa

Posterior suprapatellar fat pad

Anterior suprapatellar fat pad

Figure 5-74. Location of suprapatellar fat pads. (Reproduced with permission from Martensen K: The Knee. (In-Service Reviews in Radiologic Technology, vol 14, no 7.) Birmingham, AL: In-Service Reviews, Inc, 1991.)

- If the patient's mediolateral knee thickness measures under 5 inches (13 cm), a grid is not required. For such a patient, a high-contrast, low (60 to 70) kVp technique sufficiently penetrates the bony and soft tissue structures of the knee without causing excessive scattered radiation to reach the film and hinder contrast. If the patient's knee measures over 5 inches (13 cm), a grid should be used, because this thickness would produce enough scattered radiation to negatively affect radiographic contrast.[6, 8]
- When a grid is used, increase the kVp above 70 to penetrate the thicker knee and to provide an adequate scale of contrast. Increase the exposure (mAs) by the standard density conversion factor for the grid ratio being used to compensate for the scatter and primary radiation the grid will absorb.
- *Suprapatellar Fat Pads:*   There are two soft tissue structures of interest at the knee that are used to diagnose joint effusion and knee injury. They are the posterior and anterior suprapatellar fat pads. Both are located anterior to the patellar surface of the distal femur and are separated by the suprapatellar bursa (Fig. 5–74). Fluid that collects in the suprapatellar bursa causes the anterior and posterior suprapatellar fat pads to separate. It is a widening of this space that indicates a diagnosis of joint effusion.[14]

The bony trabecular patterns and cortical outlines of the distal femur, proximal tibia, fibula, and patella are sharply defined.

- Sharply defined recorded details are obtained when patient motion is controlled, a small focal spot is used, and a short object–image distance (OID) is maintained.

The knee is flexed 10 to 15 degrees, the patella is situated proximal to the patellar surface of the femur, and the patellofemoral joint is open.

- With less than 20 degrees of knee flexion, the patella is situated proximal to the patellar surface of the femur, the quadriceps are relaxed, and the patella is fairly mobile. In this patellar position, the anterior and posterior suprapatellar fat pads can be easily used to evaluate knee joint effusion. Conversely, when the knee is flexed 20 degrees or more, there is a tightening of the surrounding knee muscles and tendons, the patella comes into contact with the patellar surface of the femur, and the anterior and posterior suprapatellar fat pads are obscured, eliminating their usefulness in diagnosing joint effusion[14, 15] (see Rad. 63).
- *Positioning for Fracture:*   If a patellar fracture is suspected the knee should remain extended to prevent displacement of bony fragments or vascular injury.

The distal articulating surfaces of the medial and lateral femoral condyles are superimposed, and the femorotibial joint space is open.

- Take a few minutes to study a femoral bone. Place it upright with the distal femoral condylar surfaces resting against a flat surface. Notice how the femoral shaft inclines medially about 10 to 15 degrees. When a

patient is in an erect position, this is how the femurs are positioned. This femoral incline gives the body stability (Fig. 5–75). The amount of inclination a person displays depends on pelvic width and femoral shaft length. The wider the pelvis and the shorter the femoral shaft length, the more medially the femora incline.[1, 4]

- When the patient is placed in a recumbent lateral position for a lateral knee radiograph (Fig. 5–76), some of the medial femoral inclination is reduced, resulting in projection of the medial condyle distal to the lateral condyle and into the femorotibial joint space (Fig. 5–77). This can be demonstrated by laying the femoral bone on its lateral side. Note how the distal condylar surfaces are no longer on the same plane. The medial condyle is situated distal to the lateral condyle. The amount of distance demonstrated between these two condyles depends on the amount of medial femoral incline the femur displayed in the upright position, the length of the femur, and the width of the pelvis the femur originated from. If the medial

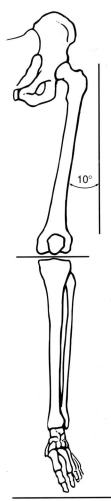

Figure 5–75. Femoral inclination in upright position. (Reproduced with permission from Martensen K: The Knee. (In-Service Reviews in Radiologic Technology, vol 14, no 7.) Birmingham, AL: In-Service Reviews, Inc, 1991.)

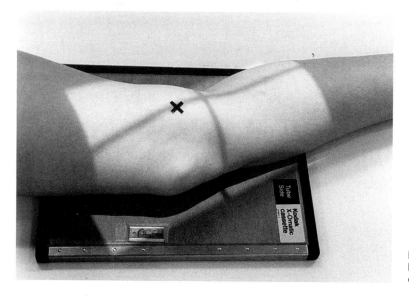

Figure 5-76. Proper patient positioning for lateral knee radiograph. *X* indicates medial femoral epicondyle.

condyle remains in this distal position, it obscures the femorotibial joint space on the radiograph. This is why a cephalic angle is needed for most lateral knee radiographs.

- **Determining Central Ray Angulation:** Because the degree of femoral inclination varies between patients, so must the degree of central ray angulation. On a patient with a wide pelvis and short femora, a 5- to 7-degree cephalad angle is the most reliable angulation to use. On a patient with a narrow pelvis and long femora, very little if any angulation is required. Although females commonly demonstrate greater pelvic width and femoral inclination and males demonstrate the narrower pelvic width and femoral inclination, there are variations in both sexes. Each patient's pelvic width and femoral length should be evaluated to determine the degree of angulation to use.

- **Effect of Central Ray Angulation on Femoral Condylar Superimposition:** If an inaccurate central ray angulation is used on a lateral knee radiograph, the distal articulating surfaces of the femoral condyles are not superimposed on the radiograph. Whenever this occurs, the femorotibial joint space is narrowed or closed. If a patient required a cephalic angulation to project the medial condyle proximally, but no angle was used, the radiograph demonstrates the distal articulating surface of the medial condyle

distal to the distal articulating surface of the lateral condyle (see Rad. 64). If a patient did not require a cephalic angulation but one was used, or if the cephalad angle was too great, the distal surface of the medial condyle is projected proximal to the distal surface of the lateral condyle (see Rad. 65).

- **Distinguishing Lateral and Medial Condyles:** The first step one should take when evaluating a radiograph on which the distal condylar surfaces are not aligned is to determine which condyle is the lateral and which is the medial. The most reliable method of identifying the medial condyle is to locate the rounded bony tubercle known as the adductor tubercle. It is located posteriorly on the medial aspect of the femur, just superior to the medial condyle. The size and shape of the tubercle are not identical on every patient, although this surface is considerably different from the same surface on the lateral condyle, which is smooth. Once the adductor tubercle is located, the medial condyle is also identified. Another difference between the medial and lateral condyles is evident on their distal articulating surfaces. The distal surface of the medial condyle is convex, and the distal surface of the lateral condyle is flat.

- **Supine Lateral Knee Radiograph:** When a lateral knee radiograph is taken with the patient supine, using a horizontal central ray, a cephalad angulation is not required, as long as the patient's femoral inclination is not reduced by shifting the distal femur laterally.

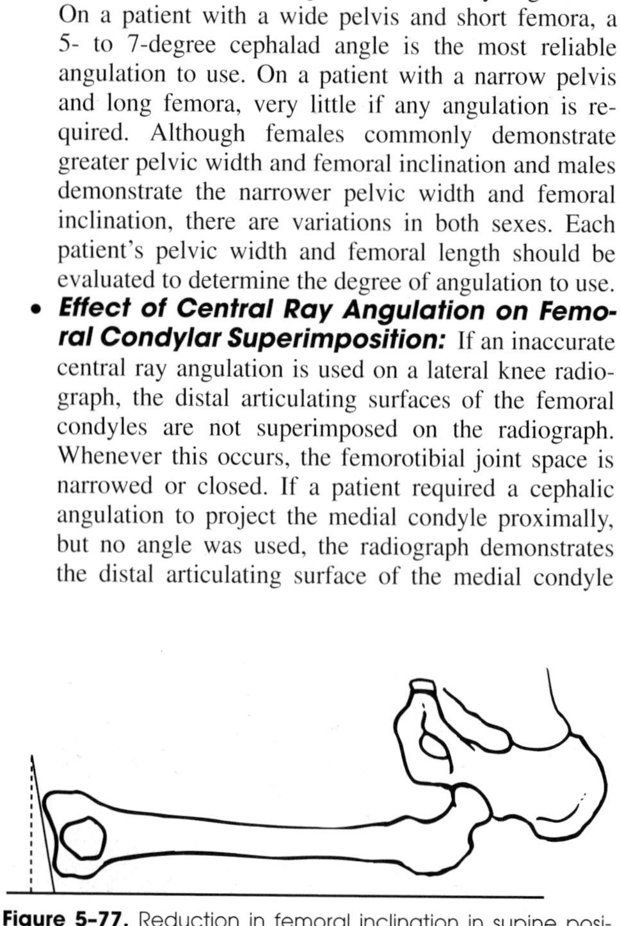

The anterior and posterior surfaces of the medial and lateral femoral condyles are superimposed, and the tibia partially superimposes the fibular head.

- How the central ray is aligned with the femur determines the relationship between the tibia and fibula, especially when a cephalic angulation is used. Study a femoral bone that is positioned in a mediolateral projection with the femoral epicondyles placed directly on top of each other. Note that in this position, the medial condyle is situated not only distal but also

Figure 5-77. Reduction in femoral inclination in supine position.

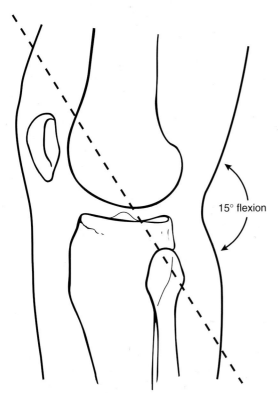

Figure 5-78. Proper central ray *(CR)* alignment for lateral knee radiograph. (Reproduced with permission from Martensen K: The Knee. (In-Service Reviews in Radiologic Technology, vol 14, no 7.) Birmingham, AL: In-Service Reviews, Inc., 1991.)

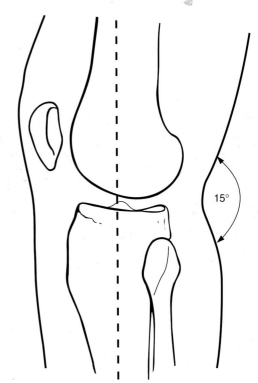

Figure 5-79. Central ray *(CR)* aligned with femur for lateral knee radiograph. (Reproduced with permission from Martensen K: The Knee. (In-Service Reviews in Radiologic Technology, vol 14, no 7.) Birmingham, AL: In-Service Reviews, Inc., 1991.)

posterior to the lateral condyle, indicating that the medial condyle must be projected proximally and anteriorly to superimpose it onto the lateral condyle.

- **Positioning to Superimpose the Anterior and Posterior Aspects of the Femoral Condyles:** Two positioning methods can be used to accomplish this goal. For the first and easier method, position the femoral epicondyles directly on top of each other, so that an imaginary line drawn between them is perpendicular to the film. Then direct the central ray across the femur, as indicated in Figure 5–78. In this method, the central ray projects the medial condyle anteriorly and proximally. This method also demonstrates the fibular head partially superimposed by the tibia, which is an accurate lateral tibiofibular relationship (Fig. 5–73).

For the second method, align the femoral epicondyles perpendicular to the film, then roll the patient's patella toward the film about 0.25 inch (0.6 cm) to move the medial condyle anteriorly, onto the lateral condyle. Finally, align the central ray with the femur as demonstrated in Figure 5–79, projecting the medial condyle proximally. This method produces a radiograph on which the condyles are superimposed but the fibular head is demonstrated without tibial superimposition (see Rad. 66). Regardless of the method your facility prefers, a true lateral knee radiograph has not been accomplished unless the condyles are superimposed.[16]

- **Effect of Patient Rotation on Femoral Condylar Superimposition:** When a radiograph is obtained that demonstrates one femoral condyle anterior to the other, the patella must be rolled closer to or farther away from the film to obtain superimposed condyles. The first step in determining which way to roll the knee is to distinguish one condyle from the other. As described previously, the most reliable method is to locate the adductor tubercle of the medial condyle. When a lateral knee radiograph is obtained that demonstrates the adductor tubercle and medial condyle posterior to the lateral condyle, the patella was situated too far from the film (Fig. 5–80 and Rad.

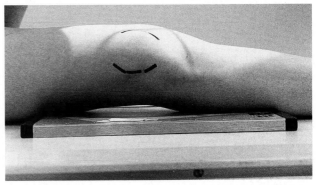

Figure 5-80. Poor knee positioning with patella too far from film.

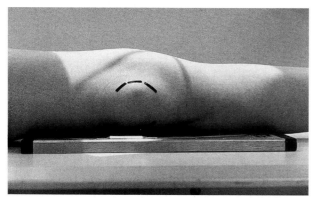

Figure 5-81. Poor knee positioning with patella too close to film.

67). When a lateral knee radiograph is obtained that demonstrates the medial condyle anterior to the lateral condyle the patella was situated too close to the film (Fig. 5–81 and Rad. 68).

Many technologists view the tibiofibular relationship to determine how to reposition for poorly superimposed condyles. If the tibia superimposes the fibular head, the patella was positioned too far from the film. If the fibular head is free of tibial superimposition, the patella was positioned too close to the film. Although this relationship is reliable for most patients, the alignment of the central ray affects the results. Radiograph 69 demonstrates such a case. Those using the adductor tubercle and medial condyle to determine how this patient should be repositioned would roll the patient's patella toward the film. Those using the tibiofibular relationship would roll the patient's patella away from the film. The adductor tubercle method is more reliable. This patient's patella needed to be rolled toward the film to superimpose the condyles.

The femorotibial joint is at the center of the collimated field. One fourth of the distal femur and proximal lower leg are included within the field.

- Center the central ray to the midline of the knee at the level of the femorotibial joint space, which is located 0.75 inch (2 cm) distal to the palpable medial epicondyle, to center the femorotibial joint in the collimated field. Open the longitudinal collimation enough to include one fourth of the distal femur and proximal lower leg. Transverse collimation should be to the knee skin-line.
- An 8 × 10 inch (18 × 24 cm) film placed lengthwise should be adequate to include all the required anatomical structures.

Critiquing Radiographs

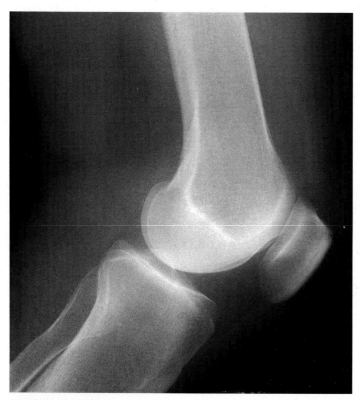

Radiograph 63.

Critique: The patient's knee is flexed beyond 20 degrees, the patella is in contact with the patellar surface of the femur, and the suprapatellar fat pads are obscured.

Correction: Decrease the amount of knee flexion to 10 to 15 degrees.

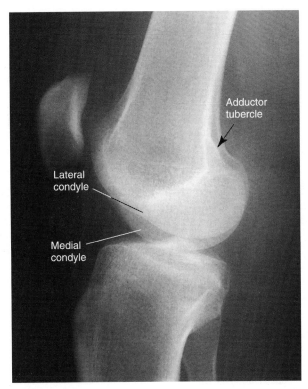

Radiograph 64.

Critique: The distal articulating surfaces of the femoral condyles are not superimposed. The medial condyle is distal to the lateral condyle.

Correction: A cephalic angulation should be used to project the medial condyle proximally. Adjust the angle about 5 degrees for every 0.25 inch (0.6 cm) of distance demonstrated between the medial and lateral distal surfaces. (This degree of angle adjustment is based on a 40-inch [102-cm] source–image distance [SID]. If a longer SID is used, the required degree of angle adjustment would be smaller, whereas if a shorter SID is used, the degree of angle adjustment would be larger.)

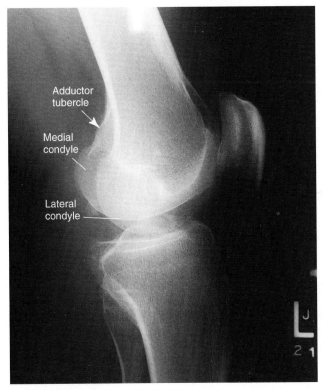

Radiograph 65.

Critique: The distal articulating surfaces of the femoral condyles are not superimposed. The medial condyle has been projected proximally to the lateral condyle. An excessively cephalad angle was used.

Correction: Decrease the central ray angulation about 5 degrees for every 0.25 inch (0.6 cm) of distance demonstrated between the medial and lateral distal surfaces. (This degree of angle adjustment is based on a 40-inch [102-cm] SID.)

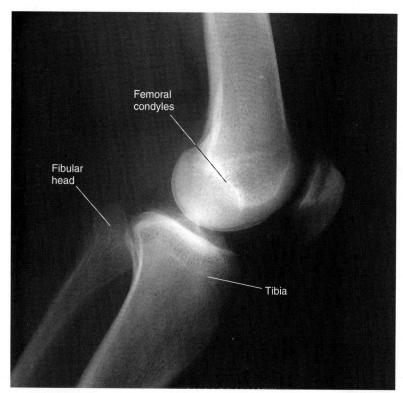

Radiograph 66.

Critique: The femoral condyles are super-imposed, and the tibiofibular articulation is demonstrated. The radiograph was taken with the central ray aligned with the femur, as demonstrated in Figure 5–79.

Correction: For a truer demonstration of the tibia and fibula, align the central ray across the femur, as demonstrated in Figure 5–78.

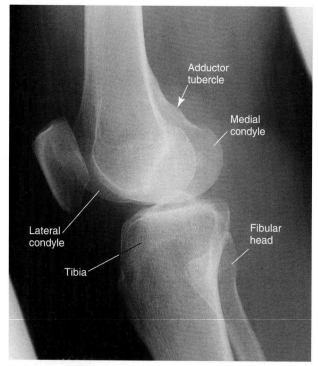

Radiograph 67.

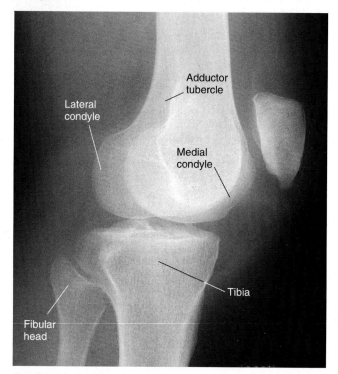

Radiograph 68.

Critique: The anterior and the posterior aspects of the femoral condyles are not superimposed. The medial condyle is situated posteriorly. The patient's patella was positioned too far from the film.

Correction: Roll the patella closer to the film. Because both condyles will move simultaneously, the amount of adjustment required is only half of the distance demonstrated between the posterior surfaces.

Critique: The anterior and the posterior aspects of the femoral condyles are not superimposed. The medial condyle is situated anteriorly. The patella was positioned too close to the film.

Correction: Roll the patella farther away from the film. Because both condyles will move simultaneously, the amount of adjustment required is only half the distance demonstrated between the posterior surfaces.

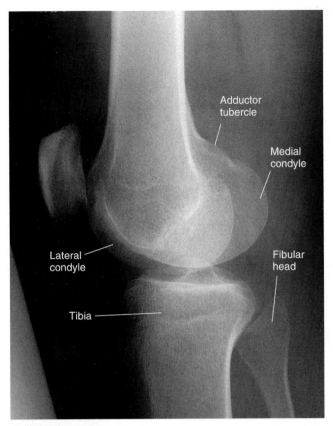

Radiograph 69.

Critique: The anteroposterior aspects of the femoral condyles are not superimposed. The medial condyle is situated posteriorly. The patella was positioned too far from the film.

Correction: Roll the patella closer to the film. Because both condyles move simultaneously, the amount of adjustment required is only half the distance demonstrated between the posterior surfaces.

Knee: PA Axial Position (Holmblad Method)

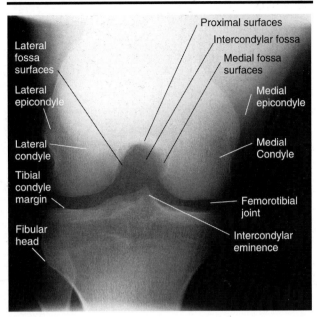

Figure 5-82. Accurately positioned Holmblad knee radiograph.

Radiographic Evaluation

Facility's patient identification requirements are visible on radiograph.
- These requirements usually are facility name, patient name, age, and hospital number, and exam time and date.
- Patient ID plate is positioned so as not to obscure anatomy of interest.

A right or left marker, identifying the correct knee, is present on the radiograph and does not superimpose anatomy of interest.
- Place the marker within the collimated light field so it does not superimpose any portion of the knee.

There is no evidence of preventable artifacts, such as bandages and splints.
- Consult with the ordering physician and the patient about whether bandages and splints can be removed.

Contrast and density are adequate to demonstrate the surrounding soft tissue and bony structures of the knee. Penetration is sufficient to visualize the bony trabecular patterns and cortical outlines of the distal femur, proximal lower leg and intercondylar eminence and fossa.
- If the patient's PA knee thickness measures under 5 inches (13 cm), a grid is not required. For such a patient, a high-contrast, low (60 to 70) kVp technique sufficiently penetrates the bony and soft tissue structures of the knee, without causing excessive scattered radiation to reach the film. If the patient's PA knee thickness measures over 5 inches (13 cm), a grid should be used, because this thickness would produce enough scattered radiation to negatively affect radiographic contrast.[6, 8]

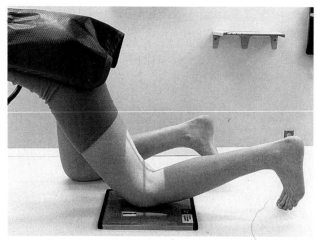

Figure 5–83. Proper patient positioning for Holmblad knee radiograph.

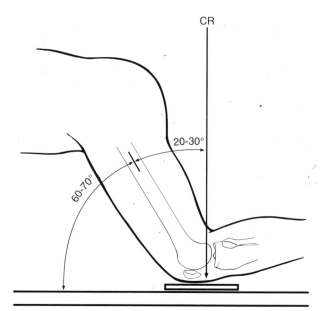

Figure 5–84. Holmblad position. *CR*, central ray.

- When a grid is used, increase the kVp above 70 to penetrate the thicker knee, and increase the exposure (mAs) by the standard density conversion factor for the grid ratio being used.

The bony trabecular patterns and cortical outlines of the intercondylar eminence and fossa are sharply defined.
- Sharply defined recorded details are obtained when patient motion is controlled, a small focal spot is used, and a short object–image distance (OID) is maintained.

The medial and the lateral surfaces of the intercondylar fossa and the femoral epicondyles are demonstrated in profile, and the fibular head partially superimposes the proximal tibia.
- The Holmblad method is performed by positioning the patient on hands and knees on the radiographic table and then requesting the patient to lean forward until the femur and the central ray form a 20- to 30-degree angle (femur–tabletop angle is 60 to 70 degrees) (Figs. 5–83 and 5–84). The cassette is positioned under the affected knee.
- ***Mechanics of Holmblad Positioning:*** To understand the way in which the femur is positioned for this view, I would suggest studying a femoral skeletal bone. Place the femoral bone upright with the distal femoral condylar surfaces resting against a flat surface. While viewing the posterior femoral surface, lean the femur anteriorly until the intercondylar fossa is positioned in profile. In this Holmblad position, note how the femoral shaft inclines medially about 10 to 15 degrees. The amount of inclination the femoral bone displays depends on the length of the femoral shaft and the width of the pelvis the femur originated from. The longer the femur and the wider the pelvis, the more femoral inclination is demonstrated.[1, 4]

  To obtain an intercondylar fossa with superimposed medial and superimposed lateral surfaces, you should not offset this inclination. If the inclination is offset by shifting the distal femur laterally or the proximal

femur medially and positioning the femur vertically, the medial and the lateral aspects of the intercondylar fossa are not superimposed and the patella is situated laterally (see Rad. 70). This fact can be demonstrated by placing the femoral skeleton bone vertically and viewing the change in the visualization of the intercondylar fossa.
- ***Effect of Foot Mispositioning:*** Mispositioning of the patient's foot may also result in rotation of the femur and demonstrate the medial and the lateral aspects of the intercondylar fossa without superimposition. The long axis of the patient's foot should be positioned perpendicular to the tabletop. If the heel was allowed to rotate medially (internally), the medial and lateral aspects of the intercondylar fossa are not superimposed, and the patella is rotated laterally (Rad. 70). If the heel was rotated laterally (externally), the medial and lateral aspects of the intercondylar fossa are not superimposed, the patella is demonstrated medially, and the tibia is demonstrated without fibular head superimposition (see Rad. 71).

The proximal surfaces of the intercondylar fossa are superimposed, and the patellar apex is demonstrated proximal to the intercondylar fossa.
- The proximal surfaces of the intercondylar fossa are superimposed when the femoral shaft is placed at a 60- to 70-degree angle with the tabletop[17, 18] (Fig. 5–84). To better study this relationship, place a femoral skeleton bone in the Holmblad position. While viewing the posterior intercondylar fossa, move the femur closer to and farther away from the tabletop. Note how the proximal surfaces of the fossa are in profile and superimposed only when the femur is at a 60- to 70-degree angle with the tabletop. The position of the femur in respect to the tabletop also determines the position of the patella. As the knee is flexed (the femur is brought away from the tabletop), the patella moves distally onto the patellar surface of the femur

and into the intercondylar fossa.[3, 12] The degree of knee flexion used for the Holmblad method situates the patella just proximal to the fossa.

- **Effect of Femur Positioning:** If a Holmblad radiograph is obtained that demonstrates the proximal intercondylar fossa's surfaces without superimposition, view the patella's position to determine whether the patient's femur was positioned too close to or too far from the tabletop. If the patellar apex is demonstrated within the fossa, the knee was overflexed (femur positioned too far away from the tabletop) (see Rad. 72). If the patella is demonstrated laterally and proximal to the fossa, the knee was underflexed (femur position too close to the table) (see Rad. 73).

The femorotibial joint space is open, and the anterior and posterior condylar margins of the tibia are superimposed. The intercondylar eminence and tubercles are demonstrated in profile.

- To obtain an open femorotibial joint space and demonstrate the eminence and tubercles in profile, dorsiflex the patient's foot and rest the foot on the toes. Because

the tibial plateau slopes downward from the anterior tibial margin to the posterior margin, this positioning is necessary to elevate the distal tibia and align the anterior and posterior tibial margins perpendicular to the film. If the foot is not dorsiflexed and resting on the toes, the femorotibial joint space is narrowed or closed, and the tibial plateau is demonstrated (see Rad. 72).

The intercondylar fossa is at the center of the collimated field. The distal femur, proximal tibia, and intercondylar fossa eminence and tubercles are included within the field.

- Center a perpendicular central ray to the midline of the knee, at a level 0.50 inch (1 cm) distal to the palpable medial femoral epicondyle, to place the intercondylar fossa in the center of the collimated field. Open the longitudinal collimation enough to include the femoral epicondyles. Transverse collimation should be to the knee skin-line.
- An 8 × 10 inch (18 × 24 cm) film placed lengthwise should be adequate to include all the required anatomical structures.

Critiquing Radiographs

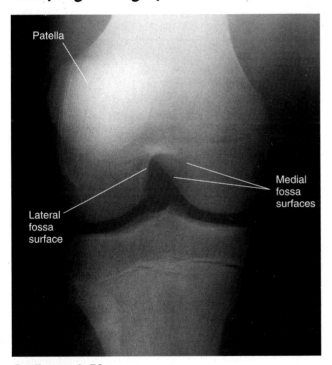

Radiograph 70.

Critique: The medial and the lateral aspects of the intercondylar fossa are not superimposed, and the patella is situated laterally. Either the femur was too vertical or the heel was rotated medially.

Correction: Position the distal femur medially or the proximal femur laterally, allowing the femur to incline medially, and align the long axis of the patient's foot perpendicular to the tabletop.

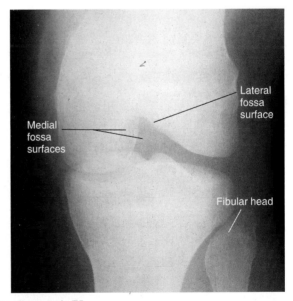

Radiograph 71.

Critique: The medial and the lateral aspects of the intercondylar fossa are not superimposed, the patella is situated medially, and the tibia is demonstrated without fibular head superimposition. The heel was laterally rotated.

Correction: Rotate the heel medially until the foot's long axis is aligned perpendicular to the tabletop.

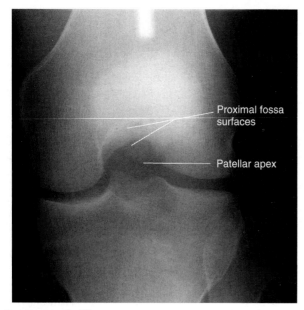

Radiograph 72.

Critique: The proximal surfaces of the intercondylar fossa are demonstrated without superimposition, and the patella is positioned within the intercondylar fossa. The knee was overflexed (femur positioned too far away from the tabletop).

Correction: Extend the knee (position the proximal femur closer to the tabletop). The amount of movement needed is half the distance demonstrated between the anterior and posterior proximal intercondylar fossa's surfaces.

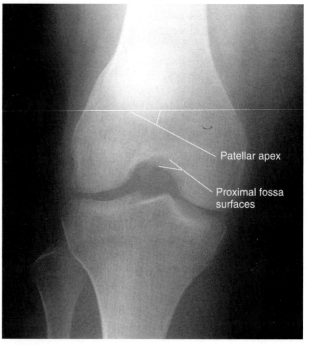

Radiograph 73.

Critique: The proximal intercondylar fossa's surfaces are demonstrated without superimposition, and the patella is positioned too far proximal to the fossa. The knee was underflexed (femur positioned too close to the tabletop). The femorotibial joint is obscured, and the tibial plateau is demonstrated. The patient's foot was not dorsiflexed and was not resting on the toes.

Correction: Flex the knee (position the femur farther away from the tabletop) and dorsiflex the foot, resting it on the toes.

PATELLA

Tangential Position (Merchant Method)

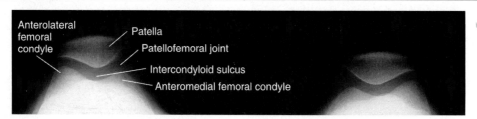

Figure 5-85. Accurately positioned Merchant knee radiograph.

Radiographic Evaluation

Facility's patient identification requirements are visible on radiograph.

- These requirements usually are facility name, patient name, age, and hospital number, and exam time and date.
- Patient ID plate is positioned at the top of the film so as not to obscure anatomy of interest.

Right and left markers, identifying the right and left knees, are present on the radiograph and do not superimpose anatomy of interest.

- Place the markers within the collimated light field so they do not superimpose any portion of the knees.

There is no evidence of preventable artifacts, such as bandages and splints.

- Consult with the ordering physician and the patient about whether bandages and splints can be removed.

Contrast and density are adequate to demonstrate the surrounding soft tissue and bony structures of the knee. Penetration is sufficient to visualize the bony trabecular patterns and cortical outlines of the patellae, anterior femoral condyles, intercondylar sulci, and patellofemoral joint spaces.

- An optimal 60 to 70 kVp technique sufficiently penetrates the bony and soft tissue structures of the knee and provides high radiographic contrast. If it is necessary to increase the kilovoltage above 70 to penetrate a thicker knee, a grid is not needed, because this exam uses a long object–image distance (OID). When a long OID is used, scattered radiation that would expose the film when a short OID is used is scattered at a direction away from the film. Because scattered radiation is not being directed toward the film, a grid is not needed to absorb the scatter. This is also referred to as the *air-gap technique*.[6]

The bony trabecular patterns and cortical outlines of the patellae, anterior femoral condyles, and intercondylar sulci are sharply defined.

- Sharply defined recorded details are obtained when patient motion is controlled and a small focal spot is used.

The knee demonstrates no rotation. The patellae, anterior femoral condyles, and intercondylar sulci are demonstrated superiorly, and the lateral femoral condyle demonstrates slightly more height than the medial condyle.[19]

- The Merchant method uses an axial viewer knee-supporting device, as demonstrated in Figure 5–86.[20] This freestanding device maintains the knees at a set degree of flexion, provides straps that restrain the patient's legs, and contains a film holder that keeps the cassette at the proper angle with the central ray.

To obtain a Merchant view of the patellae, place the patient supine on the table with the legs dangling off the end of the table. Set the axial viewer at a standard 45-degree angle, and position it at the end of the radiographic table beneath the patient's knees and calves. Situate the patient's ankles between the cassette holder, and place the cassette on the ankles so that it rests against the cassette holder (Fig. 5–86).

- To demonstrate the knees without rotation and to position the patellae, anterior femoral condyles, and intercondylar sulci superiorly, internally rotate the patient's legs until the palpable femoral epicondyles are aligned parallel with the tabletop. Then secure the legs in this position by wrapping the axial viewer's Velcro straps around the patient's calves. This positioning places the distal femora in an AP projection with the tabletop. Because the lateral condyles are situated anterior to the medial condyles, the lateral condyles demonstrate more height on a Merchant radiograph if the legs are adequately rotated. If the legs are not sufficiently rotated, the patellae are situated laterally, and either the anterior femoral condyles demonstrate equal height or the medial condyles demonstrate greater height than the lateral condyles (see Rad. 74). Both knees may not be rotated equally; often only one knee is rotated.

- ***Patellar Position on a Merchant Radiograph:*** Because this view is taken to demonstrate subluxation (partial dislocation) of the patella, the position of the patellae above the intercondylar sulci on a Merchant view may vary. In a normal knee, the patella is directly above the intercondylar sulcus on a Merchant radiograph, as shown in Figure 5–85. With patellar subluxation, the patella is lateral to the intercondylar sulcus, as demonstrated in Radiograph 75.

  Do not mistake a subluxed patella for knee rotation. Although both conditions result in a laterally positioned patella, the rotated knee demonstrates the femoral condyles at the same height, whereas with a subluxed patella, the lateral condyle is higher than the medial condyle.

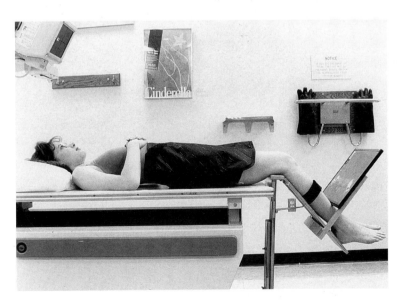

Figure 5–86. Proper patient positioning for Merchant knee radiograph.

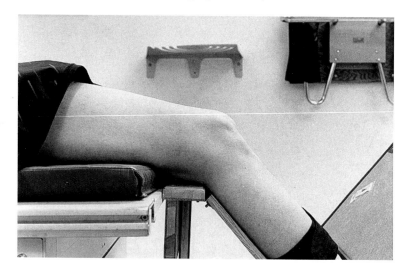

Figure 5-87. Poor femur positioning.

- ***Positioning to Demonstrate Patellar Subluxation:*** To demonstrate patellar subluxation, the quadriceps femoris (four muscles that surround the femoral bone) must be in a relaxed position. This is accomplished by instructing the patient to relax the leg muscles, allowing the calf straps to maintain the internal leg rotation. If the patient does not relax the quadriceps muscles, a patella that would be subluxed upon relaxation of the muscles will appear normal.

The patellofemoral joint spaces are open with no superimposition of the upper anterior thigh soft tissue, patellae, or tibial tuberosities.

- The position of the patient's legs on the axial viewer must be precise to obtain an open patellofemoral joint space. The height of the axial viewer is adjustable. It should be set to a height that positions the patient's femurs parallel with the table. If the distal femurs are positioned closer to the table than the proximal femurs, the angled central ray traverses the anterior thigh soft tissue, projecting it into the patellofemoral joint space (Fig. 5–87 and Rad. 76). Although the patellofemoral joint space remains open on such a radiograph, the space is underexposed.

- The relationship of the patient's posterior knee curves to the bend of the axial viewer determines whether the central ray will be parallel with the patellofemoral joint spaces. To demonstrate open patellofemoral joint spaces, position the posterior curves of the knees directly above the bend in the axial viewer, as demonstrated in Figure 5–88. If the posterior curves of the knees are situated at or below the bend of the axial viewer (causing the knees to be flexed more than what is set on the axial viewer), the central ray is not parallel with the patellofemoral joint space, and the patellae are resting against the intercondylar sulci (Fig. 5–89 and Rad. 77). If the posterior curves of the knees are situated too far above the bend of the axial viewer, (causing the knees to be extended more than what is set on the axial viewer), the tibial tuberosities are demonstrated within the patellofemoral joint space (Fig. 5–90 and Rad. 78).

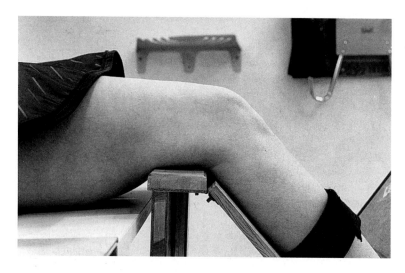

Figure 5-88. Proper posterior knee and axial viewer positioning.

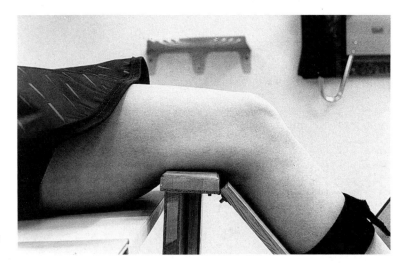

Figure 5-89. Posterior knee curve situated below bend in axial viewer.

- *Positioning and Central Ray Angulation for Large Calves:* The tibial tuberosities may also be demonstrated within the patellofemoral joint spaces on a patient with large posterior calves even when the posterior knee curves have been accurately positioned to the bend of the axial viewer. The knees of a patient with large calves are not flexed as much as the axial viewer is set. For such patients, the central ray angulation should be increased (5 to 10 degrees) or the axial viewer's angulation should be decreased until the knees are flexed 45 degrees.

- *Determining Central Ray Angulation:* The angle of the central ray and angle placed on the axial viewer also determines how well the patellofemoral joint space is demonstrated. Although 45 degrees is the standard angle, the viewer is capable of supporting the leg at 30-, 60-, or 75-degree angles as well. Each of these angles requires a predetermined central ray angulation to obtain an open patellofemoral joint.

The easiest way to determine the central ray angle to use for the different axial viewer angles is to know that the sum of the central ray angle and the axial viewer's angle must equal 105 degrees. For example, if the axial viewer is set at 30 degrees, the central ray angulation must be set at 75 degrees (30 + 75 = 105).

Evaluate the shadow of the knees that is created on the cassette when the centering light is on before exposing the film. When the patient has been accurately positioned, these shadows will display oval silhouettes with indentations on each side that outline the patellae (Fig. 5–91).

A point midway between the patellofemoral joint spaces is at the center of the collimated field. The patellae, anterior femoral condyles, and intercondylar sulci are included within the field.

- A standard 60-degree caudally angled central ray is centered between the knees at the level of the patellofemoral joint spaces, to place the patellofemoral joint spaces in the center of the collimated field (Fig. 5–91). A source–image distance (SID) of 72 inches (183 cm) is generally used to offset the magnification caused by the long OID.

- Open the longitudinal collimated field to include the patellae and the distal femurs. Transverse collimation should be to the lateral knee skin-line.

- A 10 × 12 inch (24 × 30 cm) or 11 × 14 inch (28 × 35 cm) film placed crosswise should be adequate to include all the required anatomical structures.

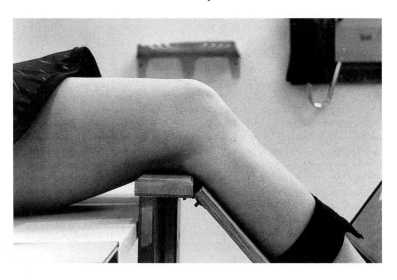

Figure 5-90. Posterior knee curve situated above bend in axial viewer.

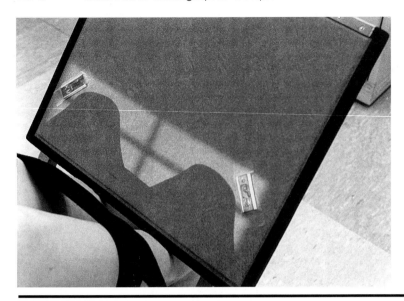

Figure 5-91. Proper knee shadows and central ray (CR) centering.

Critiquing Radiographs

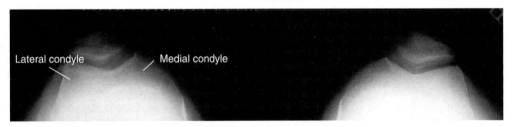

Lateral condyle   Medial condyle

Radiograph 74.

Critique: The patellae are demonstrated directly above the intercondylar sulci and are rotated laterally. The medial femoral condyles demonstrate more height than the lateral condyles. The legs were externally rotated.

Correction: Internally rotate the patient's legs until the patellae are situated superiorly, then restrain legs by wrapping the axial viewer's Velcro straps around calves.

Radiograph 75.

Critique: The femoral condyles are visualized superiorly, with the lateral femoral condyles demonstrating more height than the medial condyles. The patellae appear lateral to the intercondylar sulci and demonstrate subluxation.

Correction: No positioning movement is needed.

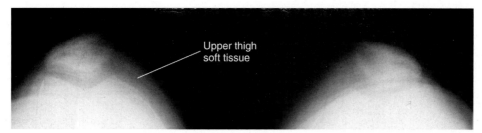

Radiograph 76.

Critique: Soft tissue from the patient's anterior thighs has been projected onto the patellae and patellofemoral joint spaces. The height of the axial viewer was not set high enough to position the femurs parallel with the table. The distal femurs were positioned closer to the table than the proximal femurs, as demonstrated in Figure 5–87.

Correction: Increase the height of the axial viewer until the femurs are positioned parallel with the table, as demonstrated in Figure 5–86.

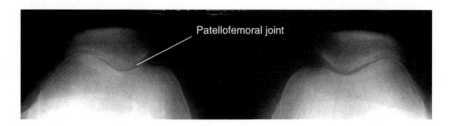

Radiograph 77.

Critique: The patellae are resting against the intercondylar sulci, obscuring the patellofemoral joint spaces. The patient's posterior knee curve was positioned at or below the bend on the axial viewer, as demonstrated in Figure 5–89.

Correction: Slide the patient's knees away from the axial viewer until the patient's posterior knee curvature is just superior to the bend of the viewer, as demonstrated in Figure 5–88.

Radiograph 78.

Critique: The tibial tuberosities are demonstrated within the patellofemoral joint spaces. Either the posterior knee curve was positioned too far above the axial viewer's bend, as demonstrated in Figure 5–90, or the patient has large posterior calves.

Correction: Slide the knees toward the axial viewer until the posterior knee curvature is just superior to the bend on the viewer, as demonstrated in Figure 5–88. If the patient was accurately positioned, but the calves are large, decrease (5 to 10 degrees) the central ray angulation or decrease the axial viewer's angulation until the knees are flexed 45 degrees. The total sum of the axial viewer's angle and the central ray angulation should be less than 105 degrees.

FEMUR

Anteroposterior Projection

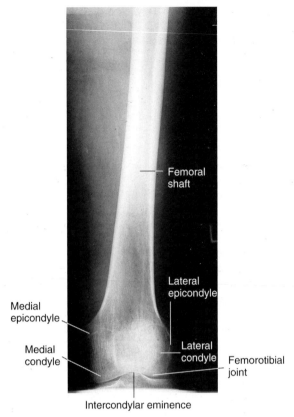

Figure 5-92. Accurately positioned AP distal femur radiograph.

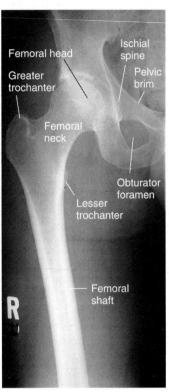

Figure 5-93. Accurately positioned AP proximal femur radiograph.

Radiographic Evaluation

Facility's patient identification requirements are visible on radiograph.

- These requirements usually are facility name, patient name, age, and hospital number, and exam time and date.
- Patient ID plate is positioned so as not to obscure anatomy of interest.

A right or left marker, identifying the correct leg, is present on the radiograph and does not superimpose anatomy of interest.

- Place the marker laterally within the collimated light field so it does not superimpose any portion of the affected femur.

There is no evidence of preventable artifacts, such as bandages and splints.

- Consult with the ordering physician and the patient about whether bandages and splints can be removed.

Contrast and density are adequate to demonstrate the surrounding soft tissue and bony structures of the femur. Penetration is sufficient to visualize the bony tra-becular patterns and cortical outlines of the knee, hip, and femoral shaft.

- An optimal 70 to 80 kVp technique sufficiently penetrates the bony and soft tissue structures of the femur and provides a high radiographic contrast.
- A grid should be used to absorb the scattered radiation produced by the femur, reducing fog and providing a higher contrast radiograph.
- The surrounding femoral soft tissue should be included to detect subcutaneous air or hematomas.
- **Anode-Heel Effect:** Another exposure factor that should be considered in positioning of the femur is the anode-heel effect. Because a long (17-inch [43-cm]) field is used for the length of the adult femur, there is a difference in the intensity of the beam on the cathode and anode ends of the film. This noticeable intensity variation is a result of increased photon absorption at the thicker, heel portion of the anode compared with the thinner, toe portion when a long field is used. Consequently, radiographic density at the anode end of the tube is less than that at the cathode end.

   Using this knowledge to our advantage can help us produce radiographs of the femur that demonstrate uniform density at both ends. Position the thicker, proximal femur at the cathode end of the tube and the thinner, distal femur at the anode end, then set an exposure (mAs) that adequately demonstrates the proximal femur. Because the anode will absorb some of the photons aimed at the anode end of the film, the distal femur, which requires less exposure than the proximal femur, will not be overexposed.

The bony trabecular patterns and cortical outlines of the femur are sharply defined.

- Sharply defined radiographic details are obtained when patient motion is controlled, a small focal spot is used, and a short object–image distance (OID) is maintained.

DISTAL FEMUR

The distal femur demonstrates a true AP projection. The medial and lateral femoral epicondyles are demonstrated in profile, the femoral condyles are symmetrical in shape, and the intercondylar eminence is centered within the intercondylar fossa.

- To obtain an AP distal femoral radiograph, place the patient in a supine position with the knee fully extended. Internally rotate the leg until an imaginary line drawn between the medial and lateral femoral epicondyles is positioned parallel with the film (Fig. 5–94). This positioning places the medial and lateral femoral epicondyles at equal distances from the film, as well as medially and laterally in profile, respectively. It also centers the intercondylar eminence within the intercondylar fossa.
- ***Effect of Mispositioning:*** If the femoral epicondyles are not positioned parallel with the film, a true AP projection has not been obtained. If the leg was not internally (medially) rotated enough to place the epicondyles at equal distances from the film, the epicondyles are not in profile, the medial femoral condyle is larger than the lateral condyle, and the intercondylar eminence is not centered within the intercondylar fossa (see Rad. 50). If the leg was internally rotated

more than needed to place the femoral epicondyles at equal distances from the film, the epicondyles are not demonstrated in profile, the lateral femoral condyle is larger than the medial condyle, and the intercondylar eminence is not centered within the intercondylar fossa (see Rad. 51).

- ***Positioning for Femoral Fracture:*** When a patient has a fractured femur, the leg should not be internally rotated, but left as is. Forced internal rotation of a fractured femur may injure the blood vessels and nerves that surround the injured area. Because the leg is not internally rotated when a fracture is in question, the distal femur demonstrates external rotation.

The femorotibial joint space is open but narrowed, and the anterior and posterior margins of the proximal tibia are superimposed.

- An open femorotibial joint space is obtained when the anterior and posterior margins of the proximal tibia are superimposed. Because these margins slope distally from the anterior condylar margin to the posterior condylar margin, and the central ray is centered proximal to the femorotibial joint, x-rays that diverge toward the proximal tibia are aligned parallel with the slope of the tibia, resulting in an open joint space. The joint space is narrower because the diverged x-rays project the distal femur partially into the joint space.

The long axis of the femoral shaft is aligned with the long axis of the collimation field.

- Aligning the long axis of the femoral shaft with the long axis of the collimated field enables you to collimate tightly without clipping any portion of the distal femur or surrounding soft tissue.

The distal femoral shaft is at the center of the collimated field. The distal femoral shaft and surrounding femoral soft tissue, the femorotibial joint, and 1 inch (2.5 cm) of the lower leg are included within the field. Any orthopedic appliances located at the knee are included in their entirety.

- A perpendicular central ray is centered to the distal femoral shaft to place the shaft in the center of the radiograph. This is accomplished by positioning the lower edge of the cassette about 2 inches (5 cm) below the femorotibial joint; the femorotibial joint is located 0.75 inch (2 cm) distal to the medial epicondyle. This lower positioning is needed to prevent the diverged x-ray beams from projecting the femorotibial joint off the film.
- The longitudinal collimation should be left open the full length of the film used. Transverse collimation should be to the lateral femoral skin-line.
- An 11 × 14 inch (28 × 35 cm) or 14 × 17 inch (35 × 43 cm) film placed lengthwise should be adequate to include all the required anatomical structures.
- ***Exam of the Entire Femur:*** If the entire femur is of interest and radiographs are taken of the distal and proximal ends of the femur, the radiographs should demonstrate at least 2 inches (5 cm) of femoral shaft overlap. Any orthopedic appliance, such as an intramedullary rod, should be included in its entirety.

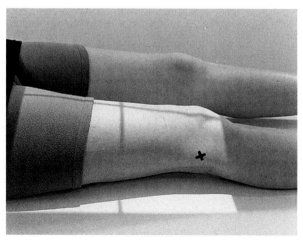

Figure 5-94. Proper patient positioning for AP distal femur radiograph. *X* indicates lateral femoral epicondyle.

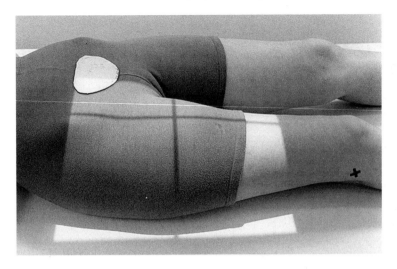

Figure 5-95. Proper patient positioning for AP proximal femur radiograph.

PROXIMAL FEMUR

The pelvis demonstrates a true AP projection. The ischial spine is aligned with the pelvic brim, and the obturator foramen is open.

- A true AP projection of the pelvis is obtained by placing the patient supine on the radiographic table with the legs extended (Fig. 5–95). To ensure that the pelvis is not rotated, judge the distance from the anterior superior iliac spine (ASIS) to the tabletop on each side of the patient. The distances should be equal.
- ***Detecting Pelvic Rotation:*** Rotation of the pelvis on a femoral radiograph is detected by evaluating the relationship of the ischial spine and the pelvic rim and visualization of the obturator foramen. When the pelvis has been rotated toward the affected femur, the ischial spine is demonstrated without pelvic brim superimposition, and visualization of the obturator foramen is decreased (see Chapter 6, Rad. 1). When the pelvis has been rotated away from the affected femur, the ischial spine is not aligned with the pelvic brim, but is demonstrated closer to the acetabulum, and visualization of the obturator foramen is increased (see Chapter 6, Rad. 2).

The femoral neck is demonstrated without foreshortening, the greater trochanter is demonstrated in profile laterally, and the lesser trochanter is superimposed by the femoral neck.

- The positions of the patient's foot and femoral epicondyle with respect to the tabletop determine how the femoral neck and trochanters are visualized on an AP femoral radiograph.
- ***Effect of Leg and Foot Rotation:*** Generally, when a patient is relaxed, the legs and feet are externally (laterally) rotated. Upon external rotation, the femoral neck inclines posteriorly (toward the tabletop) and is foreshortened on an AP femoral radiograph. Increased external rotation increases the degree of posterior incline and foreshortening of the femoral neck. If the leg was externally (laterally) rotated enough to position the foot and femoral epicondyles at a 45-degree angle with the tabletop, the femoral neck is demonstrated on end, and the lesser trochanter is demonstrated in profile (Fig. 5–96). If the leg was in partial external rotation with the femoral epicondyles positioned at about a 30-degree angle with the tabletop, the lesser trochanter is demonstrated in profile, but the femoral neck is only partially foreshortened (see Rad. 79).

  To achieve a true AP femur radiograph, which visualizes the femoral neck without foreshortening and the greater trochanter in profile, the patient's leg should be internally rotated until the foot is tilted 15 to 20 degrees from vertical and the femoral epicondyles are positioned parallel with the tabletop (see Figs. 5–93 and 5–97).
- ***Positioning for Fracture:*** When a patient has a fractured proximal femur, the leg should not be internally rotated, but left as is. Forced internal rotation of a fractured proximal femur may injure the blood vessels and nerves that surround the injured area. Because

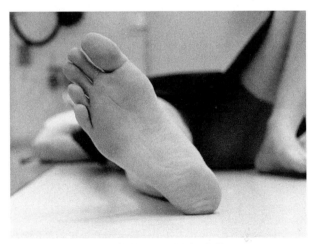

Figure 5-96. Poor foot rotation.

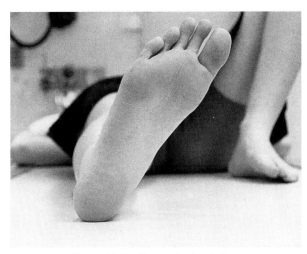

Figure 5-97. Proper foot rotation.

the patient's leg is not internally rotated when a fracture is in question, such an AP femoral radiograph demonstrates the femoral neck with some degree of foreshortening and the lesser trochanter without femoral shaft superimposition (see Rad. 80).

The proximal femoral shaft is at the center of the collimated field. The proximal femoral shaft, hip, and surrounding femoral soft tissue are included within the field. Any orthopedic appliances located at the hip are included in their entirety.

- A perpendicular central ray is centered to the proximal femoral shaft to place it in the center of the radiograph. This is accomplished by positioning the upper edge of the cassette about 2 inches (5 cm) above the hip joint; the hip joint is located 1 inch (2.5 cm) superior to the symphysis pubis.
- The longitudinal collimation should be left open the full length of the film. Transverse collimation should be to the lateral femoral skin-line.
- An 11 × 14 inch (28 × 35 cm) or 14 × 17 inch (35 × 43 cm) film placed lengthwise should be adequate to include all the required anatomical structures.
- ***Gonadal Shielding:*** Gonadal shielding should be used on all male and female patients, although it is important that no pelvic anatomy that is next to the affected femur be covered with a shield. It is not uncommon for a patient with a proximal femur fracture to have an associated pelvic fracture. Remember that the shield placed on top of the patient will greatly magnify.

Critiquing Radiographs

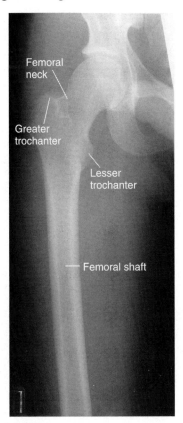

Femoral neck

Greater trochanter

Lesser trochanter

Femoral shaft

Radiograph 79.

Critique: The femoral neck is partially foreshortened, and the lesser trochanter is demonstrated in profile. The leg was in external rotation, with the femoral epicondyles positioned at about a 30-degree angle with the tabletop.

Correction: Internally rotate the patient's leg until the foot is tilted 15 to 20 degrees from vertical and the femoral epicondyles are positioned parallel with the tabletop, as demonstrated in Figure 5-97.

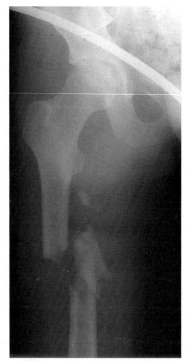

Radiograph 80.

Critique: The femoral neck is partially foreshortened, the lesser trochanter is demonstrated in profile, and the proximal femur demonstrates a fracture. The patient's leg was in external rotation.

Correction: Do not attempt to adjust the patient's leg position if a fracture of the proximal femur is suspected. No correction movement is needed.

Femur: Lateral Position (Mediolateral Projection)

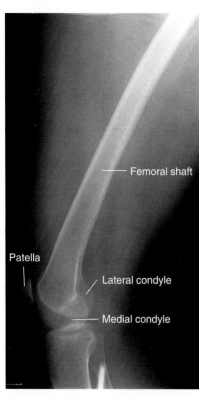

Figure 5-98. Accurately positioned lateral distal femur radiograph.

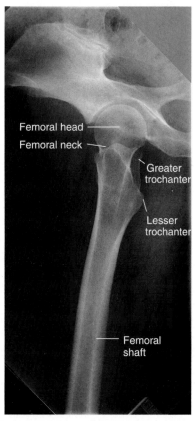

Figure 5-99. Accurately positioned lateral proximal femur radiograph.

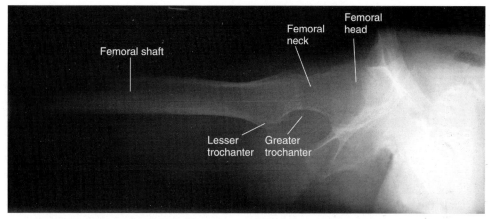

Figure 5–100. Accurately positioned cross-table lateral proximal femur radiograph.

Radiographic Evaluation

Facility's patient identification requirements are visible on radiograph.

- These requirements usually are facility name, patient name, age, and hospital number, and exam time and date.
- Patient ID plate is positioned so as not to obscure anatomy of interest.

A right or left marker, identifying the correct femur, is present on the radiograph and does not superimpose anatomy of interest.

- Place the marker laterally within the collimated light field so it does not superimpose any portion of the affected femur.

There is no evidence of preventable artifacts, such as bandages and splints.

- Consult with the ordering physician and the patient about whether bandages and splints can be removed.

Contrast and density are adequate to demonstrate the surrounding soft tissue and bony structures of the femur. Penetration is sufficient to visualize the bony trabecular patterns and cortical outlines of the knee and hip joints and the femoral shaft.

- An optimal 70 to 80 kVp technique sufficiently penetrates the bony and soft tissue structures of the femur and provides a high radiographic contrast.
- A grid should be used to absorb the scattered radiation produced by the hip, reducing fog and providing a higher contrast radiograph.
- The surrounding femoral soft tissue should be included to detect subcutaneous air or hematomas.
- ***Anode-Heel Effect:*** Another exposure factor that should be considered in positioning of the femur is the anode-heel effect. Because a long (17-inch [43-cm]) field is used for the length of the adult femur, there is a difference in the intensity of the beam on the cathode and anode ends of the film. This noticeable intensity variation is a result of increased photon absorption at the thicker, heel portion of the anode compared with the thinner, toe portion when a long

field is used. Consequently, radiographic density at the anode end of the tube is less than that at the cathode end.[1]

Using this knowledge to our advantage can help us produce radiographs of the femur that demonstrate uniform density at both ends. Position the thicker, proximal femur at the cathode end of the tube and the thinner, distal femur at the anode end. Then set an exposure (mAs) that adequately demonstrates the proximal femur. Because the anode will absorb some of the photons aimed at the anode end of the film, the distal femur, which requires less exposure than the proximal femur, will not be overexposed.

The bony trabecular patterns and cortical outlines of the femur are sharply defined.

- Sharply defined radiographic details are obtained when patient motion is controlled, a small focal spot is used, and a short object–image distance (OID) is maintained.

Distal Femur

The anterior and posterior margins of the medial and lateral femoral condyles are aligned, and the tibia partially superimposes the fibular head.

- To obtain a lateral distal femur radiograph, place the patient in a supine position with the leg extended. Then rotate the patient onto the lateral aspect of the affected femur until the femoral epicondyles are positioned perpendicular to the film (Fig. 5–101). The unaffected leg can be left posteriorly or can be flexed and drawn across the proximal femur of the affected leg. This positioning aligns the anterior and posterior margins of the medial and lateral femoral condyles and places a portion of the fibular head beneath the tibia.
- ***Effect of Mispositioning:*** If the femoral epicondyles are not positioned perpendicular to the film, the radiograph demonstrates one femoral condyle anterior to the other condyle. The patient's patella must be rolled closer to or farther from the film, by adjusting patient rotation, to align the condylar margins.

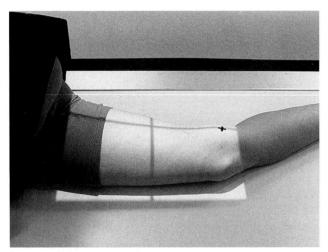

Figure 5-101. Proper patient positioning for lateral distal femur radiograph. *X* indicates medial femoral epicondyle.

The first step in determining which way to roll the patient's knee is to distinguish one condyle from the other. Because the central ray is centered proximal to the knee joint for a lateral femoral radiograph, x-ray divergence will cause the medial condyle to project distally to the lateral condyle. Consequently, the distal condyle will be the medial condyle. If a lateral distal femur radiograph is obtained that demonstrates the medial condyle posterior to the lateral condyle, the patient's patella was situated too far away from the film (see Rad. 5–81). If a lateral knee radiograph is obtained that demonstrates the medial condyle anterior to the lateral condyle, the patient's patella was situated too close to the film (see Rad. 82).

- **Cross-Table Femur Radiograph:** On patients with a suspected or known fracture, rolling onto the side may cause further soft tissue and bony injury. Consequently, a cross-table distal femur radiograph should be taken (Fig. 5–102). For this position, the

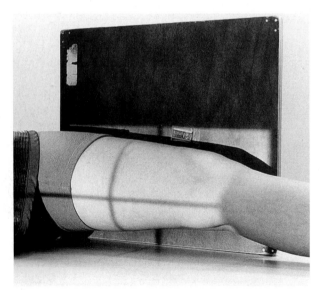

Figure 5-102. Proper patient positioning for cross-table lateral distal femur radiograph.

patient remains in a supine AP projection, a grid cassette is placed against the medial aspect of the femur, and a horizontal beam is directed perpendicular to the film.

The medial femoral condyle is projected distal to the lateral femoral condyle, closing the femorotibial joint space.

- This radiographic appearance is a result of central ray placement and x-ray divergence. Because the central ray is centered proximal to the femoral condyles, the x-rays that are used to record the images of the femoral condyles are diverged just as if a caudal angle were used. The divergence projects the medial condyle more distally than the lateral condyle because the medial condyle is situated farther from the film.

The long axis of the femoral shaft is aligned with the long axis of the collimation field.

- Aligning the long axis of the femoral shaft with the long axis of the collimated field allows you to collimate tightly without clipping the distal femur.

The distal femoral shaft is at the center of the collimated field. The distal femoral shaft, surrounding femoral soft tissue, the femorotibial joint, and 1 inch (2.5 cm) of the lower leg are included within the field. Any orthopedic appliances located at the knee are included in their entirety.

- A perpendicular central ray is centered to the distal femoral shaft to place it in the center of the radiograph. This is accomplished by positioning the lower edge of the cassette about 2 inches (5 cm) below the femorotibial joint; the femorotibial joint is located 0.75 inch (2 cm) distal to the medial epicondyle. The lower positioning is needed to prevent the diverged x-ray beams from projecting the femorotibial joint off the film.
- The longitudinal collimation should be left open the full length of the film. Transverse collimation should be to the lateral femoral skin-line.
- An 11 × 14 inch (28 × 35 cm) or 14 × 17 inch (35 × 43 cm) lengthwise film should provide adequate film size to include all the required anatomical structures.
- **Exam of the Entire Femur:** If the entire femur is of interest and radiographs are taken of the distal and the proximal ends of the femur, the radiographs should demonstrate at least 2 inches (5 cm) of femoral shaft overlap. Any orthopedic appliance, such as an intramedullary rod, should be included in its entirety.

PROXIMAL FEMUR

The lesser trochanter is demonstrated in profile medially, and the femoral neck superimposes the greater trochanter.

- To accomplish a lateral proximal femur position, begin by placing the patient supine on the radiographic table. Then flex the affected leg until the femur is placed at about a 60- to 70-degree angle with the tabletop (Fig. 5–103). This femoral position accurately places the

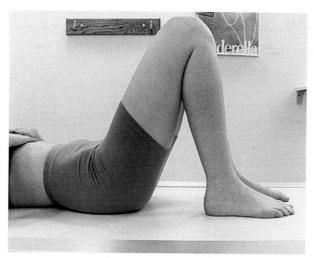

Figure 5-103. Proper leg flexion for lateral proximal femur radiograph.

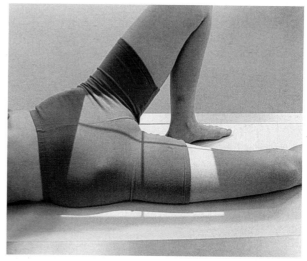

Figure 5-104. Proper patient positioning for lateral proximal femur radiograph.

greater trochanter beneath the femoral neck and puts the lesser trochanter in profile medially.

- **_Effect of Femur Positioning:_** Use a femoral skeletal bone to better understand how the relationship of the lesser and greater trochanters to the proximal femur and femoral neck changes as the distal femur is elevated upon knee flexion. Begin by placing the femoral bone on a flat surface in an AP projection. While slowly elevating the distal femur, observe how the greater trochanter rotates around the proximal femur. The greater trochanter first moves beneath the femoral neck; then, as elevation of the distal femur continues, the greater trochanter moves from beneath the femoral neck and is demonstrated on the medial side of the femur.

If the knee was not flexed enough to place the femur at a 60- to 70-degree angle with the tabletop, the greater trochanter is demonstrated laterally. If the knee was flexed too much, placing the femur at an angle greater than 60 to 70 degrees with the tabletop,

the greater trochanter is demonstrated medially (see Rad. 83).

The greater trochanter is also demonstrated medially, as shown in Radiograph 83, if the foot and ankle of the affected leg were elevated and placed on top of the extended unaffected leg. This positioning causes the femur to rotate externally. The foot of the patient's affected leg should remain resting on the tabletop.

The proximal femoral shaft is demonstrated without foreshortening, and the femoral neck is demonstrated on end.

- Once proper flexion is placed on the patient's leg, abduct the femur and roll the patient onto the affected leg until the femur rests against the tabletop (Fig. 5–104). To understand the relationship between the femoral shaft and neck, study a femoral skeletal bone placed in a lateral position. Notice that when the proximal femur rests against a flat surface in a lateral

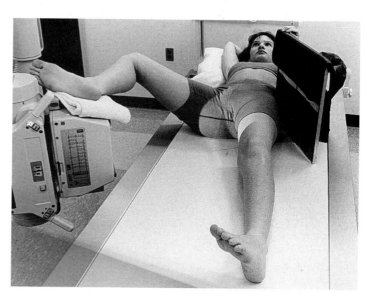

Figure 5-105. Proper patient positioning for cross-table lateral proximal femur radiograph.

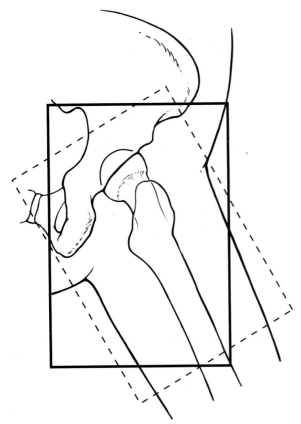

Figure 5–106. Central ray centering for proximal femur radiograph. Dotted line rectangle indicates area covered if collimator head is turned.

position, the femoral neck is on end. With this position, the femoral neck is completely foreshortened on a lateral proximal femoral radiograph. Because of this foreshortening, the femoral neck cannot be evaluated on such a lateral view. If the femoral neck is of interest, the patient's body should remain in an AP projection and the femur should be abducted no more than 45 degrees from vertical (see Rad. 84). This position demonstrates less foreshortening of the femoral neck but visualizes the proximal femur with foreshortening.

- **Positioning for Fracture:** For a patient with a suspected or known fracture, flexing or abducting the affected leg or rolling the patient onto the affected side may cause further soft tissue and bony injury. Therefore, an axiolateral position of the proximal femur should be taken (Figs. 5–100 and 5–105). Consult page 298 for positioning instructions and evaluating criteria for this position.

The long axis of the femoral shaft is aligned with the long axis of the collimated field.

- Aligning the long axis of the femoral shaft with the long axis of the collimated field allows you to collimate tightly without clipping any portion of the femur or surrounding soft tissue.
- Because the femoral shaft lies across the table when it is abducted, the patient must be rotated on the tabletop until the femur is placed as close to the long axis of the collimation field as possible, without causing the patient anxiety about being too close to the table edge.

The proximal femoral shaft is at the center of the collimated field. The proximal femoral shaft, hip joint, and surrounding femoral soft tissue are included within the field. Any orthopedic appliances located at the hip are included in their entirety.

- A perpendicular central ray is centered to the proximal femoral shaft to place it in the center of the radiograph. This is accomplished by positioning the upper edge of the cassette at the level of the anterior superior iliac spine (ASIS) (Fig. 5–106). If the collimator head can be moved, turn it until one of its axes is aligned with the long axis of the femur.
- Leave the longitudinal collimation open the full length of the film. Transverse collimation should be to the lateral femoral skin-line.
- An 11 × 14 inch (28 × 35 cm) or 14 × 17 inch (35 × 43 cm) film placed lengthwise should be adequate to include all the required anatomical structures.
- **Gonadal Shielding:** Gonadal shielding should be used on all male patients. Because the patient is rotated for this view it is difficult to place a shield on female patients without superimposing anatomy of interest.

Critiquing Radiographs

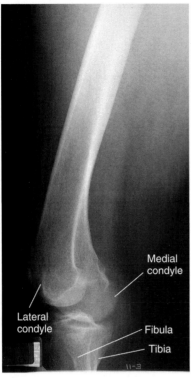

Radiograph 81.

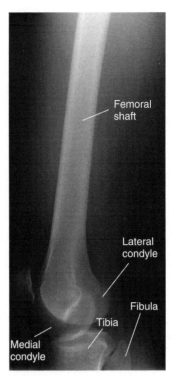

Radiograph 82.

Critique: Distal femur radiograph. The anterior and the posterior surfaces of the medial and lateral femoral condyles are not aligned. The medial condyle is posterior to the lateral condyle. The patella was too far from the film.

Correction: Roll the patient anteriorly, positioning the patella closer to the film and the femoral epicondyles perpendicular to the film. The amount of movement needed is half of the distance demonstrated between either the anterior surfaces or the posterior surfaces of the femoral condyles.

Critique: Distal femur radiograph. The anterior and the posterior surfaces of the medial and lateral femoral condyles are not aligned. The medial condyle is positioned anterior to the lateral condyle. The patella was too close to the film.

Correction: Roll the patient posteriorly, positioning the patella farther from the film and the femoral epicondyles perpendicular to the film. The amount of movement needed is half of the distance demonstrated between the anterior or the posterior surfaces of the femoral condyles.

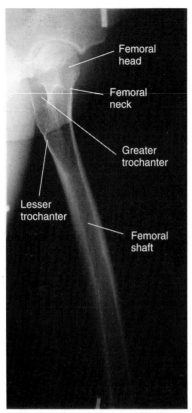

Radiograph 83.

Critique: Proximal femur radiograph. The greater trochanter is demonstrated medially next to the ischial tuberosity, and the lesser trochanter is not demonstrated in profile. Either the leg was flexed more than 60 to 70 degrees with the tabletop or the affected leg's foot and ankle were resting on top of the unaffected leg, elevating them off the tabletop.

Correction: Decrease the amount of leg flexion until the femur is positioned at a 60-degree angle with the tabletop, as demonstrated in Figure 5–103, or lower the affected leg's foot to the tabletop.

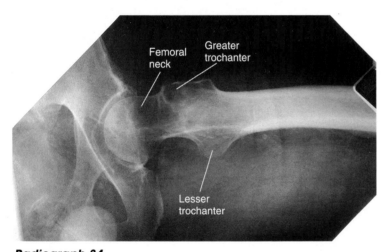

Radiograph 84.

Critique: Proximal femur radiograph. The femoral neck is demonstrated without foreshortening, and the proximal femur is foreshortened. The patient was positioned in an AP projection with the femur abducted no more than 45 degrees from vertical.

Correction: If the femoral neck is of interest, no correction movement is needed. If the proximal femur is of interest, the patient's leg should be abducted and the body rotated until the femur rests against the tabletop.

References

1. Williams P, Warwick R (eds). Gray's Anatomy, ed 36. Philadelphia: WB Saunders, 1980, pp 491–493.
2. Towbin R, Dunbar JS, Towbin J, Clark R. Teardrop sign: Plain film recognition of ankle effusion. AJR 134:985, 1980.
3. Berquist TH. Imaging of Orthopedic Trauma and Surgery. Philadelphia: WB Saunders, 1986.
4. Tortora GJ, Anagnostakos NP. Principles of Anatomy and Physiology, ed 6. New York: Harper & Row, 1990.
5. Draves DJ. Anatomy of the Lower Extremity. Baltimore: Williams & Wilkins, 1986.
6. Bushong SC. Radiologic Science for Technologists, ed 4. St. Louis: CV Mosby, 1988.
7. Frick H, Leonhardt H, Starck D. Human Anatomy 1. New York: Thieme, 1991, pp 359–360.
8. Carroll QB. Fuch's Principles of Radiographic Exposure, Processing and Quality Control, ed 4. Springfield, IL: Charles C Thomas, 1990, p 154.
9. Martensen KM. Alternate AP knee method assures open joint space. Radiol Technol 64:19–23, 1992.
10. Jacobsen K. Radiology technique for measuring instability in the knee joint. Acta Radiol 18:113–121, 1976.
11. Brower AC. Arthritis in Black and White. Philadelphia: WB Saunders, 1988, pp 82–83.
12. Hungerford DS, Barry M. Biomechanics of the patellofemoral joint. Clin Orthop 144:9–15, 1979.
13. Rogers LF. Radiology of Skeletal Trauma. New York: Churchill Livingstone, 1982, pp 751–757.
14. Hall FM. Radiographic diagnosis and accuracy in knee joint effusion. Radiology 115:49–54, 1975.
15. Bourne MH, Hazel WA, Scott SG, Sim FH. Anterior knee pain. Mayo Clin Proc 63:482–491, 1988.
16. Martensen KM. A consistent method to produce lateral knee radiographs. Radiol Technol 62:24–27, 1990.
17. Holmblad EC. Posteroanterior x-ray view of knee in flexion. JAMA 109:1196–1197, 1937.
18. Holmblad EC. Improved x-ray technic in studying knee joints. South Med J 32:240–243, 1939.
19. Merchant AC, Mercer RL, Jacobsen RH, Cool CR. Roentgenographic analysis of patellofemoral congruence. J Bone Joint Surg (Am) 56A:1391–1396, 1974.
20. The Axial Viewer: Instructions and Radiographic Technique Manual. Mountain View, CA: Orthopedic Products.

CHAPTER 6

Radiographic Critique of the Hip and Pelvis

HIP

Anteroposterior Projection

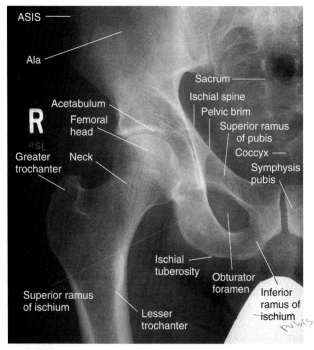

Figure 6-1. Accurately positioned AP hip radiograph.

Labels on image: ASIS, Ala, Acetabulum, Femoral head, R, RSL, Greater trochanter, Neck, Superior ramus of ischium, Ischial tuberosity, Lesser trochanter, Sacrum, Ischial spine, Pelvic brim, Superior ramus of pubis, Coccyx, Symphysis pubis, Obturator foramen, Inferior ramus of ischium, pubis

Radiographic Evaluation

Facility's patient identification requirements are visible on radiograph.

- These requirements usually are facility name, patient name, age, and hospital number, and exam time and date.

A right or left marker, identifying the correct hip, is present on the radiograph and does not superimpose anatomy of interest.

- Place the marker laterally within the collimated light field so it does not superimpose any portion of the hip.

There is no evidence of preventable artifacts, such as snaps, zippers, and objects left in patient's pockets. Patient's hand is not demonstrated beneath the hip.

- Patients often are asked to change into a gown before the hip is radiographed, and their clothes are then locked in a locker. Make certain that the locker key is not left in the patient's gown pocket. Drawing the patient's arm and hand away from the affected hip ensures that the patient will not place the hand beneath the hip in an attempt to ease the hip discomfort that results from lying on the radiographic table.

Contrast and density are adequate to demonstrate the surrounding soft tissue and bony structures of the hip. Penetration is sufficient to visualize the bony trabecular patterns and the cortical outlines of the ilium, pubis, ischium, acetabulum, and femoral head and neck.

- An optimal 75 to 85 kVp technique sufficiently penetrates the bony and soft tissue structures of the hip.
- Use a grid to absorb the scattered radiation produced by the hip, reducing fog and providing a higher-contrast radiograph.
- ***Fat Planes on AP Hip Radiograph:*** When evaluating a hip radiograph, the reviewer not only analyzes the bony structures but also studies the placement of the soft tissue fat planes. There are four fat planes of interest on an AP projection hip radiograph, and their visualization aids in the detection of intra-articular and periarticular disease: obturator internus fat plane, which lies within the pelvic inlet next to the medial brim; the iliopsoas fat plane, which lies medial to the lesser trochanter, the pericapsular fat plane, which is found superior to the femoral neck; and the gluteal fat plane, which lies superior to the pericapsular fat plane[1] (Fig. 6–2).

The bony trabecular patterns and the cortical outlines of the ilium, ischium, pubis, acetabulum, and femoral head and neck are sharply defined.

- Sharply defined recorded details are obtained when patient motion is controlled, respiration is halted, and a short object–image distance (OID) is maintained.

The pelvis demonstrates a true AP projection: The ischial spine is aligned with the pelvic brim, the sacrum and coccyx are aligned with the symphysis pubis, and the obturator foramen is open.

- A true AP projection of the hip is obtained by placing the patient supine on the radiographic table with the

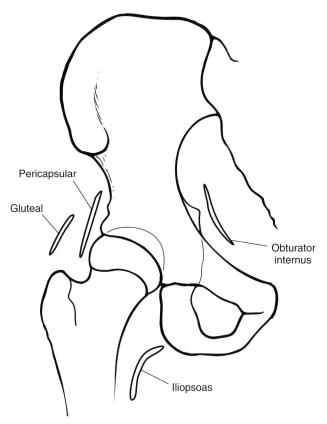

Figure 6-2. Location of fat planes.

Pericapsular

Gluteal

Obturator internus

Iliopsoas

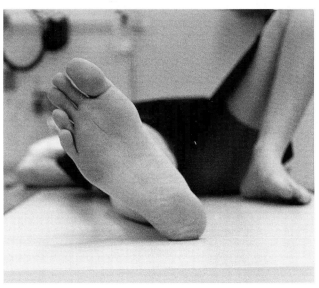

Figure 6-4. Poor foot rotation.

legs extended (Fig. 6–3). To ensure that the pelvis is not rotated, judge the distance from the anterior superior iliac spine (ASIS) to the tabletop on each side. The distances should be equal.

- ***Detecting Hip Rotation:*** Rotation on an AP hip radiograph is initially detected by evaluating the relationship of the ischial spine and the pelvic brim, the alignment of the sacrum and coccyx with the symphysis pubis, and the degree of obturator foramen visualization. If the patient was rotated toward the affected hip, the ischial spine is demonstrated without pelvic brim superimposition, the sacrum and coccyx are not aligned with the symphysis pubis, but are

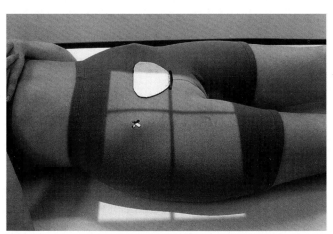

Figure 6-3. Proper patient positioning for AP hip radiograph.

rotated away from the affected hip, and the obturator foramen is narrowed (see Rad. 1). If the patient has been rotated away from the affected hip, the ischial spine is not aligned with the pelvic brim, but is demonstrated closer to the acetabulum, the sacrum and coccyx are not aligned with the symphysis pubis, but are rotated toward the affected hip, and the obturator foramen is widened (see Rad. 2).

The femoral neck is demonstrated without foreshortening, the greater trochanter is demonstrated in profile laterally, and the lesser trochanter is superimposed by the femoral neck.

- The relationship of the patient's foot and femoral epicondyles to the tabletop determines how the femoral neck and trochanters are visualized on an AP hip radiograph. Generally, when patients are relaxed, their legs and feet are externally (laterally) rotated. Upon external rotation, the femoral neck declines posteriorly (toward the table) and is foreshortened on an AP hip radiograph. Increased external rotation increases the degree of posterior decline and foreshortening of the femoral neck. If the patient's leg is externally (laterally) rotated enough to position the foot and an imaginary line connecting the femoral epicondyles at a 45-degree angle with the tabletop, the femoral neck is demonstrated "on end," and the lesser trochanter is demonstrated in profile (Fig. 6–4 and Rad. 3). If the patient's leg is in partial external rotation with the imaginary line connecting the femoral epicondyles positioned at approximately a 30-degree angle with the tabletop and the foot is vertical, the lesser trochanter remains in profile but the femoral neck is only partially foreshortened (see Rad. 4).
- ***Accurate Leg Positioning:*** To demonstrate a true AP hip, which visualizes the femoral neck without foreshortening and the greater trochanter in profile, the patient's leg should be internally rotated until the foot is tilted 15 to 20 degrees from vertical, and the femoral epicondyles are positioned parallel with the tabletop (Figs. 6–1 and 6–5). A sandbag or tape

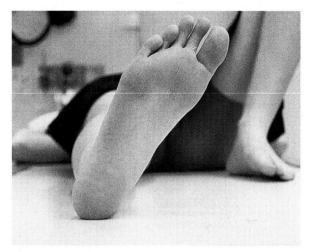

Figure 6-5. Proper internal foot rotation—15 to 20 degrees from vertical.

may be needed to help maintain this internal leg rotation.

- ***Positioning for Fractured or Dislocated Proximal Femur:*** When a patient has a dislocated or fractured proximal femur, the leg should not be internally rotated but left "as is." Forced internal rotation of a dislocated or fractured proximal femur may injure the blood supply and nerves that surround the injured area. Because the patient's leg is not internally rotated when a fracture is suspected, the resulting AP hip radiograph demonstrates the femoral

neck with some degree of foreshortening and the lesser trochanter without femoral shaft superimposition (see Rad. 5).

The femoral head and acetabulum are at the center of the collimated field. The acetabulum, greater and lesser trochanters, femoral head and neck, and half of the sacrum, coccyx, and symphysis pubis are included within the field. Any orthopedic appliances located at the hip are included in their entirety.

- A perpendicular central ray should be centered 1.5 inches (4 cm) medial to the ASIS, at the level of the symphysis pubis, to center the femoral head and acetabulum in the collimated field. Open the longitudinal collimation enough to include the ASIS and any hip orthopedic appliances. Transversely collimate to the patient's midsagittal plane and lateral hip skinline. Including half of the sacrum, coccyx and symphysis pubis within the collimated field provides a way to evaluate pelvic rotation.
- A 10 × 12 inch (24 × 30 cm) or an 11 × 14 inch (28 × 35 cm) film placed lengthwise should be adequate to include all the required anatomical structures. A larger film may be necessary to include hip orthopedic appliances.
- ***Gonadal Shielding:*** Use gonadal shielding on all male patients. Female patients should be shielded, although it is important that no pelvic anatomy is covered by the shield. It is not uncommon for patients with hip fractures to have an associated pelvic fracture. Remember that a shield placed on top of the patient will greatly magnify.

Critiquing Radiographs

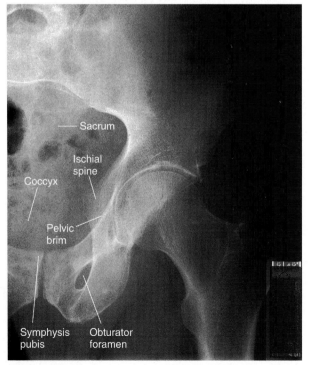

Sacrum

Ischial spine

Coccyx

Pelvic brim

Symphysis pubis

Obturator foramen

Radiograph 1.

Critique: The ischial spine is demonstrated without pelvic brim superimposition, the sacrum and coccyx are not aligned with the symphysis pubis but are rotated away from the affected hip, and the obturator foramen is narrowed. The patient was rotated toward the affected hip.

Correction: Rotate the patient away from the affected hip until the anterior superior iliac spines are positioned at equal distances from the tabletop.

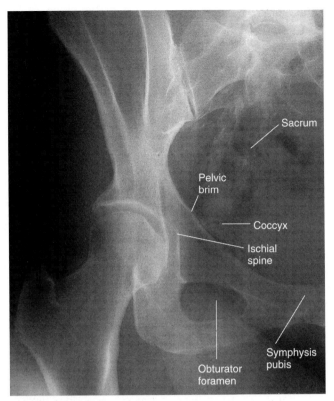

Radiograph 2.

Critique: The ischial spine is not aligned with the pelvic brim but is demonstrated closer to the acetabulum, the sacrum and coccyx are not aligned with the symphysis pubis but are rotated toward the affected hip, and the obturator foramen is clearly demonstrated. The patient was rotated away from the affected hip.

Correction: Rotate the patient toward the affected hip until the anterior superior iliac spines are positioned at equal distances from the tabletop.

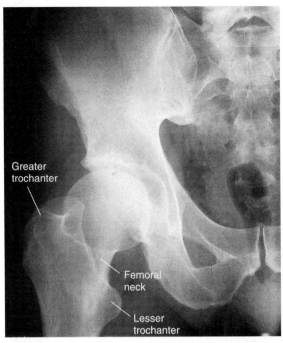

Radiograph 3.

Critique: The femoral neck is completely foreshortened, and the lesser trochanter is demonstrated in profile. The patient's leg was in external rotation with the foot and femoral epicondyles positioned at a 45-degree angle with the tabletop, as demonstrated in Figure 6–4.

Correction: Internally rotate the patient's leg until the foot is tilted 15 to 20 degrees from vertical and the femoral epicondyles are positioned parallel with the tabletop, as demonstrated in Figure 6–5.

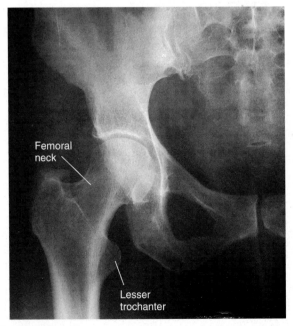

Radiograph 4.

Critique: The femoral neck is partially foreshortened, and the lesser trochanter is demonstrated in profile. The patient's leg was externally rotated with the femoral epicondyles positioned at about a 30-degree angle with the tabletop.

Correction: Internally rotate the patient's leg until the foot is tilted 15 to 20 degrees from vertical and the femoral epicondyles are positioned parallel with the tabletop, as demonstrated in Figure 6–5.

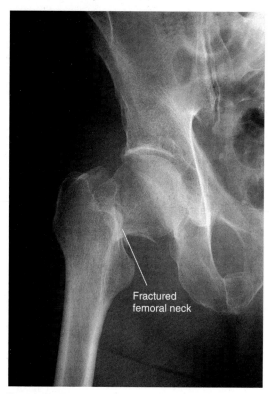

Radiograph 5.

Critique: The femoral neck is partially foreshortened and demonstrates a fracture. The lesser trochanter is demonstrated in profile. The patient's leg was in external rotation.

Correction: Do not attempt to adjust the patient's leg position if a fracture of the proximal femur is suspected. No correction movement is needed.

HIP

Frogleg Position (AP Axial Position)

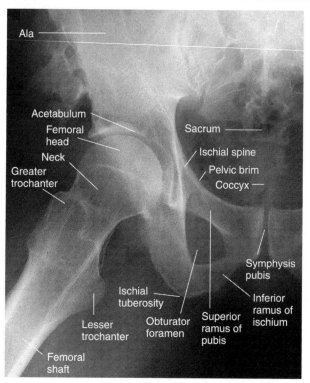

Figure 6–6. Accurately positioned frogleg hip radiograph.

Radiographic Evaluation

Facility's patient identification requirements are visible on radiograph.
- These requirements usually are facility name, patient name, age, and hospital number, and exam time and date.
- Patient ID plate does not obscure anatomy of interest.

A right or left marker, identifying the correct hip, is present on the radiograph and does not superimpose anatomy of interest.
- Place the marker laterally within the collimated light field so it does not superimpose any portion of the hip or proximal femur.

There is no evidence of preventable artifacts, such as snaps, zippers, and objects left in the patient's pockets.
- Patients often are asked to change into a gown before the hip is radiographed and their clothes are locked in a locker. Make certain a locker key is not left in the patient's gown pockets.

Contrast and density are adequate to demonstrate the surrounding soft tissue and bony structures of the hip. Penetration is sufficient to visualize the bony trabecular patterns and the cortical outlines of the ilium, pubis, ischium, acetabulum, femoral head and neck, and greater and lesser trochanters.

- An optimal 75 to 85 kVp technique sufficiently penetrates the bony and soft tissue structures of the hip.
- Use a grid to absorb the scattered radiation produced by the hip, reducing fog and providing a higher-contrast radiograph.

The bony trabecular patterns and the cortical outlines of the acetabulum, femoral head and neck, and greater and lesser trochanters are sharply defined.

- Sharply defined recorded details are obtained when patient motion is controlled, respiration is halted, and a short object to image distance (OID) is maintained.

The pelvis demonstrates a true AP projection. The ischial spine is aligned with the pelvic brim, the sacrum and coccyx are aligned with the symphysis pubis, and the obturator foramen is open.

- A frogleg radiograph of the hip is accomplished by placing the patient supine on the radiographic table with the unaffected leg extended and affected leg flexed and abducted (Fig. 6–7). To ensure that the pelvis is not rotated, judge the distance from the ASIS to the tabletop on each side. The distances should be equal.
- ***Detecting Hip Rotation:*** Rotation on a frogleg hip radiograph is detected by evaluating the relationship of the ischial spine and the pelvic brim, the alignment of the sacrum and coccyx with the symphysis pubis, and the visualization of the obturator foramen. If the patient was rotated toward the affected hip, the ischial spine is demonstrated without pelvic brim superimposition, the sacrum and coccyx are not aligned with the symphysis pubis, but are rotated away from the affected hip, and visualization of the obturator foramen is decreased (see Rad. 6). If the patient was rotated away from the affected hip, the ischial spine is not aligned with the pelvic brim but is demonstrated closer to the acetabulum, the sacrum and coccyx are not aligned with the symphysis pubis, but are rotated toward the affected hip, and visualization of the obturator foramen is increased.

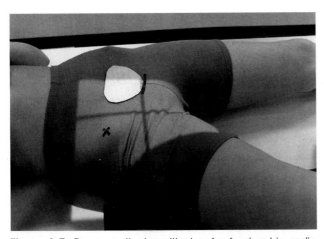

Figure 6-7. Proper patient positioning for frogleg hip radiograph.

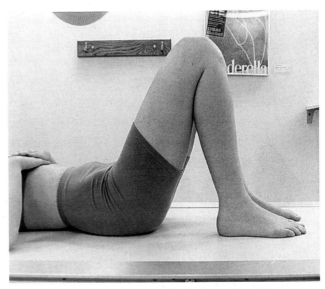

Figure 6-8. Proper knee and hip flexion—60 to 70 degrees from tabletop.

The lesser trochanter is demonstrated in profile medially, and the femoral neck superimposes the greater trochanter.

- For a frogleg hip radiograph, the position of the greater and lesser trochanters in relationship to the proximal femur is determined when the patient flexes the knee and hip.
- ***Effect of Distal Femur Elevation on Proximal Femur Visualization:*** Use a femoral skeletal bone to better understand how the relationship of the greater and lesser trochanters to the proximal femur changes as the distal femur is elevated upon knee flexion. Begin by placing the femoral bone on a flat surface in an AP projection. While slowly elevating the distal femur, observe how the greater trochanter rotates around the proximal femur. First, the greater trochanter moves beneath the proximal femur; then, as elevation of the distal femur continues, it moves from beneath the proximal femur and is demonstrated on the medial side of the femur.
- ***Femur Positioning for Frogleg Radiograph:*** To accurately position the greater trochanter beneath the proximal femur and position the lesser trochanter in profile, flex the patient's knee until the femur is angled at about 60 to 70 degrees with the tabletop (20 to 30 degrees from vertical) (Fig. 6–8). If the knee is not flexed enough to place the femur at this angle with the tabletop, the greater trochanter is demonstrated laterally, as it is on an AP projection (see Rad. 7). If the knee is flexed too much, placing the femur at an angle greater than 60 to 70 degrees with the tabletop, the greater trochanter is demonstrated medially (see Rad. 8). The greater trochanter is also demonstrated medially, as demonstrated in Radiograph 8, when the patient's affected leg's foot and ankle are elevated and placed on top of the unaffected leg. This positioning causes the femur to rotate externally. The foot of the patient's affected leg should remain resting on the tabletop.

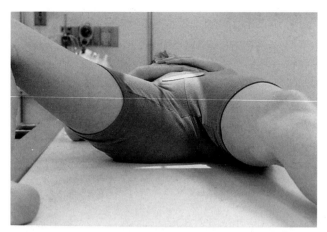

Figure 6-9. Proper leg abduction—45 degrees from tabletop.

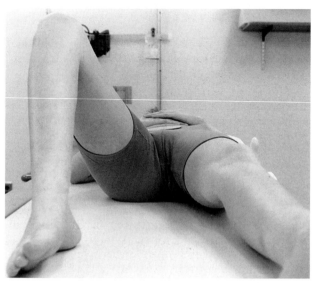

Figure 6-10. Femur in only slight abduction—20 degrees from vertical.

The femoral neck is partially foreshortened, and the greater trochanter is demonstrated at a transverse level halfway between the femoral head and the lesser trochanter.

- The degree of femoral abduction determines the amount of femoral neck foreshortening and the transverse level at which the greater trochanter is demonstrated between the femoral head and lesser trochanter.
- ***Effect of Leg Abduction:*** Use a femoral skeleton bone to understand how leg abduction determines the visualization of the femoral neck and the position of the greater trochanter. Place the femoral bone on a flat surface in an AP projection with the distal femur elevated until the greater trochanter is positioned beneath the proximal femur and the lesser trochanter is in profile (60 to 70 degrees with flat surface or 20 to 30 degrees from vertical). From this position, move the lateral surface of the femoral bone toward the flat surface, as if the femur was being abducted on a patient. As the bone moves toward the flat surface, observe how the femoral neck is positioned more on end and the greater trochanter moves proximally (toward the femoral head).

  To demonstrate the femoral neck and proximal femur with only partial foreshortening and the greater trochanter at a transverse level halfway between the femoral head and lesser trochanter, abduct the femoral shaft to a 45-degree angle with the tabletop (Figs. 6–6 and 6–9). To demonstrate the femoral neck without foreshortening and the greater trochanter at about the same transverse level as the lesser trochanter, abduct the femoral shaft to a 70-degree angle with the tabletop (20 degrees from vertical) (see Rad. 9 and Fig. 6–10). To demonstrate the proximal femoral shaft without foreshortening and the greater trochanter at the same transverse level as the femoral head, abduct the femoral shaft next to the tabletop (Rad. 10 and Fig. 6–11). This last position places the femoral neck on end.

The femoral neck is at the center of the collimated field. The acetabulum, greater and lesser trochanters, and femoral head and neck, as well as half of the sacrum, coccyx, and symphysis pubis are included within the field.

- Center a perpendicular central ray 1.5 inches (4 cm) medial to the ASIS at the level of the symphysis pubis to center the femoral neck in the collimated field. Open longitudinal collimation to include the ASIS. Transversely collimate to the patient's midsagittal plane and lateral hip skin-line.
- Including half of the sacrum, coccyx, and symphysis pubis within the collimated field provides a way to evaluate pelvic rotation.
- A 10 × 12 inch (24 × 30 cm) or an 11 × 14 inch (28 × 35 cm) film placed lengthwise should be adequate to include all the required anatomical structures.
- ***Gonadal Shielding:*** Use gonadal shielding on all male patients. Female patients should be shielded, although it is important that no pelvic anatomy is covered with shield. Remember that the shield placed on top of patient will greatly magnify.

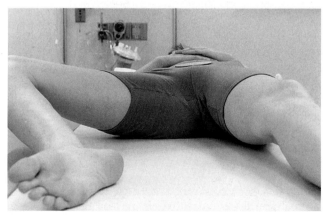

Figure 6-11. Femur in maximum abduction—20 degrees from tabletop.

Critiquing Radiographs

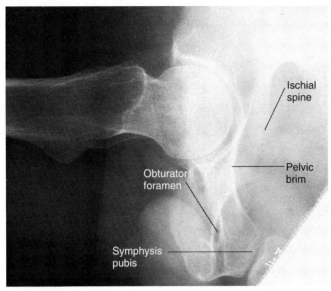

Radiograph 6.

Critique: The ischial spine is demonstrated without pelvic brim superimposition, the sacrum and coccyx are not aligned with the symphysis pubis but are rotated away from the affected hip, and the obturator foramen is not well demonstrated. The patient was rotated toward the affected hip.

Correction: Rotate the patient away from the affected hip until the anterior superior iliac spines are positioned at equal distances from the tabletop.

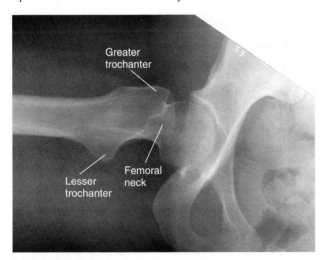

Radiograph 7.

Critique: The greater trochanter is positioned laterally. The patient's knee was not flexed enough to align the femur at a 60- to 70-degree angle with the tabletop (20 to 30 degrees from vertical), or the affected leg's foot and ankle were resting on top of the unaffected leg, elevating them off the tabletop.

Correction: Increase the knee flexion until the femur is aligned at a 60- to 70-degree angle with the tabletop, as demonstrated in Figure 6–8, or lower the affected leg's foot to the tabletop.

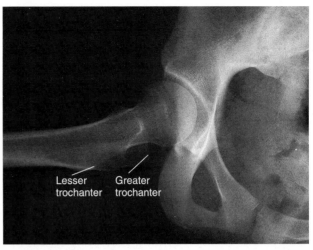

Radiograph 8.

Critique: The greater trochanter is positioned medially. The patient's knee was flexed more than needed, positioning the femur at an angle greater than 60 to 70 degrees with the tabletop (20 to 30 degrees from vertical).

Correction: Decrease the knee flexion until the femur is aligned at a 60- to 70-degree angle with the tabletop, as demonstrated in Figure 6–8.

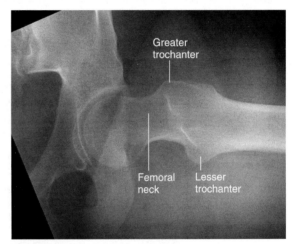

Radiograph 9.

Critique: The femoral neck is demonstrated without foreshortening, and the greater and lesser trochanters are demonstrated at about the same transverse level. The femur was in only slight abduction, at about a 70-degree angle with the tabletop (20 degrees from vertical), as demonstrated in Figure 6–10.

Correction: Consult with reviewers in your facility to determine whether this is an acceptable radiograph. If the proximal femoral shaft demonstrates too much foreshortening, have the patient abduct the femur to a 45-degree angle with the tabletop.

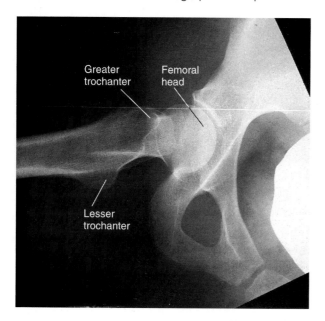

Radiograph 10.

Critique: The femoral neck is demonstrated on end. The greater trochanter is demonstrated on the same transverse level as the femoral head. The femur was positioned next to the tabletop, as demonstrated in Figure 6–11.

Correction: Consult with the reviewers in your facility to determine whether this is an acceptable radiograph. If the femoral neck is of interest, decrease the degree of femoral abduction.

HIP

Axiolateral Position (Inferosuperior Projection)

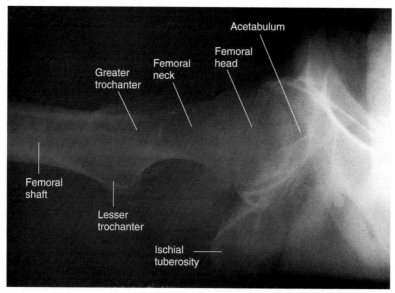

Figure 6-12. Accurately positioned axiolateral hip radiograph.

Radiographic Evaluation

Facility's patient identification requirements are visible on radiograph.

- These requirements usually are facility name, patient name, age, and hospital number, and exam time and date.
- Patient ID is positioned toward the femoral shaft so as not to obscure anatomy of interest.

A right or left marker, identifying the correct hip, is present on the radiograph and does not superimpose anatomy of interest.

- Place the marker anteriorly within the collimated light field so it does not superimpose any portion of the hip.

There is no evidence of preventable artifacts.

- It is recommended patient changes into a hospital gown before procedure.

Contrast and density are adequate to demonstrate the surrounding soft tissue and bony structures of the hip and proximal femur. Penetration is sufficient to visualize the bony trabecular patterns and the cortical outlines of the acetabulum, femoral head, neck, and proximal shaft, and greater and lesser trochanters.

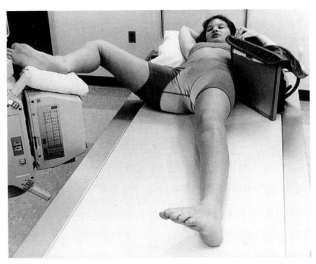

Figure 6-13. Proper patient positioning for axiolateral hip radiograph.

- An optimal 85 to 95 kVp technique sufficiently penetrates the bony and soft tissue structures of the hip and proximal femur.
- Use a grid to absorb the scattered radiation produced by the hip and proximal femur, providing a higher-contrast radiograph and increasing the visibility of the recorded details.
- Tight collimation and placement of a flat lead contact strip or the straight edge of a lead apron over the top, unused half of the cassette, as demonstrated in Figure 6–13, also prevents scattered radiation from reaching the film.
- ***Compensating Filter:*** Frequently, when an exposure (mAs) is set that adequately demonstrates the hip joint, the proximal femur is overexposed, because of the difference in body thickness in these two regions. A wedge-type compensating filter attached to the x-ray tube can be used to obtain uniform radiographic density of the hip joint and proximal femur. Align the thin end of the filter with the femoral neck and the thicker end with the proximal femur.

The bony trabecular patterns and cortical outlines of the acetabulum, femoral neck and head, and greater and lesser trochanters are sharply defined.

- Sharply defined recorded details are obtained when patient motion is controlled and a short object–image distance (OID) is maintained.

The femoral neck is demonstrated without foreshortening, and the greater and lesser trochanters are demonstrated at about the same transverse level.

- An axiolateral radiograph of the hip is obtained by placing the patient on the radiographic table in a true AP projection, with the unaffected hip positioned next to the lateral edge of the table. Flex the patient's unaffected leg until the femur is as close to a vertical position as the patient can manage and then abduct the leg as far as the patient will allow. Support this leg position by using a specially designed leg holder or by placing the foot on the collimator head. If the patient's foot is rested on the collimator head, place a

pad between the foot and collimator to avoid possible heat injury from the collimator.
- Flexion and abduction of the unaffected leg moves its bony and soft tissue structures away from the affected hip. Inadequate flexion or abduction of the unaffected leg results in superimposition of soft tissue onto the affected hip, preventing visualization of the affected hip (see Rad. 11).
- ***Film Placement:*** Once the patient's unaffected hip has been positioned, place the grid-cassette against the patient's affected side at the level of the iliac crest (Fig. 6–13). To demonstrate the affected femoral neck without foreshortening, align the x-ray tube horizontally with the central ray perpendicular to the femoral neck, and adjust the distal end of the film until the film's long axis is perpendicular to the central ray and parallel with the femoral neck.
- ***Localizing the Femoral Neck:*** To localize the affected femoral neck, first find the center of an imaginary line drawn between the symphysis pubis and the anterior superior iliac spine (ASIS). Then palpate the greater trochanter, and find a point 1 inch (2.5 cm) distal to it. (The greater trochanter can be palpated only after the leg has been internally rotated.) Finally, draw an imaginary line between this point and the center of the first line drawn[2] (Fig. 6–14). This imaginary line parallels the long axis of the femoral neck regardless of the degree of femoral abduction.

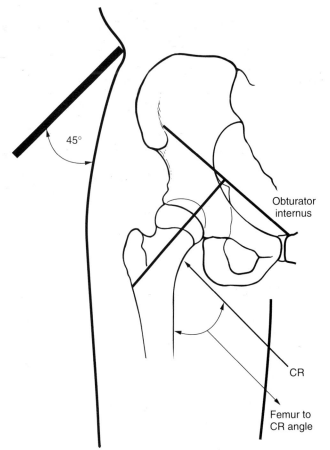

Figure 6-14. Locating the femoral neck and proper cassette placement for small and average patients. *CR,* central ray.

Once the long axis of the femoral neck has been located, align the central ray perpendicular to it and the film parallel with it. For the small to average patient, the film is placed at about a 45-degree angle with the patient's lateral body surface.

- **Alternative Method of Locating Symphysis Pubis:** If the greater trochanter cannot be palpated because of a fracture that prevents internal leg rotation, or if the patient has thick thigh soft tissue, one can predict the location of the greater trochanter by palpating the symphysis pubis. The greater trochanter lies at a level 1 to 1.5 inches (2.5 to 4 cm) superior to the symphysis pubis.

- **Effect of Film and Central Ray Misalignment:** Misalignment of the central ray and film with the femoral neck results in femoral neck foreshortening and a shift in the transverse level at which the greater trochanter is located. If the angle formed between the femur and the central ray is too large, the greater trochanter is demonstrated proximal to the transverse level of the lesser trochanter and is superimposed by a portion of the femoral neck (see Rad. 12). If the angle between the femur and the central ray is too small, the greater trochanter is demonstrated distal to the transverse level of the lesser trochanter. This mispositioning seldom occurs, because the table and tube position prevents such a small angle.

The lesser trochanter is demonstrated in profile posteriorly, and the greater trochanter is superimposed by the femoral shaft.

- Rotation of the patient's affected leg determines the relationship of the lesser and greater trochanter to the proximal femur on an axiolateral hip radiograph. Generally, when a patient is placed on the radiographic table and the affected leg is allowed to rotate freely, it is laterally (externally) rotated.

- **Effect of Leg Rotation on Proximal Femur Visualization:** To position the proximal femur in a true lateral position (90 degrees from the AP projection), demonstrating the lesser trochanter in profile posteriorly and superimposing the greater trochanter by the femoral shaft, the affected leg must be internally rotated until an imaginary line drawn between the femoral epicondyles is positioned parallel with the tabletop. The patient's foot is tilted internally 15 to 20 degrees from a vertical position (Fig. 6–15). If the affected leg is not rotated internally, the greater trochanter is demonstrated posteriorly and the lesser trochanter superimposes the femoral shaft (see Rad. 13). How much greater trochanter is demonstrated without femoral shaft superimposition depends on the degree of external rotation. Greater external rotation increases amount of greater trochanter visualized.

- **Positioning for Proximal Femoral Fracture or Dislocation:** When a patient has a dislocated hip or a suspected or known proximal femoral frac-

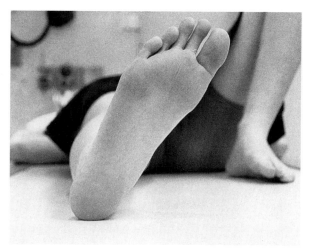

Figure 6-15. Proper foot position—15 to 20 degrees from vertical.

ture, the leg should not be internally rotated, but left "as is." Forced internal rotation of a dislocated hip or fractured proximal femur may injure the blood supply and nerves that surround the injured area. Because the patient's leg is not internally rotated in such cases, it is acceptable for the greater trochanter to be demonstrated posteriorly and the lesser trochanter to superimpose the femoral shaft (see Rad. 14).

The femoral neck is at the center of the collimated field. The acetabulum, femoral head and neck, greater and lesser trochanters, and ischial tuberosity are included within the field. Any orthopedic appliance should be included in its entirety.

- Center a perpendicular central ray to the femoral neck at a level halfway between the anterior and posterior aspects of the upper thigh to place the femoral neck in the center of the collimated field. Open longitudinal collimation the full length of the film. Transverse collimation should be to the proximal femoral skinline.

- An 8 × 10 inch (18 × 24 cm) or 10 × 12 inch (24 × 30 cm) film placed crosswise should be adequate to include all the required anatomical structures.

- **Film Placement Alternative:** The level at which the cassette is placed along the patient's lateral body surface determines whether the acetabulum and femoral head are included on the film. On patients with minimal lateral soft tissue thickness, the upper cassette edge should be firmly placed in the crease formed at the patient's waist, just superior to the iliac crest (Fig. 6–14). On patients with ample lateral soft tissue thickness, the film needs to be positioned superior to the iliac crest (Fig. 6–16). This superior positioning will result in magnification due to the increase in OID, but is necessary to include the acetabulum and femoral head on the axiolateral hip radiograph.

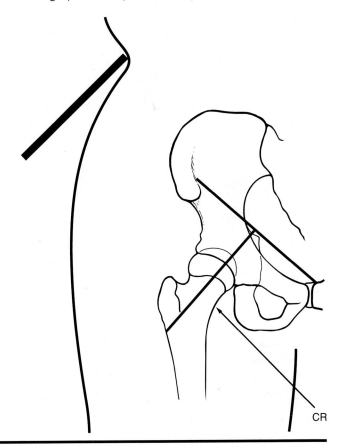

Figure 6-16. Proper cassette placement for large patients. *CR*, central ray.

CR

Critiquing Radiographs

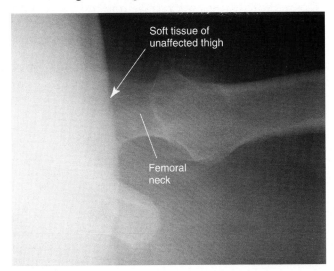

Soft tissue of unaffected thigh

Femoral neck

Radiograph 11.

Critique: Soft tissue from the unaffected thigh is superimposing the acetabulum and femoral head of the affected hip. The unaffected leg was not adequately flexed or abducted.

Correction: Flex and abduct the unaffected leg, drawing it away from the affected acetabulum and femoral head. If the patient is unable to further adjust the unaffected leg, the kVp and mAs can be increased to demonstrate this area. A wedge-type compensating filter may also be added to prevent overpenetration of the femoral neck and shaft.

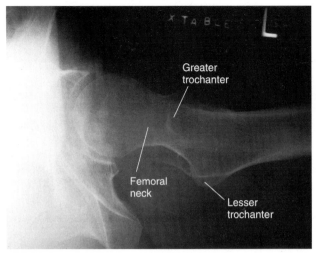

Radiograph 12.

Critique: The greater trochanter is demonstrated at a transverse level proximal to the lesser trochanter, and the femoral neck is partially foreshortened. The angle between the central ray and femur was too large.

Correction: Localize the femoral neck. Position the film parallel with the femoral neck and the central ray perpendicular to the film and femoral neck, as demonstrated in Figure 6–14.

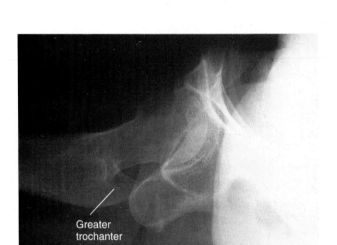

Radiograph 13.

Critique: The greater trochanter is demonstrated posteriorly, and the lesser trochanter superimposes the femoral shaft. The patient's affected leg was in external rotation.

Correction: Internally rotate the patient's leg, until the femoral epicondyles are aligned parallel with the tabletop and the foot is tilted internally 15 to 20 degrees from vertical, as demonstrated in Figure 6–15.

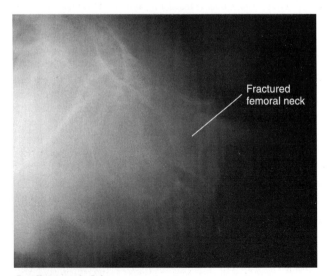

Radiograph 14.

Critique: There is a fracture of the femoral neck. The greater trochanter is demonstrated posteriorly, and the lesser trochanter superimposes the femoral shaft. The patient's leg was in external rotation.

Correction: Do not attempt to adjust the patient's leg position if a fracture of the proximal femur is suspected. No correction movement is needed.

PELVIS

Anteroposterior Projection

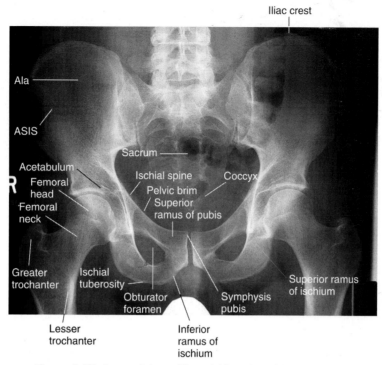

Figure 6-17. Accurately positioned AP male pelvis radiograph.

Radiographic Evaluation

Facility's patient identification requirements are visible on radiograph.
- These usually are facility name, patient name, age, and hospital number, and exam time and date.
- Patient ID plate does not obscure anatomy of interest.

A left or right marker, identifying the correct hip, is present on the radiograph and does not superimpose anatomy of interest.
- Place the marker laterally within the collimated light field so it does not superimpose any portion of the pelvis or proximal femurs.

There is no evidence of preventable artifacts, such as snaps, zippers, and objects left in the patient's pockets. Patient's hands are not demonstrated beneath the hips.
- Patients often are asked to change into a gown before the pelvis is radiographed, and their clothes are stored in a locker. Make certain that the locker key is not left in the patient's gown pocket.
- Drawing the patient's arms and hands away from the pelvis prevents hand visualization on a pelvis radiograph.

Contrast and density are adequate to demonstrate the surrounding soft tissue and bony structures of the pelvis and proximal femurs. Penetration is sufficient to visualize the bony trabecular patterns and the cortical outlines of the ischial spines, ilia, pubis, ischia, acetabula, and femoral heads and necks.

- An optimal 75 to 85 kVp technique sufficiently penetrates the bony and soft tissue structures of the pelvis and proximal femurs.
- Use a grid to absorb the scattered radiation produced by the pelvis and proximal femurs, reducing fog and providing a higher contrast radiograph.
- ***Soft Tissue Fat Planes on a Pelvis Radiograph:*** When evaluating a pelvis radiograph, the reviewer not only analyzes the bony structures but also studies the placement of the soft tissue fat planes. There are four bilateral fat planes of interest on an AP pelvis radiograph, and their visualization aids in the detection of intra-articular and periarticular disease: the obturator internus fat planes, which lie within the pelvic inlet, next to the medial brims; the iliopsoas fat planes, which lie medial to the lesser trochanters; the pericapsular fat planes, which are found superior to the femoral necks, and the gluteal fat planes, which lie superior to the pericapsular fat planes[1] (Fig. 6–18).

The bony trabecular patterns and the cortical outlines of the ilia, ischia, pubis, acetabula, and femoral heads and necks are sharply defined.
- Sharply defined recorded details are obtained when respiration is halted, patient motion is controlled, and a short object–image distance (OID) is maintained.

The pelvis demonstrates a true AP projection: The ischial spines are aligned with the pelvic brim, the sacrum and coccyx are aligned with the symphysis pu-

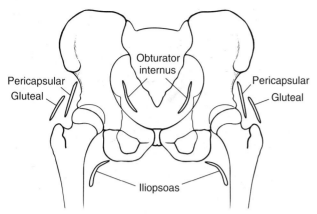

Figure 6-18. Location of fat planes.

bis, and the ilia and the obturator foramina are uniform in size and shape.

- A true AP projection of the pelvis is accomplished by placing the patient supine on the radiographic table with the legs extended and the arms drawn away from the pelvic area (Fig. 6–19). To ensure that the pelvis is not rotated, judge the distance from the anterior superior iliac spine (ASIS) to the tabletop on each side. The distances should be equal.

- ***Detecting Pelvic Rotation:*** Radiographically, a nonrotated pelvis demonstrates symmetrical ilia and obturator foramina. Rotation is initially detected by evaluating the relationships of the ischial spines with the pelvic brim and of the sacrum and coccyx with the symphysis pubis. The ischial spines should be aligned with the pelvic brim, and the sacrum and coccyx should be in alignment with the symphysis pubis on a nonrotated pelvis.

  If the pelvis is rotated into a left posterior oblique (LPO) position, the left ilium is wider than the right, the left obturator foramen is narrower than the right, the left ischial spine is demonstrated without pelvic brim superimposition, and the sacrum and coccyx are

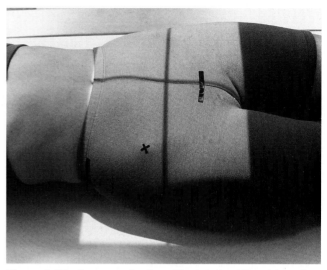

Figure 6-19. Proper patient positioning for AP pelvis radiograph.

not aligned with the symphysis pubis but are rotated toward the right hip (Rad. 15).

If the patient was rotated into a right posterior oblique (RPO) position, the opposite is true. The right ilium is wider than the left, the right obturator foramen is narrower than the left, the right ischial spine is demonstrated without pelvic brim superimposition, and the sacrum and coccyx are rotated toward the left hip.

- ***Male versus Female Pelvis:*** One should also be aware of the bony architectural differences that exist between the male and female pelvis. The differences are due to the need for the female pelvis to accommodate fetal growth during pregnancy and fetal passage during delivery. Figure 6–17 shows a male pelvis, and Figure 6–20 a female pelvis. Note that the male pelvis is larger and bulkier, the male obturator foramina and the acetabula are larger, and the male

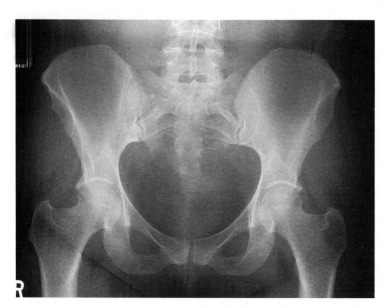

Figure 6-20. Accurately positioned AP female pelvis radiograph.

pelvic cavity is more heart shaped whereas the female cavity is oval.[3]

The femoral necks are demonstrated without foreshortening, and the greater trochanters are demonstrated in profile laterally, whereas the lesser trochanters are superimposed by the femoral necks.

- The relationship of the patient's feet and femoral epicondyles to the tabletop determines how the femoral necks and trochanters are visualized on an AP pelvis radiograph. Generally when patients are relaxed, their legs and feet are externally (laterally) rotated. Upon external rotation, the femoral necks incline posteriorly (toward the table) and are foreshortened on an AP pelvis radiograph. Greater external rotation increases the posterior incline and foreshortening of the femoral necks. If the patient's legs are externally (laterally) rotated enough to position the feet and femoral epicondyles at a 45-degree angle with the tabletop, the femoral necks are demonstrated on end and the lesser trochanters are demonstrated in profile (Fig. 6–21 and Rad. 16). If the patient's legs are in partial external rotation with the femoral epicondyles positioned at about a 30-degree angle with the tabletop, the lesser trochanters are demonstrated in profile, but the femoral necks are only partially foreshortened (see Rad. 17).

- ***Accurate Leg Positioning:*** To visualize the femoral necks without foreshortening and the greater trochanters in profile on an AP pelvis radiograph, the patient's legs should be internally rotated until the feet are tilted 15 to 20 degrees from vertical and the femoral epicondyles are positioned parallel with the tabletop (Figs. 6–17 and 6–22). Sandbags or tape may be needed to help maintain this internal leg rotation. A pelvic radiograph may not demonstrate the proximal femurs with exactly the same degree of internal rotation. How each proximal femur will appear depends on the degree of internal rotation placed on that leg.

- ***Positioning for Proximal Femoral Fracture:*** Often, when a fracture of a proximal femur is sus-

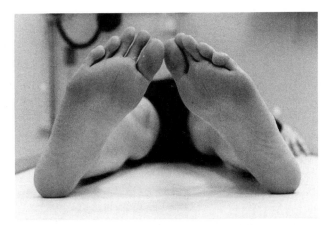

Figure 6-22. Proper internal foot positioning—15 to 20 degrees from vertical.

pected, a pelvic radiograph is ordered instead of a view demonstrating just the affected hip. This is because pelvic fractures are frequently associated with proximal femur fractures. If a patient has a suspected or fractured proximal femur, the leg should not be internally rotated, but should be left "as is." Forced internal rotation of a fractured proximal femur may injure the blood supply and nerves that surround the injured area. Because the patient's leg is not internally rotated when a fracture is in question, such a pelvic radiograph demonstrates the affected femoral neck with some degree of foreshortening and the lesser tuberosity without femoral shaft superimposition.

The inferior sacrum is at the center of the collimated field. The ilia, symphysis pubis, ischia, acetabula, femoral necks and heads, and greater and lesser trochanters are included within the field.

- Center a perpendicular central ray to the midsagittal plane at a level halfway between the symphysis pubis and an imaginary line connecting the ASIS, to place the inferior sacrum in the center of the collimated field. Open the longitudinal collimation the full 14-inch (35-cm) film length for most adult patients. Transverse collimation should be to the lateral skinline.

- A 14 × 17 inch (35 × 43 cm) film placed crosswise should be adequate to include all the required anatomical structures.

- ***Central Ray Centering for Evaluation of Hip Joint Mobility:*** When an AP pelvis radiograph is being taken specifically to evaluate hip joint mobility, the central ray should be centered to the midsagittal plane at a level 1 inch (2.5 cm) superior to the symphysis pubis. Such positioning centers the hip joints on the radiograph, but may result in clipping of the superior ilia.

- ***Gonadal Shielding:*** Use gonadal shielding on all male patients. Female patients should be shielded, although it is important that no pelvic anatomy is covered by the shield. Remember that a shield placed on top of the patient will greatly magnify.

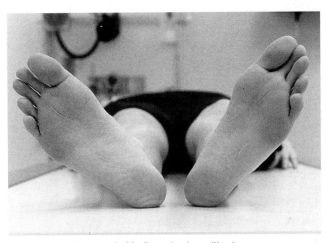

Figure 6-21. Poor foot positioning.

Critiquing Radiographs

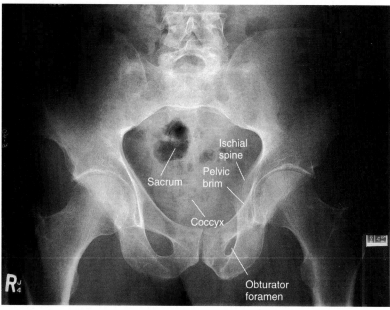

Radiograph 15.

Critique: The left obturator foramen is narrower than the right foramen, the left ischial spine is demonstrated without pelvic brim superimposition, and the sacrum and coccyx are rotated toward the right hip. The pelvis was rotated onto the left hip (LPO).

Correction: Rotate the patient toward the right hip until the anterior superior iliac spines are positioned at equal distances from the tabletop.

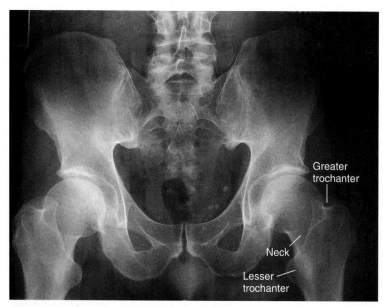

Radiograph 16.

Critique: The femoral necks are completely foreshortened, and the lesser trochanters are demonstrated in profile. The patient's legs were externally rotated, with the patient's feet and femoral epicondyles positioned at a 45-degree angle with the tabletop, as demonstrated in Figure 6–21.

Correction: Internally rotate the patient's legs until the feet are tilted 15 to 20 degrees from vertical and the femoral epicondyles are positioned parallel with the tabletop, as demonstrated in Figure 6–22.

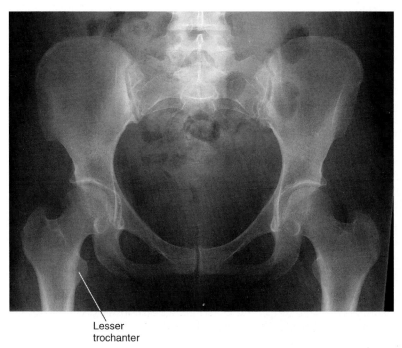

Radiograph 17.

Critique: The femoral necks are partially foreshortened, and the lesser trochanters are demonstrated in profile. The patient's legs were externally rotated, with the femoral epicondyles at about a 30-degree angle with the tabletop.
Correction: Internally rotate the patient's legs until the feet are tilted 15 to 20 degrees from vertical and the femoral epicondyles are positioned parallel with the tabletop, as demonstrated in Figure 6–22.

Lesser trochanter

Frogleg Position (AP Axial Position)

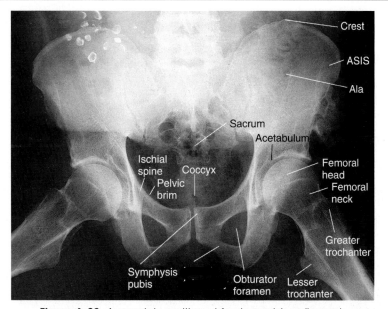

Figure 6–23. Accurately positioned frogleg pelvis radiograph.

Radiographic Evaluation

Facility's patient identification requirements are visible on radiograph.

- These requirements usually are facility name, patient name, age, and hospital number, and exam time and date.
- Patient ID plate does not obscure anatomy of interest.

A right or left marker, identifying the correct hip, is present on the radiograph and does not superimpose anatomy of interest.

- Place the marker laterally within the collimated light field so it does not superimpose any portion of the pelvis or proximal femur.

There is no evidence of removable artifacts, such as snaps, zippers, and objects left in patient's pockets.

- Patients often are asked to change into a gown before the pelvis is radiographed, and their clothes are stored in a locker. Make certain that the locker key is not left in the patient's gown pocket.
- Drawing the patient's arms and hands away from the pelvis prevents hand visualization on a pelvis radiograph.

Contrast and density are adequate to demonstrate the surrounding soft tissue and bony structures of the pelvis and proximal femurs. Penetration is sufficient to visualize the bony trabecular patterns and the cortical out-

lines of the ischial spines, ilia, pubis, ischia, acetabula, and femoral heads and necks.

- An optimal 75 to 85 kVp technique sufficiently penetrates the bony and soft tissue structures of the pelvis.
- Use a grid to absorb the scattered radiation produced by the pelvis, reducing fog and providing a higher-contrast radiograph.

The bony trabecular patterns and the cortical outlines of the ilia, ischia, pubis, acetabula, and femoral heads and necks are sharply defined.

- Sharply defined recorded details are obtained when respiration is halted, patient motion is controlled, and a short object–image distance (OID) is maintained.

The pelvis demonstrates a true AP projection: The ischial spines are aligned with the pelvic brim, the sacrum and coccyx are aligned with the symphysis pubis, and the ilia and the obturator foramina are uniform in size and shape.

- A true AP projection of the pelvis is accomplished by placing the patient on the radiographic table with the legs flexed and abducted (Fig. 6–24). To ensure that the pelvis is not rotated, judge the distance from the anterior superior iliac spine (ASIS) to the tabletop on each side. The distances should be equal.
- ***Detecting Pelvic Rotation:*** Radiographically a non-rotated pelvis will demonstrate symmetrical ilia and obturator foramina. Rotation can be detected by evaluating the relationships of the ischial spines with the pelvic brim and of the sacrum and coccyx with the symphysis pubis. The ischial spines should be aligned with the pelvic brim, and the sacrum and coccyx should align with the symphysis pubis on a nonrotated pelvis. If the pelvis is rotated into a left posterior oblique (LPO) position, the left ilium is wider than the right, the left obturator foramen is narrower than the right, the left ischial spine is demonstrated without pelvic brim superimposition, and the sacrum and coccyx are not aligned with the symphysis pubis, but are rotated toward the right hip (see Rad.

18). If the patient is rotated into a right posterior oblique (RPO) position, the opposite is true. The right ilium is wider than the left, the right obturator foramen is narrower closed than the left, the right ischial spine is demonstrated without pelvic brim superimposition, and the sacrum and coccyx are rotated toward the left hip.

The lesser trochanters are demonstrated in profile medially, and the femoral necks superimpose the adjacent greater trochanters.

- For a frogleg pelvis radiograph, the relationship of the greater and the lesser trochanters with the proximal femurs is determined when the patient flexes the knees and hips.
- ***Effect of Distal Femur Elevation on Proximal Femur Visualization:*** Use a femoral skeletal bone to better understand how the relationship of the greater and lesser trochanters with the proximal femur changes as the distal femur is elevated upon knee flexion. Begin by placing the femoral bone on a flat surface in an AP projection. While slowly elevating the distal femur, observe how the greater trochanter rotates around the proximal femur. First, the greater trochanter moves beneath the proximal femur; then, as elevation of the distal femur continues, it moves from beneath the proximal femur and is demonstrated on the medial side of the femur.
- ***Femur Positioning for Frogleg Radiograph:*** To accurately position the greater trochanters beneath the proximal femurs for a frogleg pelvic radiograph, flex the patient's knees until the femurs are placed at about a 60- to 70-degree angle with the tabletop (20 to 30 degrees from vertical) (Fig. 6–25). If the knees are not flexed enough to place the femurs at this angle with the tabletop, the greater trochanters are demonstrated laterally, as they would on an AP projection (see Rad. 7, page 297). If the knees are flexed too much, placing the femurs at an angle greater than 70 degrees with the tabletop, the greater trochanters are demonstrated medially (see Rad. 8, page 297).

The femoral necks are partially foreshortened, and the greater trochanters are demonstrated at a transverse

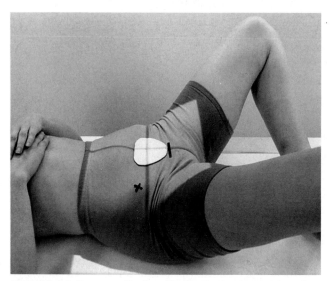

Figure 6-24. Proper patient positioning for frogleg pelvis radiograph.

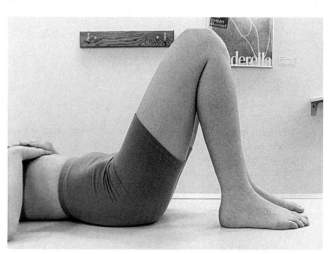

Figure 6-25. Proper knee and hip flexion—60 to 70 degrees from tabletop.

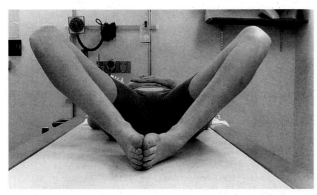

Figure 6-26. Proper femoral abduction—45 degrees from tabletop.

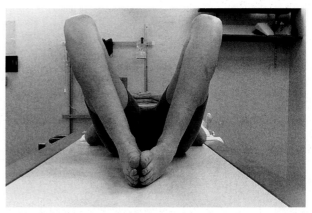

Figure 6-27. Femurs in only slight abduction—20 degrees from vertical.

level halfway between the femoral heads and lesser trochanters.

- The degree of femoral abduction determines the amount of femoral neck foreshortening and the transverse level at which the greater trochanters are demonstrated between the femoral heads and lesser trochanters.
- ***Effect of Leg Abduction:*** Use a femoral skeleton bone to understand how leg abduction determines the visualization of the femoral neck and the position of the greater trochanter. Place the femoral bone on a flat surface in an AP projection, with the distal femur elevated until the greater trochanter is positioned beneath the proximal femur and the lesser trochanter is in profile (60- to 70-degree angle with flat surface or 20 to 30 degrees from vertical). From this position, move the lateral surface of the femoral bone toward the flat surface, as if the femur was being abducted on a patient. As the bone moves toward the flat surface, observe how the femoral neck is positioned more on end and the greater trochanter moves proximally (toward the femoral head).

  To demonstrate the femoral necks and proximal femora with only partial foreshortening, the femoral shafts should be abducted to a 45-degree angle with the tabletop (Figs. 6–23 and 6–26). To demonstrate the femoral necks without foreshortening, abduct the femoral shafts to a 70-degree angle with the tabletop (20 degrees from vertical) (see Rad. 19 and Fig. 6–27). To demonstrate the proximal femoral shafts without foreshortening, abduct the femoral shafts close to the tabletop (see Rad. 20 and Fig. 6–28). This position places the femoral necks "on-end."
- ***Importance of Symmetrical Femoral Abduction:*** A frogleg pelvic radiograph may not demonstrate the proximal femurs with exactly the same degree of femoral abduction. How each proximal femur appears depends on the degree of femoral abduction placed on that leg. As a standard, unless the radiograph is ordered to evaluate hip mobility, both femurs should be abducted equally for the radiograph. This symmetrical abduction helps prevent pelvic rotation. It may be necessary to position an angled sponge beneath the patient's femurs to maintain the desired femoral abduction.

The inferior sacrum is at the center of the collimated field. The ilia, symphysis pubis, ischia, acetabula, femoral necks and heads, and greater and lesser trochanters are included within the field.

- Center a perpendicular central ray to the midsagittal plane at a level halfway between the symphysis pubis and an imaginary line connecting the anterior superior iliac spines to place the inferior sacrum in the center of the collimated field. Open the longitudinal collimation the full 14-inch (35-cm) length for most adult patients. Transverse collimation should be to the lateral skin-line.
- A 14 × 17 inch (35 × 43 cm) film placed crosswise should be adequate to include all the required anatomical structures.
- ***Central Ray Centering for Evaluation of Hip Joint Mobility:*** When the a frogleg pelvis radiograph is being taken to evaluate hip joint mobility, the central ray should be centered to the midsagittal plane at a level 1 inch (2.5 cm) superior to the symphysis pubis. Such positioning centers the hip joints on the radiograph but may result in clipping of the superior ilia.
- ***Gonadal Shielding:*** Use gonadal shielding on all male patients. Female patients should be shielded, although it is important that no pelvic anatomy is covered by the shield. Remember that the shield placed on top of the patient will greatly magnify.

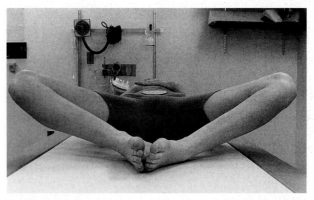

Figure 6-28. Femurs in maximum abduction—20 degrees from tabletop.

Critiquing Radiographs

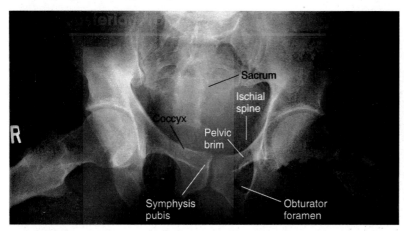

Radiograph 18.

Critique: The left obturator foramen is narrower than the right foramen, the left ischial spine is demonstrated without pelvic brim superimposition, and the sacrum and coccyx are rotated toward the right hip. The patient was rotated onto the left hip (LPO).

Correction: Rotate the patient toward the right hip until the anterior superior iliac spines are positioned at equal distances from the tabletop.

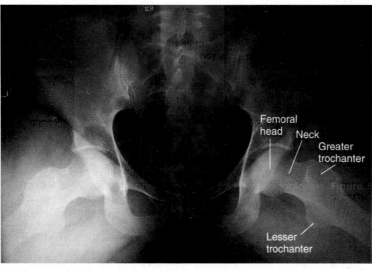

Radiograph 19.

Critique: The femoral necks are demonstrated without foreshortening, and the greater and lesser trochanters are demonstrated at about the same transverse level. The patient's femurs were in only slight abduction, at about a 70-degree angle with the tabletop (20 degrees from vertical), as demonstrated in Figure 6–27.

Correction: Consult with reviewers in your facility to determine whether this is an acceptable radiograph. If the proximal femoral shafts demonstrate too much foreshortening, have the patient abduct the femurs to a 45-degree angle with the tabletop.

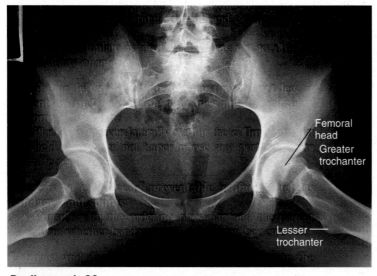

Radiograph 20.

Critique: The femoral necks are demonstrated "on end." The greater trochanters are demonstrated on the same transverse level as the femoral heads. The patient's femurs were positioned next to the tabletop, as demonstrated in Figure 6–28.

Correction: Consult with reviewers in your facility to determine whether this is an acceptable radiograph. Because the femoral necks cannot be evaluated because of foreshortening, it may be necessary to have the patient position the femurs at a 45-degree angle with the tabletop.

SACROILIAC JOINTS

Anteroposterior Projection

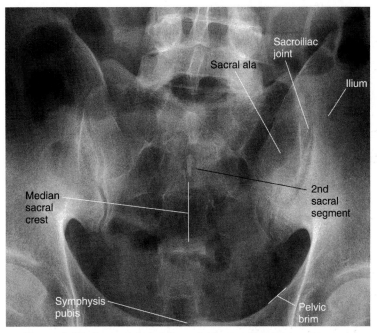

Figure 6-29. Accurately positioned AP sacroiliac joint radiograph.

Radiographic Evaluation

Facility's patient identification requirements are visible on radiograph.

- These requirements usually are facility name, patient name, age, and hospital number, and exam time and date.
- Patient ID plate is positioned toward the feet so it does not obscure anatomy of interest.

A right or left marker, identifying the correct side of the patient, is present on the radiograph and does not superimpose anatomy of interest.

- Place the marker laterally within the collimated light field so it does not superimpose any portion of the sacroiliac joints.
- Because the transversely collimated field is coned to about a 9-inch (22-cm) area, make certain that the marker is positioned within 4.5 inches (11 cm) of the center of the film to guarantee that it will not be collimated off.

There is no evidence of removable artifacts, such as buttons and zippers.

- It is recommended that the patient be instructed to change into a hospital gown before the procedure.

Contrast and density are adequate to demonstrate the bony structures of the sacroiliac joints. Penetration is sufficient to visualize the bony trabecular patterns and cortical outlines of the sacroiliac joints and the first through third sacral segments.

- An optimal 75 to 85 kVp technique sufficiently penetrates the bony structures of the sacrum.
- To obtain a high-contrast radiograph and increase the visibility of recorded details, use tight collimation to reduce the amount of scattered radiation produced, and a high-ratio grid to absorb scattered radiation before it reaches the film.

The bony trabecular patterns and the cortical outlines of the sacroiliac joints are sharply defined.

- Sharply defined recorded details are obtained when patient motion is controlled, respiration is halted, and a short object–image distance (OID) is maintained.
- Using a small focal spot also improves the sharpness of the recorded details but may result in motion on radiographs of larger patients because of the long exposure time that would be required.

The sacroiliac joints are demonstrated in a true AP projection: The median sacral crest is aligned with the symphysis pubis, and the sacrum is at equal distance from the lateral wall of the pelvic brim on either side.

- An AP projection of the sacroiliac joints is obtained by positioning the patient supine on the radiographic table with the legs extended. Position the patient's shoulders and anterior superior iliac spines at equal distances from the tabletop to prevent rotation (Fig. 6–30).
- **Detecting Sacroiliac Joint Rotation:** Rotation is detected on an AP sacroiliac joint radiograph by evaluating the alignment of the long axis of the

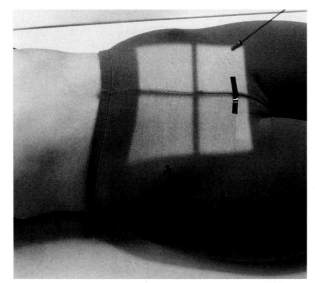

Figure 6-30. Proper patient positioning for AP sacroiliac joint radiograph.

median sacral crest with the symphysis pubis and the distance from the sacrum to the lateral pelvic brim. When the patient is rotated away from the AP projection, the sacrum moves in a direction opposite from the movement of the symphysis pubis and is positioned next to the lateral pelvic brim situated farther from the tabletop. If the patient is rotated into a left posterior oblique (LPO) position, the sacrum is rotated toward the patient's right pelvic brim. If the patient is rotated into a right posterior oblique (RPO) position, the sacrum rotates toward the patient's left pelvic brim.

The sacroiliac joints are visualized without foreshortening, and the sacrum is elongated, with the symphysis pubis superimposing the inferior sacral segments.

- When the patient is positioned supine with the legs extended, the lumbosacral curve causes the proximal sacrum and sacroiliac joints to be angled 25 to 30 degrees with the tabletop and film. To demonstrate the sacroiliac joints without foreshortening, a 25 to 30 degree cephalic central ray angulation needs to be used. The smaller angulation should be used on patients who have less lumbosacral curvature, whereas those with greater curvature require the larger angulation. If an AP sacroiliac joint radiograph is taken with a perpendicular central ray or without enough cephalad angulation, the sacroiliac joints and the first through third sacral segments are foreshortened (see Rad. 21).

The long axis of the median sacral crest is aligned with the long axis of the collimated field.

- Aligning the long axis of the median sacral crest with the long axis of the collimated field allows for tight

collimation and ensures that the central ray is angled directly into the sacroiliac joints. To obtain proper alignment, find the point halfway between the patient's palpable anterior superior iliac spines (ASISs); then align this point and the palpable symphysis pubis with the center of the collimator's longitudinal light line.

The second sacral segment is at the center of the collimated field. The sacroiliac joints and the first through fourth sacral segments are included within the field.

- Center the central ray to the patient's midsagittal plane at a level halfway between an imaginary line connecting the ASISs and the symphysis pubis. Open the longitudinally collimated field to the symphysis pubis. Transversely collimate to about a 9-inch (22-cm) field size.
- A 10 × 12 inch (24 × 30 cm) film placed lengthwise should be adequate to include all the required anatomical structures.
- **Gonadal Shielding:** Use gonadal shielding on all male patients. Female patients cannot be shielded, or sacral information will be obscured.

Critiquing Radiograph

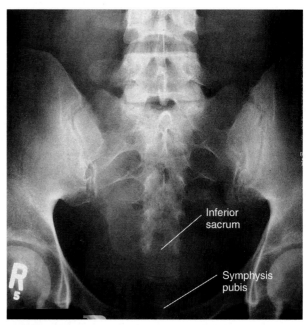

Inferior sacrum

Symphysis pubis

Radiograph 21.

Critique: The sacroiliac joints are foreshortened, and the inferior sacrum is demonstrated without symphysis pubis superimposition. The central ray was inadequately angled.
Correction: Angle the central ray 25 to 30 degrees cephalad.

Sacroiliac Joints: Posterior Oblique Position

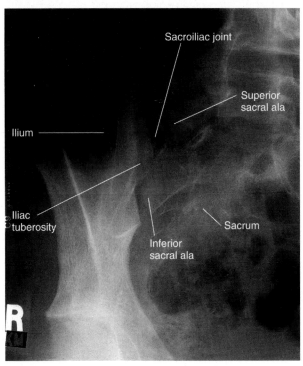

Figure 6-31. Accurately positioned oblique sacroiliac joint radiograph.

Radiographic Evaluation

Facility's patient identification requirements are visible on radiograph.

- These requirements usually are facility name, patient name, age, and hospital number, and exam time and date.
- Patient ID plate does not obscure anatomy of interest.

A right or left marker, identifying the correct side of the patient, is present on the radiograph and does not superimpose anatomy of interest.

- Place the marker laterally within the collimated light field so it does not superimpose any portion of the sacroiliac joints.
- Because the sacroiliac joint of interest is situated farther from the film when posterior oblique radiographs are taken, the marker used should identify the sacroiliac joint situated farther from the film. This is different from the way most oblique radiographs are marked; routinely, the side marked is the one positioned closer to the film.

There is no evidence of removable artifacts such as buttons and zippers.

- It is recommended that the patient be instructed to change into a hospital gown before the procedure.

Contrast and density are adequate to demonstrate the bony structures of the sacrum and ilium, which articulate to form the sacroiliac joints. Penetration is suffi- cient to visualize the bony trabecular patterns and the cortical outlines of the sacroiliac joints, ilium, and first through third sacral segments.

- An optimal 70 to 80 kVp technique sufficiently penetrates the articulating surfaces of the sacrum and the ilium.
- Tight collimation and a high-ratio grid should be used to reduce the amount of scattered radiation that reaches the film, providing higher contrast and better visibility of recorded details.

The bony trabecular patterns and the cortical outlines of the sacroiliac joints are sharply defined.

- Sharply defined recorded details are obtained when patient motion is controlled, respiration is halted, and a short object–image distance (OID) is maintained.
- Using a small focal spot also improves sharpness of the recorded details but may result in motion on larger patients because of the long exposure time that would be required.
- ***Advantage of Posterior Oblique Position:*** Precise positioning and centering for the oblique sacroiliac joint is best accomplished when the patient is placed in a posterior oblique position, even though an anterior oblique position would place the joint of interest closest to the film, resulting in less magnification.

The ilium and sacrum are demonstrated without superimposition, and the sacroiliac joint is open.

- An oblique sacroiliac joint radiograph is obtained by beginning with the patient positioned supine on the radiographic table with the legs extended. From this position, rotate the patient toward the unaffected side until the midcoronal plane is at a 25 to 30 degree angle with the tabletop and film. The sacral ala and ilium are positioned in profile. Place a radiolucent angled sponge beneath the patient's elevated hip and thorax to help maintain the position (Fig. 6–32). Both posterior oblique positions (RPO and LPO) must be taken to demonstrate the right and left sacroiliac joints. When posterior oblique radiographs are performed, the elevated sacroiliac joint is the joint of interest.
- ***Determining Accuracy of Obliquity:*** The accuracy of an oblique sacroiliac joint can be determined by the lack of ilium and sacral superimposition. The

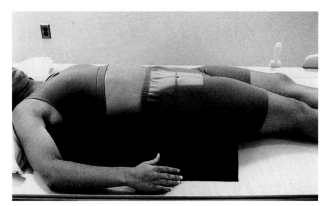

Figure 6-32. Proper patient positioning for oblique sacroiliac joint radiograph.

degree of separation or cavity demonstrated between the ilium and sacrum, which represents the sacroiliac joint, varies from patient to patient. The ilia and sacrum fit very snugly together, and in older patients, the joint spaces between them may be reduced in size or even nonexistent because of fibrous adhesions or synostosis.[4] If the patient was not rotated enough to place the ilium and sacral ala in profile, the inferior and superior sacral ala are demonstrated without ilium superimposition, whereas the lateral sacral ala superimposes the iliac tuberosity (see Rad. 22). The lateral sacrum is also demonstrated without ilium superimposition. If the patient was rotated more than needed to position the ilium and sacral ala in profile, the ilium superimposes the lateral sacral ala and the inferior sacrum (see Rad. 23).

The long axis of the sacroiliac joint is aligned with the long axis of the collimated field.
- Aligning the long axis of the sacroiliac joint with the long axis of the collimated field allows for tight collimation without clipping any portion of the joint. To obtain proper alignment, align the collimator's longitudinal light line parallel with the elevated anterior superior iliac spine (ASIS).

The sacroiliac joint of interest is at the center of the collimated field. The sacroiliac joint, sacral ala, and ilium are included within the field.
- Center the central ray 1 to 1.5 inches (2.5 to 4 cm) medial to the elevated ASIS to position the sacroiliac joint of interest in the center of the collimated field.
- Open the longitudinal collimation to the elevated iliac crest. Transverse collimation should be to the elevated ASIS.
- An 8 × 10 inch (18 × 24 cm) film placed lengthwise should be adequate to include all the required anatomical structures.
- ***Gonadal Shielding:*** Use gonadal shielding on all male patients. Female patients cannot be shielded, or sacral information will be obscured.

Critiquing Radiographs

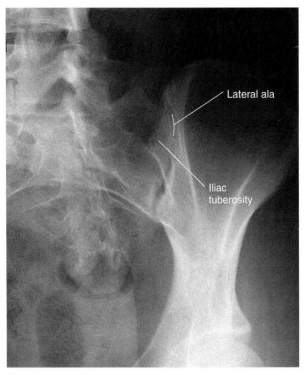

Radiograph 22.

Critique: The sacroiliac joint is closed. The superior and inferior sacral alae are demonstrated without iliac superimposition, and the lateral sacral ala superimposes the iliac tuberosity. The patient was not rotated enough.
Correction: Increase the pelvic obliquity. Because both the sacral ala and the ilium move simultaneously, the adjustment made should be only half the amount of superimposition of the sacral ala and iliac tuberosity.

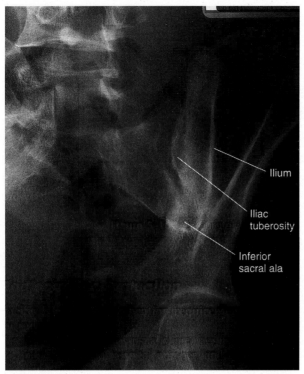

Ilium

Iliac
tuberosity

Inferior
sacral ala

Radiograph 23.

Critique: The sacroiliac joint is closed. The ilium superimposes the inferior sacral ala and the lateral sacrum. Pelvic obliquity was excessive.

Correction: Decrease the pelvic obliquity. Because both the sacral ala and ilium move simultaneously, the amount of adjustment made should be only half of the amount of ilium and sacral superimposition.

References

1. Berquist TH. Imaging of Orthopedic Trauma Surgery. Philadelphia: W. B. Saunders, 1986, pp 181–200.
2. Ballinger PW. Merrill's Atlas of Radiographic Positions and Radiologic Procedures, ed 7. St Louis: Mosby Year Book, 1991, pp 260–261.
3. Draves DJ. Anatomy of the Lower Extremity. Baltimore: Williams & Wilkins, 1986, pp 33–47.
4. Clemente CD. Gray's Anatomy, ed 30. Philadelphia: Lea & Febiger, 1984, pp 360–361.

CHAPTER 7

Radiographic Critique of the Cervical and Thoracic Vertebrae

CERVICAL VERTEBRAE

Anteroposterior Projection

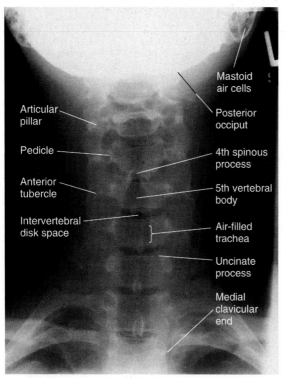

Figure 7-1. Accurately positioned AP cervical vertebral radiograph.

Articular pillar

Pedicle

Anterior tubercle

Intervertebral disk space

Mastoid air cells

Posterior occiput

4th spinous process

5th vertebral body

Air-filled trachea

Uncinate process

Medial clavicular end

Radiographic Evaluation

Facility's patient identification requirements are visible on radiograph.

- These requirements usually are facility name, patient name, age, and hospital number, and exam time and date.
- Patient ID plate is positioned caudally so as not to obscure anatomy of interest.

A right or left marker, identifying the correct side of the patient, is present on the radiograph and does not superimpose anatomy of interest.

- Place the marker laterally within the collimated light field so it does not superimpose any portion of the cervical vertebrae or its surrounding soft tissue.
- Because the transversely collimated field can be coned to about a 6-inch (15-cm) area, make certain the marker is positioned within 3 inches (7.5 cm) of the film's center to guarantee that it is not cut off.

There is no evidence of preventable artifacts, such as snaps, zippers, and jewelry.

- Evaluate the patient's neck for any radiopaque objects that may obstruct visualization of the cervical vertebrae. It may be necessary to have a patient with a high buttoned collar change into a snapless hospital gown.

Contrast and density are adequate to demonstrate the surrounding soft tissue, air-filled trachea, and bony structures of the cervical vertebrae. Penetration is sufficient to visualize the bony trabecular patterns and cortical outlines of the vertebral bodies, uncinate processes, spinous processes, and anterior tubercles.

- An optimal 75 to 80 kVp technique sufficiently penetrates the bony and soft tissue structures of the cervical vertebrae.
- Use a grid to absorb the scattered radiation produced by the cervical vertebrae, reducing fog and providing a higher-contrast radiograph.

The bony trabecular patterns and cortical outlines of the cervical vertebrae are sharply defined.

- Sharply defined recorded details are obtained when patient motion is controlled, respiration is halted, and a short object–image distance (OID) is maintained.

The cervical vertebrae demonstrate a true AP projection: The spinous processes are aligned with the midline of the cervical bodies, the mandibular angles and mastoid tips are at equal distances from the cervical vertebrae, the articular pillars and pedicles are symmetrically visualized lateral to the cervical bodies, and the distances from the vertebral column to the medial (sternal) ends of the clavicles are equal.

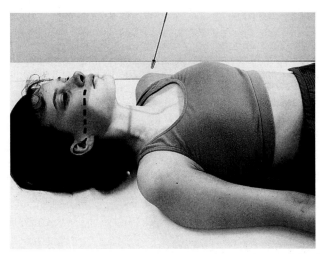

Figure 7-2. Proper patient positioning for AP cervical vertebral radiograph.

- An AP projection of the cervical vertebrae is obtained by placing the patient in a supine or upright AP projection, with the shoulders positioned at equal distances from the tabletop or upright grid holder (Fig. 7–2). The patient's face should be positioned so it is forward, placing the mandibular angles and mastoid tips at equal distances from the tabletop or upright grid holder.
- *Effect of Cervical Rotation:* When the patient and cervical vertebrae are rotated away from the AP projection, the vertebral bodies move toward the side positioned closer to the film, and the spinous processes move toward the side positioned farther from the film. The upper (C1–C4) and lower (C5–C7) cervical vertebrae can demonstrate rotation independently or simultaneously, depending on which part of the body is rotated. If the head is rotated but the thorax remains in an AP projection, the upper cervical vertebrae demonstrate rotation and the lower cervical vertebrae remain in an AP projection. If the thorax is rotated but the head remains in an AP projection, the lower cervical vertebrae demonstrate rotation and the upper cervical vertebrae remain in an AP projection. If the patient's head and thorax are rotated simultaneously the entire cervical column demonstrates rotation (see Rad. 1).
- *Detecting Rotation:* Radiographically, rotation is present if (1) the mandibular angles and mastoid tips are not demonstrated at equal distances from the cervical vertebrae, (2) the spinous processes are not demonstrated in the midline of the cervical bodies, (3) the pedicles and articular pillars are not symmetrically demonstrated lateral to the vertebral bodies, and (4) the medial ends of the clavicles are not demonstrated at equal distances from the vertebral column. The side of the patient positioned closer to the tabletop or upright grid holder is the side the mandible is rotated toward and also the side that visualizes less of articular pillars and less clavicular and vertebral column superimposition.
- *Positioning for Trauma:* When cervical vertebral radiographs are taken on a trauma patient in whom

subluxation or fracture is suspected, take the AP projection with the patient positioned as is. *Do not attempt to remove the cervical collar or adjust the head or body rotation, mandible position, or cervical column tilting. To do so might result in greater injury to the vertebrae or spinal cord.* Five to ten percent of spinal cord injuries occur from the mishandling of the patient after injury has taken place.[1]

The intervertebral disk spaces are open, the vertebral bodies are demonstrated without distortion, and each vertebra's spinous process is visualized at the level of its inferior intervertebral disk space.

- The cervical vertebral column demonstrates a lordotic curvature. This curvature and the shape of the vertebral bodies cause the disk articulating surfaces of the vertebral bodies to slant upward anteriorly to posteriorly.
- *Importance of Central Ray Angulation:* To obtain open intervertebral disk spaces and undistorted vertebral bodies, the central ray must be angled in the same direction as the slope of the vertebral bodies. This can be easily discerned by viewing the lateral cervical radiograph in Figure 7–3. Studying this lateral cervical radiograph, you can see that when the correct central ray angulation is used, each vertebra's spinous process is located within its inferior intervertebral disk space. The degree of central ray angulation needed to obtain open intervertebral disk spaces and to accurately align the spinous processes within them depends on the degree of cervical lordotic curvature.

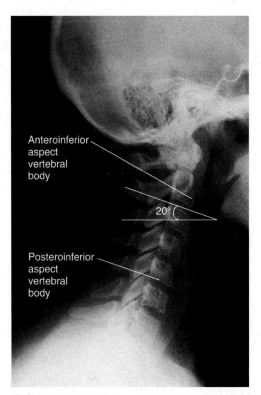

Figure 7-3. Lateral cervical vertebral radiograph taken with patient upright.

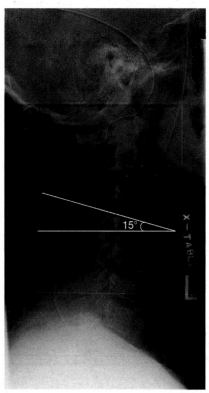

Figure 7-4. Lateral cervical vertebral radiograph taken with patient supine.

If the AP cervical vertebrae exam is taken with the patient in an upright position, the cervical vertebrae demonstrate more lordotic curvature than if the exam is taken with the patient supine. In a supine position, the gravitational pull placed on the middle cervical vertebrae results in straightening of the cervical curvature. Figure 7–3 demonstrates a lateral cervical radiograph taken on a patient in an upright position, and Figure 7–4 demonstrates a lateral cervical radiograph taken on a supine patient. Notice the difference in lordotic curvature between these two radiographs. Because of this difference, the central ray angulation should be varied when an AP cervical vertebral radiograph is taken erect rather than supine. In the erect position, a 20-degree cephalad central ray angulation is needed to align the central ray parallel with the intervertebral disk spaces. In a supine position, a 15-degree cephalad central ray angulation sufficiently aligns the central ray parallel with the intervertebral disk spaces.

- **Effect of Central Ray Misalignment:** Misalignment of the central ray and the intervertebral disk spaces results in closed disk spaces, distorted vertebral bodies, and the projection of the spinous processes into the vertebral bodies. If the central ray angulation is not used or is insufficient, the resulting radiograph demonstrates closed intervertebral disk spaces, and each vertebra's spinous process is demonstrated within its vertebral body (see Rad. 7–2). This anatomical relationship also results if the patient's head is tilted toward the x-ray tube for the exam, causing the cervical vertebrae to tilt anteriorly. If the central ray is angled more than needed to align the central ray parallel with the intervertebral disk spaces, or if the patient's cervical vertebral column was extended posteriorly for the exam, the resulting radiograph demonstrates closed intervertebral disk spaces, each vertebra's spinous process is demonstrated within the inferior adjoining vertebral body, and the uncinate processes are elongated (see Rad. 7–3).

The third cervical vertebra is demonstrated in its entirety, and the posterior occiput and mandibular mentum are superimposed.

- Accurate positioning of the occiput and mandibular mentum is achieved when an imaginary line connecting the upper occlusal plane (chewing surface of maxillary teeth) and the posterior occiput's inferior edge is aligned perpendicular to the tabletop or upright grid holder. This positioning also aligns the acanthiomeatal line (an imaginary line connecting the point where upper lip and nose meet with the external ear opening) perpendicular to the tabletop or upright grid holder. In this position, you might expect the patient's mandible to superimpose the upper cervical vertebrae, but it will not do so because the cephalad central ray angulation used will project the mandible superiorly.
- **Effect of Occiput-Mentum Mispositioning:** Mispositioning of the posterior occiput and the upper occlusal plane results in an obstructed view of the upper cervical vertebrae. If the occlusal plane is positioned superior to the posterior occiput's inferior edge, the upper cervical vertebrae superimpose the occiput (see Rad. 4). If the upper occlusal plane is positioned inferior to the posterior occiput's inferior edge, the mandibular mentum superimposes the superior cervical vertebrae (see Rad. 5).

The long axis of the cervical column is aligned with the long axis of the collimated field.

- Aligning the long axis of the cervical column with the long axis of the collimated field ensures that there is no lateral flexion of the cervical column and allows for tight collimation. This alignment is obtained by aligning the midline of the patient's neck with the collimator's longitudinal light line. When the patient's head and upper cervical vertebrae are allowed to lean to one side, lateral flexion results (see Rad. 6).

The fifth cervical vertebra is centered within the collimated field. The third through seventh cervical vertebrae, the first thoracic vertebra, and the surrounding soft tissue are included within the field.

- Center the central ray to the patient's midsagittal plane at a level halfway between the external auditory meatus (EAM) and the jugular notch to place the fifth cervical vertebra in the center of the collimated field.
- Open the longitudinal collimation to the EAM and the jugular notch. Transverse collimation should be to the lateral neck skin-line.
- An 8 × 10 inch (18 × 24 cm) film placed lengthwise should be adequate to include all the required anatomical structures.

Critiquing Radiographs

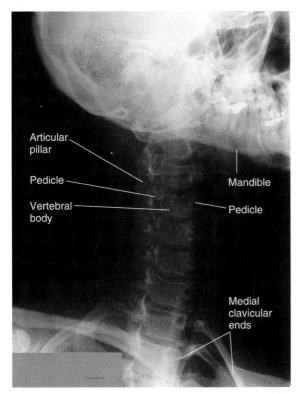

Radiograph 1.

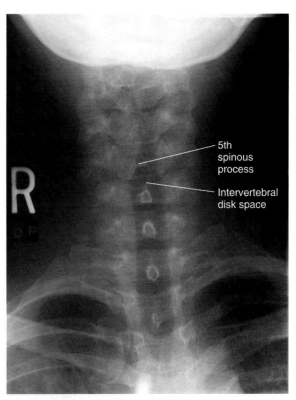

Radiograph 2.

Critique: The spinous processes are not demonstrated within the midline of the cervical bodies, and the pedicles and articular pillars are not symmetrically demonstrated lateral to the vertebral bodies. The mandible is rotated toward the patient's left side and the medial end of the left clavicle demonstrates no vertebral column superimposition. The patient was rotated onto the left side (LPO).

Correction: Rotate the patient toward the right side until the shoulders are at equal distances from the tabletop or upright grid holder, and turn the head toward the right side until the mandibular angles and mastoid tips are at equal distances from the tabletop or upright grid holder.

Critique: The anteroinferior aspects of the cervical bodies (see Fig. 7–3 for identification) are obscuring the intervertebral disk spaces, and each vertebra's spinous process is demonstrated within its vertebral body. The central ray angulation either was not used or was insufficient to align the central ray parallel with the intervertebral disk spaces.

Correction: Angle the central ray more cephalically.

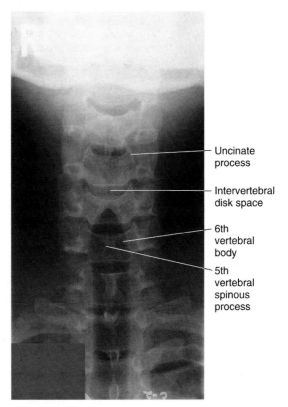

Radiograph 3.

Critique: The posteroinferior aspects of the cervical bodies (see Fig. 7–3 for identification) are obscuring the intervertebral disk spaces, the uncinate processes are elongated, and each vertebra's spinous process is demonstrated within the inferior adjoining vertebral body. The central ray was angled too cephalically to align the central ray parallel with the intervertebral disk spaces.

Correction: Decrease the amount of cephalic central ray angulation.

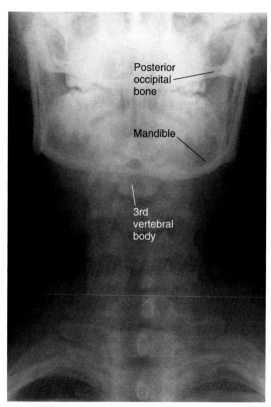

Radiograph 5.

Critique: The mandible superimposes a portion of the third cervical vertebra. The upper occlusal plane was positioned inferior to the base of the occiput.

Correction: Raise the chin half the distance demonstrated between the base of the skull and the mandibular mentum, or until an imaginary line connecting the upper occlusal plane and the inferior base of the posterior occiput is aligned perpendicular to the tabletop or upright grid holder.

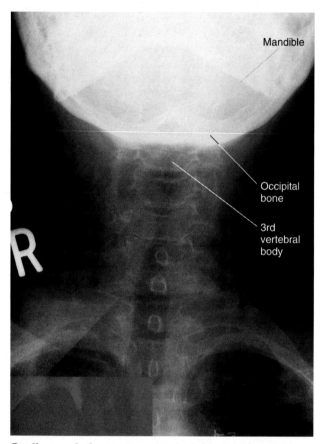

Radiograph 4.

Critique: A portion of the third cervical vertebra superimposes the posterior occipital bone, preventing a clear visualization of the third cervical vertebra. The upper occlusal plane was positioned superior to the posterior occiput's inferior edge.

Correction: Tuck the chin half the distance demonstrated between the base of the skull and the mandibular mentum, or until an imaginary line connecting the upper occlusal plane and the posterior occiput's inferior edge is aligned perpendicular to the tabletop or upright grid holder. For this patient, the movement should be about 1 inch (2.5 cm).

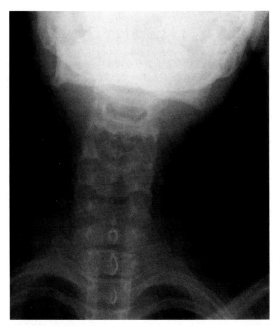

Radiograph 6.

Critique: The head is tilted toward the left side, causing the upper cervical vertebrae to flex laterally. The long axis of the cervical vertebral column was not aligned with the long axis of the collimated field.

Correction: Tilt the head toward the right side, until the midline of the patient's upper and lower neck is aligned with the collimator's longitudinal light line.

Cervical Vertebrae: Anteroposterior Projection, Atlas (C1) and Axis (C2) Open-Mouth Position

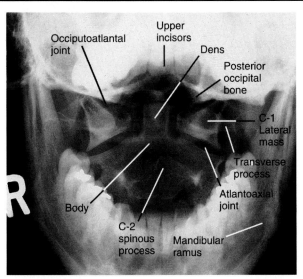

Figure 7–5. Accurately positioned AP atlas and axis radiograph.

Radiographic Evaluation

Facility's patient identification requirements are visible on radiograph.

- These requirements usually are facility name, patient name, age, and hospital number, and exam time and date.
- Patient ID plate is positioned so as not to obscure anatomy of interest.

A right or left marker, identifying the correct side of the patient, is present on the radiograph and does not superimpose anatomy of interest.

- Place the marker laterally within the collimated light field so it does not superimpose any portion of the atlas or axis.
- Because the transversely collimated field can be coned to about a 5-inch (12.5-cm) area, make certain that the marker is positioned within 2.5 inches (6.25 cm) of the film's center to guarantee that it will not be cut off.

There is no evidence of preventable artifacts, such as hairpins, hair ornaments, and removable dental structures.

- Instruct the patient to remove dental structures, such as false teeth or retainers, and any radiopaque objects located within the hair that may obstruct visualization of the atlas and axis.

Contrast and density are adequate to demonstrate the bony structures of the atlas and axis. Penetration is sufficient to visualize the bony trabecular patterns and cortical outlines of the atlas's lateral masses and transverse processes and the axis's dens, spinous process, and body.

- An optimal 75 to 80 kVp technique sufficiently penetrates the bony and soft tissue structures of the atlas and axis.
- Use a grid and tight collimation to decrease the amount of scattered radiation that reaches the film, increasing the visibility of the recorded details and providing a higher-contrast radiograph.

The bony trabecular patterns and cortical outlines of the cervical vertebrae are sharply defined.

- Sharply defined recorded details are obtained when patient motion is controlled, respiration is halted, and a short object–image distance (OID) is maintained.

The atlas and axis demonstrate a true AP projection. The atlas is symmetrically seated on the axis, with the atlas's lateral masses at equal distances from the dens. The spinous process of the axis is aligned with the midline of the axis's body, and the mandibular rami are demonstrated at equal distances from the lateral masses.

- An AP projection of the atlas and axis is obtained by placing the patient in either a supine or upright AP projection with the shoulders, mandibular angles, and mastoid tips positioned at equal distances from the tabletop or upright grid holder (Fig. 7–6).
- **Effect of Rotation:** Rotation of the atlas and axis occurs when the head is turned away from an AP projection. Upon head rotation, the atlas pivots around

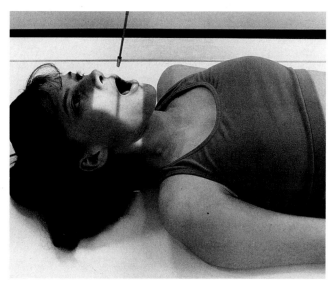

Figure 7-6. Proper patient positioning for AP atlas and axis radiograph.

the dens, so the lateral mass located on the side the face is turned away from is displaced anteriorly, and the mass located on the side the face is turned toward is displaced posteriorly. This displacement causes the space between the lateral mass and the dens to narrow on the side the face is turned away from and to enlarge on the side the face is turned toward (see Rad. 7). As the amount of head rotation increases, the axis rotates in the same direction as the atlas, resulting in a shift in the position of its spinous process, in the direction opposite from the direction in which the patient's face is turned.[2]

- **Detecting Direction of Rotation:** Radiographically, one can determine which way the patient's face was turned by judging the distance between the mandibular rami and the lateral masses. The side that demonstrates the greater distance is the side toward which the face was rotated.

- **Positioning for Trauma:** When cervical vertebral radiographs are taken on a trauma patient in whom subluxation or fracture is suspected, take the AP projection with the patient's position left as is. *Do not* attempt to remove the cervical collar or to adjust head or body rotation, mandible position, or cervical vertebral column tilting. To do so might result in increased injury to the vertebrae or spinal cord. Five to ten percent of spinal cord injuries occur from the mishandling of the patient after injury.[1]

The upper incisors and the posterior occiput's inferior edge are demonstrated superior to the dens and the atlantoaxial joint.

- The dens and the atlantoaxial joint are located at the midsagittal plane, at a level 0.50 inch (1 cm) inferior to an imaginary line connecting the mastoid tips. To visualize them without upper incisor (front teeth) or posterior occiput superimposition, instruct the patient to open the mouth as wide as possible. Then have the patient tuck the chin until an imaginary line connect-

ing the upper occlusal plane (chewing surface of maxillary teeth) and the posterior occiput's inferior edge is aligned perpendicular to the tabletop or upright grid holder. If the patient does not have upper teeth, one should imagine where the occlusal plane would be if the patient had teeth. This positioning also aligns the acanthiomeatal line (an imaginary line drawn between the point where the upper lip and nose meet the external ear opening) perpendicular with the tabletop or upright grid holder. It may be necessary to position a small angled sponge beneath the patient's head to maintain accurate head positioning, especially if the patient's chin has to be tucked so much that it is difficult to adequately open the mouth. The sponge causes the upper occlusal plane and posterior occiput's inferior edge to align perpendicularly without requiring as much chin tucking.

- **Relationship of Central Ray Angulation and Patient Position:** The lateral cervical radiograph in Figure 7–7 demonstrates how the occlusal plane and the posterior occiput's inferior edge should be aligned for an accurate open-mouth radiograph. After studying this radiograph, you might conclude that the atlantoaxial joint will be free of upper incisor or occiput superimposition if the patient maintains this head position and simply drops the jaw. Because the upper incisors are positioned at a long OID, however, they are greatly magnified, causing them to be projected onto the dens and atlantoaxial joint. On most patients, when the upper occlusal plane and posterior occiput's inferior edge are superimposed, magnification causes the upper incisors to be projected

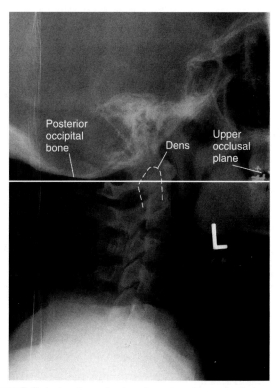

Figure 7-7. Lateral cervical vertebral radiograph demonstrating upper incisor, dens, and posterior occiput relationship.

about 1 inch (2.5 cm) inferior to the posterior occiput's inferior edge (see Rad. 8). To project these incisors superiorly, a 5-degree cephalic angle should be placed on the central ray. The upper incisors will be projected about 1 inch (2.5 cm) for every 5 degrees of angulation. This angle adjustment is based on a 40-inch (102-cm) source–image distance (SID); if a longer SID is used, the required angle adjustment would be less, whereas if a shorter SID is used, the angulation adjustment would be greater. If, instead of using an angle, the patient's chin was tilted upward in an attempt to shift the upper incisors superiorly, the posterior occiput would simultaneously be shifted inferiorly. This inferior shift of the occiput would obscure the dens and possibly the atlantoaxial joint.

The dens and atlantoaxial joint space may also be obscured if a 5-degree cephalad central ray angle was used but the occlusal plane and posterior occiput's inferior edge were not superimposed. When the posterior occiput's inferior edge is positioned inferior to the upper occlusal plane, the radiograph demonstrates the dens and, depending on the degree of misposition, the atlantoaxial joint space superimposed onto the posterior occiput (see Rad. 9). When the occlusal plane is positioned inferior to the posterior occiput's inferior edge, the posterior occiput is demonstrated superior to the dens, and the upper incisors superimposes a portion of the superior dens (see Rad. 10).

- ***Positioning for Trauma:*** To demonstrate the dens and atlantoaxial joint without incisor or occiput superimposition in a trauma patient, the degree and direction of the central ray angle must be changed from the standard position. The patient's head or neck cannot be adjusted on a trauma patient, so you must angle the central ray until it is aligned parallel with the infraorbitomental line (imaginary line connecting the inferior orbital rim and the external ear opening). This line is easily accessible on a patient wearing a cervical collar. The exact degree of angulation needed depends on the amount of chin elevation. Most patients in a cervical collar require about a 10-degree caudal angle.

Once the angle is set, attempt to get the patient to drop the lower jaw. *Do not* adjust head rotation or tilting. If the cervical collar allows the lower jaw to move without elevating the upper jaw, instruct patient to drop the lower jaw. If the cervical collar prevents lower jaw movement without elevating the upper jaw, instruct the patient about the importance of holding the head and neck perfectly still. Then have the ordering physician remove the front of the cervical collar so the patient can drop the jaw without adjusting the head or neck position (Fig. 7–8).

After the patient's jaw is dropped, align the central ray to the midsagittal plane at a level 0.50 inch (1 cm) inferior to the occlusal plane. Immediately after the radiograph is taken, the physician should return the front of the cervical collar to its proper position.

For trauma positioning, insufficient caudal angulation causes upper incisors to be demonstrated superior

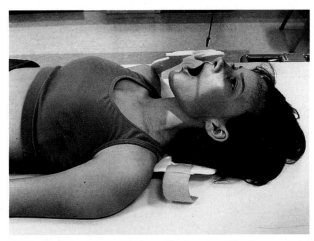

Figure 7–8. Proper patient positioning for AP atlas and axis radiograph taken to evaluate trauma.

to the dens and the dens to superimpose the posterior occiput (see Rad. 11). If the central ray was angled too caudally, the posterior occiput is demonstrated superior to the dens and the upper incisors superimpose the dens (see Rad. 12).

The atlantoaxial joint is open, and the axis's spinous process is demonstrated in the midline and inferior to the dens.

- Anteroposterior neck extension and flexion determine the alignment of the atlantoaxial joint with the tabletop and the position of the axis's spinous process to the dens. When the occlusal plane and posterior occiput's inferior edge are aligned perpendicular to the tabletop, the atlantoaxial joint should be open.

- ***Effect of Head Flexion or Extension:*** If the head is extended backward or flexed forward, as it is when the occlusal plane and posterior occiput's inferior edge are not aligned perpendicular to the tabletop, the cervical vertebral column is extended or flexed, respectively. This extension or flexion results in a closed atlantoaxial joint and a superior or increased inferior location of the axis's spinous process in respect to the dens (see Rad. 9). Neck extension causes the axis's spinous process to move inferiorly, whereas neck flexion moves it superiorly.

The dens is centered within the collimated field. The atlantoaxial and occiputoatlantal joints, the atlas's lateral masses and transverse processes, and the axis's dens and body are included within the field.

- Centering the central ray to the midsagittal plane at a level 0.50 inch (1 cm) inferior to an imaginary line connecting the mastoid tips centers the dens within the collimated field.

- Open the longitudinally collimated field to the patient's external ear opening. Transverse collimation should be to a 5-inch (12.5-cm) field size.

- An 8 × 10 inch (18 × 24 cm) film placed lengthwise should be adequate to include all the required anatomical structures.

Critiquing Radiographs

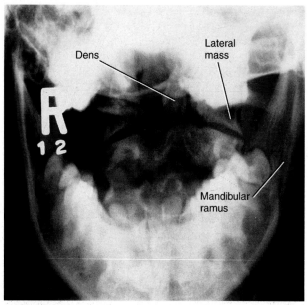

Radiograph 7.

Critique: The distances from the atlas's lateral masses to the dens and from the mandibular rami to the dens are narrower on the left side than on the right side, and the axis's spinous process is shifted from the midline toward the left. The face was rotated toward the right side.

Correction: Rotate the face toward the left side, until the mandibular angles and mastoid tips are positioned at equal distances from the tabletop or upright grid holder.

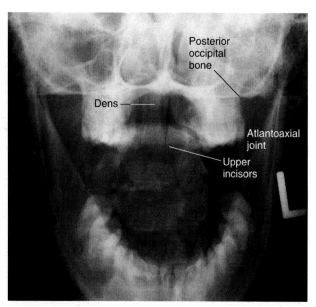

Radiograph 8.

Critique: The upper incisors are demonstrated about 1 inch (2.5 cm) inferior to the posterior occiput's inferior edge, obscuring the dens and atlantoaxial articulation. The posterior occiput's inferior edge is demonstrated directly superior to the dens.

Correction: If the upper occlusal plane and the posterior occiput's inferior edge were aligned perpendicular to the tabletop and a perpendicular central ray was used for this radiograph, do not adjust patient positioning; simply direct the central ray 5 degrees cephalad. If a 5-degree cephalad angulation was used for this radiograph, do not adjust patient positioning; simply increase the cephalad angulation by 5 degrees. The incisors will shift about 1 inch (2.5 cm) for every 5 degrees of central ray angulation. (This angle adjustment is based on a 40-inch [102-cm] SID; if a longer SID is used, less angle adjustment is required, and if a shorter SID is used, more angle adjustment is required.)

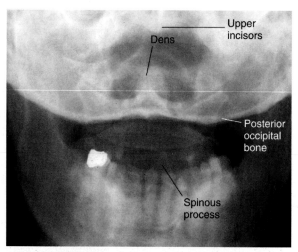

Radiograph 9.

Critique: The dens is superimposing the posterior occiput. The upper incisors are demonstrated about 1 inch (2.5 cm) superior to the posterior occiput's inferior edge.

Correction: Tuck the chin toward the chest until an imaginary line connecting the upper occlusal plane with the posterior occiput's inferior edge is aligned perpendicular to the film. The needed movement is equal to half the distance demonstrated between the upper incisors and the posterior occiput's inferior edge. For this patient, the chin should be tucked about 0.50 inch (1 cm).

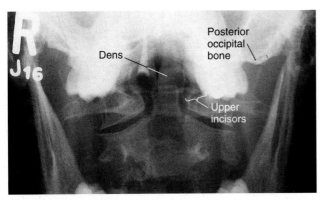

Radiograph 10.

Critique: The upper incisors are superimposing the dens. The posterior occiput's inferior edge is demonstrated about 0.50 inch (1 cm) superior to the upper incisors and 0.25 inch (0.6 cm) superior to the dens. The upper occlusal plane was positioned inferior to the posterior occiput's inferior edge.

Correction: Elevate the upper jaw until an imaginary line connecting the upper occlusal plane with the posterior occiput's inferior edge is aligned perpendicular to the film. The needed movement is equal to half of the distance demonstrated between the upper incisors and the posterior occiput's inferior edge. For this patient, the upper occlusal plane should be elevated about 0.25 inch (0.6 cm).

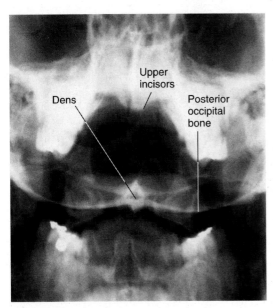

Radiograph 11.

Critique: This radiograph displays trauma positioning. The upper incisors are demonstrated superior to the dens and the posterior occiput's inferior edge, and the dens superimposes the posterior occiput. The central ray angulation was not directed enough caudally.

Correction: Angle the central ray about 5 degrees caudad for every 1 inch (2.5 cm) demonstrated between the upper incisors and the posterior occiput's inferior edge. (This angle adjustment is based on a 40-inch [102-cm] SID.) Because about 1 inch (2.5 cm) is demonstrated between the upper incisors and posterior occiput's inferior edge on this radiograph, the central ray angulation should be adjusted about 5 degrees caudally.

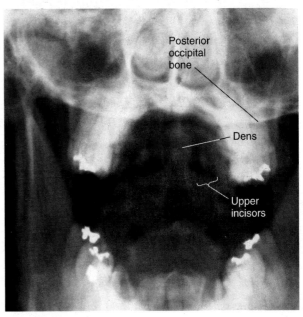

Radiograph 12.

Critique: This radiograph displays trauma positioning. The upper incisors are superimposing the dens, and the posterior occiput's inferior edge is situated superior to the dens and upper incisors. The central ray was angled too caudally.

Correction: Angle the central ray about 5 degrees cephalically for every 1 inch (2.5 cm) demonstrated between the upper incisors and the posterior occiput's inferior edge.

Cervical Vertebrae: Lateral Position

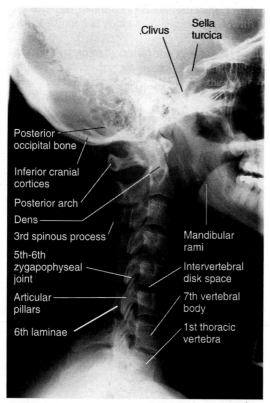

Figure 7-9. Accurately positioned lateral cervical vertebral radiograph.

Radiographic Evaluation

Facility's patient identification requirements are visible on radiograph.

- These requirements usually are facility name, patient name, age, and hospital number, and exam time and date.
- Patient ID plate is positioned caudally so as not to obscure the sella turcica and clivus.

A left or right marker, identifying the side of the patient positioned closer to the film, is present on the radiograph and does not superimpose anatomy of interest.

- Place the marker anteriorly within the collimated light field so it does not superimpose any portion of the cervical vertebrae or its surrounding soft tissue.
- If the lateral position is taken with the patient in flexion or extension, an arrow should be included to indicate the direction of neck movement.
- Because the transversely collimated field is coned to about a 7-inch (18-cm) area, make certain that the marker is positioned within 3.5 inches (8.5 cm) of the film's center to guarantee that it will not be cut off.

There is no evidence of preventable artifacts, such as snaps, buttons, necklaces, earrings, and hairpins.

- Removing any radiopaque objects from the neck and head prevents them from obscuring any anatomy of interest.

Contrast and density are adequate to demonstrate the surrounding soft tissue, air filled trachea, prevertebral fat stripe, and bony structures of the cervical vertebrae. Penetration is sufficient to visualize the bony trabecular patterns and cortical outlines of the vertebral bodies, zygapophyseal joints, spinous processes, mandibular rami, sella turcica, clivus, and posterior occiput.

- An optimal 75 to 80 kVp technique sufficiently penetrates the bony and soft tissue structures of the cervical vertebrae.
- **_Prevertebral Fat Stripe:_** The soft tissue structure of interest on a lateral cervical radiograph is the prevertebral fat stripe. It is located in front of the anterior surfaces of the vertebrae and is visualized on accurately positioned and exposed lateral cervical radiographs (Fig. 7–10). The reviewer evaluates the distance between the anterior surface of the cervical vertebrae and the prevertebral fat stripe. Abnormal widening of this space is used for the detection and localization of fractures, masses, and inflammation.[3]
- **_Air-Gap Technique:_** Because this exam uses a long object–image distance (OID), a grid is optional. When the OID is long, scattered radiation that would expose the film at a short OID is scattered away from the film. Because much of the scattered radiation is not being directed toward the film, a grid is not needed to absorb the scatter. This is also referred to as the *air-gap technique.*[4]

The bony trabecular patterns and cortical outlines of the cervical vertebrae are sharply defined.

- Sharply defined recorded details are obtained when patient motion is controlled, respiration is halted, and the smallest OID is maintained.

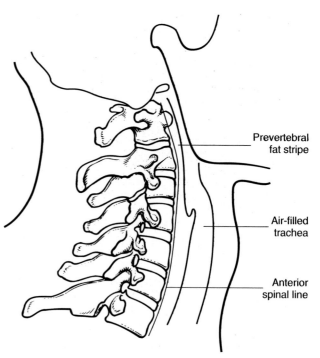

Figure 7-10. Location of prevertebral fat stripe.

- In the lateral position, the patient's shoulder prevents the cervical vertebrae from being positioned close to the film. A long OID will result in magnification and loss of recorded detail unless a 72-inch (183-cm) source–image distance (SID) is used to offset the magnification. This decrease in image magnification provides an increase in recorded detail.

The cervical vertebrae demonstrate a true lateral position: The right and left articular pillars and zygapophyseal joints of each cervical vertebra are superimposed, the vertebral bodies are demonstrated without pillar superimposition, and the spinous processes are demonstrated in profile.

- A lateral cervical vertebral radiograph is obtained by placing the patient in an upright position with the midcoronal plane positioned perpendicular to the film (Fig. 7–11). In this position, the right and left sides of each cervical vertebra are superimposed, demonstrating the spinous processes and vertebral bodies in profile. To prevent rotation superimpose the patient's shoulders, mastoid tips and mandibular rami.

- **Effect of Rotation:** The upper and lower cervical vertebrae can demonstrate rotation simultaneously or separately, depending on which part of the body is rotated. If the head was rotated and the thorax remained in a lateral position, the upper cervical vertebrae demonstrate rotation. If the patient's thorax was rotated and the head remained in a lateral position, the lower cervical vertebrae demonstrate rotation. If the patient's head and thorax were rotated simultaneously, the entire cervical column demonstrates rotation.

- **Detecting Rotation:** Radiographically, rotation of the cervical vertebrae can be initially detected by evaluating each vertebra for pillar superimposition and for zygapophyseal joint superimposition. When the patient is rotated, the pillars and zygapophyseal joints on one side of the vertebra move anterior to

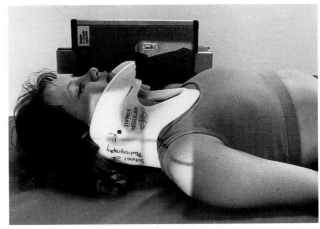

Figure 7–12. Proper patient positioning for lateral cervical vertebral radiograph taken to evaluate trauma.

those on the other side (see Rad. 13). Because the two sides of the vertebrae are mirror images, it is very difficult to determine from a rotated lateral cervical radiograph which side of the patient is rotated anteriorly and which posteriorly. The magnification of the side situated farther from the film may give a moderately reliable clue at the articular pillar regions.

- **Positioning for Trauma:** When cervical vertebral radiographs are taken on a trauma patient in whom subluxation or fracture is suspected, take the lateral projection with the patient's position left as is. *Do not attempt to remove the cervical collar or to adjust head or body rotation, mandible position, or vertebral tilting. To do so might result in increased injury to the vertebrae or spinal cord.* Five to ten percent of spinal cord injuries occur from the mishandling of the patient after injury.[1]

  A trauma lateral cervical vertebral radiograph is obtained by placing a lengthwise film against the patient's shoulder and directing a horizontal beam to the cervical vertebrae (Fig. 7–12). Such a radiograph should meet as many of the evaluation requirements listed for a nontrauma lateral radiograph as possible without moving the patient.

The posterior arch of C1 and the spinous process of C2 are demonstrated in profile without posterior occiput superimposition, and their bodies are demonstrated without mandibular superimposition. The cranial cortices and the mandibular rami are superimposed, and the intervertebral disk spaces are open.

- When the patient is positioned for a lateral cervical radiograph, place the head in a true lateral position with the midsagittal plane aligned parallel with the film, and the chin elevated until the acanthiomeatal line (an imaginary line connecting the point where upper lip and nose meet with the external ear opening) is aligned parallel with the floor and the interpupillary line is aligned perpendicular to the film. This positioning accomplishes three goals: alignment of the cervical vertebral column parallel with the film, demonstration of C1 and C2 without occiput or mandibular superimposition, and superimposition of the anterior, posterior,

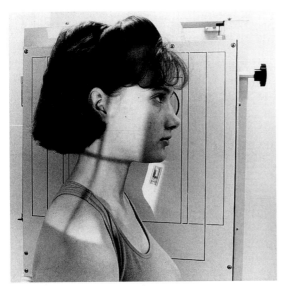

Figure 7–11. Proper patient positioning for lateral cervical vertebral radiograph.

superior, and inferior aspects of the cranial and mandibular cortices.

- **Effect of Head Positioning on Mandible Demonstration:** The position of the mandible on a lateral cranial radiograph is affected by head positioning. The posterior cortices of the mandibular rami are superimposed when the head's midsagittal plane was aligned parallel with the film. If the cortices are not superimposed on a lateral cervical vertebral radiograph, one mandibular ramus superimposes the bodies of C1 and C2 and the other is situated anteriorly (see Rad. 14). If the chin was elevated adequately to place the acanthiomeatal line parallel with the floor, the mandibular rami are demonstrated anterior to the vertebral column. If the patient's chin was not adequately elevated, the mandibular rami superimpose the bodies of C1 and C2 (see Rad. 15).

- **Detecting Head Tilting:** If the patient's head and upper cervical column are tilted toward or away from the film, the upper cervical vertebral column is no longer aligned parallel with the film. Radiographically, head tilting can be identified as an inferosuperior separation between the cranial cortices and between the mandibular rami. If the head was tilted toward the film, which is the more common error, neither the superior or inferior cortices of the cranium nor the mandibular rami are superimposed, and the vertebral foramen of C1 is visualized (see Rad. 16). If the head and upper cervical vertebral column were tilted away from the film, neither the inferior cortices of the cranium nor the mandibular rami are superimposed, and the posterior arch of C1 remains in profile (see Rad. 14).

The long axis of the cervical vertebral column is aligned with the long axis of the collimated field.

- Aligning the long axis of the cervical vertebral column with the long axis of the collimated field ensures against flexion or extension of the cervical column and allows for tight collimation. This alignment is

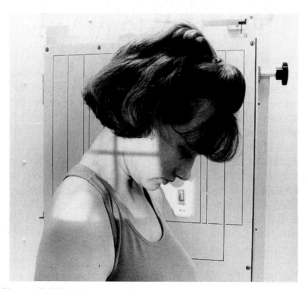

Figure 7-13. Patient positioning for lateral cervical vertebral radiograph with hyperflexion.

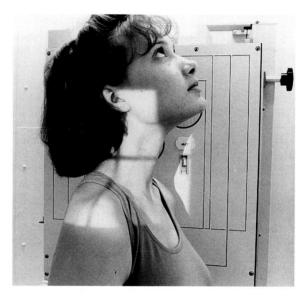

Figure 7-14. Patient positioning for lateral cervical vertebral radiograph with hyperextension.

obtained by positioning the patient's neck vertically and aligning the midline of the patient's neck with the collimator's longitudinal light line. This alignment places the cervical column in a neutral position.

- **Positioning to Evaluate AP Mobility of Cervical Vertebrae:** If the cervical vertebrae are being radiographed in the lateral position to demonstrate anteroposterior vertebral mobility, two lateral radiographs should be taken with the patient placed in a lateral position, one with the neck in maximum flexion and the other with the neck in maximum extension. For maximum flexion, instruct the patient to tuck the chin into the chest as far as possible (Fig. 7-13).

  For patients who demonstrate extreme degrees of flexion, it may be necessary to place the film crosswise to include the entire cervical column on the same radiograph. Such a radiograph should meet all the evaluation requirements listed for a neutral lateral radiograph, except that the long axis demonstrates forward bending (see Rad. 17).

  For maximum extension, instruct the patient to extend the chin up and backward as far as possible (Fig. 7-14). Such a radiograph should meet all the evaluation requirements listed for a neutral lateral radiograph, except that the long axis demonstrates backward bending (see Rad. 18).

The fourth cervical vertebra is centered within the collimated field. The sella turcica, clivus, first through seventh cervical vertebrae, and superior half of the first thoracic vertebra and the surrounding soft tissue are included within the field.

- Center a perpendicular central ray to the midcoronal plane at a level halfway between the external ear meatus (EAM) and the jugular notch in order to center the fourth cervical vertebra in the collimated field.
- Open the longitudinally and transversely collimated field enough to include the clivus and sella turcica,

which is at a level 0.75 inch (2 cm) anterosuperior to the EAM. (The clivus, a slanted structure that extends posteriorly off the sella turcica, and the dens are used to determine cervical injury. A line drawn along the clivus should point to the tip of the dens on the normal upper cervical vertebral radiograph.[5])

- A 10 × 12 inch (24 × 30 cm) film placed lengthwise should be adequate to include all the required anatomical structures.

- ***Visualization of C7 and T1 Vertebrae:*** The seventh cervical vertebra and first thoracic vertebra are located between the patient's shoulders. This location makes it difficult to visualize them because of the great difference in lateral thickness between the neck and the shoulders. The best method to demonstrate C7 is to have the patient hold 5 or 10 lb weights on each arm, to depress the shoulders and attempt to move them inferior to C7. Without weights, it is often difficult to demonstrate more than six cervical

vertebrae (see Rad. 19). Taking the radiograph in expiration also aids in lowering the shoulders.

- ***Visualization of C7 and T1 in Trauma or Recumbency:*** On trauma or recumbent patients, depress the shoulders by having someone pull down on the patient's arms while the radiograph is taken. To accomplish this, instruct an assistant to wear a protection apron and stand at the end of the radiographic table, with the patient's feet resting against the assistant's abdomen and the assistant's hands wrapped around the patient's wrists. The assistant should slowly pull on the patient's arms until the shoulders are moved inferiorly as much as possible.

- ***Swimmer's Position Radiograph:*** If even after using weights to depress the patient's shoulders C7 cannot be demonstrated in its entirety, a special view known as the swimmer's position should be taken. Refer to page 337 for specifics.

Critiquing Radiographs

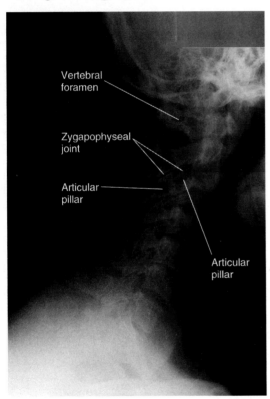

Radiograph 13.

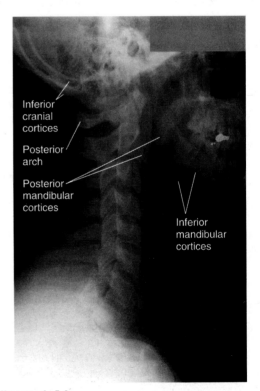

Radiograph 14.

Critique: The articular pillars and zygapophyseal joints on one side of the patient are situated anterior to those on the other side. The patient was rotated. The inferior cortices of the cranium and mandible are demonstrated without superimposition, and the vertebral foramen of C1 is visualized. The patient's head and upper cervical vertebral column were tilted toward the film.

Correction: Rotate the patient until the midcoronal plane is aligned perpendicular to the film, and tilt the head away from the film until the interpupillary line is perpendicular to the film.

Critique: Neither the inferior, superior, posterior, or anterior cortices of the cranium nor the mandible is superimposed. The posterior arch of C1 is demonstrated in profile. The patient's head was rotated and tilted away from the film.

Correction: Rotate the head until the midsagittal plane is aligned parallel with the film, and then tilt the head toward the film until the interpupillary line is perpendicular to the film.

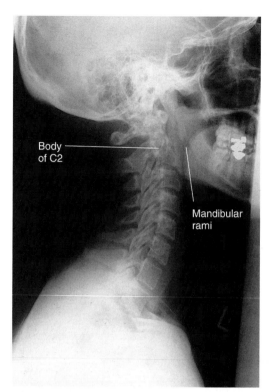

Radiograph 15.

Critique: The cranial and mandibular cortices are accurately aligned, and the mandibular rami are superimposing the body of C2. The patient's chin was not adequately elevated.
Correction: Elevate the chin until the acanthiomeatal line is aligned parallel with the floor.

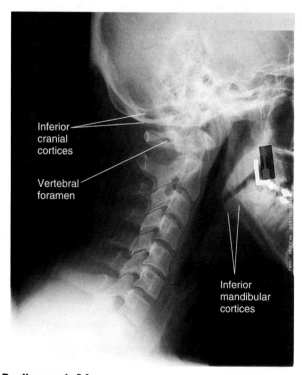

Radiograph 16.

Critique: The inferior cortices of the cranium and mandible are demonstrated without superimposition, and the vertebral foramen of C1 is visualized. The patient's head and upper cervical vertebrae were tilted toward the film.
Correction: Tilt the head away from the film until the interpupillary line is aligned perpendicular to the film.

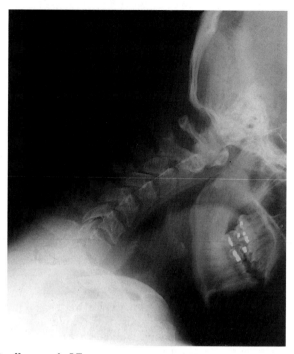

Radiograph 17.

Critique: The long axis of the cervical vertebral column is not aligned with the long axis of the collimated field. The cervical vertebral column is tilted forward. The patient was in hyperflexion.
Correction: Extend the patient's chin until the eyes are facing forward and the long axis of the neck is aligned with the long axis of the collimated field. If this exam is being performed to evaluate anteroposterior mobility, no correction movement is required.

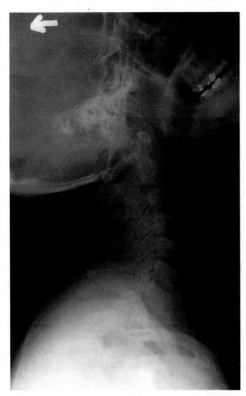

Radiograph 18.

Critique: The long axis of the cervical vertebral column is not aligned with the long axis of the collimated field. The cervical vertebral column is tilted backward. The patient was in hyperextension.

Correction: Tuck the patient's chin until the eyes are facing forward and the long axis of the neck is aligned with the long axis of the collimated field. If this exam is being performed to evaluate anteroposterior mobility, no correction movement is required.

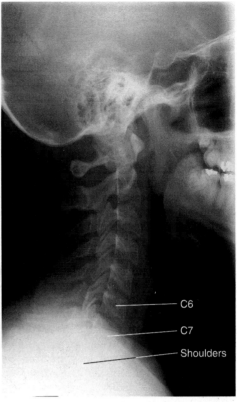

Radiograph 19.

Critique: The vertebral body of C7 is not demonstrated in its entirety, and the superior body of T1 is not demonstrated. The shoulders were not adequately depressed.

Correction: If possible, have the patient hold 5 to 10 lb weights on each arm to depress the shoulders. If the patient cannot hold weights or if the weights do not sufficiently drop shoulders, a special view known as the "swimmer's" position should be taken to demonstrate this area (see page 337).

Cervical Vertebrae: Anterior and Posterior Oblique Positions

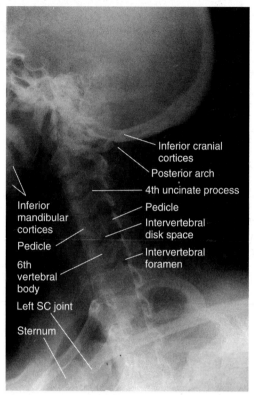

Inferior cranial cortices

Posterior arch

4th uncinate process

Inferior mandibular cortices

Pedicle

Intervertebral disk space

Pedicle

Intervertebral foramen

6th vertebral body

Left SC joint

Sternum

Figure 7-15. Accurately positioned oblique cervical vertebral radiograph.

Radiographic Evaluation

Facility's patient identification requirements are visible on radiograph.
- These requirements usually are facility name, patient name, age, and hospital number, and exam time and date.
- Patient ID plate is positioned cephalically so as not to obscure anatomy of interest.

A right or left marker, identifying the side of the patient positioned closer to the film, is present on the radiograph and does not superimpose any anatomy of interest.
- Place the marker laterally within the collimated field so it does not superimpose any portion of the cervical vertebrae or its surrounding soft tissue.
- Because the transversely collimated field is coned to about a 7-inch (18-cm) area, make certain the marker is positioned within 3.5 inches (8.5 cm) of the center of the film to guarantee that it will not be cut off.
- Anteriorly obliqued radiographs are hung on the view box as if the patient is facing the viewer; therefore, the marker will appear backward when the radiograph is correctly hung.

There is no evidence of preventable artifacts, such as snaps, buttons, necklaces, earrings, and hairpins.

- Removing any radiopaque objects from the neck and head prevents them from obscuring any anatomy of interest.

Contrast and density are adequate to demonstrate the surrounding soft tissue and bony structures of the cervical vertebrae. Penetration is sufficient to visualize the bony trabecular patterns and cortical outlines of the vertebral bodies, uncinate processes, and pedicles.
- An optimal 75 to 80 kVp technique sufficiently penetrates the bony and soft tissue structures of the cervical vertebrae.
- ***Air-Gap Technique:*** Because this exam uses a long object–image distance (OID), a grid is optional. When the OID is long, scattered radiation that would expose the film at a short OID is scattered away from the film. Consequently, much of the scattered radiation is not being directed toward the film, and a grid is not needed to absorb the scatter. This is also referred to as the *air-gap technique*.[4]

The bony trabecular patterns and cortical outlines of the cervical vertebrae are sharply defined.
- Sharply defined recorded details are obtained when patient motion is controlled, respiration is halted, and the shortest OID is maintained.
- This exam can be taken using anterior or posterior oblique positions. The anterior oblique positions place the intervertebral foramina of interest closer to the film, whereas the posterior oblique positions place the intervertebral foramina of interest farther from the film. Even when anterior oblique positions are used, some OID remains. Any amount of OID results in magnification and loss of recorded detail. To offset some of this magnification, a 72-inch (183-cm) source–image distance (SID) can be used. This decrease in image magnification provides an increase in recorded detail.

The cervical vertebrae have been rotated 45 degrees. The second through seventh intervertebral foramina

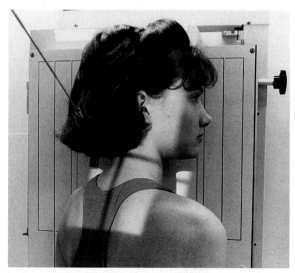

Figure 7-16. Proper patient positioning for anterior oblique cervical vertebral radiograph.

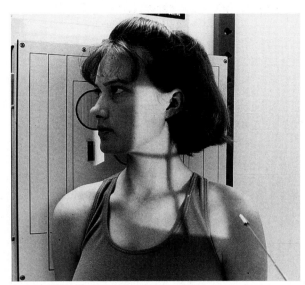

Figure 7-17. Proper patient positioning for posterior oblique cervical vertebral radiograph.

are clearly demonstrated, the pedicles of interest are visualized in profile, and the opposite pedicles are aligned with the anterior vertebral bodies. The sternum and sternoclavicular joints are demonstrated without vertebral column superimposition.

- To position the intervertebral foramina and pedicles of interest in profile, begin by placing the patient in a recumbent or upright PA/AP projection. From this projection, rotate the patient until the midcoronal plane is at a 45-degree angle to the tabletop or upright film holder. To demonstrate the foramina and pedicles on each side of the cervical vertebrae, right and left oblique radiographs must be taken. When anterior oblique radiographs (Fig. 7–16) are obtained, the foramina and pedicles situated closer to the film are visualized, whereas posterior oblique radiographs (Fig. 7–17) visualize the foramina and pedicles situated farther from the film.

- **Effect of Incorrect Rotation:** If the cervical vertebral rotation is insufficient, the intervertebral foramina are narrowed or obscured, the pedicles are foreshortened, and a portion of the sternum, one sternoclavicular joint, and the vertebral column are superimposed (see Rad. 20). If the cervical vertebrae are rotated more than 45 degrees, one side of the pedicles is partially foreshortened but the other side is aligned with the midline of the vertebral bodies, and the zygapophyseal joints demonstrated without vertebral body superimposition are open (see Rad. 21).

- **Positioning for Trauma:** When radiographing the cervical vertebrae of a trauma patient in whom subluxation or fracture is suspected, obtain the trauma AP projection and lateral position and have them evaluated by the radiologist before the patient is moved for the oblique position.

The trauma oblique position of the cervical vertebrae is accomplished by elevating the supine patient's head, neck, and thorax enough to place a lengthwise cassette beneath the neck. If the right vertebral foram-

ina and pedicles are of interest, the film should be shifted to the left enough to align the left mastoid tip with the longitudinal axis of the film and inferior enough to position the right gonion (C3) with the transverse axis of the film. Direct the central ray 45 degrees medial to the right side of the patient's neck and 15 degrees cephalically, then center it halfway between the anteroposterior surfaces of the neck at the level of the thyroid cartilage (C4) (Fig. 7–18). If the left vertebral foramina and pedicles are of interest, shift the film to the right enough to align the right mastoid tip with the longitudinal axis of the film and inferior enough to position the left gonion with the transverse axis of the film. The central ray should be angled and centered as previously described, except that it should be directed to the left side of the patient's neck. A trauma oblique cervical radiograph should meet all the evaluation requirements listed for a regular oblique cervical radiograph, except for the cranium, which is not in a lateral position (Fig. 7–19).

The intervertebral disk spaces are open, and the cervical bodies and intervertebral foramina are demonstrated without distortion.

- The cervical vertebral column demonstrates a lordotic curvature. This curvature, and the shape of the cervical bodies and intervertebral foramina, cause the disk articulating surfaces of the vertebral bodies to slant downward posteriorly to anteriorly.

- **Importance of Central Ray Angulation:** To obtain open intervertebral disk spaces and undistorted vertebral bodies, the central ray must be angled in the same direction as the slope of the vertebral bodies. This is accomplished by angling the central ray 15 degrees caudally for anterior oblique radiographs and 15 degrees cephalically for posterior oblique radiographs.

- **Effect of Inaccurate Central Ray Angulation:** If the central ray is not accurately angled with intervertebral disk spaces, they are closed and the

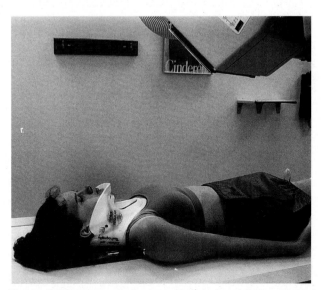

Figure 7-18. Proper patient positioning for oblique cervical vertebral radiograph taken to evaluate trauma.

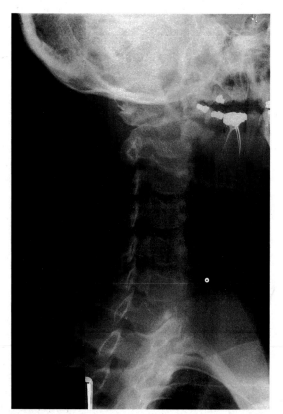

Figure 7-19. Accurately positioned oblique cervical vertebral radiograph taken to evaluate trauma.

cervical bodies and intervertebral foramina are distorted (see Rads. 22 and 23). Because this exam can be taken using anterior or posterior oblique positions, and because the direction of angulation varies between the two positions, you should be able to identify a radiograph that was taken with the angle directed in the wrong direction. If an anterior oblique position of the cervical vertebrae was taken with a cephalic angulation or a posterior oblique position was taken with a caudal angulation, the intervertebral foramina and pedicles are still visualized, but the cervical bodies are distorted, the intervertebral disk spaces are closed, and the zygapophyseal joints situated farther from the film on an anterior oblique radiograph and closer to the film on a posterior oblique radiograph are demonstrated within the cervical bodies.

- **Positioning for Kyphosis:** On patients with severe kyphosis, the lower cervical vertebrae are angled toward the film because of the greater lordotic curvature of this area. To better align these cervical vertebrae parallel with the film, the upper thorax should be tilted away from the film (posteriorly) for an anterior oblique and toward the film for a posterior oblique radiograph. Even with this tilt, place the patient's head in a true lateral position, without tilting. If the cervical vertebrae are not brought parallel with the film for the oblique position, the intervertebral disk spaces are closed, the zygapophyseal joints situated farther from the film on anterior oblique radiographs and closer to the film on posterior oblique radiographs are demonstrated within the vertebral bodies, and the vertebral

bodies and intervertebral foramina are distorted (see Rad. 22).

The cranium is in a lateral position. The upper cervical vertebrae are demonstrated without occipital or mandibular superimposition, and the posterior cortices of the cranium and mandible are superimposed.

- Turning the patient's face away from the side of interest until the head's midsagittal plane is aligned parallel with the film superimposes the posterior cortices of the cranium and mandible, preventing them from superimposing the upper cervical vertebrae. If these posterior cortices are demonstrated without superimposition, the posterior occiput superimposes the posterior arch of C1, and one of the mandibular rami superimposes the vertebral bodies of C1 and C2 (see Rad. 24).
- Once the head is adequately turned, adjust chin elevation until the acanthiomeatal line is aligned parallel with the floor. This positioning places the mandibular rami anterior to the bodies of C1 and C2. If the patient's chin is not properly elevated, the mandibular rami superimpose the bodies of C1 and C2 (similar to Rad. 15).

The posterior arch of the atlas is demonstrated without self-superimposition, demonstrating the vertebral foramen. The inferior outline of the outer cranial cortices and the mandibular rami are demonstrated without superimposition.

- The distances demonstrated between the inferior cortical outlines of the cranium and the mandibular rami are a result of the angulation placed on the central ray. On anterior oblique cervical radiographs, the caudal angle projects the cranial cortex situated farther from the film about 0.25 inch (0.6 cm) inferiorly and the mandibular ramus situated farther from the film about 0.50 inch (1 cm) inferiorly. This distance difference is based on a 40-inch (102-cm) SID; if a longer SID is used, the distance between the cranial and mandibular cortices is less, whereas if a shorter SID is used, the distance is greater. The ramus is projected farther inferiorly because it is located at a larger OID than the cranial cortex. On posterior oblique radiographs, the cephalic angle projects the cranial cortex and mandibular rami situated farther from the film superiorly.

  The distance between these two cortical outlines will be increased or decreased if the patient's head is allowed to tilt toward or away from the film. Such tilting also causes the upper cervical vertebrae to lean toward or away from the film. To avoid head and cervical column tilting, position the interpupillary line (imaginary line connecting the outer corners of the eyelids) perpendicular to the film and the long axis of the cervical column parallel with the film.

- **Detecting Head Tilting:** On anterior oblique radiographs, if the head and upper cervical column were allowed to tilt, the atlas and its posterior arch are distorted. From such a radiograph, one can determine whether the head and upper cervical vertebrae were tilted toward or away from the film by evaluating the distance demonstrated between the inferior cranial cortices and the inferior mandibular rami. If these distances are increased, the head and upper cervical vertebrae were tilted away from the film (see Rad. 25). If these distances are decreased, the head and upper cervical vertebrae were tilted toward the film.

The long axis of the cervical vertebral column is aligned with the long axis of the collimated field.

- Aligning the long axis of the cervical column with the long axis of the collimated field ensures against lateral flexion of the cervical column and allows for tight collimation. This alignment is obtained by aligning the midline of the patient's neck with the collimator's longitudinal light line.

The fifth cervical vertebra is centered within the collimated field. The first through seventh cervical vertebrae and the first thoracic vertebra, and the surrounding soft tissue are included within the field.

- Center the central ray to the patient's midsagittal plane at a level halfway between the external ear meatus (EAM) and the jugular notch.
- Open the longitudinal collimation to the EAM and the jugular notch. Transverse collimation should be to the lateral neck skin-line.
- A 10 × 12 inch (24 × 30 cm) film placed lengthwise should be adequate to include all the required anatomical structures.

Critiquing Radiographs

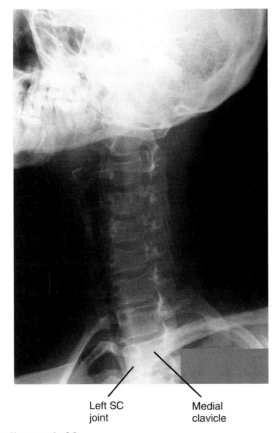

Left SC joint   Medial clavicle

Radiograph 20.

Critique: This patient was in an LAO position. The pedicles and intervertebral foramina are obscured, and portions of the left sternoclavicular joint and medial clavicular end are superimposed by the vertebral column. The patient was not rotated the required 45 degrees.

Correction: Increase the patient obliquity until the midcoronal plane is placed at a 45-degree angle with the film.

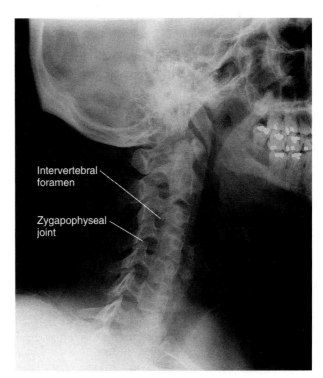

Intervertebral foramen

Zygapophyseal joint

Radiograph 21.

Critique: This patient was in an RAO position. The intervertebral foramina are demonstrated, the right pedicles are visualized although they are not in true profile, the left pedicles are demonstrated in the midline of the vertebral bodies, and the right zygapophyseal joints are demonstrated. The patient was rotated more than 45 degrees.

Correction: Decrease the patient rotation until the midcoronal plane is placed at a 45-degree angle with the film.

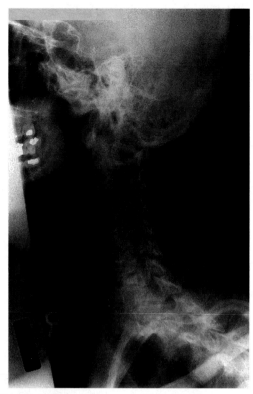

Radiograph 22.

Critique: This patient is in an LAO position. The intervertebral disk spaces are obscured, and the vertebral bodies and intervertebral foramina are distorted. Either the central ray was not aligned parallel with the disk spaces or the patient is kyphotic and the upper thorax was tilting toward the film.

Correction: Angle the central ray 15 degrees caudally for an anterior oblique radiograph. If the patient is kyphotic, tilt the upper thorax away from the film until the lower cervical vertebrae are aligned parallel with the film.

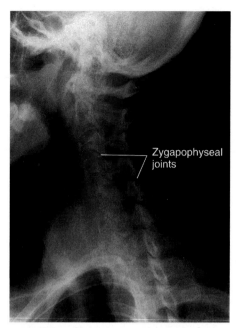

Radiograph 23.

Critique: This patient was in an RPO position. The intervertebral disk spaces are closed, the vertebral bodies are distorted, and the zygapophyseal joints superimposed by the cervical bodies are demonstrated. The central ray was angled 15 degrees caudally.

Correction: Angle the central ray 15 degrees cephalically for posterior oblique radiographs.

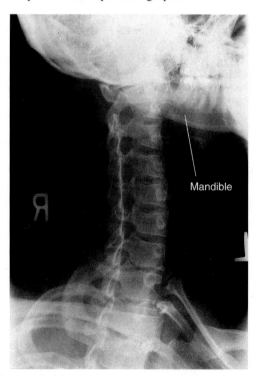

Radiograph 24.

Critique: This patient was in an RAO position. The upper cervical vertebrae are obscured by the patient's cranium and mandible. The patient's head was not turned into a lateral position.

Correction: Rotate the head into a lateral position, placing its midsagittal plane parallel with the film.

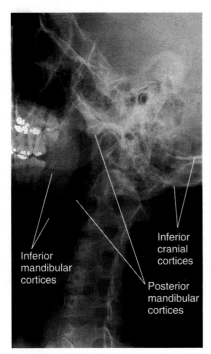

Radiograph 25.

Critique: This patient was in an LAO position. The atlas and its posterior arch are obscured. The inferior cranial cortices demonstrate more than 0.25 inch (0.6 cm) between them, and the inferior cortices of the mandibular rami demonstrate more than 0.50 inch (1 cm) between them. The first thoracic vertebra is not included. The head and the upper cervical vertebrae were tilted away from the film, and the central ray and film were positioned too superiorly.

Correction: Tilt the patient's head toward the film until the interpupillary line is aligned perpendicular to the film, and move the central ray and film inferiorly.

CERVICOTHORACIC VERTEBRAE

Swimmer's Lateral Position

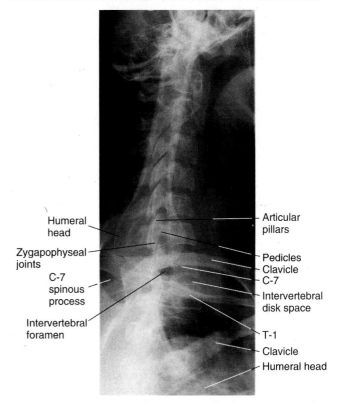

Figure 7-20. Accurately positioned lateral cervicothoracic vertebral radiograph.

This exam is performed when the routine lateral cervical radiograph does not adequately demonstrate the seventh cervical vertebra or when the routine lateral thoracic radiograph does not demonstrate the first through third thoracic vertebrae.

Radiographic Evaluation

Facility's patient identification requirements are visible on radiograph.

- These requirements usually are facility name, patient name, age, and hospital number, and exam time and date.
- Patient ID plate is positioned so as not to obscure anatomy of interest.

A right or left marker, identifying the side of the patient positioned closer to the film, is present on the radiograph and does not superimpose anatomy of interest.

- Place the marker anteriorly within the collimated light field, along the lower cassette edge, so it does not superimpose any portion of the cervicothoracic vertebral area.

There is no evidence of preventable artifacts, such as gown snaps and jewelry.

- It is recommended that the patient be instructed to change into a snapless hospital gown before the procedure.

Contrast and density are adequate to demonstrate the bony structures of the cervicothoracic vertebrae. Penetration is sufficient to visualize the bony trabecular patterns and cortical outlines of the lower cervical and upper thoracic vertebral bodies, pedicles, spinous processes, and intervertebral foramina.

- An optimal 80 to 90 kVp technique sufficiently penetrates the bony structures of the cervicothoracic vertebral area.
- The higher kilovoltage used to penetrate the vertebrae results in an increase in the amount of scattered radiation with enough energy to reach the film. Use tight collimation, a high-ratio grid, and a lead protection shield, placed on the tabletop at the edge of the posteriorly collimated field, to reduce the amount of scattered radiation that reaches the film, providing higher contrast and better visibility of recorded details.

The bony trabecular patterns and cortical outlines of the lower cervical and upper thoracic vertebrae are sharply defined.

- Sharply defined recorded details are obtained when patient motion is controlled, respiration is halted, and a short object–image distance (OID) is maintained.
- Using a small focal spot also improves the sharpness of recorded details, but may result in motion on larger patients owing to the long exposure time that would be required.

The cervicothoracic vertebrae are demonstrated in a true lateral position. The humerus elevated above the patient's head is aligned with the vertebral column, the right and left cervical zygapophyseal joints and articular pillars are superimposed, and the posterior ribs are superimposed.

- Position the patient in an erect or a lateral recumbent position. Whether the right or left side of the patient is positioned against the radiographic table or upright grid holder is not significant, although left-side positioning is easier for the technologist. For the recum-

bent position, flex the patient's knees and hips for support. For the erect position, instruct the patient to evenly distribute weight on both feet. Elevate the arm positioned closer to the film above the patient's head as high as the patient allows. The forearm and hand may be rested on the head for support in the erect position. Place the other arm against the patient's side, and instruct the patient to depress (drop toward the feet) this shoulder (Fig. 7–21).

- This supplementary swimmer's position moves the shoulders in opposite directions, overlapping one onto the upper cervical region and the other onto the lower thoracic region, allowing visualization of the cervicothoracic area without shoulder superimposition. If the patient can shift one shoulder posteriorly and the other anteriorly without rotating the thorax, doing so can also help to move the shoulders away from the cervicothoracic area.
- Once the shoulders are positioned, adjust patient head and body rotation to obtain a true lateral position. You can avoid cervical rotation by placing the head in a true lateral position, and thoracic rotation by resting your extended flat palm against the patient's shoulders and the inferior posterior ribs, and then adjusting patient rotation until your hand is positioned perpendicular to the tabletop and film, respectively.
- ***Detecting Rotation:*** If the patient is rotated, the articular pillars, posterior ribs, zygapophyseal joints, and humeri move away from each other, obscuring the pedicles and distorting the vertebral bodies. When rotation is demonstrated on a swimmer's radiograph, you can determine which side was rotated anteriorly or posteriorly by evaluating the position of the humeral head positioned closer to the film. If the patient was rotated anteriorly, the humeral head farther from the film is positioned anteriorly (see Rad. 26). If the patient was rotated posteriorly, the humeral head closer to the film is positioned anteriorly, and the humeral head farther from the film is positioned posteriorly (see Rad. 27).
- ***Positioning for Trauma:*** When routine cervical radiographs taken on a trauma patient in whom a subluxation or fracture is suspected do not visualize

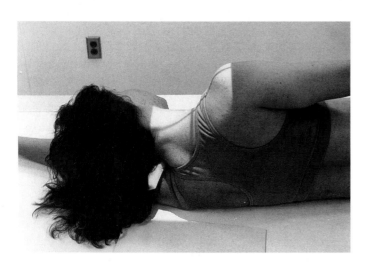

Figure 7-21. Proper patient positioning for recumbent lateral cervicothoracic vertebral radiograph.

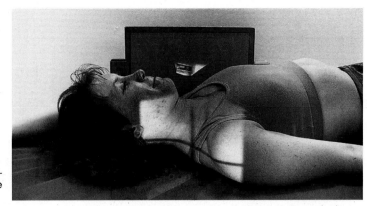

Figure 7-22. Proper patient positioning for lateral cervicothoracic vertebral radiograph taken to evaluate trauma.

the seventh lateral cervical vertebra, take the swimmer's position with the patient's head, neck, and body trunk left as is. Instruct the patient to elevate the arm farther from the x-ray tube and to depress the arm closer to the tube. Then place a grid-cassette against the patient's lateral body surface, centering its transverse axis at a level 1.5 inches (4 cm) superior to the jugular notch (Fig. 7–22). Position the central ray horizontal to the posterior neck surface at the level of the transverse axis of the grid-cassette.

The intervertebral disk spaces are open, and the vertebral bodies are demonstrated without distortion.

- To obtain open disk spaces and undistorted vertebral bodies, position the head in a true lateral position, with the interpupillary line perpendicular to, and the midsagittal plane parallel with, the upright grid holder or tabletop.
- If the patient is in a recumbent lateral position, it may be necessary to elevate the head on a sponge to place it in a lateral position, preventing cervical column tilting (see Rad. 28).

The long axis of the cervicothoracic column is aligned with the long axis of the collimated field.

- Aligning the long axis of the cervicothoracic vertebral column with the long axis of the collimated field allows for tight collimation.
- The cervical and thoracic vertebrae are located in the posterior half of the patient's body. To obtain proper alignment, align the collimator's longitudinal light line

with the coronal plane located about 2 inches (5 cm) anterior to the C7 vertebral prominens.

The first thoracic vertebra is centered within the collimated field. The fifth through seventh cervical vertebrae and the first through third thoracic vertebrae are included within the field.

- Center a perpendicular central ray to the coronal plane located about 2 inches (5 cm) anterior to the palpable vertebral prominens at a level 1.5 inches (4 cm) superior to the jugular notch. Radiographically, the seventh cervical vertebra can be identified on a swimmer's radiograph by locating the elevated clavicle, which is normally seen traversing the seventh cervical vertebra.
- Open the longitudinal collimated field to the patient's mandibular angle. Transverse collimation should be to the cervical skin-line.
- An 8 × 10 inch (18 × 24 cm) film placed lengthwise should be adequate to include all the required anatomical structures.
- ***Depressing the Shoulder Positioned Away from the Film:*** To demonstrate the fifth through seventh cervical vertebrae and the first through third thoracic vertebrae without shoulder superimposition, the shoulder positioned away from the film is depressed. Taking the radiograph on expiration will also aid in lowering the shoulder.

  A 5-degree caudal central ray angulation may be used for a patient who is unable to adequately depress the shoulder positioned farther from the film. This angle projects the shoulder inferiorly.

Critiquing Radiographs

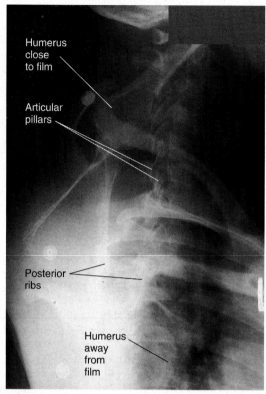

Radiograph 26.

Critique: The right and left articular pillars, zygapophyseal joints, and posterior ribs are demonstrated without superimposition. The humerus that was raised and situated closer to the film is demonstrated posterior to the vertebral column. The shoulder that was depressed and positioned farther from the film was rotated anteriorly.

Correction: Rotate the shoulder positioned farther from the film posteriorly, until your flat palms placed against the shoulders and the posterior ribs, respectively, are aligned perpendicular to the tabletop and upright grid holder.

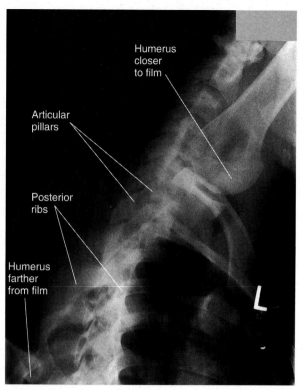

Radiograph 27.

Critique: The right and left articular pillars, zygapophyseal joints, and posterior ribs are demonstrated without superimposition. The humerus that was raised and situated closer to the film is demonstrated anterior to the vertebral column. The shoulder that was depressed and positioned farther from the film was rotated posteriorly.

Correction: Rotate the shoulder positioned farther from the film anteriorly until your flat palms placed against the shoulders and the posterior ribs, respectively, are aligned perpendicular to the tabletop and upright grid holder.

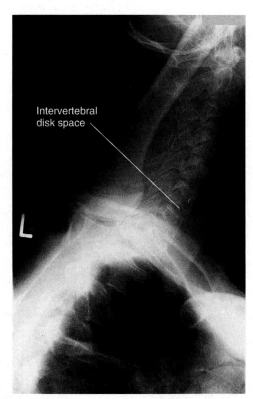

Radiograph 28.

Critique: The intervertebral disk spaces are closed, and the vertebral bodies are distorted. The patient's cervical vertebral column was not positioned parallel with the film.
Correction: Position the midsagittal plane of the head and cervical vertebral column parallel with the film. It may be necessary to prop the head on a sponge to help the patient maintain the position.

THORACIC VERTEBRAE

Anteroposterior Projection

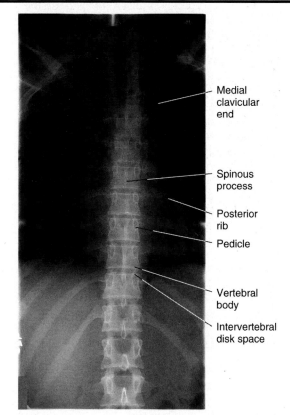

Figure 7-23. Accurately positioned AP thoracic vertebral radiograph.

Radiographic Evaluation

Facility's patient identification requirements are visible on radiograph.
- These requirements usually are facility name, patient name, age, and hospital number, and exam time and date.
- Patient ID plate is positioned so as not to obscure anatomy of interest.

A right or left marker, identifying the correct side of the patient, is present on the radiograph and does not superimpose anatomy of interest.
- Place the marker laterally within the collimated light field so it does not superimpose any portion of the thoracic vertebrae.
- Because the transversely collimated field is coned to about an 8-inch (20-cm) area, make certain that the marker is positioned within 4 inches (10 cm) of the center of the film to guarantee that it will not be cut off.

There is no evidence of preventable artifacts, such as buttons, zippers, undergarments, and necklaces.
- It is recommended that the patient be instructed to change into a snapless hospital gown before the procedure.

Contrast and density are adequate to demonstrate the surrounding mediastinum soft tissue and the bony structures of the thoracic vertebrae and connecting posterior ribs. Penetration is sufficient to visualize the bony trabecular patterns and cortical outlines of the vertebral bodies, pedicles, spinous processes, posterior ribs, and transverse processes.

- An optimal 75 to 85 kVp technique sufficiently penetrates the bony and soft tissue structures of the mediastinum and thoracic vertebrae.

- Use a high-ratio grid and tight collimation to decrease the scattered radiation that reaches the film, reducing fog, improving the visibility of recorded details, and providing a higher-contrast radiograph.

- When an exposure (mAs) is set that adequately demonstrates the lower thoracic vertebrae (T6–T12), the upper thoracic vertebrae (T1–T5) are often overexposed, because of the difference in AP body thickness between these two regions. There are two methods of obtaining uniform density in spite of this difference in thickness. The first method uses a wedge compensating filter and the second method uses the anode-heel effect.

- ***Wedge Filter:*** The wedge filter absorbs x-ray photons before they reach the patient, thus decreasing the number of photons exposing the film where the filter is located. The thicker end of a wedge filter absorbs more photons than the thinner end. When a wedge compensating filter is used, attach it to the x-ray collimator head with the thick end positioned toward the patient's head and the thin end toward the patient's feet. The collimator light projects a shadow of the compensating filter onto the patient's midsagittal plane (Fig. 7–24). The number of the upper thoracic vertebrae that should be covered by the filter's shadow depends on the slope of the patient's sternum and upper thorax. Position the thin edge of the compensating filter's shadow at the inferior sternum and thorax, at the level where they begin to decline (Fig. 7–25).

  Set a technique that adequately exposes the lower thorax. If the filter has been accurately positioned, it

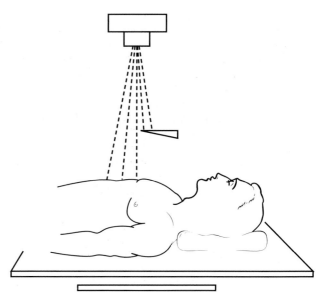

Figure 7–25. Proper placement of compensating filter.

will absorb the excessive radiation directed toward the upper thorax, thus obtaining uniform radiographic density throughout the thoracic column. If the filter was inaccurately positioned, there will be a definite density difference defining where the filter was and was not placed. Positioning the filter too inferiorly on the patient results in an underexposed area where the filter was misplaced (see Rad. 29). Positioning the filter too superiorly results in an overexposed area where the filter should have been placed.

- ***Anode-Heel Effect:*** The anode-heel effect works similar to a filter because it decreases the number of photons reaching the upper thoracic vertebrae and results in decreased density in this area. This method works sufficiently on patients who have very little difference in AP body thickness between their upper and lower thoracic vertebrae, but does not provide an adequate density decrease on patients with larger thickness differences. For the latter patients, use the anode-heel effect in combination with a wedge compensating filter.

  To utilize the anode-heel effect, position the patient's head and upper thoracic vertebrae at the anode end of the tube and the feet and lower thoracic vertebrae at the cathode end. Then set an exposure (mAs) that adequately demonstrates the lower thoracic vertebrae. Because the anode will absorb some of the photons aimed at the anode end of the film, the upper thoracic vertebrae will receive less exposure than the lower vertebrae.

- ***Expiration versus Inspiration Radiograph:*** Patient respiration determines the amount of contrast and density difference demonstrated between the mediastinum and the vertebral column. These differences are a result of the variation in density (number of atoms per given area) that exists between the thoracic cavity and the vertebrae. The thoracic cavity is largely composed of air, which contains very few atoms in a given area; the same area of bone, as in the vertebrae, contain many compacted atoms. As radiation goes

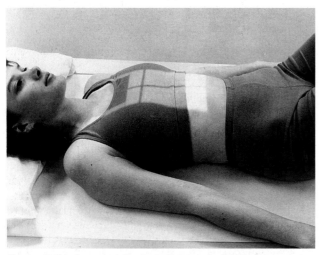

Figure 7–24. Proper patient positioning for AP thoracic vertebral radiograph with compensating filter.

through the patient's body, fewer photons are absorbed in the thoracic cavity than in the vertebral column, because there are fewer atoms in the thoracic cavity for the photons to interact with. Consequently, more photons will penetrate the thoracic cavity to expose the film than penetrate the vertebral column.

Taking the exposure on expiration can help to decrease the thoracic cavity's radiographic density by reducing the air volume and compressing the tissue in this area. This decreased radiographic density allows better visualization of the posterior ribs and mediastinum region. If the AP thoracic vertebral radiograph is exposed while the patient is in full inspiration, the thoracic cavity demonstrates increased radiographic density compared with the vertebral column (see Rad. 30). It should be noted, however, that the contrast created on an AP thoracic vertebral radiograph taken on inspiration can be valuable in detecting thoracic tumors or disease.

The bony trabecular patterns and cortical outlines of the thoracic vertebrae and posterior ribs are sharply defined.

- Sharply defined recorded details are obtained when patient motion is controlled, respiration is halted, and a short object–image distance (OID) is maintained.

The thoracic vertebral column demonstrates a true AP projection: The spinous processes are aligned with the midline of the vertebral bodies, the distances from the vertebral column to the medial (sternal) ends of the clavicles are equal, and the distances from the pedicles to the spinous processes are equal on the two sides.

- An AP thoracic vertebral radiograph is obtained by placing the patient supine on the radiographic table. Position the shoulders and anterior superior iliac spines (ASISs) at equal distances from the tabletop to prevent rotation, and draw the patient's arms away from the thoracic area to keep them from being tucked beneath the patient (Fig. 7–26).
- ***Effect of Rotation:*** The upper and lower thoracic vertebrae can demonstrate rotation independently or simultaneously, depending on which section of the

body is rotated. If the patient's shoulders and upper thorax were rotated and the pelvis and lower thorax remained in an AP projection, the upper thoracic vertebrae demonstrate rotation. If the patient's pelvis and lower thorax were rotated and the thorax and shoulders remained in an AP projection, the lower thoracic vertebrae demonstrate rotation. If the patient's thorax and pelvis are rotated simultaneously, the entire thoracic column demonstrates rotation.

- ***Detecting Rotation:*** Rotation is effectively detected on an AP thoracic radiograph by comparing the distances between pedicles and spinous processes on the same vertebra and the distances between the vertebral column and the sternal ends of the clavicles. When no rotation is present, the comparable distances are equal. If one side demonstrates a greater distance, vertebral rotation is present. The side demonstrating a greater distance is the side of the patient positioned closer to the tabletop and film.
- ***Distinguishing Rotation from Scoliosis:*** In patients with spinal scoliosis, the thoracic bodies may appear rotated because of the lateral twisting of the vertebrae. Scoliosis of the vertebral column can be very severe, demonstrating a large amount of lateral deviation, or can be subtle, demonstrating only a small amount of deviation. Severe scoliosis is very obvious and is seldom mistaken for patient rotation, whereas subtle scoliotic changes may be easily mistaken for rotation.

Although both conditions demonstrate unequal distances between the pedicles and spinous processes, certain clues can be used to distinguish subtle scoliosis from rotation. The long axis of a rotated vertebral column remains straight, whereas the scoliotic vertebral column demonstrates lateral deviation. When the thoracic vertebrae demonstrate rotation, it has been caused by the rotation of the upper or lower torso. Rotation of the middle thoracolumbar vertebrae does not occur unless the upper and lower thoracic vertebrae also demonstrate rotation. On a scoliosis radiograph, the thoracolumbar vertebrae may demonstrate rotation without corresponding upper or lower vertebral rotation. Familiarity with the difference between a rotated thoracic vertebral column and a scoliotic one prevents unnecessary repeats on patients with spinal scoliosis.

The intervertebral disk spaces are open, and the vertebral bodies are demonstrated without distortion.

- The thoracic vertebral column demonstrates a kyphotic curvature. Because the thoracic vertebrae have very limited flexion and extension movements, it is difficult to achieve a significant reduction of this curvature. A small reduction can be obtained by placing the patient's head on a thin pillow or sponge and flexing the hips and knees until the lower back rests firmly against the tabletop; both procedures improve the relationship of the upper and lower vertebral disk spaces and bodies with the x-ray beam. The head position reduces the upper vertebral curvature, and the hip and knee position reduces the lower vertebral curvature. If the disk spaces are not aligned parallel with the x-ray beam and the vertebral bodies are not aligned

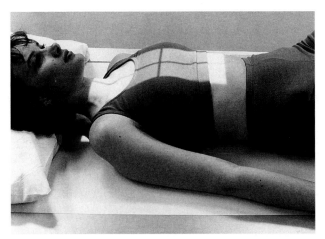

Figure 7–26. Proper patient positioning for AP thoracic vertebral radiograph without compensating filter.

perpendicular to the x-ray beam, it is difficult for the reviewer to evaluate the height of the disk spaces and vertebral bodies (see Rad. 31).

- *Positioning for Kyphosis:* To demonstrate open disk spaces and undistorted vertebral bodies on a patient with excessive spinal kyphosis, it may be necessary to angle the central ray until it is perpendicular to the vertebral area of interest. Because it is painful for such a patient to lie supine on the radiographic table, it is best to perform the exam with the patient upright, or in a lateral recumbent position with use of a horizontal beam.

The long axis of the thoracic vertebral column is aligned with the long axis of the collimated field.

- Aligning the long axis of the thoracic vertebral column with the long axis of the collimated field ensures against lateral flexion and allows tight collimation. To obtain good vertebral column alignment, align the

long axis of the sternum with the collimator's longitudinal light line.

The seventh thoracic vertebra is centered within the collimated field. The seventh cervical vertebra, 1st through 12th thoracic vertebrae, first lumbar vertebra, and 2.5 inches (6.25 cm) of the posterior ribs and mediastinum on each side of the vertebral column are included within the field.

- Center a perpendicular central ray to the patient's midsagittal plane at a level halfway between the sternal angle and the xiphoid to position the seventh thoracic vertebra in the center of the collimated field.
- Open the longitudinal collimation the full 17-inch (43-cm) film length for adult patients. Transverse collimation should be to about an 8-inch (20 cm) field.
- A 14 × 17 inch (35 × 43 cm) film placed lengthwise should be adequate to include all the required anatomical structures.

Critiquing Radiographs

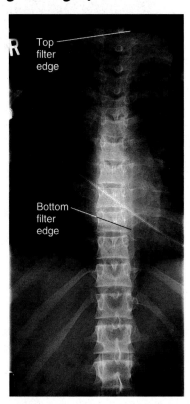

Radiograph 29.

Critique: The sixth through ninth thoracic vertebrae are underexposed. The wedge compensating filter was positioned too inferiorly.
Correction: Position the shadow of the compensating filter's thin edge at the beginning of the downward slope of the patient's sternum and upper thorax, as demonstrated in Figure 7–25.

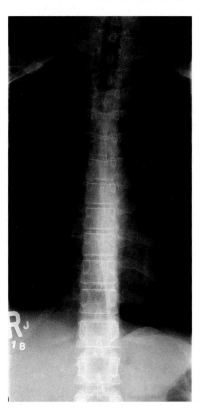

Radiograph 30.

Critique: The thoracic cavity is overexposed. The radiograph was taken on inspiration.
Correction: To demonstrate the posterior ribs, take the radiograph with the patient in full expiration. If a mediastinal tumor or disease is in question, however, no correction is needed.

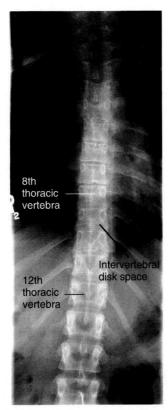

Radiograph 31.

Critique: The eighth through twelfth intervertebral disk spaces are obscured and the vertebral bodies distorted. The patient's legs were extended.
Correction: Flex the patient's hips and knees, placing the feet and back firmly against the tabletop.

Thoracic Vertebrae: Lateral Position

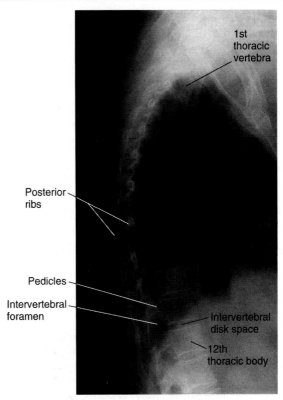

Figure 7-27. Accurately positioned lateral thoracic vertebral radiograph.

Radiographic Evaluation

Facility's patient identification requirements are visible on radiograph.

- These requirements usually are facility name, patient name, age, and hospital number, and exam time and date.
- Patient ID plate is positioned so as not to obscure anatomy of interest.

A right or left marker, identifying the side of the patient positioned closer to the film, is present on the radiograph and does not superimpose anatomy of interest.

- Place the marker anteriorly within the collimated light field, along the lower cassette edge, so it does not superimpose any portion of the thoracic vertebrae.
- Because the transversely collimated field is coned to about an 8-inch (20-cm) area, make certain that the marker is positioned within 4 inches (10 cm) of the center of the film to guarantee that it will not be cut off.

There is no evidence of preventable artifacts, such as buttons, zippers, and jewelry.

- It is recommended the patient be instructed to change into a snapless hospital gown before the procedure.

Contrast and density are adequate to demonstrate the bony structures of the thoracic vertebrae. Penetration

is sufficient to visualize the bony trabecular patterns and cortical outlines of the vertebral bodies, pedicles, and intervertebral foramina.

- An optimal 80 to 90 kVp technique sufficiently penetrates the bony structures of the thoracic vertebrae; this value should not exceed 90 kVp, or an overpenetrated radiograph may result. The thoracic cavity is largely composed of air, which has low density (contains very few atoms per given area). As the radiation goes through the air-filled thorax, few photons are absorbed, because there are few atoms in the thoracic cavity for the photons to interact with, resulting in a radiograph demonstrating high density and a low contrast.

- Use tight collimation, a high-ratio grid, and a lead protection shield placed on the tabletop at the edge of the posteriorly collimated field to reduce the amount of scattered radiation that reaches the film, providing higher contrast and better visibility of recorded details.

- *Breathing Technique:* The thoracic vertebrae have many overlying structures, including the axillary ribs and lungs. Using a long exposure time (3 to 4 seconds) and requiring the patient to breathe shallowly (costal breathing) during the exposure forces a slow and steady, upward and outward movement of the ribs and lungs. This technique is often referred to as *breathing technique.* This movement causes blurring of the ribs and lung markings on the radiograph, providing greater thoracic vertebral visualization.[6] Deep breathing, which requires movement (elevation) of the sternum and a faster and expanded upward and outward movement of the ribs and lungs, should be avoided during the breathing technique, because deep breathing results in motion of the thoracic cavity and vertebrae (see Rad. 32).

  Note: If patient motion cannot be avoided when using the extended 3 to 4 seconds for breathing technique, take the radiograph on expiration to reduce the air volume within the thoracic cavity.

The bony trabecular patterns and cortical outlines of the thoracic vertebrae are sharply defined.

- Sharply defined recorded details are obtained when patient motion is controlled and a short object–image distance (OID) is maintained.

The thoracic vertebrae demonstrate a true lateral position: The intervertebral foramina are clearly visualized, the pedicles are in profile, the posterior surfaces of each vertebral body are superimposed, and no more than 0.5 inch (1 cm) of space is demonstrated between the posterior ribs.

- To obtain a lateral thoracic vertebral radiograph, place the patient on the radiographic table in a lateral recumbent position. Whether the patient is lying on the right or left side is not significant, although left-side positioning is easier for the technologist (Fig. 7–28). Abduct the patient's arms to a 90-degree angle with the body, to prevent the humeri or their soft tissue from obscuring the thoracic vertebrae. Flex the patient's knees and hips for support, and position a pillow or sponge between the knees. The thickness of the pillow or sponge should be enough to prevent the side of the pelvis situated farther from the film from rotating anteriorly but not so thick as to cause posterior rotation. To avoid vertebral rotation, align the shoulders, the posterior ribs, and the posterior pelvic wings perpendicular to the tabletop and film by resting an extended flat palm against each, respectively, then adjusting patient rotation until the hand is positioned perpendicular to the film.

- *Effect of Rotation:* The upper and lower thoracic vertebrae can demonstrate rotation independently or simultaneously, depending on which section of the torso was rotated. If the shoulders and the superoposterior ribs were not placed on top of each other but the posterior pelvic wings and inferoposterior ribs were aligned, the upper thoracic vertebrae demonstrate rotation and the lower thoracic vertebrae demonstrate a true lateral position. If the posterior pelvic wings and inferoposterior ribs were rotated but the shoulders and superoposterior ribs were placed on top of each other, the lower thoracic vertebrae demon-

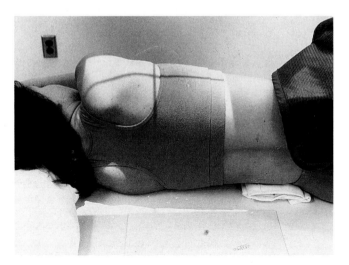

Figure 7-28. Proper patient positioning for lateral thoracic vertebral radiograph.

strate rotation and the upper vertebrae demonstrate a true lateral position.

- **Detecting Rotation:** Rotation can be detected on a lateral thoracic vertebral radiograph by evaluating the superimposition of the right and left posterior surfaces of the vertebral bodies and the amount of posterior rib superimposition. On a nonrotated lateral thoracic radiograph, the posterior surfaces are superimposed and the posterior ribs are nearly superimposed. Because the posterior ribs positioned farther from the film were placed at a greater OID than the other side, they demonstrate more magnification. This magnification prevents the posterior ribs from being directly superimposed, but positions them about 0.50 inch (1 cm) apart. This distance is based on a 40-inch (102-cm) source–image distance (SID). If a longer SID is used, the distance between the posterior ribs is decreased, and if a shorter SID is used, the distance is increased. Upon rotation, the right and left posterior surfaces of the vertebral bodies are radiographically demonstrated one anterior to the other.

Because the two sides of the thorax and vertebrae are mirror images, it is very difficult to determine from a rotated lateral thoracic radiograph which side of the patient was rotated anteriorly and which posteriorly. If the patient was only slightly rotated, one way of determining which way the patient was rotated is to evaluate the amount of posterior rib superimposition. If the patient's elevated side was rotated posteriorly, the posterior ribs demonstrate more than 0.50 inch (1 cm) of space between them (see Rad. 33). If the patient's elevated side was rotated anteriorly, the posterior ribs are superimposed on slight rotation (see Rad. 34) and demonstrate greater separation as rotation of the patient increases.

- **Distinguishing Rotation from Scoliosis:** On the radiograph of a patient with spinal scoliosis, the lung field may appear rotated owing to the lateral deviation of the vertebral column (see Rad. 12, page 51). On such a radiograph, the posterior ribs demonstrate differing degrees of separation depending on the severity of the scoliosis. View the accompanying AP thoracic radiograph to confirm this patient condition. Familiarizing yourself with the lateral radiographs obtained on patients with scoliosis prevents unnecessary repeats taken when scoliosis is mistaken for rotation.

The intervertebral disk spaces are open, and the vertebral bodies are demonstrated without distortion.

- The thoracic vertebral column is capable of lateral flexion. When the patient is placed in a lateral recumbent position, the vertebral column may not be aligned parallel with the tabletop and film, but may sag at the level of the lower thoracic vertebrae, especially in a patient who has wide hips and a narrow waist (Fig. 7–29). If the patient's thoracic column is allowed to sag, the diverging x-ray beams are not aligned parallel with the intervertebral disk spaces and perpendicular with the vertebral bodies. Radiographically, lateral flexion is most evident at the lower thoracic vertebral bodies where there are closed disk spaces and distorted vertebral bodies (see Rad. 35). For a patient who has

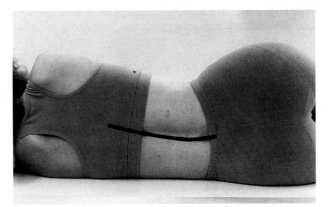

Figure 7-29. Poor alignment of vertebral column with table-top.

a sagging thoracic column, it may be necessary to tuck a radiolucent sponge between the lateral body surface and the tabletop just superior to the iliac crest, elevating the sagging area. The sponge should be thick enough to bring the thoracic vertebral column parallel with the tabletop and film (see Fig. 7–28).

- An alternative method of obtaining open disk spaces and undistorted vertebral bodies on a patient whose thoracic column is sagging is to angle the central ray 5 to 10 degrees cephalically. The degree of cephalic angulation used should align the central ray perpendicular to the thoracic vertebral column.

The long axis of the thoracic vertebral column is aligned with the long axis of the collimated field.

- Aligning the long axis of the thoracic vertebral column with the collimator's longitudinal light allows for tight collimation, which is important in the reduction of scattered radiation.

The 7th thoracic vertebra is centered within the collimated field. The seventh cervical vertebra, the 1st through 12th thoracic vertebrae, and the first lumbar vertebrae are included within the field.

- Center a perpendicular central ray to a point 1 inch (2.5 cm) superior to the inferior angle of the elevated scapula, with the patient's arm positioned at a 90-degree angle with the body, to place T7 at the center of the collimated field.
- Open the longitudinal collimation the full 17-inch (43-cm) film length for adult patients. Transverse collimation should be to an 8-inch (20-cm) field.
- A 14 × 17 inch (35 × 43 cm) film placed lengthwise should be adequate to include all the required anatomical structures.
- **Verifying Inclusion of All Thoracic Vertebrae:** When, viewing a lateral thoracic radiograph, you can be sure the 12th thoracic vertebra has been included by locating the vertebra that has the last rib attached to it; this is the 12th vertebra. To confirm this finding, follow the posterior vertebral bodies of the lower thoracic and upper lumbar vertebrae, watching for the subtle change in curvature from kyphotic to lordotic. The twelfth thoracic vertebra is located just above it.

The first thoracic vertebra can be identified radiographically by counting up from the twelfth thoracic vertebra or by locating the seventh cervical vertebral prominens. The first thoracic vertebra is at the same level as this prominens.

- **Swimmer's Position Radiograph:** Because of shoulder thickness and the superimposition of the shoulders over the first through third thoracic vertebrae, it may be necessary to take a supplementary view of this area to demonstrate the thoracic vertebrae. Refer to page 337 for specifics.

Critiquing Radiographs

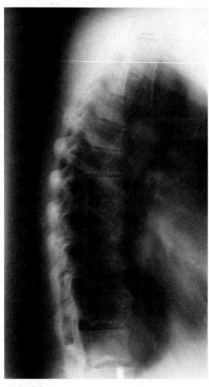

Radiograph 32.

Critique: The thoracic vertebrae, ribs, and lung markings demonstrate a blurring of the recorded details. The radiograph was exposed using deep breathing technique during the exposure, causing patient motion.

Correction: Instruct the patient to breath shallowly. If the patient is unable to perform costal breathing, take the exposure on expiration.

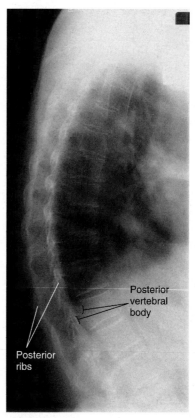

Radiograph 33.

Critique: The posterior surfaces of the vertebral bodies are demonstrated without superimposition, and more than 0.50 inch (1 cm) of space is visualized between the posterior ribs. The elevated side of the thorax was rotated posteriorly.

Correction: Rotate the elevated thorax anteriorly until a flat palm placed against the shoulders, posterior ribs, and posterior pelvic wings is aligned perpendicular to the tabletop. The amount of rotation required is half the distance demonstrated between the posterior surfaces of the vertebral bodies.

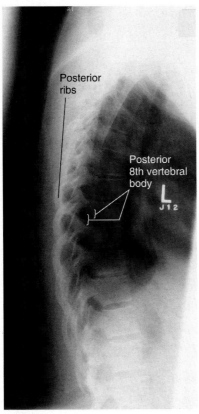

Radiograph 34.

Critique: The posterior surfaces of the vertebral bodies are demonstrated without superimposition, and the posterior ribs are superimposed. The elevated side of the thorax was rotated anteriorly.

Correction: Rotate the elevated thorax posteriorly until a flat palm placed against the shoulder, posterior ribs, and posterior pelvic wings is aligned perpendicular to the tabletop. The amount of rotation required is half the distance demonstrated between the posterior surfaces of the vertebral bodies.

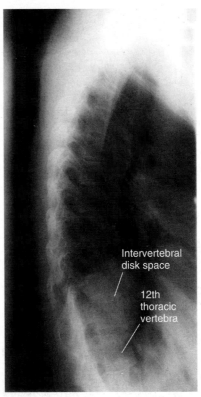

Radiograph 35.

Critique: The T8 through T12 intervertebral disk spaces are obscured and vertebral bodies distorted. The thoracic vertebral column was not aligned parallel with the tabletop.

Correction: Position a radiolucent sponge between the lateral body surface and tabletop just superior to the iliac crest. The sponge should be thick enough to align the thoracic vertebral column parallel with the tabletop. If a sponge cannot be used, the central ray can be angled cephalically until it is perpendicular to the thoracic vertebral column.

References

1. Roger LF. Radiology of Skeletal Trauma. New York: Churchill Livingstone, 1982, p 273.
2. Harris JH Jr. Acute injuries of the spine. Semin Roentgenol 13:53–68, 1978.
3. Whalen JP, Woodruff CL. The cervical prevertebral fat stripe. AJR 109:445–451, 1970.
4. Bushong SC. Radiologic Science for Technologists, ed 5. St. Louis: CV Mosby, 1993, pp 263–264.
5. Berquist TH. Imaging of Orthopedic Trauma and Surgery. Philadelphia: WB Saunders, 1986, pp 105–108.
6. Anagnostakos NP, Tortora GJ. Principles of Anatomy and Physiology, ed 6. New York: Harper & Row, 1990, pp 702–704.

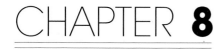

CHAPTER 8

Radiographic Critique of the Lumbar Vertebrae, Sacrum, and Coccyx

LUMBAR VERTEBRAE

Anteroposterior Projection

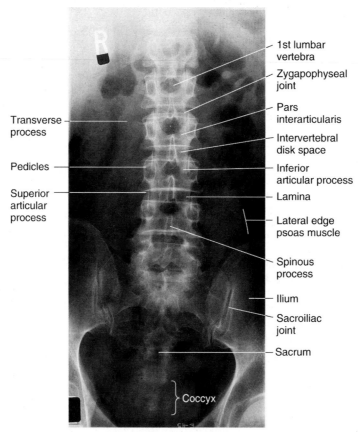

Figure 8-1. Accurately positioned AP lumbar vertebral radiograph.

Radiographic Evaluation

Facility's patient identification requirements are visible on radiograph.

- These requirements usually are facility name, patient name, age, and hospital number, and exam time and date.
- Patient ID plate is positioned so as not to obscure anatomy of interest.

A right or left marker, identifying the correct side of the patient, is present on the radiograph and does not superimpose anatomy of interest.

- Place the marker laterally within the collimated light field so it does not superimpose any portion of the lumbar vertebrae.
- Because the transversely collimated field is coned to about an 8-inch (20-cm) area, make certain the marker is positioned within 4 inches (10 cm) of the center of the film to guarantee it will not be cut off.

350

There is no evidence of preventable artifacts, such as buttons and zippers.

- It is recommended that the patient be instructed to change into a snapless hospital gown before the procedure.

Contrast and density are adequate to demonstrate the psoas muscle and the bony structures of the lumbar vertebrae. Penetration is sufficient to visualize the bony trabecular patterns and cortical outlines of the vertebral bodies, pedicles, spinous processes, laminae, and pars interarticulari.

- An optimal 75 to 85 kVp technique sufficiently penetrates the soft tissue and bony structures of the lumbar vertebrae.
- Use a high-ratio grid and tight collimation to reduce the scattered radiation that reaches the film, reducing fog, increasing the visibility of recorded details and providing a higher-contrast radiograph.
- ***Soft Tissue Structures of Lumbar Vertebrae:*** The soft tissue structures that should be visualized on AP lumbar vertebral radiographs are the psoas muscles. They are located lateral to the lumbar vertebrae, originating at the first lumbar vertebra on each side and extending to the corresponding side's lesser trochanter. They are used in lateral flexion and rotation of the thigh and in flexion of the vertebral column. Radiographically, they are visualized on an AP lumbar radiograph on each side of the vertebral bodies as long triangular soft tissue shadows.[1]

The bony trabecular patterns and cortical outlines of the lumbar vertebrae are sharply defined.

- Sharply defined recorded details are obtained when patient motion is controlled, respiration is halted, and a short object–image distance (OID) is maintained.

The lumbar vertebrae demonstrate a true AP projection: The spinous processes are aligned with the midline of the vertebral bodies, and the distances from the pedicles to the spinous processes and from the sacroiliac joints to the spinous processes are equal on either side. When demonstrated, the sacrum and coccyx should be centered within the inlet pelvis and aligned with the symphysis pubis.

- An AP lumbar vertebral radiograph is obtained by placing the patient supine on the radiographic table. Position the shoulders and anterior superior iliac spines at equal distances from the tabletop to prevent rotation, and draw the arms away from the abdominal area to prevent them from being tucked beneath the body (Fig. 8–2).
- ***Effect of Rotation:*** The upper and lower lumbar vertebrae can demonstrate rotation independently or simultaneously, depending on which section of the body is rotated. If the patient's thorax was rotated and the pelvis remained in an AP projection, the upper lumbar vertebrae demonstrate rotation. If the patient's pelvis was rotated and the thorax remained in an AP projection, the lower lumbar vertebrae demonstrate rotation. If the patient's thorax and pelvis were rotated simultaneously, the entire lumbar column demonstrates rotation.

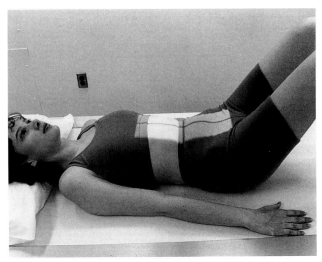

Figure 8–2. Proper patient positioning for AP lumbar vertebral radiograph.

- ***Detecting Rotation:*** Rotation is effectively detected on an AP lumbar radiograph by comparing the distances between each pedicle and the spinous processes on the same vertebra and by comparing the distances between each sacroiliac joint and the spinous processes. If no rotation was present, the comparable distances are equal. If one side demonstrates a greater distance, vertebral rotation was present (see Rad. 1). The side demonstrating the greater distance was the side of the patient positioned closer to the tabletop and film. Lower lumbar rotation can be easily detected by evaluating the position of the sacrum and coccyx within the pelvic inlet. If no rotation was present, they are centered within the pelvic inlet. Upon rotation, the sacrum and coccyx rotate toward the side of the pelvic inlet positioned farther from the film.
- ***Distinguishing Rotation from Scoliosis:*** On patients with spinal scoliosis, the lumbar bodies may appear rotated owing to the lateral twisting of the vertebrae. Scoliosis of the vertebral column can be very severe, demonstrating a large amount of lateral deviation, or can be subtle, demonstrating only a small amount of deviation. Severe scoliosis is very obvious and is seldom mistaken for patient rotation (see Rad. 2), whereas subtle scoliotic changes can be easily mistaken for rotation (see Rad. 3).

  Although both conditions demonstrate unequal distances between the pedicles and spinous processes, certain clues can be used to distinguish subtle scoliosis from rotation. The long axis of a rotated vertebral column remains straight, whereas the scoliotic vertebral column demonstrates lateral deviation. If the lumbar vertebrae demonstrate rotation, it has been caused by the rotation of the upper or lower torso. Rotation of the middle lumbar vertebrae (L3–L4) does not occur unless the lower thoracic or upper or lower lumbar vertebrae also demonstrate rotation. On a scoliotic radiograph, the middle lumbar vertebrae may demonstrate rotation without corresponding upper or lower vertebral rotation. Familiarity with the differences between a rotated lumbar vertebral column and a scoliotic one prevents unnecessary repeats on patients with spinal scoliosis.

The intervertebral disk spaces are open, and the vertebral bodies are demonstrated without distortion.

- When the patient is in a supine position with the legs extended, the lumbar vertebrae have an exaggerated lordotic curvature. Taking an AP lumbar radiograph with the patient in this position results in closed intervertebral disk spaces and distorted vertebral bodies, because of the way the x-ray beams are directed at the disk spaces and vertebral bodies (Fig. 8–3). To straighten the lumbar vertebral column—thereby aligning the intervertebral disk spaces parallel with and the vertebral bodies perpendicular to the x-ray beam—flex the patient's knees and hips until the lower back rests firmly against the tabletop (Fig. 8–4).
- **_Effect of Lordotic Curvature:_** Radiographically, one can determine how well the central ray paralleled the intervertebral disk spaces by evaluating the openness of the T12 through L3 intervertebral disk spaces and the visualization of the iliac spines without pelvic brim superimposition. If the lordotic curvature was adequately reduced, the disk spaces are open and the iliac spines are only partially demonstrated without pelvic brim superimposition. If the lordotic curvature was not adequately reduced, the intervertebral disk spaces are closed and the iliac spines are demonstrated without pelvic brim superimposition (see Rad. 4).

The long axis of the lumbar vertebral column is aligned with the long axis of the collimated field.

- Aligning the long axis of the lumbar vertebral column with the long axis of the collimated field ensures

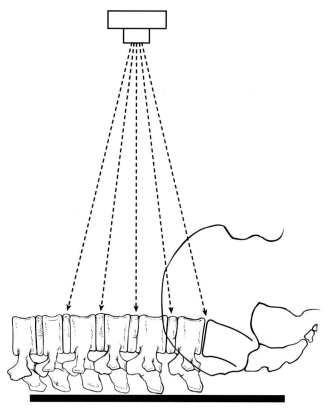

Figure 8-4. Alignment of central ray and lumbar vertebrae when legs are flexed.

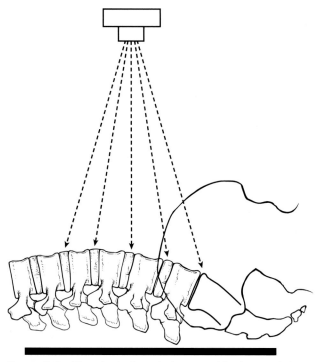

Figure 8-3. Alignment of central ray and lumbar vertebrae when legs are not flexed.

against lateral lumbar flexion and allows tight collimation. To obtain proper upper vertebral alignment, align the xiphoid with the collimator's longitudinal light line. To obtain proper lower vertebral column alignment, find the point halfway between the patient's palpable anterior superior iliac spines. Then align this point with the collimator's longitudinal light line. Do not assume that the patient's navel is positioned directly above the vertebral column; often, it is shifted to one side.

If a 14 × 17 inch (35 × 43 cm) film placed lengthwise was used, the L4–L5 intervertebral disk space and the iliac crest are centered within the collimated field. The 12th thoracic vertebra, 1st through 5th lumbar vertebrae, sacroiliac joints, sacrum, coccyx, and psoas muscles are included within the field. If an 11 × 14 inch (28 × 35 cm) film placed lengthwise was used, the L3–L4 intervertebral disk space is centered within the collimated field. The 12th thoracic vertebra, 1st through 5th lumbar vertebrae, sacroiliac joints, and psoas muscles are included within the field.

- Center a perpendicular central ray to the patient's midsagittal plane at the level of the iliac crest for a 14 × 17 inch (35 × 43 cm) film and at a level 1 to 1.5 inches (2.5 to 4 cm) superior to the iliac crest for 11 × 14 inch (28 × 35 cm) film. The superior centering point is needed for slender patients; patients with greater body thickness require the inferior centering point.

- Open the longitudinal collimation the full 17-inch (43-cm) or 14-inch (35-cm) film length for adult patients. Transverse collimation should be to about an 8-inch (20-cm) field.
- **_Gonadal Shielding:_** Use gonadal protection shielding on all male and female patients. If the sacrum and coccyx are of interest, female patients should not be shielded, since the shield will obscure the lower sacrum and coccyx.

Critiquing Radiographs

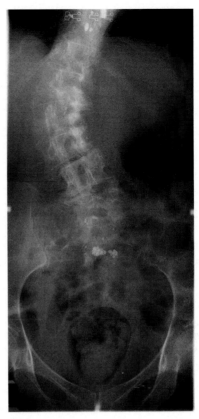

Radiograph 2.

Critique: The vertebral column demonstrates severe spinal scoliosis.

Correction: No correction movement is required. An AP lumbar radiograph of a patient with scoliosis appears rotated.

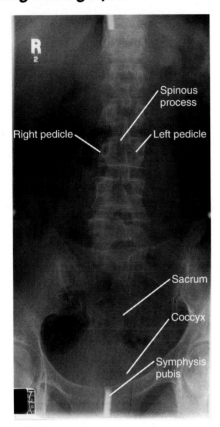

Radiograph 1.

Critique: The distances from the left pedicles to the spinous processes are less than the distances from the right pedicles to the spinous processes, and the sacrum and coccyx are rotated toward the left lateral inlet pelvis. The patient was rotated onto the right side (RPO).

Correction: Rotate the patient toward the left side until the shoulders and the anterior superior iliac spines are positioned at equal distances from the film.

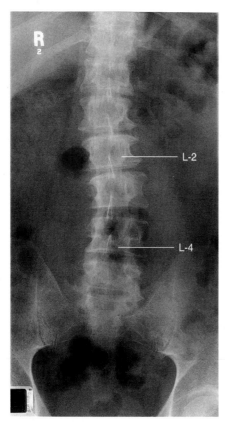

Radiograph 3.

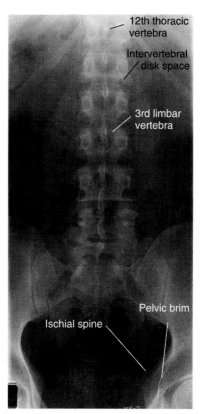

Radiograph 4.

Critique: The vertebral column deviates laterally at the level of second through fourth lumbar vertebrae, the sacrum is centered within the pelvic inlet, and the distances from the pedicles to the spinous processes of the eleventh thoracic vertebra and fifth lumbar vertebra are nearly equal. The vertebral column demonstrates subtle spinal scoliosis.

Correction: No correction movement is required. An AP lumbar radiograph of a patient with scoliosis appears rotated.

Critique: The T12 to L3 intervertebral disk spaces are closed, and the lumbar bodies are distorted. The iliac spines are demonstrated without pelvic brim superimposition. The lordotic curvature of the spine was not reduced, as demonstrated in Figure 8–3.

Correction: Flex the hips and knees until the lower back rests firmly against the tabletop, restraightening the lumbar vertebrae as demonstrated in Figure 8–4.

Lumbar Vertebrae: Posterior Oblique Position

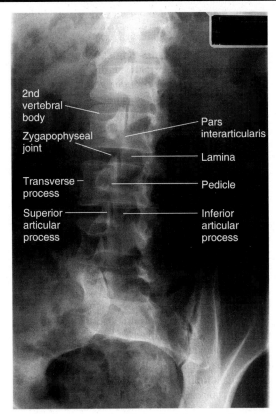

2nd vertebral body

Zygapophyseal joint

Transverse process

Superior articular process

Pars interarticularis

Lamina

Pedicle

Inferior articular process

Figure 8-5. Accurately positioned oblique lumbar vertebral radiograph.

Radiographic Evaluation

Facility's patient identification requirements are visible on radiograph.

- These requirements usually are facility name, patient name, age, and hospital number, and exam time and date.
- Patient ID plate is positioned toward the upper lumbar region so as not to obscure anatomy of interest.

A right or left marker, identifying the side of the patient situated closer to the film, is present on the radiograph and does not superimpose anatomy of interest.

- Place the marker laterally within the collimated light field, along the upper edge of the cassette, so it does not superimpose any portion of the lumbar vertebrae.
- Because the transversely collimated field is coned to about an 8-inch (20-cm) area, make certain that the marker is positioned within 4 inches (10 cm) of the center of the film to guarantee that it will not be cut off.

There is no evidence of preventable artifacts, such as buttons and zippers.

- It is recommended that the patient be instructed to change into a snapless hospital gown before the procedure.

Contrast and density are adequate to demonstrate the surrounding soft tissue and bony structures of the lumbar vertebrae. Penetration is sufficient to visualize the bony trabecular patterns and cortical outlines of the vertebral bodies, pedicles, pars interarticulari, zygapophyseal joints, and superior and inferior articular processes.

- An optimal 75 to 85 kVp technique sufficiently penetrates the bony and soft tissue structures of the lumbar vertebrae.
- Use tight collimation and a high-ratio grid to reduce the amount of scattered radiation that reaches the film, providing higher contrast and better visibility of recorded detail.

The bony trabecular patterns and cortical outlines of the lumbar vertebrae are sharply defined.

- Sharply defined recorded details are obtained when patient motion is controlled, respiration is halted, and a short object–image distance (OID) is maintained.
- This exam can be performed using either a posterior or anterior oblique position. In the posterior oblique position (Fig. 8–6), the zygapophyseal joints of interest are placed closer to the film, and in the anterior oblique position, the zygapophyseal joints of interest are positioned farther from the film, resulting in greater magnification.

The lumbar vertebrae have been adequately rotated: The superior and inferior articular processes are in profile, the zygapophyseal joints are clearly visualized, and the pedicles are demonstrated in the center of the vertebral bodies. The ears, necks, eyes, feet, and bodies of the "Scottie dogs" are well defined.

- A posterior oblique lumbar vertebral radiograph is obtained by placing the patient supine on the radiographic table, then rotating the patient toward the side until the superior and inferior articular processes are positioned in profile. The knees should be flexed as needed for support.

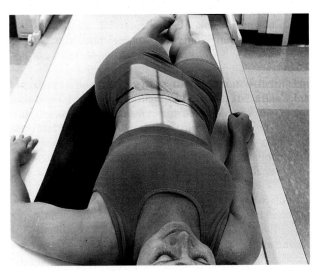

Figure 8-6. Proper patient positioning for posterior oblique lumbar vertebral radiograph.

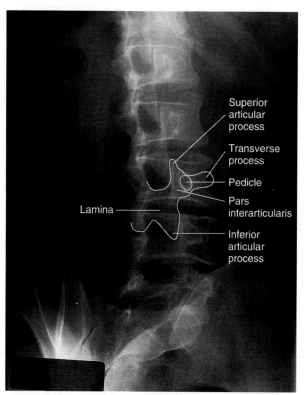

Figure 8–7. Identifying "Scottie dogs" and lumbar anatomy.

Labels on figure: Superior articular process, Transverse process, Pedicle, Pars interarticularis, Inferior articular process, Lamina

- The articular processes are placed in profile by rotating the thorax until the midcoronal plane is at a 40- to 45-degree angle with the film and rotating the pelvis until the midcoronal plane is at a 55- to 60-degree angle with the film (see Fig. 8–6). The difference in the degree of obliquity needed for the upper lumbar vertebrae (L1–L2) and lower lumbar vertebrae (L5–S1) is a result of the gradual increase in vertebral body width and corresponding increase in separation between the right and left articular processes from the first through fifth lumbar vertebrae. To demonstrate the right and the left articular processes and zygapophyseal joints of each vertebra, both right and left posterior oblique radiographs must be taken.
- **"Scottie Dogs" on Oblique Lumbar Radiographs:** The accuracy of an oblique lumbar radiograph is often judged by the visualization of five "Scottie dogs" that are stacked on top of one another. Figure 8–7 is a close-up of an accurately positioned oblique lumbar vertebra with the "Scottie dog" parts outlined and labeled. It should be noted that the

"Scottie dogs" can be identified even on poorly positioned oblique lumbar radiographs. One should always judge the openness of each zygapophyseal joint to determine whether the lumbar vertebrae have been adequately rotated.

Because different degrees of patient obliquity are required to demonstrate the upper and lower zygapophyseal joints, they may not be demonstrated as open joints simultaneously. If a lumbar vertebra was not rotated enough to position the superior and inferior articular processes (ear and front leg of "Scottie dog") in profile, the corresponding zygapophyseal joint is closed, the pedicle (eye of "Scottie dog") is situated closer to the lateral vertebral body surface than the vertebral body midline, and more of the lamina (body of "Scottie dog") is demonstrated (see Rad. 5). If a lumbar vertebra was rotated more than needed to position the superior and inferior articular processes in profile, the corresponding zygapophyseal joint is closed, the pedicle and transverse process (nose of "Scottie dog") are distorted, and less of the lamina is visualized (see Rad. 6).

The long axis of the lumbar vertebral column is aligned with the long axis of the collimated field.
- Aligning the long axis of the lumbar vertebral column with the long axis of the collimated field allows for tighter collimation.

The third lumbar vertebra is centered within the collimated field. The 12th thoracic vertebra, 1st through 5th lumbar vertebrae, 1st and 2nd sacral segments, and sacroiliac joints are included within the field.
- Center a perpendicular central ray 2 inches (5 cm) medial to the elevated anterior superior iliac spine (ASIS) at a level 1 to 1.5 inches (2.5 to 4 cm) superior to the iliac crest. The superior centering point is needed on slender patients, whereas patients with greater body thickness require the inferior centering point.
- Open the longitudinally collimated field the full 14-inch (35-cm) film length for adult patients. Transverse collimation should be to an 8-inch (20-cm) field.
- An 11 × 14 inch (28 × 35 cm) film placed lengthwise should be adequate to include all the required anatomical structures.
- **Gonadal Shielding:** Use gonadal protection shielding on all male patients. Female patients should be shielded, although it is important that no sacral information is covered by the shield. Remember that a shield placed on top of the patient greatly magnifies.

Critiquing Radiographs

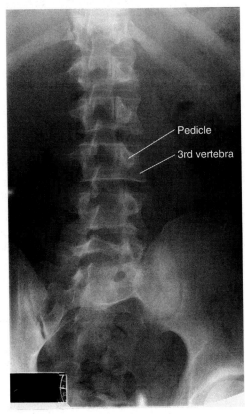

Radiograph 5.

Critique: The third, fourth, and fifth lumbar vertebrae's superior and inferior articular processes are not demonstrated in profile, their corresponding zygapophyseal joint spaces are closed, and their pedicles (eyes of "Scottie dog") are visualized closer to the vertebrae's lateral vertebral body surfaces than to their midlines. The patient's inferior lumbar vertebrae and pelvis were in insufficient obliquity.

Correction: While maintaining the degree of thoracic and upper lumbar vertebral obliquity, increase the lower lumbar vertebral and pelvic rotation.

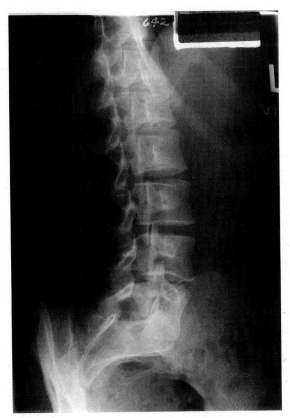

Radiograph 6.

Critique: This patient has six lumbar vertebrae. The first through third lumbar vertebrae's superior and inferior articular processes are not demonstrated in profile, their corresponding zygapophyseal joint spaces are closed, their laminae are obscured, and their pedicles and transverse processes (nose of "Scottie dog") are distorted. The patient's upper lumbar vertebrae and thorax were in excessive obliquity.

Correction: While maintaining the degree of pelvic and lower lumbar vertebral obliquity, decrease the upper lumbar vertebral and thoracic rotation.

Lumbar Vertebrae: Lateral Position

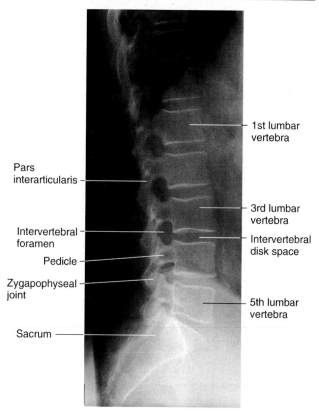

Pars interarticularis

1st lumbar vertebra

3rd lumbar vertebra

Intervertebral foramen

Intervertebral disk space

Pedicle

Zygapophyseal joint

5th lumbar vertebra

Sacrum

Figure 8–8. Accurately positioned lateral lumbar vertebral radiograph.

Radiographic Evaluation

Facility's patient identification requirements are visible on radiograph.

- These requirements usually are facility name, patient name, age, and hospital number, and exam time and date.
- Patient ID plate is positioned so as not to obscure anatomy of interest.

A right or left marker, identifying the side of the patient positioned closer to the film, is present on the radiograph and does not superimpose anatomy of interest.

- Place the marker anteriorly within the collimated light field, along the upper edge of the film, so it does not superimpose any portion of the lumbar vertebrae.
- Because the transversely collimated field is coned to about an 8-inch (20-cm) area, make certain the marker is positioned within 4 inches (10 cm) of the center of the film to guarantee that it will not be cut off.

There is no evidence of preventable artifacts, such as buttons and zippers.

- It is recommended the patient be instructed to change into a snapless hospital gown before the procedure.

Contrast and density are adequate to demonstrate the bony structures of the lumbar vertebrae. Penetration is sufficient to visualize the bony trabecular patterns and cortical outlines of the vertebral bodies, pedicles, intervertebral foramina, and spinous processes.

- An optimal 85 to 95 kVp technique sufficiently penetrates the bony structures of the lumbar vertebrae.
- Use tight collimation, a high-ratio grid, and a flat contact shield, placed on the tabletop at the edge of the posteriorly collimated field, to reduce the amount of scattered radiation that reaches the film, providing higher contrast and better visibility of recorded details.

The bony trabecular patterns and cortical outlines of the lumbar vertebrae are sharply defined.

- Sharply defined recorded details are obtained when patient motion is controlled, respiration is halted, and a short object–image distance (OID) is maintained.

The lumbar vertebrae demonstrate a true lateral position: The intervertebral foramina are clearly visualized, and the spinous processes are in profile. The right and left pedicles and the posterior surfaces of each vertebral body are superimposed.

- To obtain a lateral lumbar radiograph, place the patient on the radiographic tabletop in a lateral recumbent position.
- Whether the patient is lying on the right or left side is insignificant, although left-side positioning is easier for the technologist. One exception to this guideline is the scoliotic patient, who should be placed on the table so the central ray is directed into the spinal curve (Fig. 8–9). You can determine how the patient's curve is directed by viewing the back and following the curve of the vertebral column.
- Once the patient has been placed on the table, flex the knees and hips for support, and position a pillow or sponge between the knees. The thickness of the pillow or sponge should be enough to prevent the side of the pelvis situated farther from the film from rotating anteriorly, without being so thick as to cause this side to rotate posteriorly (Fig. 8–10).
- To avoid vertebral rotation, align the shoulders, the posterior ribs, and the posterior pelvic wings perpendicular to the tabletop and film. This is accomplished by resting your extended flat hand against each structure, individually, then adjusting the patient's rotation until your hand is perpendicular to the film.
- **Effect of Rotation:** The upper and lower lumbar vertebrae can demonstrate rotation independently or simultaneously depending on which section of the torso is rotated. If the thorax was rotated but the pelvis remained in a true lateral position, the upper lumbar vertebrae demonstrate rotation. If the pelvis was rotated but the thorax remained in a lateral position, the lower lumbar vertebrae demonstrate rotation.
- **Detecting Rotation:** Rotation can be detected on a lateral lumbar radiograph by evaluating the superimposition of the right and left posterior surfaces of the vertebral bodies. On a nonrotated lateral lumbar radiograph, these posterior surfaces are superimposed, appearing as one. Upon rotation, these posterior surfaces are not superimposed, but are demonstrated one anterior to the other (see Rad. 7).

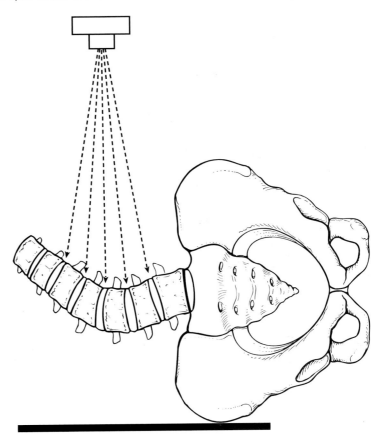

Figure 8-9. Alignment of central ray and scoliotic lumbar vertebral column.

Because the two sides of the vertebrae, thorax, and pelvis are mirror images, it is very difficult to determine from a rotated lateral lumbar radiograph which side of the patient was rotated anteriorly and which posteriorly, unless the 12th posterior ribs are demonstrated. The 12th posterior rib that demonstrates the greatest magnification and is situated inferiorly, is adjacent to the side of the patient positioned farther from the film.

The intervertebral disk spaces are open, and the vertebral bodies are demonstrated without distortion.

- The lumbar vertebral column is capable of lateral flexion. Thus, when the patient is placed in a lateral

recumbent position, the vertebral column may not be aligned parallel with the tabletop and film, but may sag at the level of the iliac crest, especially in a patient with wide hips and a narrow waist (Fig. 8–11). If the patient's lumbar column is allowed to sag, the diverging x-ray beams are not aligned parallel with the intervertebral disk spaces and perpendicular to the vertebral bodies. Radiographically, lateral lumbar flexion is most evident at the lower lumbar region, where there are closed disk spaces and distorted vertebral bodies (see Rad. 8). For a patient who has a sagging lumbar column, it may be necessary to tuck a radiolucent sponge between the lateral body surface and the tabletop just superior to the iliac crest, elevat-

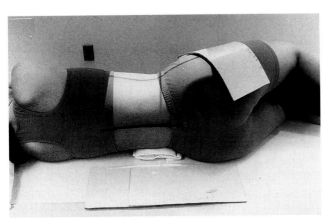

Figure 8-10. Proper patient positioning for lateral lumbar vertebral radiograph.

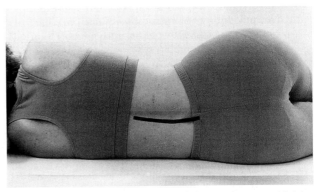

Figure 8-11. Poor alignment of vertebral column and tabletop.

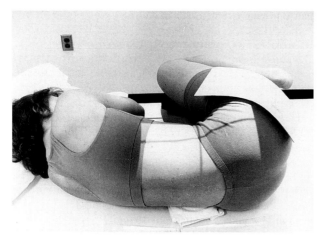

Figure 8-12. Proper patient positioning for lateral (flexion) lumbar vertebral radiograph.

ing the sagging area. The sponge should be only thick enough to bring the lumbar vertebral column parallel with the tabletop and film (see Fig. 8–10).

- An alternative method of obtaining open disk spaces and undistorted vertebral bodies for a patient whose lumbar column is sagging is to angle the central ray 5 to 8 degrees caudally. This caudal angulation should align the central ray perpendicular to the vertebral column.

The lumbar vertebral column is in a neutral position, without anteroposterior flexion or extension. There is a lordotic curvature.

- A neutral position of the lumbar vertebrae is obtained when the long axis of the patient's body is aligned with the long axis of the tabletop. The thoracic and pelvic regions are aligned.
- ***Positioning to Evaluate AP Mobility of Lumbar Vertebrae:*** If the lumbar vertebrae are being radiographed in the lateral position to demonstrate anteroposterior vertebral mobility, two lateral radiographs should be taken, one with the patient in maximum flexion and one in maximum extension. For maximum flexion, instruct the patient to flex the

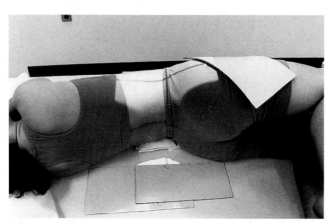

Figure 8-13. Proper patient positioning for lateral (extension) lumbar vertebral radiograph.

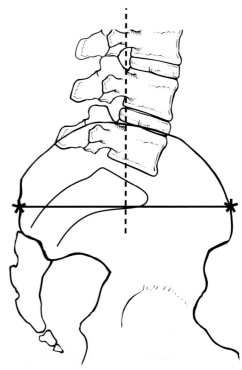

Figure 8-14. Proper central ray centering and long axis placement. Asterisks identify the posterior iliac wing and ASIS.

shoulders, upper thorax, and knees anteriorly, rolling into a tight ball (Fig. 8–12). The resulting radiograph should meet all the requirements listed for an accurately positioned lateral radiograph, except that the lumbar vertebral column demonstrates a very straight longitudinal axis without lordotic curvature (see Rad. 9).

For maximum extension, instruct the patient to arch the back by extending the shoulders, upper thorax, and legs as far posteriorly as possible (Fig. 8–13). The resulting radiograph should meet all the requirements listed for an accurately positioned lateral radiograph, except that the lumbar vertebral column demonstrates an increased lordotic curvature (see Rad. 10).

The long axis of the lumbar vertebral column is aligned with the long axis of the collimated field.

- Aligning the long axis of the lumbar vertebral column with the collimator's longitudinal light line allows tight collimation, which is necessary to reduce the production of scattered radiation.
- The lumbar vertebrae are located in the posterior half of the torso. Their exact posterior location can be determined by palpating the ASIS and posterior iliac wing (at the level of the sacroiliac joint) of the side of the patient situated farther from the film. The long axis of the lumbar vertebral column is aligned with the coronal plane that is situated halfway between these two structures (Fig. 8–14).

If a 14 × 17 inch (35 × 43 cm) film placed lengthwise was used, **the iliac crest and the 4th lumbar vertebra are centered within the collimated field. The 11th and**

12th thoracic vertebrae, 1st through 5th lumbar vertebrae, and sacrum are included within the field. *If an 11 × 14 inch (28 × 35 cm) film placed lengthwise was used,* the 3rd lumbar vertebra is centered within the collimated field. The 12th thoracic vertebra, 1st through 5th lumbar vertebrae, and L5–S1 intervertebral disk space are included within the field.

- Center a perpendicular central ray to the coronal plane located halfway between the elevated ASIS and posterior wing, at the level of the iliac crest for a 14 × 17 inch (35 × 43 cm) film, and at a level 1 to 1.5 inches (2.5 to 4 cm) superior to the iliac crest for an 11 × 14 inch (28 × 35 cm) film. The superior centering point is needed on slender patients, whereas patients with greater body thickness require the inferior centering point.
- Open the longitudinal collimation the full 17- or 14-inch (43- or 35-cm) film length for adult patients. Transverse collimation should be to an 8-inch (20-cm) field.

- ***Supplementary View of the L5–S1 Lumbar Region:*** A coned-down view of the L5–S1 lumbar region is required when a lateral lumbar radiograph is obtained that demonstrates insufficient radiographic density in this area or the L5–S1 joint space is closed.

  On patients with wide hips, it is often difficult to set an exposure that adequately demonstrates the upper and lower lumbar regions concurrently. For these patients, set an exposure that adequately demonstrates the upper lumbar region. Then take a tightly collimated lateral view of the L5–S1 lumbar region to demonstrate the lower lumbar area. Follow the procedure and evaluating criteria given in this text for the L5–S1 spot view (see page 363).
- ***Gonadal Shielding:*** Use gonadal protection shielding on all patients. This can be accomplished by positioning the edge of a lead protection strip or apron against an imaginary line drawn from the coccyx to a point 1 inch (2.5 cm) posterior to the elevated ASIS. (See discussion of radiation protection in Chapter 1.)

Critiquing Radiographs

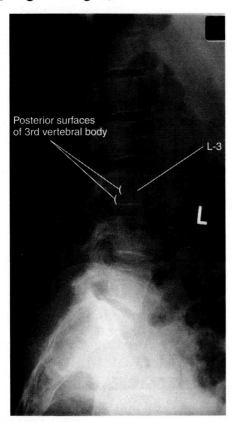

Radiograph 7.

Critique: The posterior surfaces of the first through fourth vertebral bodies and the posterior ribs are demonstrated one anterior to the other. The posterior ribs demonstrating the greater magnification were positioned posteriorly.

Correction: Rotate the side positioned farther from the film anteriorly until the posterior ribs are superimposed, while maintaining posterior pelvic wing superimposition.

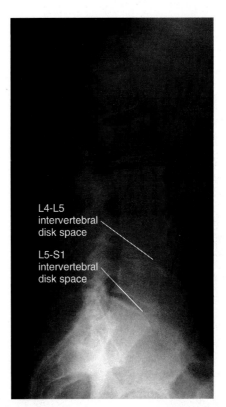

Radiograph 8.

Critique: The L4–L5 and L5–S1 intervertebral disk spaces are closed, and the third through fifth vertebral bodies are distorted. The lumbar vertebral column was not aligned parallel with the tabletop or film.

Correction: Position a radiolucent sponge between the patient's lateral body surface and the tabletop just superior to the iliac crest. The sponge should be only thick enough to align the lumbar column parallel with the tabletop and film.

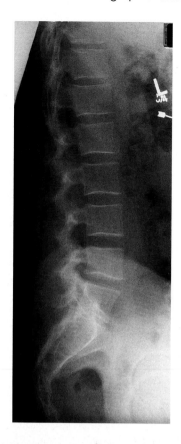

Radiograph 9.

Critique: The lumbar column demonstrates no lordotic curvature. The patient was in a flexed position, as demonstrated in Figure 8–12.

Correction: If a neutral lateral position is desired, extend the shoulders, upper thorax, and legs posteriorly until the posterior thorax and pelvic wings are aligned with the long axis of the tabletop. If a flexion lumbar radiograph is being performed to evaluate anteroposterior mobility, no correction movement is required.

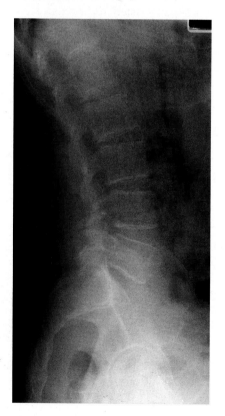

Radiograph 10.

Critique: The lumbar vertebral column demonstrates excess lordotic curvature. The patient was in an extended position, as demonstrated in Figure 8–13.

Correction: If a neutral lateral position is desired, flex the shoulders, upper thorax, and legs anteriorly until the posterior thorax and pelvic wings are aligned with the long axis of the tabletop. If an extended position is desired to evaluate anteroposterior mobility, no correction movement is required.

Lumbar Vertebrae: L5–S1 Spot Lateral Position

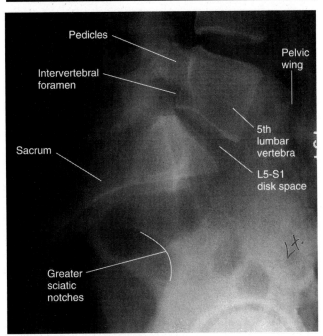

Figure 8-15. Accurately positioned lateral L5–S1 spot radiograph.

Radiographic Evaluation

Facility's patient identification requirements are visible on radiograph.

- These requirements usually are facility name, patient name, age, and hospital number, and exam time and date.
- Patient ID plate is positioned so as not to obscure anatomy of interest.

A right or left marker, identifying the side of the patient positioned closer to the film, is present on the radiograph and does not superimpose anatomy of interest.

- Place the marker anteriorly within the collimated light field, along the upper edge of the film, so it does not superimpose any portion of the fifth lumbar vertebra or superior sacral segments.
- Because the transversely collimated field is coned to about an 8-inch (20-cm) area, make certain the marker is positioned within 4 inches (10 cm) of the center of the film to guarantee that it will not be cut off.

There is no evidence of preventable artifacts, such as buttons and zippers.

- It is recommended that the patient be instructed to change into a snapless hospital gown before the procedure.

Contrast and density are adequate to demonstrate the bony structures of the fifth lumbar vertebra and superior sacrum. Penetration is sufficient to visualize the bony trabecular patterns and cortical outlines of the fifth vertebral body, pedicles, intervertebral foramina, and the first and second sacral segments.

- An optimal 90 to 100 kVp technique sufficiently penetrates the bony structures of L5–S1.
- Use tight collimation, a high-ratio grid, and a lead protection shield, placed on the tabletop at the edge of the posteriorly collimated field, to reduce the amount of scattered radiation that reaches the film, providing higher contrast and better visibility of recorded details.

The bony trabecular patterns and cortical outlines of the fifth lumbar vertebra and first and second sacral segments are sharply defined.

- Sharply defined recorded details are obtained when patient motion is controlled, respiration is halted, and a short object–image distance (OID) is maintained.

The fifth lumbar vertebra and sacrum demonstrate a true lateral position: The intervertebral foramina are clearly visualized, the right and left pedicles are superimposed and visualized in profile, and the greater sciatic notches and pelvic wings are nearly superimposed.

- To obtain a lateral L5–S1 spot radiograph, place the patient on the radiographic table in a lateral recumbent position. Whether the patient is lying on the right or left side is not significant, although the left-side positioning is easier for the technologist.

  Flex the patient's knees and hips for support, and position a pillow or sponge between the knees. The thickness of the pillow or sponge should be enough to prevent the side of the pelvis situated farther from the film from rotating anteriorly, without being so thick as to cause this side to rotate posteriorly (Fig. 8–16).
- To avoid vertebral rotation, align the shoulders, posterior ribs, and posterior pelvic wings perpendicular to the tabletop and film. This is accomplished by resting your extended flat palm against each structure, individually, then adjusting the patient's rotation until your hand is perpendicular to the tabletop.
- ***Detecting Rotation:*** Rotation can be detected on a lateral L5–S1 spot radiograph by evaluating the superimposition of the greater sciatic notches and the pelvic wings. On a nonrotated lateral L5–S1 radiograph, the greater sciatic notches and the pelvic wings

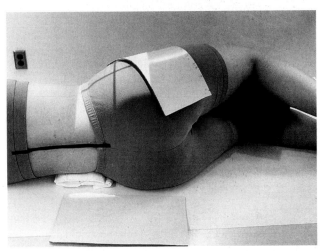

Figure 8-16. Proper lateral L5–S1 spot positioning.

are superimposed. Upon rotation, neither the greater sciatic notches nor the pelvic wings are superimposed, but are demonstrated one anterior to the other (see Rad. 11). Because the two sides of the pelvis are mirror images, it is difficult to determine which side of the patient was rotated anteriorly and which posteriorly on a poorly positioned lateral sacral radiograph. When rotation has occurred, it is most common for the side of the patient situated farther from the film to be rotated anteriorly, owing to the gravitational forward and downward pull on this side's arm and leg, if a sponge is not placed between the patient's knees.

The L5–S1 intervertebral disk space is open, and the sacrum is demonstrated without foreshortening.

- The inferior lumbar vertebral column is capable of lateral flexion. This lateral flexion also affects the position of the sacrum. Thus, when the patient is placed in a lateral recumbent position, the vertebral column may not be aligned parallel with the tabletop and film, but may sag at the level of the iliac crest, especially true in a patient with wide hips and a narrow waist. If the patient's lumbar column is allowed to sag, the diverging x-ray beams are not aligned parallel with the L5–S1 disk space and perpendicular to the long axis of the sacrum. Radiographically, lateral flexion is most evident at the L5–S1 disk space, which is closed and the sacrum, which is foreshortened (see Rad. 12). For a patient who has a sagging lumbar column, it may be necessary to tuck a radiolucent sponge between the patient's lateral body surface and the tabletop just superior to the iliac crest, elevating the sagging area. The sponge should be just thick enough to bring the lumbar vertebral column parallel with the tabletop (Fig. 8–16).
- An alternative method of obtaining an open L5–S1 disk space and an unforeshortened sacrum in a patient whose lumbar column is sagging is to angle the central ray caudally about 5 degrees for a male patient and 8 degrees for a female patient. The caudal angulation used should align the central ray parallel with the L5–S1 disk space and perpendicular to the long axis of the sacrum.

The long axis of the lumbar vertebral column is aligned with the long axis of the collimated field.

- Aligning the long axis of the lumbar vertebral column with the collimator's longitudinal light line allows for tight collimation, which is necessary to reduce the production of scattered radiation.
- The lumbar vertebrae are located in the posterior half of the torso. Their exact posterior location can be determined by palpating the ASIS and posterior wing (at the level of the sacroiliac joint) on the side of the patient situated farther from the film. The long axis of the lumbar vertebral column is aligned with the coronal plane that is situated halfway between these two structures.

The L5–S1 intervertebral disk space is at the center of the collimated field. The fifth lumbar vertebra and the first and second sacral segments are included within the field.

- Center a perpendicular central ray to a point halfway between the elevated ASIS and the posterior wing at a level 1.5 inches (4 cm) inferior to the iliac crest.
- Longitudinally collimate 1 inch (2.5 cm) superior to the iliac crest. Transverse collimation should be to an 8-inch (20-cm) field.
- An 8 × 10 inch (18 × 24 cm) film placed lengthwise should be adequate to include all the required anatomical structures.
- **Gonadal Shielding:** Use gonadal protection shielding on all patients. This can be accomplished by positioning the edge of a lead protection strip or apron against an imaginary line drawn from the coccyx to a point 1 inch (2.5 cm) posterior to the elevated ASIS. (See discussion of radiation protection in Chapter 1.)

Critiquing Radiographs

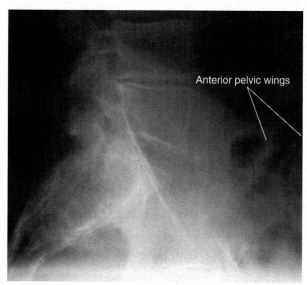

Anterior pelvic wings

Radiograph 11.

Critique: The L5–S1 intervertebral foramen is obscured, and the anterior iliac wings are not closely superimposed. The patient was rotated.

Correction: It is difficult to determine whether the left or right side of the patient was rotated anteriorly, although it is most common for the elevated side to have been anterior if a pillow or sponge was not placed between the patient's knees. Rotate the thorax and pelvis until the posterior ribs and the posterior pelvic wings are superimposed.

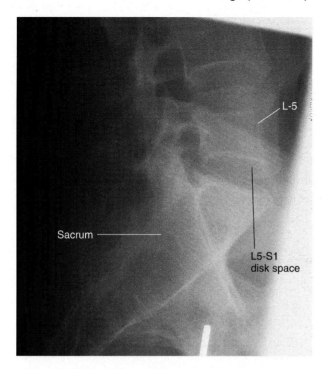

Radiograph 12.

Critique: The L5–S1 intervertebral disk space is closed, and the fifth lumbar vertebra and sacrum are foreshortened. Neither the long axis of the lumbar vertebral column nor the sacrum was aligned parallel with the tabletop.

Correction: Position a radiolucent sponge between the patient's lateral body surface and the tabletop just superior to the patient's iliac crest. The sponge should be just thick enough to align the long axis of the vertebral column and sacrum parallel with the tabletop.

SACRUM

Anteroposterior Projection

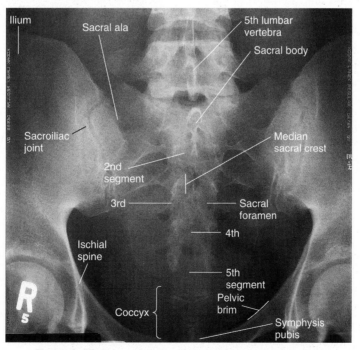

Figure 8-17. Accurately positioned AP sacral radiograph.

Radiographic Evaluation

Facility's patient identification requirements are visible on radiograph.

- These requirements usually are facility name, patient name, age, and hospital number, and exam time and date.
- Patient ID plate is positioned so as not to obscure anatomy of interest.

A right or left marker is present on the radiograph and does not superimpose anatomy of interest.

- Place the marker laterally within the collimated light field so it does not superimpose any portion of the sacrum.
- Because the transversely collimated field is coned to about an 8-inch (20-cm) area, make certain that the marker is positioned within 4 inches (10 cm) of the center of the film to guarantee that it will not be cut off.

There is no evidence of preventable artifacts, such as buttons and zippers.

- It is recommended that the patient be instructed to change into a snapless hospital gown before the procedure.

  The patient's urinary bladder should be emptied prior to the procedure. It is also recommended that the colon be free of gas and fecal material. Elimination of urine, gas, and fecal material from the area superimposing the sacrum improves its visualization.

Contrast and density are adequate to demonstrate the bony structures of the sacrum. Penetration is sufficient to visualize the bony trabecular patterns and cortical outlines of the sacral segments and sacroiliac joints.

- An optimal 75 to 85 kVp technique sufficiently penetrates the bony structures of the sacrum.
- Use tight collimation and a high-ratio grid to reduce the amount of scattered radiation that reaches the film.

The bony trabecular patterns and cortical outlines of the sacrum are sharply defined.

- Sharply defined recorded details are obtained when patient motion is controlled, respiration is halted, and a short object–image distance (OID) is maintained.
- Using a small focal spot also improves the sharpness of the recorded detail, but may result in motion on larger patients, owing to the long exposure time that would be required.

The sacrum demonstrates a true AP projection: The ischial spines are equally demonstrated and are aligned with the pelvic brim, and the median sacral crest and coccyx are aligned with the symphysis pubis.

- An AP sacrum radiograph is obtained by positioning the patient supine on the radiographic table with the legs extended. Position the shoulders and anterior superior iliac spines (ASISs) at equal distances from the tabletop to prevent rotation (Fig. 8–18).
- *Detecting Rotation:* Rotation is effectively detected on an AP sacral radiograph by comparing the amount of iliac spine visualization without pelvic brim superimposition and by evaluating the alignment of

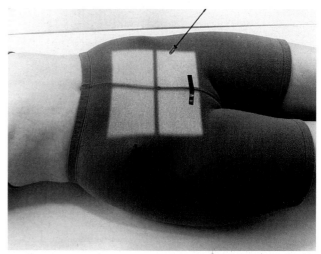

Figure 8-18. Proper patient positioning for AP sacral radiograph.

the median sacral crest and coccyx with the symphysis pubis. If the patient was rotated away from the AP projection, the sacrum shifts toward the side positioned farther from the tabletop and film, and the pelvic brim and symphysis shift toward the side positioned closer to the tabletop and film. If the patient was rotated into a left posterior oblique (LPO) position, the left ischial spine is demonstrated without pelvic brim superimposition, and the median sacral crest and coccyx are not aligned with the symphysis pubis, but are rotated toward the patient's right side (see Rad. 13). If the patient is rotated into a right posterior oblique (RPO) position, the opposite is true; the right ischial spine is demonstrated without pelvic brim superimposition, and the median sacral crest and coccyx are rotated toward the patient's left side (see Rad. 14).

The first through fifth sacral segments are visualized without foreshortening, the sacral foramina demonstrate equal spacing, and the symphysis pubis does not superimpose any portion of the sacrum.

- When the patient is in a supine position with the legs extended, the lumbar vertebral column demonstrates a lordotic curvature, and the sacrum demonstrates a kyphotic curvature (Fig. 8–19). To demonstrate the sacrum without foreshortening, a 15-degree cephalad central ray angulation is used. This angle will align the central ray perpendicular to the long axis of the sacrum and parallel with the L5–S1 intervertebral disk space.
- *Effect of Misalignment or Mispositioning:* If an AP sacral radiograph was taken with a perpendicular central ray, the first, second, and third sacral segments are foreshortened (see Rad. 14). If the radiograph was taken with the patient's legs flexed, the lordotic curvature of the lumbar vertebral column is reduced, and the long axis of the sacrum is positioned closer to parallel with the tabletop and film. For this positioning, a 15-degree cephalad angulation causes

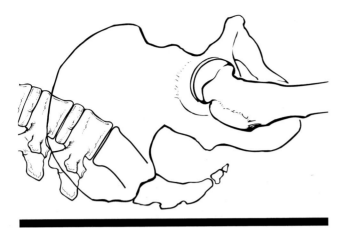

Figure 8–19. Sacral curvature.

elongation of the sacrum and superimposition of the symphysis pubis onto the inferior sacral segments (see Rad. 15). The same elongation results if the patient's legs remain extended and the central ray is angled more than 15 degrees cephalad.

The long axis of the median sacral crest is aligned with the long axis of the collimated field.

- Aligning the long axis of the median sacral crest with the long axis of the collimated field allows for tight collimation and ensures that the central ray is angled directly into the sacrum.
- To obtain proper alignment, find the point halfway between the palpable anterior superior iliac spines. Then align this point and the palpable symphysis pubis with the collimator's longitudinal light line.

The third sacral segment is at the center of the collimated field. The fifth lumbar vertebra, first through fifth sacral segments, first coccygeal vertebra, symphysis pubis, and the sacroiliac joints are included within the field.

- Center the central ray to the patient's midsagittal plane at a level halfway between an imaginary line connecting the anterior superior iliac spines and the symphysis pubis. Open the longitudinally collimated field to the symphysis pubis. Transverse collimation should be to about an 8-inch (20-cm) field size.
- A 10 × 12 inch (24 × 30 cm) film placed lengthwise should be adequate to include all the required anatomical structures.
- **Gonadal Shielding:** Use gonadal protection shielding on all male patients. Female patients cannot be shielded or sacral information will be obscured.

Critiquing Radiographs

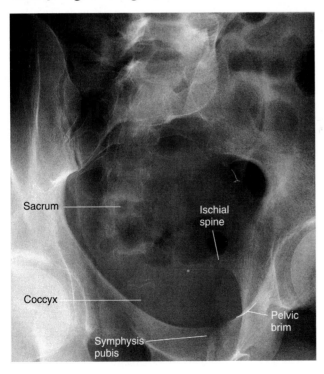

Sacrum

Ischial spine

Coccyx

Pelvic brim

Symphysis pubis

Radiograph 13.

Critique: The left ischial spine is demonstrated without pelvic brim superimposition, and the median sacral crest and coccyx are rotated toward the right hip. The patient was rotated onto the left side (LPO).
Correction: Rotate the patient toward the right hip until the anterior superior iliac spines are positioned at equal distances from the tabletop.

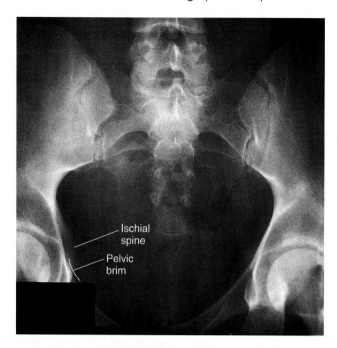

Ischial
spine

Pelvic
brim

Radiograph 14.

Critique: The right ischial spine is demonstrated without pelvic brim superimposition, and the first, second, and third sacral segments are foreshortened. The patient was rotated onto the right side (RPO), and the central ray was not angled cephalically enough to align it perpendicular to the long axis of the sacrum.

Correction: Rotate the patient toward the left hip until the anterior superior iliac spines are positioned at equal distances from the tabletop and the patient's legs are fully extended, then angle the central ray 15 degrees cephalad.

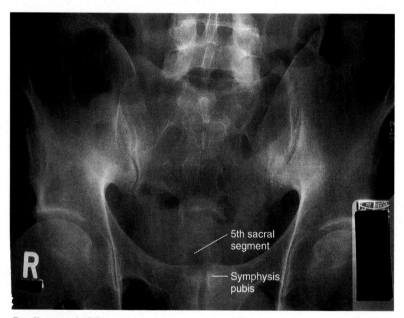

5th sacral
segment

Symphysis
pubis

R

Radiograph 15.

Critique: The sacrum is elongated, and the symphysis pubis is superimposing the fifth sacral segment. Either the central ray was angled too cephalically or the patient's legs were not fully extended and a 15-degree central ray angle was used.

Correction: If the patient's legs were extended, decrease the central ray angulation about 5 degrees for every 1 inch (2.5 cm) you wish to move the symphysis pubis. This angulation adjustment is based on a 40-inch (102-cm) source–image distance (SID); if a shorter SID is used, the angle adjustment needs to be increased, and if a longer SID is used, the angle adjustment needs to be decreased. For this patient, the angulation should be decreased 5 degrees. If the patient's legs were flexed and a 15-degree central ray angle was used, fully extend the patient's legs and use the same angulation.

Sacrum: Lateral Position

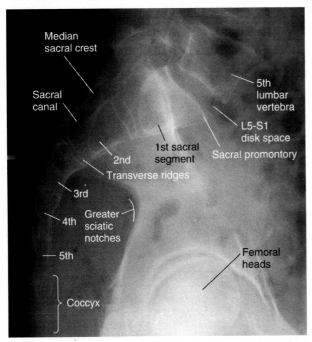

Figure 8–20. Accurately positioned lateral sacral radiograph.

Radiographic Evaluation

Facility's patient identification requirements are visible on radiograph.
- These requirements usually are facility name, patient name, age, and hospital number, and exam time and date.
- Patient ID plate is positioned so as not to obscure anatomy of interest.

A right or left marker, identifying the side of the patient positioned closer to the film, is present on the radiograph and does not superimpose anatomy of interest.
- Place the marker anteriorly within the collimated light field, along the upper edge of the film, so it does not superimpose any portion of the sacrum.
- Because the transversely collimated field is coned to about an 8-inch (20-cm) area, make certain that the marker is positioned within 4 inches (10 cm) of the center of the film to guarantee that it will not be cut off.

There is no evidence of preventable artifacts.
- It is recommended that the patient be instructed to change into a hospital gown before the procedure.

Contrast and density are adequate to demonstrate the bony structures of the sacrum. Penetration is sufficient to visualize the bony trabecular patterns and cortical outlines of the sacral segments, sacral canal, median sacral crest, promontory, and transverse ridges.
- An optimal 80 to 85 kVp technique sufficiently penetrates the bony structures of the sacrum.
- Use tight collimation, a high-ratio grid, and a lead protection shield, placed on the tabletop at the edge of the posteriorly collimated field, to reduce the amount of scattered radiation that reaches the film, providing higher contrast and better visibility of recorded details.

The bony trabecular patterns and cortical outlines of the sacrum are sharply defined.
- Sharply defined recorded details are obtained when patient motion is controlled, respiration is halted, and a short object–image distance (OID) is maintained.
- Using a small focal spot can improve the sharpness of the recorded details but may result in motion on larger patients, owing to the long exposure time that would be required.

The sacrum demonstrates a true lateral position: The median sacral crest is demonstrated in profile, and the greater sciatic notches and the pelvic wings are nearly superimposed.
- To obtain a lateral sacral radiograph, place the patient on the radiographic table in a lateral recumbent position. Whether the patient is lying on the right or left side is not significant, although the left-side positioning is easier for the technologist.

  Flex the patient's knees and hips for support, and position a pillow or sponge between the knees. The thickness of the pillow or sponge should be enough to prevent the side of the pelvis situated farther from the film from rotating anteriorly, without being so thick as to cause this side to rotate posteriorly (Fig. 8–21).
- To avoid vertebral rotation, align the shoulders, posterior ribs, and posterior pelvic wings perpendicular to the tabletop and film. This is accomplished by resting your extended flat palm against each structure, individually, then adjusting the patient's rotation until your hand is positioned perpendicular to the tabletop.
- **Detecting Rotation:** Rotation can be detected on a lateral sacral radiograph by evaluating the superimposition of the greater sciatic notches and pelvic wings. On a nonrotated lateral sacral radiograph, the greater sciatic notches and pelvic wings are superim-

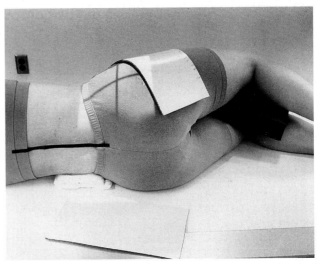

Figure 8–21. Proper patient positioning for lateral sacral radiograph.

posed. Upon rotation, neither the greater sciatic notches nor the pelvic wings are superimposed, but are demonstrated one anterior to the other (Rad. 16).

Because the two sides of the pelvis are mirror images, it is often difficult to determine which side of the patient was rotated anteriorly and which posteriorly on a poorly positioned lateral sacral radiograph. When rotation has occurred and the patient's femoral heads are visualized on the radiograph, the hip that is projected more inferiorly was the one situated farther from the film.

The L5–S1 intervertebral disk space is open, and the sacrum is demonstrated without foreshortening.
- The inferior lumbar vertebral column is capable of lateral flexion. This lateral flexion also affects the position of the sacrum. Thus, when the patient is placed in a lateral recumbent position, the long axis of the vertebral column may not be aligned parallel with the tabletop and film, but may sag at the level of the iliac crest, especially in a patient with wide hips and a narrow waist. If the patient's lumbar column is allowed to sag, the diverging x-ray beams are not aligned parallel with the L5–S1 disk space and perpendicular to the long axis of the sacrum. Radiographically, lateral flexion is most evident at the L5–S1 disk space, which is closed, and the sacrum, which is foreshortened (see Rad. 17). For a patient with a sagging lumbar column, it may be necessary to tuck a radiolucent sponge between the patient's lateral body surface and the tabletop just superior to the iliac crest, elevating the sagging area. The sponge should be just thick enough to bring the lumbar vertebral column parallel with the tabletop (Fig. 8–21).
- An alternative method of obtaining an open L5–S1 disk space and an unforeshortened sacrum for a patient whose lumbar column is sagging is to angle the central ray caudally, about 5 degrees for a male patient and 8 degrees for a female patient. The degree of caudal angulation used should align the central ray parallel with the L5–S1 disk space and perpendicular to the long axis of the sacrum.

The long axis of the sacrum is aligned with the long axis of the collimated field.
- Aligning the long axis of the sacrum with the long axis of the collimated field allows for tight collimation, which is necessary to reduce the production of scattered radiation.
- To obtain good sacral alignment, align the long axis of the sacrum with the collimator's longitudinal light line. The sacrum is located about 5 inches (12.5 cm) posterior to the elevated ASIS.

The third sacral segment is at the center of the collimated field. The fifth lumbar vertebra, first through fifth sacral segments, promontory, and first coccygeal vertebra are included within the field.
- Center a perpendicular central ray to the coronal plane located 5 inches (12.5 cm) posterior to the elevated ASIS at a level halfway between the elevated ASIS and coccyx.
- Open the longitudinal collimation the full 12-inch (30-cm) film length for adult patients. Transverse collimation should be to an 8-inch (20-cm) field.
- A 10 × 12 inch (24 × 30 cm) film placed lengthwise should be adequate to include all the required anatomical structures.
- ***Gonadal Shielding:*** Use gonadal protection shielding on all patients. This can be accomplished by positioning the edge of a lead protection strip or apron against an imaginary line drawn between the coccyx and 1 inch (2.5 cm) posterior to the elevated ASIS. (See the radiation protection section of Chapter 1.)

Critiquing Radiographs

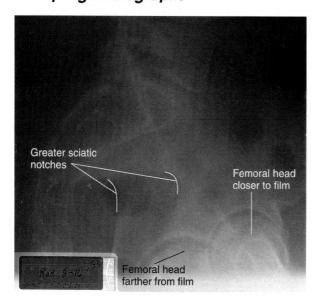

Greater sciatic notches

Femoral head closer to film

Femoral head farther from film

Radiograph 16.

Critique: The greater sciatic notches are demonstrated one anterior to the other, and the median sacral crest is not in profile. The pelvis and sacrum were rotated. The femoral head situated farther from the film, which is identified by its more inferior position, was rotated posteriorly.
Correction: Rotate the elevated pelvic wing anteriorly until the posterior pelvic wings are aligned perpendicular to the film.

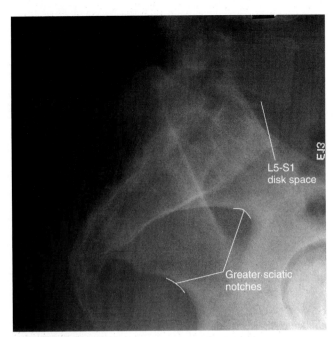

Radiograph 17.

Critique: The L5–S1 intervertebral disk space is closed, the fifth lumbar vertebra and the sacrum are foreshortened, and the greater sciatic notches are demonstrated without superimposition. The patient's long axis was not parallel with the tabletop.

Correction: Position the long axis of the lumbar vertebral column and sacrum parallel with the film. It may be necessary to place a radiolucent sponge between the patient's lateral body surface and the tabletop just superior to the iliac crest. The sponge should be just thick enough to align the lumbar column parallel with the tabletop.

COCCYX

Anteroposterior Projection

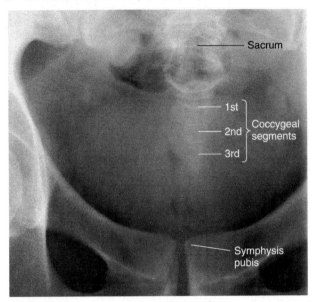

Figure 8–22. Accurately positioned AP coccygeal radiograph.

Radiographic Evaluation

Facility's patient identification requirements are visible on radiograph.

- These requirements usually are facility name, patient name, age, and hospital number, and exam time and date.
- Patient ID plate is positioned so as not to obscure anatomy of interest.

A right or left marker, identifying the correct side of the patient, is present on the radiograph and does not superimpose anatomy of interest.

- Place the marker laterally within the collimated light field so it does not superimpose any portion of the coccyx.
- Because the collimated field is coned to about a 6-inch (15-cm) area, make certain the marker is positioned within 3 inches (7.5 cm) of the center of the film to guarantee that it will not be cut off.

There is no evidence of preventable artifacts, such as buttons and zippers.

- It is recommended that the patient be instructed to change into a hospital gown before the procedure.
- The patient's urinary bladder should be emptied prior to the procedure. It is also suggested that the colon be free of gas and fecal material. Both procedures will prevent overlap of these materials onto the coccyx, thereby improving its visualization (see Rad. 18).

Contrast and density are adequate to demonstrate the bony structures of the coccyx. Penetration is sufficient to visualize the bony trabecular patterns and cortical outlines of the coccygeal vertebrae.

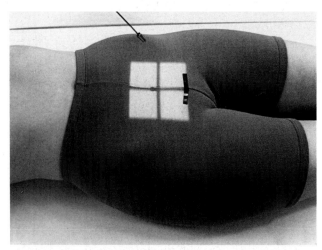

Figure 8-23. Proper patient positioning for AP coccygeal radiograph.

- An optimal 75 to 85 kVp technique sufficiently penetrates the bony structures of the coccyx.
- Use tight collimation and a high-ratio grid to reduce the amount of scattered radiation that reaches the film.

The bony trabecular patterns and cortical outlines of the coccyx are sharply defined.
- Sharply defined recorded details are obtained when patient motion is controlled, respiration is halted, and a short object–image distance (OID) is maintained.
- Using a small focal spot also improves the sharpness of the recorded details but may result in motion on larger patients, owing to the long exposure time that would be required.

The coccyx demonstrates a true AP projection: The coccyx is aligned with the symphysis pubis and is at equal distances from the lateral walls of the inlet pelvis.
- An AP coccyx radiograph is obtained by positioning the patient supine on the radiographic table with the legs extended. Position the patient's shoulders and anterior superior iliac spines (ASISs) at equal distances from the tabletop to prevent rotation (Fig. 8–23).
- **Detecting Rotation:** Rotation is detected on an AP coccyx radiograph by evaluating the alignment of the long axis of the coccyx with the symphysis pubis and by comparing the distances from the coccyx to the lateral walls of the inlet pelvis. If the patient was

rotated away from the AP projection, the coccyx moves in a direction opposite to the direction of the symphysis pubis and is positioned closer to the lateral pelvic wall situated farther from the tabletop and film. If the patient was rotated into a left posterior oblique (LPO) position, the coccyx is rotated toward the patient's right side (see Rad. 18). If the patient was rotated into a right posterior oblique (RPO) position, the coccyx is rotated toward the patient's left side.

The first through third coccygeal vertebrae are demonstrated without foreshortening and without symphysis pubis superimposition.
- When the patient is in a supine position with the legs extended, the coccyx curves anteriorly and is located beneath the symphysis pubis. To demonstrate the coccyx without foreshortening and without overlap by the symphysis pubis, a 10-degree caudal central ray angulation is used. This angle aligns the central ray perpendicular to the coccyx and projects the symphysis pubis inferiorly. If the AP projection of the coccyx is taken with a perpendicular central ray, the second and third coccygeal vertebrae are foreshortened and are superimposed by the symphysis pubis (see Rad. 19).

The long axis of the coccyx is aligned with the long axis of the collimated field.
- Aligning the long axis of the coccyx with the long axis of the collimated field allows for tight collimation and ensures that the central ray is angled directly into the coccyx.

The coccyx is at the center of the collimated field. The fifth sacral segment, the three coccygeal vertebrae, the symphysis pubis, and the pelvic brim are included within the field.
- Center the central ray to the patient's midsagittal plane at a level 2 inches (5 cm) superior to the symphysis pubis.
- Open the longitudinal collimation to the symphysis pubis. Transverse collimation should be to about a 6-inch (15-cm) field size.
- An 8 × 10 inch (18 × 24 cm) film placed lengthwise should be adequate to include all the required anatomical structures.
- **Gonadal Shielding:** Use gonadal protection shielding on all male patients. Female patients cannot be shielded or coccygeal information will be obscured.

Critiquing Radiographs

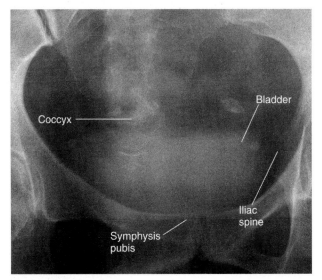

Radiograph 18.

Critique: The urinary bladder is dense and creating a shadow over the coccyx. The coccyx is not aligned with the symphysis pubis, but is situated closer to the right lateral wall of the inlet pelvis. The patient did not empty the urinary bladder and was rotated onto the left side (LPO). **Correction:** Have the patient empty the urinary bladder, and rotate the patient toward the right side until the anterior superior iliac spines are positioned at equal distances from the tabletop and film.

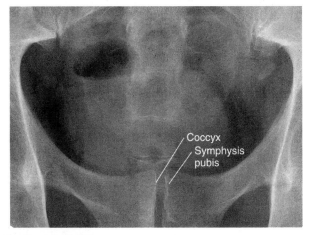

Radiograph 19.

Critique: The symphysis pubis superimposes the coccyx, and the second and third coccygeal vertebrae are foreshortened. The central ray was not angled caudally. **Correction:** Angle the central ray about 5 degrees for every 1 inch (2.5 cm) you wish to move the symphysis pubis. This angulation adjustment is based on a 40-inch (102-cm) source–image distance (SID); if a shorter SID is used, the angle adjustment needs to be increased, and if a longer SID is used, the angle adjustment needs to be decreased. For this patient, the angulation should be angled 10 degrees caudally.

Coccyx: Lateral Position

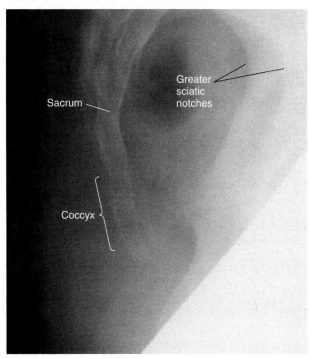

Figure 8-24. Accurately positioned lateral coccygeal radiograph.

Radiographic Evaluation

Facility's patient identification requirements are visible on radiograph.

- These requirements usually are facility name, patient name, age, and hospital number, and exam time and date.
- Patient ID plate is positioned so as not to obscure anatomy of interest.

A right or left marker, identifying the side of the patient positioned closer to the film, is present on the radiograph and does not superimpose anatomy of interest.

- Place the marker anteriorly within the collimated light field, along the upper edge of the film, so it does not superimpose any portion of the coccyx.
- Because the transversely collimated field is coned to about a 4-inch (10-cm) area, make certain that the marker is positioned within 2 inches (5 cm) of the center of the film to guarantee that it will not be cut off.

There is no evidence of preventable artifacts.

- It is recommended that the patient be instructed to change into a hospital gown before the procedure.

Contrast and density are adequate to demonstrate the bony structures of the coccyx. Penetration is sufficient to visualize the bony trabecular patterns and cortical outlines of the fifth sacral segment, the three coccygeal vertebrae, and the sacral and coccygeal cornua.

- An optimum 75 to 80 kVp technique sufficiently penetrates the bony structures of the coccyx. Use tight collimation, a high-ratio grid, and a lead protection shield, placed on the tabletop at the edge of the posteriorly collimated field, to reduce the amount of scattered radiation that reaches the film, providing higher contrast and better visibility of recorded details.

The bony trabecular patterns and cortical outlines of the coccyx are sharply defined.

- Sharply defined recorded details are obtained when patient motion is controlled and a short object–image distance (OID) is maintained.
- Using a small focal spot also improves the sharpness of the recorded details but may result in motion on larger patients owing to the long exposure time that would be required.

The coccyx demonstrates a true lateral position: The median sacral crest is demonstrated in profile, and the greater sciatic notches are nearly superimposed.

- To obtain a lateral coccyx radiograph, place the patient on the radiographic table in a lateral recumbent position. Whether the patient is lying on the right or left side is not significant, although the left-side positioning is easier for the technologist.

  Flex the patient's knees and hips for support, and position a pillow or sponge between the knees. The thickness of the pillow or sponge should be enough to prevent the side of the pelvis situated farther from the film from rotating anteriorly, without being so thick as to cause this side to rotate posteriorly (Fig. 8–25).

- To avoid vertebral rotation, align the shoulders, posterior ribs, and posterior pelvic wings perpendicular to the film. This is accomplished by resting your extended flat palm against each structure, individually, then adjusting the patient's rotation until your hand is perpendicular to the tabletop and film.
- **Detecting Rotation:** Rotation can be detected on a lateral coccyx radiograph by evaluating the superimposition of the greater sciatic notches. On a nonrotated lateral coccygeal radiograph, the greater sciatic notches are superimposed. Upon rotation, the greater sciatic notches are not superimposed, but are demonstrated one anterior to the other, and the coccyx and posteriorly situated ischium are nearly superimposed on slight rotation and truly superimposed on severe rotation (see Rad. 20).

  Because the two sides of the pelvis are mirror images, it is difficult to determine which side of the patient was rotated anteriorly and which posteriorly on a poorly positioned lateral coccygeal radiograph. When rotation has occurred, it is most common for the side of the patient situated farther from the film to have been rotated anteriorly, if a sponge was not

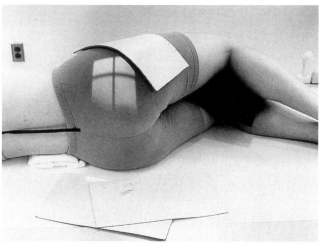

Figure 8–25. Proper patient positioning for lateral coccygeal radiograph.

placed between the patient's knees, owing to the gravitational forward and downward pull on this side's arm and leg.

The first coccygeal vertebra is at the center of the collimated field. The fifth sacral segment, first through third coccygeal vertebrae, and inferior median sacral crest are included within the field.

- Center a perpendicular central ray to the coccyx to position it in the center of the collimated field. Palpate along the median sacral crest until you reach the most inferior palpable portion. It is here that the last sacral segment is located. Center a perpendicular central ray about 0.50 inch (1 cm) anterior to this area to place the coccyx in the center of the collimated field.
- Because tight collimation is essential to obtain optimal recorded detail visibility, collimate longitudinally and transversely to a 4-inch (10-cm) field.
- The third coccygeal vertebra is situated slightly more anteriorly than the first coccygeal vertebra. Upon injury, this anterior position may be increased, causing the coccyx to align transversely (see Rad. 21). When this condition is suspected, transverse collimation should not be too tight.
- An 8 × 10 inch (18 × 24 cm) film placed lengthwise should be adequate to include all the required anatomical structures.
- **Gonadal Shielding:** Use gonadal protection shielding on all patients. This can be accomplished by positioning the edge of a lead protection strip or apron against an imaginary line drawn between the coccyx and a point 1 inch (2.5 cm) posterior to the elevated ASIS.

Critiquing Radiographs

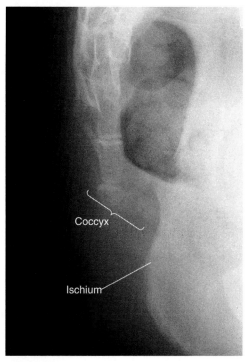

Radiograph 20.

Critique: The greater sciatic notches are demonstrated one anterior to the other, and the ischium nearly superimposes the third coccygeal segment. The pelvis, sacrum, and coccyx were rotated.

Correction: When rotation has occurred, it is most common for the elevated side of the patient to have been rotated anteriorly. Rotate the elevated pelvic wing posteriorly until the posterior pelvic wings are aligned perpendicular to the film. It may be necessary to position a sponge or pillow between the patient's knees to help maintain this positioning.

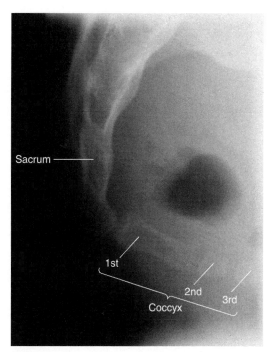

Radiograph 21.

Critique: The coccyx is aligned transversely, and the third coccygeal vertebra is not included within the collimated field. The transversely collimated field was collimated too tightly.

Correction: Open the transversely collimated field enough to include the third coccygeal vertebra.

Reference

1. Anagnostakos NP, Tortora GJ. Principles of Anatomy and Physiology, ed 6. New York: Harper & Row, 1990, pp 309–310.

CHAPTER 9

Radiographic Critique of the Sternum and Ribs

STERNUM

Right Anterior Oblique Position

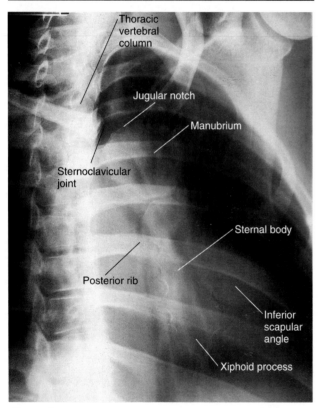

Thoracic vertebral column

Jugular notch

Manubrium

Sternoclavicular joint

Sternal body

Posterior rib

Inferior scapular angle

Xiphoid process

Figure 9-1. Accurately positioned RAO sternum radiograph.

Radiographic Evaluation

Facility's patient identification requirements are visible on radiograph.
- These requirements usually are facility name, patient name, age, and hospital number, and exam time and date.
- Patient ID plate is positioned so as not to obscure anatomy of interest.

A right marker, identifying the side of the patient positioned closer to the film, is present on the radiograph and does not superimpose anatomy of interest.
- Place a right marker on the film to coincide with the right side of the patient. The marker should be placed within the collimation borders so it does not superimpose anatomy of interest.

There is no evidence of preventable artifacts such as undergarments, necklaces, and gown snaps.
- It is recommended that the patient be instructed to remove all clothing above the waist and change into a snapless hospital gown prior to the procedure.

Contrast, density, and penetration are adequate to visualize the bony trabecular patterns and cortical outlines of the jugular notch, manubrium, sternal body, and xiphoid process.
- An optimal 60 to 70 kVp technique sufficiently penetrates the bony structures of the sternum.
- The right anterior oblique (RAO) position is employed to rotate the sternum from behind the thoracic vertebrae.
- ***Importance of Choosing the RAO Position:*** The RAO position is chosen over the LAO position because the RAO position superimposes the heart shadow over the sternum (see Rad. 1). Because the air-filled lungs and the heart shadow have different densities, they demonstrate distinctly different degrees of darkness on a radiograph produced using the same exposure factors. The air-filled lungs demonstrate more radiographic density than the heart shadow. Positioning the sternum in the heart shadow ensures homogeneous darkness across the entire sternum. Any portion of the sternum that is positioned outside the heart shadow demonstrates a darker density than the portion positioned within the heart shadow.
- Use a grid to absorb the scattered radiation produced by the body, reducing fog and providing a higher-contrast radiograph.

The sternum is demonstrated without motion or distortion. The ribs and lung markings are blurred, and the posterior ribs and left scapulae are magnified.

- In the RAO position, the sternum has many overlying structures—the posterior ribs, lung markings, heart shadow, and left inferior scapula. Specific positioning techniques should be followed to visualize a sharply defined sternum while magnifying and blurring these overlying structures.
- ***Blurring Overlying Sternal Structures:*** A short (30-inch [76-cm]) source–image distance (SID) magnifies and blurs the posterior ribs and left scapula.

  Using a long exposure time (3 to 4 seconds) and requiring the patient to breathe shallowly (costal breathing) during the exposure forces upward and outward, and downward and inward movements of the ribs and lungs, thus blurring the posterior ribs and lung markings on the radiograph. Deep breathing requires movement (elevation) of the sternum to provide deep lung expansion and should be avoided during breathing technique because this sternal motion would blur the sternum on the radiograph[1] (see Rad. 2).

  If a shorter SID or breathing technique is not employed, the details and cortical outlines of the posterior ribs, left scapula and lung markings are sharply defined, and the increased recorded detail obscures the details of the sternum (see Rad. 3).

The manubrium, sternoclavicular (SC) joints, sternal body, and xiphoid process are demonstrated within the heart shadow without vertebral superimposition.

- Rotating the patient until the midcoronal plane is angled 15 to 20 degrees to the film draws the sternum from beneath the thoracic vertebrae (Fig. 9–2). This degree of obliquity provides the reviewer a PA projection of the sternum with only a small amount of rotation.

  To sufficiently evaluate an anatomical structure, two views of the area of interest, taken 90 degrees from each other, should be obtained. The RAO and lateral positions are taken to fulfill this requirement for the sternum. Though these are not exactly 90 degrees from each other, it is necessary to slightly rotate the patient for the RAO radiograph to demonstrate the sternum without vertebral superimposition.

- ***Determining the Required Obliquity:*** To determine the exact obliquity needed to rotate the sternum away from the thoracic vertebral column on a prone patient, place the fingertips of one hand on the right SC joint and the fingertips of your other hand on the spinous processes of the upper thoracic vertebrae. Rotate the patient until your fingers on the SC joint are positioned just to the left of your fingers on the spinous processes.

- ***Evaluating Accuracy of Obliquity:*** When evaluating a RAO sternal radiograph, one can be certain that patient obliquity was sufficient when the sternum is located within the heart shadow and the manubrium and right SC joint are visualized without vertebral superimposition. If the patient was not adequately rotated, the right SC joint and manubrium are positioned beneath the vertebral column (see Rad. 4). If patient obliquity was excessive, the sternum is rotated and situated beyond the heart shadow. When the sternum is rotated beyond the heart shadow, a radiographic density variation between the superior and inferior sternum exists, because part of the sternum is in the heart shadow but another portion is in the lung field (see Rad. 3).

The midsternum is at the center of the collimated field. The jugular notch, sternoclavicular joints, sternal body, and xiphoid process are included within the field.

- Centering a perpendicular central ray about 3 inches (7.5 cm) to the left of the thoracic spinous processes, at a level halfway between the jugular notch and the xiphoid process, places the midsternum in the center of the radiograph. Increase patient obliquity until the jugular notch and xiphoid process can be easily palpated. Once the midsternum is found, place the central ray at this longitudinal level, restore the 15 to 20 degrees of patient obliquity, and shift the patient transversely until the central ray is about 3 inches (7.5 cm) to the left of the spinous processes.

- ***Determining Film Size and Collimation:*** The size of film and amount of collimation used for a RAO sternum radiograph depends on the age and sex of the patient. The adult male sternum is about 7 inches (18 cm) long, but the female sternum is considerably shorter.[2] A 10 × 12 inch (24 × 30 cm) film should sufficiently accommodate both male and female patients. Because there is less chest depth from the thoracic vertebrae to the manubrium than from the thoracic vertebrae to the xiphoid process, the manubrium remains closer to the thoracic vertebrae than the xiphoid process when the patient is rotated. The sternum, then, is not aligned with the longitudinal plane but is slightly tilted. Because of this sternal tilt, the transverse collimation should be confined to the thoracic spinous processes and the left inferior angle of the scapula.

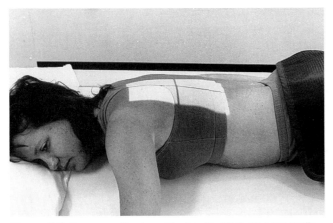

Figure 9–2. Proper patient positioning for RAO sternum radiograph.

Critiquing Radiographs

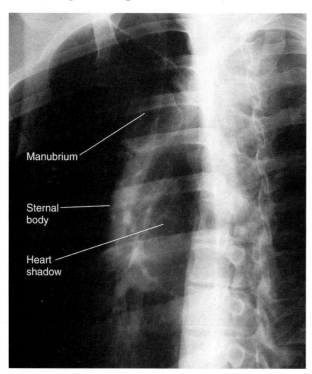

Radiograph 1.

Critique: The patient was positioned in a LAO position. The thoracic vertebrae superimpose the heart shadow, and the sternum is demonstrated to the right of the heart shadow.

Correction: Place the patient in a RAO position.

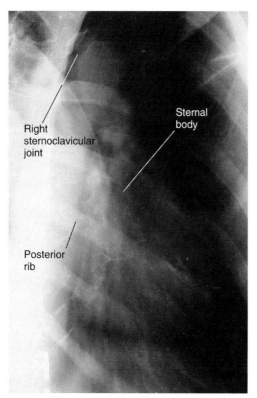

Radiograph 2.

Critique: The right SC joint is sharply defined, but the sternal body, posterior ribs, and lung markings are blurry. Breathing technique was used for this radiograph, but the patient was breathing deeply instead of shallowly, causing the sternum to move and blur.

Correction: Instruct the patient to breathe shallowly.

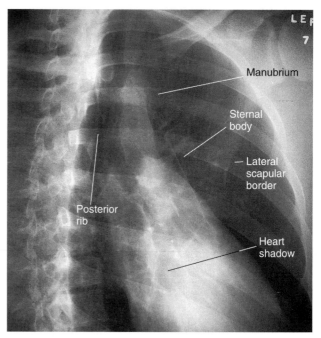

Radiograph 3.

Critique: The lung markings, posterior ribs, and left scapula are demonstrated without magnification or blurring, making it difficult to distinguish the sternum through these overlying structures. The SID was not shortened, and the patient's breathing was halted for this radiograph. Also, patient obliquity was excessive, as indicated by the position of the sternum beyond the heart shadow and by the amount of sternum rotation.

Correction: Shorten the SID to 30 inches (76 cm), take the exposure while the patient is breathing shallowly, and decrease the patient obliquity.

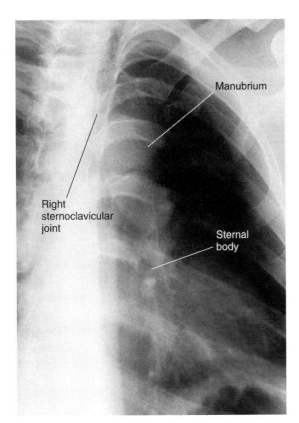

Radiograph 4.

Critique: The right SC joint and the right side of the manubrium are superimposed by the thoracic vertebrae. The patient was not rotated enough to move the entire manubrium from beneath the thoracic vertebrae.

Correction: Increase the patient obliquity. Rotate the patient until the palpable right SC joint is positioned to the left of the thoracic vertebrae.

Sternum: Lateral Position

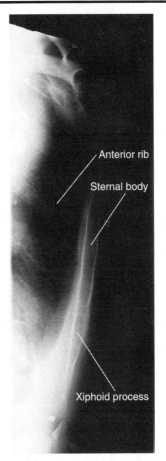

Figure 9-3. Accurately positioned lateral sternum radiograph.

Radiographic Evaluation

Facility's patient identification requirements are visible on radiograph.

- These requirements usually are facility name, patient name, age, and hospital number, and exam time and date.
- Patient ID plate is positioned so as not to obscure anatomy of interest.

A left or right marker, identifying the side of the patient positioned closer to the film, is present on the radiograph and does not superimpose anatomy of interest.

- Place a left or right marker identifying the side of the patient positioned closer to the film, anterosuperiorly in the collimated light field.

There is no evidence of removable artifacts such as undergarments, necklaces or gown snaps.

- It is recommended the patient remove all clothing above the waist and change into a snapless hospital gown prior to the procedure.

Contrast, density, and penetration are adequate to visualize the bony trabecular patterns and cortical outlines of the jugular notch, manubrium, sternal body, and xiphoid process.

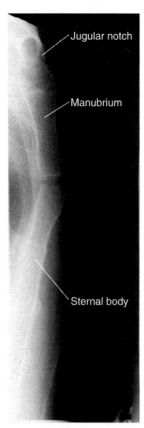

Figure 9-4. Accurately positioned superior lateral sternum radiograph.

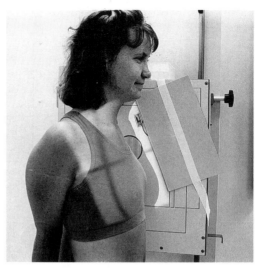

Figure 9-5. Proper patient positioning for lateral sternum radiograph.

- An optimal 70 to 75 kVp technique sufficiently penetrates the bony structures of the sternum.
- An even density is difficult to obtain over the entire sternum region, because the lower sternum is superimposed by the pectoral (chest) muscles or by the female breast tissue whereas the upper sternum is free of this superimposition. The amount of density difference between the two halves of the sternum depends on the development of the patient's pectoral muscles and the amount of female breast tissue. Enlargement of either tissue requires an increase in exposure to obtain sufficient density to visualize the sternum through them. This increase may overexpose the upper sternum region on the radiograph, requiring an additional radiograph to be taken with a lower exposure so the entire sternum can be demonstrated (Fig. 9–4).
- **Reduce Scattered Radiation:** Use a high-ratio grid to absorb the scattered radiation produced by the body, reducing fog and providing a higher-contrast radiograph.

  A remarkable amount of scattered radiation is evident on a lateral sternal radiograph anterior to the sternum. One can be certain that if scatter is demonstrated here, it is also overlying the image of the sternum, decreasing the overall radiographic contrast. To eliminate some of this scattered radiation and produce a higher-contrast image, tightly collimate and place a flat lead contact strip anterior to the sternum

close to the patient's skin-line (Fig. 9–5). This strip will absorb patient and table surface scattered radiation.

The lung markings, ribs, and sternum are sharply defined.

- Halting patient respiration and body movements during the exposure prevents motion and poorly defined outlines of the lung markings, ribs, and sternum. Detail sharpness is also increased by using a small focal spot.

The sternum and chest demonstrate no rotation, the manubrium, sternal body, and xiphoid process are demonstrated in profile, and the anterior ribs do not superimpose the sternum.

- To obtain a lateral sternum radiograph, place the patient in an upright position with the right or left lateral aspect of the body against the upright film holder (Fig. 9–5).
- Avoid chest rotation by aligning the shoulders, posterior ribs, and the posterior pelvic wings perpendicular to the film. This alignment, which superimposes each of these posterior body parts on the radiograph, and is accomplished by resting your extended flat hand against each structure, individually, and then adjusting the patient's rotation until your hand is perpendicular to the film. When the thorax is demonstrated without rotation, the sternum is in profile and the anterior ribs are superimposed over each other instead of over the sternum.
- Elevation of the sternum, resulting from deep inspiration, aids in better sternal visualization by drawing the sternum away from the anterior ribs.
- **Lateral Sternal Radiograph in Supine Position:** If the patient is unable to be positioned upright, a lateral sternum radiograph can be accomplished with the patient supine. In this position, rest the patient's arms against the sides, and position a grid-cassette vertically against the patient's arm. All other position-

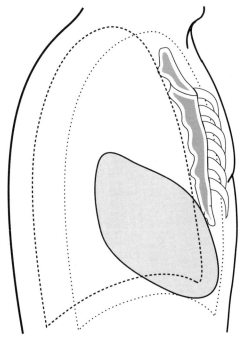

Figure 9-6. Rotation—left lung anterior.

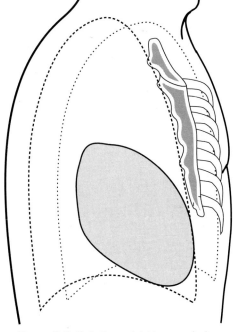

Figure 9-7. Rotation—right lung anterior.

ing and critiquing aspects of the position are the same as for an upright radiograph.

- **Detecting Rotation and Determining How to Reposition the Rotated Patient:** Rotation is effectively detected on a lateral sternum radiograph by evaluating the degree of anterior rib and sternal superimposition. If a lateral sternum radiograph demonstrates rotation, the right and left anterior ribs are not superimposed; one side is positioned anterior to the sternum and the other posterior to the sternum.

Determine how to reposition after obtaining a rotated radiograph by using the heart shadow to identify the right and left anterior ribs. Because the heart shadow is located in the left chest cavity and extends anteroinferiorly, outlining the superior border of the heart shadow enables you to recognize the left side of the chest. If the left lung and ribs were positioned anterior to the sternum, as demonstrated in Figure 9–6, the outline of the superior heart shadow continues beyond the sternum and into the anteriorly located lung (see Rad. 5). If the right lung and ribs were positioned anterior to the sternum, as demonstrated in Figure 9–7, the superior heart shadow does not continue into the anteriorly situated lung, but ends at the sternum (see Rad. 6). Once the right and left sides of the chest have been identified, reposition the patient by rotating the thorax. If the left lung and ribs were anteriorly positioned, rotate the left thorax posteriorly. If the right lung and ribs were anteriorly positioned, rotate the right thorax posteriorly.

There is no superimposition of humeral soft tissue over the sternum.

- Extending the patient's arms behind the back with the hands clasped positions the humeral soft tissue away from the sternum (see Rad. 5).

The midsternum is at the center of the collimated field. The jugular notch, sternal body, and xiphoid process are included within the field.

- Directing a horizontal central ray perpendicular to a point about 1 inch (2.5 cm) posterior to the sternal skin surface, at a level halfway between the palpable jugular notch and xiphoid process, places the midsternum in the center of the radiograph. Because a lateral sternum radiograph is taken with the patient in full inspiration, centering should be performed after the patient has inhaled. Make sure to use the sternal skin surface when determining posterior central ray placement. Do not be thrown off by the vastness of the patient's pectoral muscles or breast tissue; these structures are situated anterior to the sternum and its skin surface. With accurate posterior centering, transverse collimation can be safely executed without fear of clipping the posteriorly slanted manubrium.
- Once the central ray is centered to the patient's sternum, center the film to the central ray.
- Check to make sure the film size you are using is large enough to accommodate the entire sternum. Because the distance from the sternum to the film is quite large, the sternum is unavoidably magnified. To accommodate for this magnification, the long axis of the film should extend about 2 inches (5 cm) beyond the jugular notch and the xiphoid process. For most adult lateral sternum radiographs, an 11 × 14 inch (28 × 35 cm) film placed lengthwise should be adequate to include all the required anatomical structures.

Critiquing Radiographs

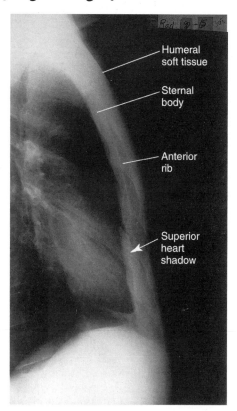

Radiograph 5.

Critique: The anterior ribs are not superimposed, and the sternum is not in profile, indicating that the chest was rotated. The superior heart shadow is seen extending anterior to the sternum and into the anteriorly situated lung, verifying it as the left lung. The patient was positioned with the left thorax rotated anteriorly and the right thorax rotated posteriorly. The humeral soft tissue is superimposing the manubrium, causing it to be underexposed.

Correction: Position the right thorax slightly anteriorly, and extend the patient's arms behind the back, with hands clasped.

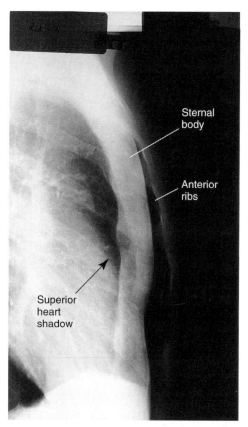

Radiograph 6.

Critique: The anterior ribs are not superimposed, and the sternum is not in profile, indicating that the chest was rotated. The superior heart shadow does not extend beyond the sternum, verifying that the right lung is situated anterior to the sternum, and the left lung is situated posterior. The patient was positioned with the right thorax rotated anteriorly and the left thorax rotated posteriorly.

Correction: Position the left thorax posteriorly.

RIBS

AP and PA Projections

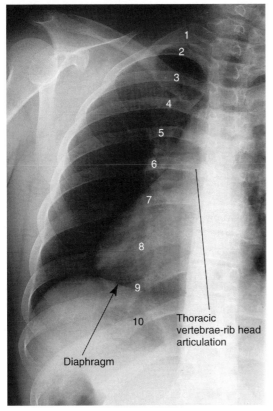

Figure 9-8. Accurately positioned PA above-diaphragm rib radiograph.

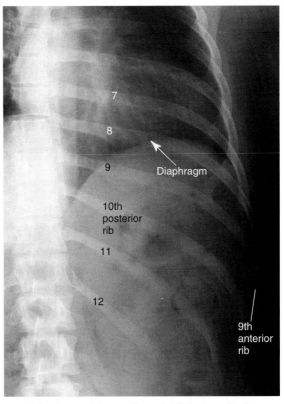

Figure 9-9. Accurately positioned AP below-diaphragm rib radiograph.

Radiographic Evaluation

Facility's patient identification requirements are visible on radiograph.

- These requirements usually are facility name, patient name, age, and hospital number, and exam time and date.
- Patient ID plate is positioned away from the affected ribs.

A right or left marker, identifying the correct side of the patient, is present on the radiograph and does not superimpose anatomy of interest.

- Mark the side of the patient that is being examined. Place the marker laterally within the collimated light field so it does not superimpose any portion of the affected ribs.

There is no evidence of preventable artifacts, such as undergarments, necklaces, belts, buttons, and gown snaps.

- It is recommended the patient remove all clothing above the waist and change into a snapless hospital gown prior to the procedure.

Contrast, density, and penetration are adequate to demonstrate the surrounding chest and intra-abdominal soft tissue, the cortical outline of the anterior and posterior ribs, and the vertebral column.

- A lower (65 to 70) kVp, high-contrast technique best defines the upper ribs that surround the lung field without overpenetrating the air-filled lungs. When the posterior ribs that overlap the heart shadow are of interest, it may be necessary to use a higher kVp to penetrate the heart enough to visualize these ribs. A slightly higher (75 to 80) kVp is also needed when the lower ribs are of interest, to penetrate the denser abdominal structures while maintaining relatively high radiographic contrast.
- Use tight collimation and a high-ratio grid to reduce the amount of scattered radiation that reaches the film, providing higher contrast and better visibility of recorded details.
- ***Soft Tissue Structures of Interest:*** The visualization of the soft tissue structures that surround the ribs is also very important. When an upper rib fracture is suspected, the surrounding upper thorax, axillary, and neck soft tissues and vascular lung markings are carefully studied for signs (hematoma, a presence of air, etc.) that indicate associated lung pathology

(pneumothorax, interstitial emphysema, etc.) or rupture of the trachea, bronchus, or aorta. When a lower rib fracture is suspected, the upper abdominal tissue is examined for signs of associated injury to the kidney, liver, spleen, or diaphragm.[3]

The lung markings, diaphragm borders, and cortical outlines of the ribs are sharply defined.

- Halting patient respiration and body movements during the exposure prevents poorly defined structural outlines of the lung markings, diaphragm, and rib borders.
- Maintaining a short object–image distance (OID) also helps provide sharp rib details.
- *AP versus PA Projection:* When the patient complains of anterior rib pain, take the radiograph in a PA projection, to place the anterior ribs closer to the film. When the posterior ribs are the affected ribs, take the radiograph in an AP projection, to place the posterior ribs closer to the film.

  Compare the difference in posterior rib detail sharpness in Figures 9–8 and 9–9. Figure 9–8 was taken in a PA projection and Figure 9–9 in an AP projection. Note how the posterior ribs in Figure 9–8 are magnified, demonstrating less detail sharpness than the posterior ribs in Figure 9–9, which were positioned closer to the film for the radiograph.

The thorax demonstrates no rotation. The thoracic vertebrae–rib head articulations are demonstrated, the sternum and vertebral column are superimposed, and the distances from the vertebral column to the sternal ends of the clavicles, when demonstrated, are equal.

- Thorax and rib rotation are avoided on the AP projection by flexing the patient's knees and placing the feet flat against the table (Fig. 9–10). The shoulders should also be positioned at equal distances from the tabletop.

  For the kyphotic patient, it may be necessary to place a sponge under each shoulder or take the radiograph in an upright position to avoid rotation of the

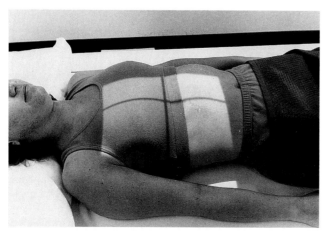

Figure 9-10. Proper patient positioning for AP below-diaphragm rib radiograph.

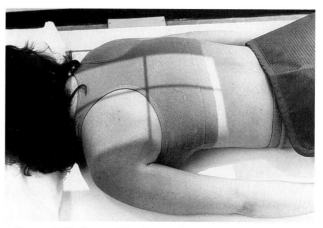

Figure 9-11. Proper PA, above diaphragm rib positioning.

upper thorax. Preventing rotation in the PA projection is slightly more difficult. It is best accomplished by placing the patient's chin on a sponge so he or she can look straight ahead and still be able to breathe, as well as by positioning shoulders and anterosuperior iliac spines (ASISs) at equal distances from the table (Fig. 9–11).

  For the patient who has excessive abdominal tissue and has a tendency to roll to one side in the PA projection, it may be necessary to place an angled sponge under the side of the lower abdomen the patient is leaning toward or to take the radiograph in an upright position to avoid thoracic rotation.

- *Detecting Rotation:* Rotation is effectively detected on an AP or PA rib radiograph by evaluating the sternum and vertebral column superimposition and by comparing the distances between the vertebral column and the sternal ends of the clavicles. When a rib radiograph demonstrates rotation and the patient was in an AP projection, the side of the patient positioned closer to the film demonstrates the sternum and the sternoclavicular (SC) joint with less vertebral column superimposition (see Rad. 7). The opposite is true for a PA projection. The side of the chest positioned farther from the film demonstrates the sternum and the SC joint with less vertebral column superimposition (see Rad. 8).
- *Rotation versus Scoliosis:* On patients with spinal scoliosis, the ribs and vertebral column will appear rotated due to the lateral deviation of the vertebrae (see Rad. 2, Chapter 2). Become familiar with this condition to prevent unnecessary repeats on these patients.

AP AND PA PROJECTIONS OF RIBS ABOVE THE DIAPHRAGM

The scapulae are located outside the lung field.

- For the AP projection, position the scapulae outside the lung field by placing the back of the patient's hands on the hips and rotating the elbows and shoulders anteriorly.

- For the PA projection, position the scapulae outside the lung field by internally rotating the patient's arms, forcing the shoulders to rotate anteriorly.
- To avoid rotation, it is best to position the two arms alike even when only one side of the thorax is being radiographed. If the scapula is not drawn away from the lung field, it is demonstrated in the upper ribs (see Rad. 9).

Nine posterior ribs are demonstrated above the diaphragm, indicating full lung aeration.

- The number of ribs demonstrated above the diaphragm is determined by the depth of patient inspiration. In full inspiration, when the patient is recumbent, about 9 posterior ribs are demonstrated above the diaphragm. When the patient is in an upright position, 10 or 11 posterior ribs will be demonstrated. If the patient does not fully inhale, the inferior ribs are demonstrated below the diaphragm. Any ribs situated below the diaphragm are not well visualized, because an increase in exposure would be needed to penetrate the abdominal tissue they surround. To maximize the number of ribs located above the diaphragm, the exposure should be taken with the patient in full inspiration.

The seventh posterior rib is at the center of the collimated field. The affected side's first through ninth ribs and the vertebral column are included within the field.

- In the AP projection, to place the seventh posterior rib at the center of the radiograph, center a perpendicular central ray halfway between the sternum and the affected lateral body surface at a level halfway between the jugular notch and the xiphoid process.
- In the PA projection, center a perpendicular central ray halfway between the palpable thoracic spinous processes and the affected lateral body surface at the level of the inferior scapular angle. Palpate the scapular angle with the arm next to the patient's body. After accurate centering has been accomplished, abduct the arm to position it out of the collimated field. Abducting the arm shifts the inferior scapular angle laterally and inferiorly, so centering should be accomplished before arm abduction.
- Once the central ray is centered, collimate transversely to the thoracic vertebral column and the patient's lateral skin-line. Because above-diaphragm ribs are radiographed on inspiration, causing the thorax to expand transversely, perform the transverse collimation with the patient in deep inspiration.
  Open the longitudinal collimation the full 17-inch (43-cm) film length.
- A 14 × 17 inch (35 × 43 cm) film placed lengthwise should be adequate to include all the required anatomical structures.

AP AND PA PROJECTIONS OF RIBS BELOW THE DIAPHRAGM

The 9th through 12th posterior ribs are demonstrated below the diaphragm.

- The number of ribs visualized below the diaphragm is determined by the depth of patient inspiration. In full inspiration, up to 10 posterior ribs may be demonstrated above the diaphragm (see Rad. 10). In expiration, only 7 or 8 posterior ribs are clearly visualized above the diaphragm, and 4 or 5 ribs are demonstrated below the diaphragm. When below-diaphragm ribs are radiographed, it is necessary to use a higher kVp and exposure than needed for the above-diaphragm ribs, to penetrate the denser abdominal tissue. Any ribs situated above the diaphragm for this radiograph may be too dark to evaluate. To maximize the number of ribs located below the diaphragm that can be evaluated, the exposure should be taken on expiration.

The 9th or 10th posterior rib is at the center of the collimated field. A portion of the thoracic and lumbar vertebral column and the 7th through 12th ribs of affected side of patient are included within the field.

- In the AP projection, to place the ninth or tenth posterior ribs at the center of the radiograph, center a perpendicular central ray halfway between the sternum and the affected lateral body surface at the level of the xiphoid process.
- In the PA projection, centering is accomplished by positioning the lower border of the cassette at the patient's iliac crest, centering a perpendicular central ray to the center of the film, then moving the patient transversely until the longitudinal centering is halfway between the palpable thoracic spinous processes and the lateral body surface.
  For a hypersthenic patient with a short, wide thorax, the centering needs to be positioned slightly higher. Place the lower border of the cassette about 2 inches (5 cm) above the crest, center the central ray to the film, then move the patient transversely until the longitudinal collimator's light line is positioned halfway between the vertebral column and the lateral body surface of the affected side.
- After the patient has been properly centered to the film, collimate transversely to the vertebral column and the patient's lateral skin-line. Open the longitudinal collimation the full 17-inch (43-cm) field size.
- A 14 × 17 inch (35 × 43 cm) film placed lengthwise should be adequate to include all the anatomical structures.

Critiquing Radiographs

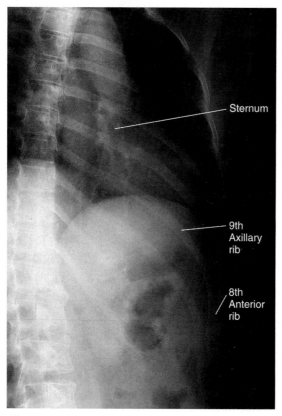

Radiograph 7.

Critique: This is an AP projection. The sternum is demonstrated to the left of the patient's vertebral column. The patient was rotated. In an AP projection, the sternum is rotated toward the side that was positioned closer to the film. For this radiograph, the patient was rotated toward the left side.

Correction: Position the patient in a true AP projection by flexing the knees and placing the shoulders at equal distances from the tabletop.

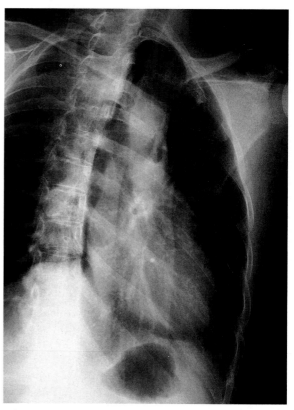

Radiograph 8.

Critique: This is a PA projection. The sternum and the SC joints are demonstrated to the left of the patient's vertebral column. The patient was rotated. In a PA projection, the sternum and SC joints are rotated toward the side that was positioned farther from the film. For this radiograph, the patient was rolled toward the right side, away from the left side.

Correction: Position the patient in a true PA projection by having the patient look straight ahead with the chin elevated on a sponge. The shoulders and the anterior superior iliac spines should be positioned at equal distances from the tabletop.

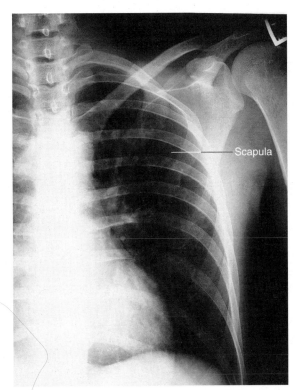

Radiograph 9.

Critique: This an AP projection. The left scapula is superimposing the upper lateral rib field. The left elbow and shoulder were not rotated anteriorly.

Correction: If the patient's condition allows, place the back of the patient's hands on the hips, and rotate the elbows and shoulders anteriorly.

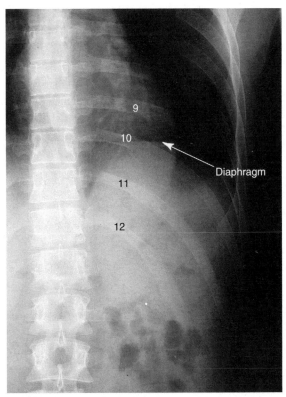

Radiograph 10.

Critique: For this below-diaphragm rib radiograph, only three posterior ribs are demonstrated below the diaphragm. The radiograph was exposed after the patient had taken a deep breath.

Correction: To demonstrate more posterior ribs below the diaphragm, the radiograph should be exposed after the patient exhales.

Ribs: Posterior and Anterior Oblique Positions

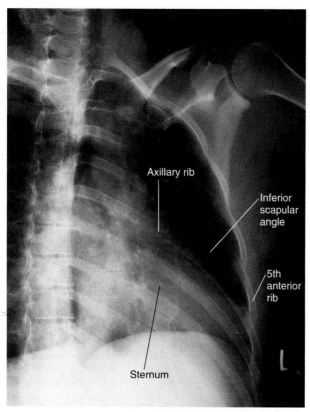

Figure 9-12. Accurately positioned posterior oblique, above-diaphragm rib radiograph.

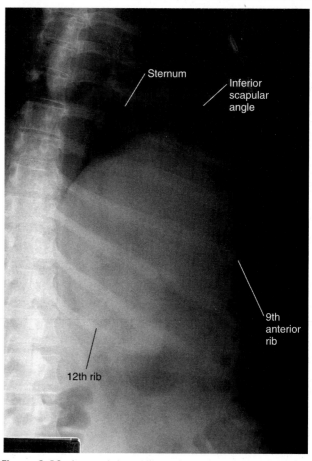

Figure 9-13. Accurately positioned posterior oblique, below-diaphragm rib radiograph.

The posterior oblique position should be the position performed routinely, because it positions the axillary (lateral) ribs closer to the film.

Radiographic Evaluation

Facility's patient identification requirements are visible on radiograph.
- These requirements usually are facility name, patient name, age, and hospital number, and exam time and date.
- Patient ID plate is positioned away from the affected ribs.

A right or left marker, identifying the side of the patient positioned closer to the film, is present on the radiograph and does not superimpose anatomy of interest.
- Mark the patient's side being examined. Place the marker laterally within the collimated light field so it does not superimpose any portion of the ribs.

There is no evidence of preventable artifacts, such as undergarments, necklaces, belts, buttons, and gown snaps.

- It is recommended the patient remove all clothing above the waist and change into a snapless hospital gown prior to the procedure.

Contrast, density, and penetration are adequate to demonstrate the surrounding chest and intra-abdominal soft tissue, the cortical outlines of the anterior, posterior, and axillary ribs, and the vertebral column.
- A lower (65 to 70) kVp, high-contrast technique would best define the upper axillary ribs that surround the lateral portion of the lung field without overpenetrating the air-filled lungs. When the lower axillary ribs are of interest, a slightly higher (75 to 80) kVp is needed to penetrate the denser abdominal structures and visualize the ribs while still maintaining a relatively high radiographic contrast.
- Use tight collimation and a high ratio grid to reduce the amount of scattered radiation that reaches the film, providing higher contrast and better visibility of recorded details.
- **Soft Tissue Structures of Interest:** The visualization of the soft tissue structures that surround the ribs is also very important. When an upper rib fracture is suspected, the surrounding upper thorax, axillary,

and neck soft tissues and vascular lung markings are carefully studied for signs (hematoma, a presence of air, etc.) that indicate associated lung pathology (pneumothorax, interstitial emphysema, etc.) or rupture of the trachea, bronchus, or aorta. When a lower rib fracture is suspected, the upper abdominal tissue is examined for signs of associated injury to the kidney, liver, spleen, or diaphragm.[3]

The lung markings, diaphragm borders, and cortical outlines of the ribs are sharply defined.

- Halting patient respiration and body movements during the exposure prevents poorly defined structural outlines of the lung markings, diaphragm and rib borders.
- ***Posterior versus Anterior Oblique:*** The degree of sharpness the rib details demonstrate is also increased by maintaining a short object–image distance (OID). To provide maximum axillary rib detail, posterior oblique positions should be routinely performed. This positioning places the axillary ribs close to the film, preventing magnification and radiographic detail loss. Another advantage of the posterior oblique position over the anterior oblique position is the better visualization of the sternum. In the anterior and posterior oblique positions, the sternum and the axillary ribs are superimposed, making evaluation of axillary ribs difficult. When the sternum is at a long OID, as is achieved with posterior oblique positions, it becomes less visible owing to magnification. Radiograph 11 demonstrates below-diaphragm ribs exposed with the patient in an anterior oblique position. Compare this radiograph with the posterior oblique rib radiograph in Figure 9–12. Note the greater magnification and loss of detail of the ribs and the increased visualization of the sternum in Radiograph 11.

The thorax has been rotated 45 degrees. The inferior sternal body is located halfway between the lateral body surface and the vertebral column, overlapping the axillary ribs. The axillary ribs are layered out and are located in the center of the collimated field, and the anterior ribs are layered out and are located at the lateral edge.

- Rotating the patient until the midcoronal plane is angled 45 degrees with the film provides the reviewer with an additional perspective of the axillary ribs, without the self-superimposition demonstrated on the AP or PA projection.

  To layer out the axillary ribs, rotate the patient toward the affected side for a posterior oblique position and away from the affected side for an anterior oblique position (Figs. 9–14 and 9–15). If the patient is rotated the opposite way, the axillary ribs demonstrate greater self-superimposition (see Rad. 12).
- ***Determining Accuracy of Rotation:*** Because the sternum rotates toward the affected axillary ribs upon thorax rotation, the position of the sternum can be used to identify accuracy of patient rotation. If the inferior sternum is positioned halfway between the vertebral column and the anterior ribs, the patient was rotated 45 degrees and the axillary ribs are layered out. When the desired 45-degree obliquity has not

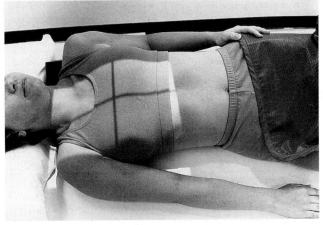

Figure 9-14. Proper patient positioning for posterior oblique, above-diaphragm rib radiograph.

been obtained, view the position of the inferior sternum to determine how to reposition the patient. If the sternal body is demonstrated next to the vertebral column, the patient was not rotated enough (see Rad. 13). If the inferior sternal body is demonstrated laterally, the patient was rotated more than 45 degrees.

POSTERIOR AND ANTERIOR OBLIQUE RADIOGRAPHS OF RIBS ABOVE THE DIAPHRAGM

Nine axillary ribs are demonstrated above the diaphragm, indicating full lung aeration.

- The number of ribs demonstrated above the diaphragm is determined by the depth of patient inspiration. In full inspiration, when the patient is recumbent, 9 axillary ribs are usually demonstrated above the diaphragm. When the patient is in an upright position, 10 or 11 axillary ribs are demonstrated. If the patient does not fully inhale, the inferior axillary ribs are positioned below the diaphragm. Any ribs situated below the diaphragm are not well visualized, because an increase in exposure would be needed to penetrate the abdominal tissue they surround. To maximize the number of ribs located above the diaphragm, take the exposure with the patient in full inspiration.

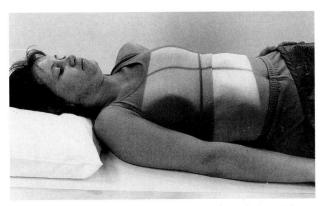

Figure 9-15. Proper patient positioning for posterior oblique, below-diaphragm rib radiograph.

The seventh axillary rib is at the center of the collimated field. The first through ninth axillary ribs of the affected side and the thoracic vertebral column are included within the field.

- For posterior oblique axillary rib radiographs (RPO or LPO), the seventh posterior rib is placed at the center of the radiograph by centering a perpendicular central ray at a level halfway between the jugular notch and the xiphoid process, then moving the patient transversely until the longitudinal collimator's light line is aligned with the inferior sternum.

- For anterior oblique axillary rib radiographs (RAO or LPO), center a perpendicular central ray halfway between the thoracic vertebral column and the affected lateral body surface, at a level 1 inch (2.5 cm) superior to the inferior scapular angle. The scapular angle should be palpated with the arm next to the body. After accurate centering has been accomplished, abduct the arm to position it out of the collimated field. Because abducting the arm shifts the inferior scapular angle laterally and inferiorly, centering should be accomplished before arm abduction.

- Once the central ray is centered, collimate transversely to the thoracic vertebral column and the patient's lateral skin-line. Because above-diaphragm ribs are radiographed on inspiration, causing the thorax to expand transversely, transverse collimation should be performed with the patient in deep inspiration. Open the longitudinal collimation the full 17-inch (43-cm) field size.

- A 14 × 17 inch (35 × 43 cm) lengthwise film placed should be adequate to include all the required anatomical structures.

POSTERIOR AND ANTERIOR OBLIQUE RADIOGRAPHS OF RIBS BELOW THE DIAPHRAGM

The 9th through 12th axillary ribs are demonstrated below the diaphragm.

- The number of ribs located below the diaphragm is determined by the depth of patient inspiration. In full inspiration, up to ten axillary ribs may be demonstrated above the diaphragm. In expiration only seven or eight axillary ribs are clearly visualized above the diaphragm, and four or five ribs are demonstrated below the diaphragm. When below-diaphragm ribs are radiographed, it is necessary to use a higher kVp and exposure than needed for the above-diaphragm ribs, to penetrate the denser abdominal tissue. Any ribs situated above the diaphragm for this radiograph may be too dark to evaluate. To maximize the number of ribs located below the diaphragm, take the exposure on expiration.

The 9th or 10th axillary rib is at the center of the collimated field. A portion of the thoracic and lumbar vertebral column and the 7th through 12th axillary ribs of the affected side of patient are included within the field.

- For posterior oblique axillary rib radiographs, the 9th axillary rib is centered to the radiograph by centering a perpendicular central ray at the level of the xiphoid process, then moving the patient transversely until the longitudinal collimator's light line is aligned with the inferior sternum.

- For anterior oblique axillary rib radiographs position the lower border of the cassette at the patient's iliac crest, center a perpendicular central ray to the center of the film, and then move the patient transversely until the longitudinal collimator's light line is positioned halfway between the vertebral column and the lateral body surface.

  For a hypersthenic patient with a short, wide thorax, this centering needs to be slightly higher. Place the lower border of the cassette about 2 inches (5 cm) superior to the iliac crest, center the central ray to the film, and move the patient transversely until the longitudinal collimator's light line is positioned halfway between the palpable thoracic spinous processes and the affected lateral body surface.

- After the patient has been properly centered to the film, collimate transversely to the vertebral column and the lateral skin-line. Open the longitudinal collimation the full 17-inch (43-cm) field size.

- A 14 × 17 inch (34 × 43) film placed lengthwise should be adequate to include all the required anatomical structures.

Critiquing Radiographs

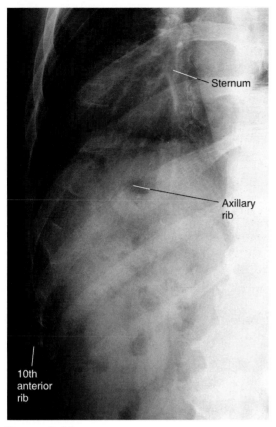

Radiograph labels: Sternum, Axillary rib, 10th anterior rib

Radiograph 11.

Critique: This is an anterior oblique radiograph of the lower ribs. The sternum demonstrates sharply defined cortical outlines, but the axillary ribs are magnified and demonstrate little definition.

Correction: The axillary ribs would demonstrate greater definition if a posterior oblique had been taken instead. Replace a RAO position with a LPO position to demonstrate the left axillary ribs. Replace a LAO position with a RPO position to demonstrate the right axillary ribs.

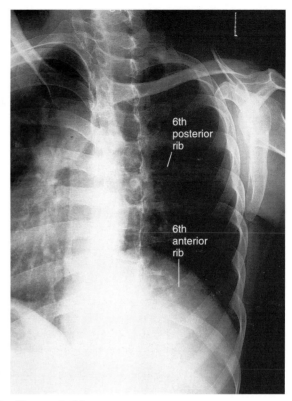

Radiograph labels: 6th posterior rib, 6th anterior rib

Radiograph 12.

Critique: The axillary ribs demonstrate greater self-superimposition, and the sternum is rotated away from the affected ribs. The patient was rotated the wrong way.

Correction: For posterior oblique positions, rotate the patient toward the affected side. For anterior oblique positions, rotate the patient away from the affected side.

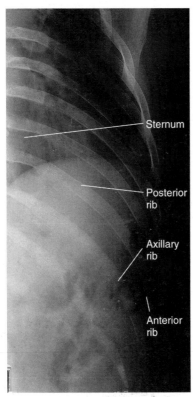

Sternum

Posterior rib

Axillary rib

Anterior rib

Radiograph 13.

Critique: The sternal body is not positioned halfway between the vertebral column and the affected lateral body surface. The sternum is situated next to the vertebral column. The patient was rotated less than 45 degrees.

Correction: Increase the patient obliquity until the midcoronal plane is angled 45 degrees with the film.

References

1. Anagnostakos NP, Tortora GJ. Principles of Anatomy and Physiology, ed 6. New York: Harper & Row, 1990, pp 702–704.
2. Williams PL, Warwick R. Gray's Anatomy, ed 36. Philadelphia: WB Saunders, 1980, pp 286–288.
3. Rogers LF. Radiology of Skeletal Trauma. New York: Churchill Livingstone, 1982, pp 339–373.

CHAPTER 10

Radiographic Critique of the Cranium

CRANIUM

Posteroanterior Projection and Trauma Anteroposterior Projection

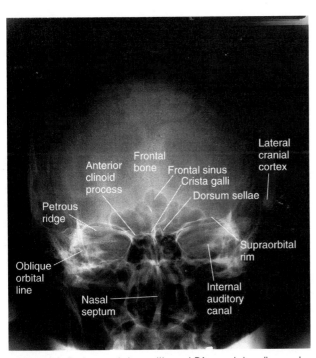

Figure 10-1. Accurately positioned PA cranial radiograph.

Labels on figure: Anterior clinoid process; Frontal bone; Frontal sinus; Crista galli; Lateral cranial cortex; Dorsum sellae; Petrous ridge; Supraorbital rim; Oblique orbital line; Internal auditory canal; Nasal septum

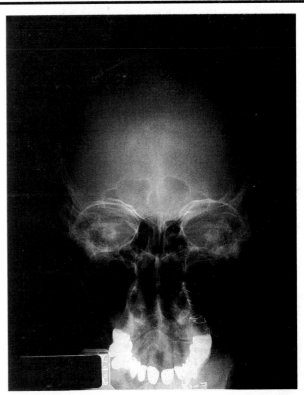

Figure 10-2. Accurately positioned trauma AP cranial radiograph.

Radiographic Evaluation

Facility's patient identification requirements are visible on radiograph.
- These requirements usually are facility name, patient name, age, and hospital number, and exam time and date.
- Patient ID plate is positioned caudally so as not to obscure any portion of the skull.

A right or left marker, identifying the correct side of the patient, is present on the radiograph and does not superimpose anatomy of interest.
- Place the marker laterally within the collimated light field so it does not superimpose any portion of the cranium.
- PA projection radiographs are hung on the view box as if you are facing the patient; therefore, the marker will appear backward when the radiograph is correctly hung.

393

There is no evidence of preventable artifacts, such as hairpins, hair ornaments, removable dental structures, earrings, and hearing aids.

- These structures might overlap needed information.

Contrast and density are adequate to demonstrate the air-filled cavities of the frontal sinuses and the bony structures of the cranium. Penetration is sufficient to visualize the bony trabecular patterns and cortical outlines of the cranium, crista galli, petrous ridges, and dorsum sellae.

- An optimal 70 to 80 kVp technique sufficiently penetrates the soft tissue and bony structures of the cranium.
- Use a high-ratio grid and tight collimation to reduce the amount of scattered radiation that reaches the film, providing a high-contrast radiograph and improving visibility of recorded details.

The bony trabecular patterns and cortical outlines of the cranium as well as the soft tissue structures of the internal auditory canal and frontal sinuses are sharply defined.

- Sharply defined recorded details are obtained when patient motion is controlled, a small focal spot is used, and a short object to image distance (OID) is maintained.

The cranium demonstrates a true PA projection. The distances from the oblique orbital lines to the lateral cranial cortices and from the crista galli to the lateral cranial cortices on either side are equal.

- A PA projection of the cranium is obtained by positioning the patient in an upright or recumbent prone position with the nose and forehead resting against the upright film holder or tabletop (Fig. 10–3).
- Positioning the midsagittal plane perpendicular to the film prevents skull rotation. The best method of accomplishing this goal is to place an extended flat palm next to each lateral parietal bone. Then adjust the head

rotation until your hands are perpendicular to the film and parallel with each other.

- **Detecting Head Rotation:** Radiographically, head rotation is present if the distance from the oblique orbital line to the lateral cranial cortex on one side is greater than on the other side and the distance from the crista galli to the lateral cranial cortex on one side is greater than on the other side (see Rad. 1). The patient's face was rotated away from the side demonstrating the greater distance.
- **Trauma AP Projection of Cranium:** For the trauma AP projection of the cranium, the patient is placed supine on the radiographic table. If injury to cervical vertebrae is suspected, do not adjust the patient's head rotation. Take the radiograph with the head positioned as is. If a cervical vertebral injury is not in question, adjust the patient's head until the midsagittal plane is perpendicular to the film, to prevent rotation.

  An AP skull radiograph should meet all the requirements listed for the PA cranial radiograph, although some features of the cranium appear different. The AP projection demonstrates increased orbital magnification and less distance from the oblique orbital line to the lateral cranial cortices than the PA projection. These differences result from greater magnification of the anatomy situated farther from the film. In the AP projection, the orbits are positioned farther from the film than the lateral parietal bones, whereas in the PA projection, the lateral parietal bones are farther from the film.

The anterior clinoids and dorsum sellae are demonstrated superior to the ethmoid sinuses. The petrous ridges superimpose the supraorbital rims, and the internal auditory canals are demonstrated horizontally through the center of the orbits.

- To position the anterior clinoids and dorsum sellae superior to the ethmoid sinuses, lower or tuck the patient's chin toward the chest until the orbitomeatal line (OML) (imaginary line connecting the outer eye canthus and the external auditory opening) is perpendicular to the film. This positioning moves the frontal bone inferiorly, until it is parallel with the film, and the orbits inferiorly, until the supraorbital rims are situated beneath the petrous ridges, and places the petrous pyramids and internal auditory canals within the orbits.
- **Adjusting Central Ray for Poor OML Alignment:** If the patient is unable to tuck the chin adequately to position the OML perpendicular to the film, the central ray angle may be adjusted to compensate. Instruct the patient to tuck the chin to place the OML as close as possible to perpendicular to the film. Then angle the central ray parallel with the patient's OML (this is easily accomplished by aligning the collimator's transverse light line with the patient's OML).
- **Detecting Poor OML Alignment:** Poor OML alignment can be detected radiographically by evaluating the relationship of the petrous ridges and supraorbital rim. If the patient's chin was not adequately tucked to bring the OML perpendicular to the film,

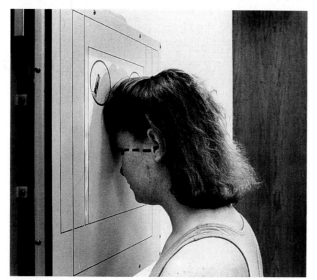

Figure 10-3. Proper patient positioning for PA cranial radiograph.

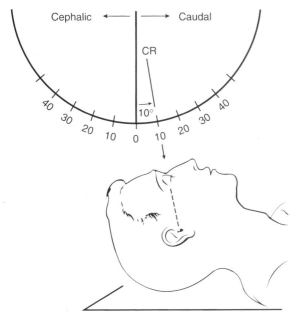

Figure 10-4. Proper patient positioning for AP cranial radiograph. *CR*, central ray. (Reproduced with permission from Martensen K: Trauma Skulls. (In-Service Reviews in Radiologic Technology, vol 15, no 5.) Birmingham, AL: Educational Reviews, 1991.)

the petrous ridges are demonstrated inferior to the supraorbital rims, the internal auditory canals are obscured by the infraorbital rims, and the dorsum sellae and anterior clinoids are demonstrated within the ethmoid sinuses (see Rad. 2). If the patient's chin was tucked more than needed to bring the OML perpendicular to the film, the petrous ridges are demonstrated superior to the supraorbital rims, the internal auditory canals are distorted, and there is greater visualization of the dorsum sellae and anterior clinoids superior to the ethmoid sinuses (see Rad. 3). When adjusting for poor OML alignment, adjust the patient's head the full distance demonstrated between the petrous ridges and supraorbital rims.

- **Trauma AP Projection:** For a trauma AP projection of the cranium when a cervical vertebrae injury is not in question, adjust the patient's head as described for the PA projection. If a cervical vertebrae injury is suspected, do not adjust the patient's head position, or greater cervical injury may result. Instead, angle the central ray through the OML, as demonstrated in Figure 10–4. The angulation required varies according to the chin elevation provided by the cervical collar, but is most often between 10 and 15 degrees caudad.
- **Correcting the Central Ray Angulation for a Trauma AP Projection:** For the trauma AP projection, the central ray angulation determines the relationship of the petrous ridges and the supraorbital rims. For a trauma AP skull radiograph that demonstrates poor supraorbital rim and petrous ridge superimposition, adjust the angulation in the direction you want the orbits to move. If the petrous ridges are demonstrated inferior to the supraorbital rims, the central ray was angled too cephalically and should be adjusted caudally (see Rad. 4). If the petrous ridges

are demonstrated superior to the supraorbital rims, the central ray was angled too caudally and should be adjusted cephalically (see Rad. 5).

The crista galli and nasal septum are aligned with the long axis of the film, and the supraorbital rims are visualized on the same horizontal plane.
- Aligning the head's midsagittal plane with the long axis of the film ensures that the cranium is demonstrated without tilting. Head tilting does not change any anatomical relationships for this position, although severe tilting prevents tight collimation and makes viewing the radiograph slightly more awkward.

The dorsum sellae is centered within the collimated field. The outer cranial cortex and the maxillary sinuses are included within the field.
- Center a perpendicular central ray 0.5 inch (1 cm) superior to the glabella (area located on the midsagittal plane at the level of the eyebrows) to place the dorsum sellae in the center of the collimated field and include the top of the cranium.
- Open the longitudinal and transverse collimation to the head skin-line, or use a circle diaphragm.
- A 10 × 12 inch (24 × 30 cm) film placed lengthwise should be adequate to include all the required anatomical structures.

Critiquing Radiographs

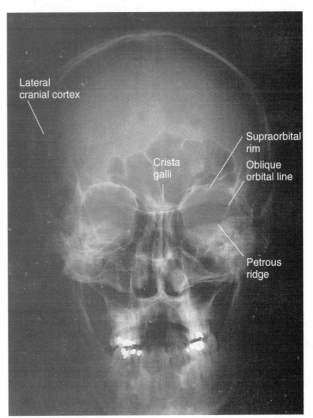

Radiograph 1.

Critique: The distances from the oblique orbital line to the lateral cranial cortex and from the crista galli to the lateral cranial cortex on the right side are greater than the same distances on the left side. The patient's face was rotated toward the left side. The petrous ridges are demonstrated inferior to the supraorbital rims, and the dorsum sellae and anterior clinoids are demonstrated within the ethmoid sinuses. The patient's chin was not tucked enough to position the OML perpendicular to the film.

Correction: Place an extended flat palm next to each lateral parietal bone. Rotate the patient's face toward the right side until your hands are perpendicular to the film. Tuck the patient's chin until the OML is perpendicular to the film.

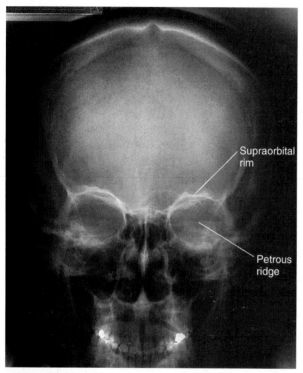

Radiograph 2.

Critique: The petrous ridges are demonstrated inferior to the supraorbital rims, and the dorsum sellae and anterior clinoids are demonstrated within the ethmoid sinuses. The patient's chin was not tucked enough to position the OML perpendicular to the film.

Correction: You need to move the orbits toward the petrous ridges until the ridges superimpose the supraorbital rims. For a nontrauma PA or AP projection, this is accomplished by tucking the patient's chin toward the chest. The amount of movement needed is the full distance demonstrated between the petrous ridges and the supraorbital rims. For this patient, the movement would be about 0.5 inch (1 cm). If the patient is unable to tuck the chin any farther, leave the chin positioned as is, and angle the central ray cephalad for a PA projection and caudad for an AP projection about 5 degrees for every 0.25 inch (0.6 cm) of distance demonstrated between the petrous ridges and the supraorbital rims. This angulation adjustment is based on a 40-inch (102-cm) source–image distance (SID). If a longer SID is used, the angulation adjustment needed is less, whereas if a shorter SID is used, the angulation adjustment needed is more.

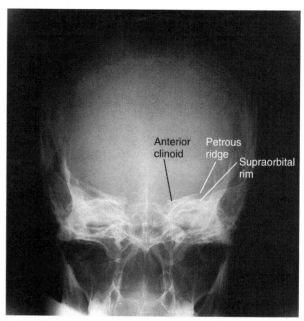

Radiograph 3.

Critique: The petrous ridges are demonstrated superior to the supraorbital rims, and the internal auditory canals are distorted. The patient's chin was tucked more than needed to position the OML perpendicular to the film.

Correction: You need to move the orbits toward the petrous ridges until they are superimposed. For a nontrauma PA or AP projection, this is accomplished by elevating the patient's chin. The amount of movement needed is the full distance demonstrated between the petrous ridges and the supraorbital rims. If this was an AP trauma cranial projection, the central ray angulation would need a cephalic adjustment. The amount of adjustment needed is about 5 degrees for every 0.25 inch (0.6 cm) of distance demonstrated between the petrous ridges and the supraorbital rims. This angulation adjustment is based on a 40-inch (102 cm) SID.

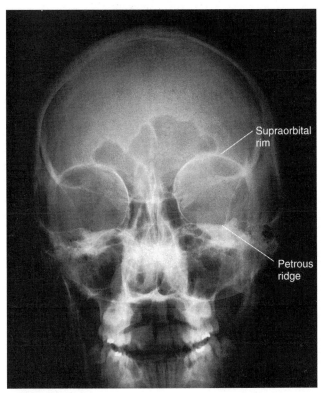

Radiograph 4.

Critique: This is a trauma AP projection. The petrous ridges are demonstrated inferior to the supraorbital rims, and the dorsum sellae and anterior clinoids are demonstrated within the ethmoid sinuses. The central ray was angled too cephalically.

Correction: You need to move the orbits toward the petrous ridges until the supraorbital rims superimpose the petrous ridges. To accomplish this, the angulation needs to be adjusted caudally. The amount of adjustment needed is about 5 degrees for every 0.25 inch (0.6 cm) of distance demonstrated between the petrous ridges and the supraorbital rims. This angulation adjustment is based on a 40-inch (102-cm) SID.

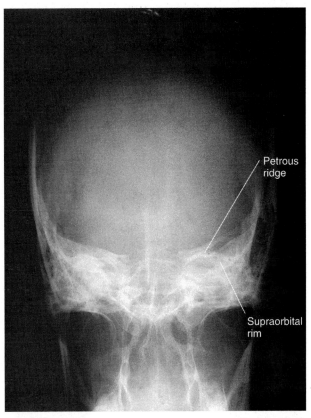

Radiograph 5.

Critique: This is a trauma AP projection. The petrous ridges are demonstrated superior to the supraorbital rims, and the internal auditory canals are obscured. The central ray was angled too caudally.

Correction: You need to move the orbits toward the petrous ridges. To accomplish this, adjust the central ray cephalically. The amount of adjustment needed is about 5 degrees for every 0.25 inch (0.6 cm) of distance demonstrated between the petrous ridges and the supraorbital rims. This angulation adjustment is based on a 40-inch (102-cm) SID.

CRANIUM/FACIAL BONES/SINUSES

Posteroanterior Projection (Caldwell Method) and Trauma Anteroposterior (Caldwell) Projection

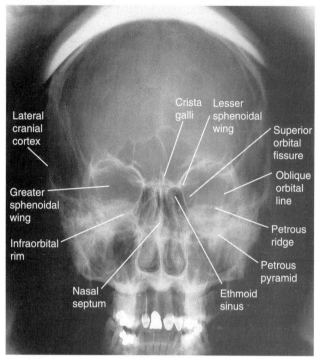

Figure 10-5. Accurately positioned PA (Caldwell) cranial radiograph.

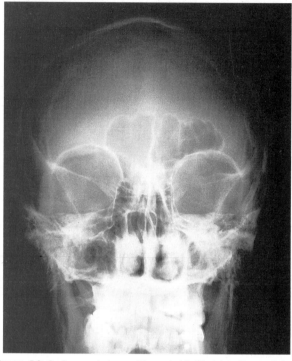

Figure 10-6. Accurately positioned AP (Caldwell) cranial radiograph.

Radiographic Evaluation

Facility's patient identification requirements are visible on radiograph.

- These requirements usually are facility name, patient name, age, and hospital number, and exam time and date.
- Patient ID plate is positioned so as not to obscure anatomy of interest.

A right or left marker, identifying the correct side of the patient, is present on the radiograph and does not superimpose anatomy of interest.

- Place the marker laterally within the collimated light field so it does not superimpose any portion of the cranium.
- PA projection radiographs are hung on the view box as if you are facing the patient; therefore, the marker will appear backward when the radiograph is correctly hung.

There is no evidence of preventable artifacts, such as earrings, hairpins, hair ornaments, removable dental structures, and hearing aids.

- These structures might overlap needed information.

Contrast and density are adequate to demonstrate the air-filled cavities of the frontal and ethmoid sinuses

and the bony structures of the cranium. Penetration is sufficient to visualize the bony trabecular patterns and cortical outlines of the cranium, crista galli, petrous ridges, superior orbital fissures, greater and lesser wings of sphenoid, and orbital rims.

- An optimal 70 to 80 kVp technique sufficiently penetrates the soft tissue and bony structures of the cranium.
- Use a high-ratio grid and tight collimation to reduce the amount of scattered radiation that reaches the film, providing a high-contrast radiograph and improving visibility of recorded details.

The bony trabecular patterns and cortical outlines of the cranium, as well as the soft tissue structures of the frontal and ethmoid sinuses, are sharply defined.

- Sharply defined recorded details are obtained when patient motion is controlled, a small focal spot is used, and a short object–image distance (OID) is maintained.

The cranium demonstrates a true PA projection. The distances from the oblique orbital line to the lateral cranial cortices on each side and from the crista galli to the lateral cranial cortices on each side are equal.

- A PA (Caldwell) projection of the cranium is obtained by positioning the patient in an upright or recumbent

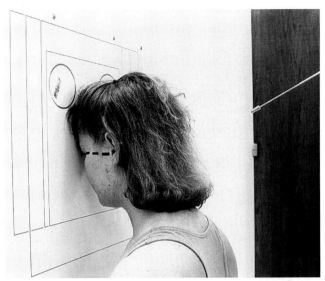

Figure 10-7. Proper patient positioning for PA (Caldwell) cranial radiograph.

prone position with the nose and forehead resting against the upright film holder or tabletop (Fig. 10–7).

- To prevent cranial rotation, position the midsagittal plane perpendicular to the film. The best method of accomplishing this goal is to place an extended flat palm next to each lateral parietal bone. Then adjust the patient's head rotation until your hands are positioned perpendicular to the film and parallel with each other.
- ***Detecting Rotation:*** Radiographically, head rotation is present if the distance from the oblique orbital line to the lateral cranial cortex on one side is greater than that on the other side and if the distance from the crista galli to the lateral cranial cortex on one side is greater than on the other side (Rad. 6). The patient's face was rotated away from the side demonstrating the greater distance.
- ***Positioning for Trauma AP (Caldwell) Projection:*** For the trauma AP (Caldwell) projection of the cranium, the patient is placed supine on the radiographic table. If a cervical vertebral injury is suspected, do not adjust the patient's head rotation. Take the radiograph with the head positioned as is. If a cervical vertebral injury is not in question, adjust the patient's head until the midsagittal plane is perpendicular to the film to prevent rotation.

An AP (Caldwell method) radiograph should meet all the requirements listed for a PA (Caldwell method) radiograph, although some features of the cranium appear different. The AP projection demonstrates greater orbital magnification and less distance from the oblique orbital lines to the lateral cranial cortices than the PA projection. (Compare Figures 10–5 and 10–6.) These differences result from greater magnification of the anatomy situated farther from the film. In an AP projection, the orbits are situated farther from the film than the lateral parietal bones, whereas in a PA projection, the lateral parietal bones are positioned farther from the film.

The petrous ridges are demonstrated horizontally through the lower third of the orbits, the petrous pyramids superimpose the infraorbital rims, and the superior orbital fissures are demonstrated within the orbits.

- Accurate petrous ridge and pyramid placement within the lower third of the orbits is accomplished when the patient's chin is lowered or tucked toward the chest until the orbitomeatal line (OML; imaginary line connecting the outer eye canthus and the external auditory opening) is aligned perpendicular to the film. This positioning moves the frontal bone inferiorly until it is parallel with the film, and the orbits inferiorly until the supraorbital rims are situated beneath the petrous ridges, and places the pyramids and internal auditory canals within the orbits just as they are positioned for a PA skull projection.

For the PA (Caldwell) projection, a 15-degree caudal central ray angulation is then used to align the central ray perpendicular to the frontal and ethmoid sinuses, orbital rims, superior orbital fissures, nasal septum, and anterior nasal spine. This angulation also projects the petrous ridges and pyramids inferiorly, onto the lower third of the orbits.

- ***Adjusting the Central Ray for Poor OML Alignment:*** For a patient who is unable to tuck the chin adequately to position the OML perpendicular to the film, the central ray angulation may be adjusted to compensate. Instruct the patient to tuck the chin to position the OML as close as possible to perpendicular to the film. Angle the central ray parallel with the patient's OML (this is easily accomplished by aligning the collimator's transverse light line with the patient's OML). Then adjust the central ray 15 degrees caudally from the angle obtained when the central ray was parallel with the OML.
- ***Detecting Poor OML-Central Ray Alignment:*** Poor OML and central ray alignment can be detected radiographically by evaluating the relationship of the petrous ridges and the orbits. If the patient's chin was not adequately tucked to bring the OML perpendicular to the film, or if the OML was adequately positioned but the central ray was angled more than 15 degrees caudally, the petrous ridges are demonstrated inferior to the infraorbital rims (see Rad. 7). If the patient's chin was tucked more than needed to bring the OML perpendicular to the film, or if the OML was adequately positioned but the central ray was angled less than 15 degrees caudally, the petrous ridges and pyramids are demonstrated in the upper half of the orbits (see Rad. 8).
- ***Central Ray Angulation for a Trauma AP (Caldwell) Projection:*** For a trauma AP (Caldwell) projection of the cranium if a cervical vertebrae injury is not in question, adjust the patient's head as described for the PA (Caldwell) projection. If a cervical vertebrae injury is suspected, do not adjust the patient's head position, or increased cervical injury may result. Instead, begin by angling the central ray parallel with the OML, as demonstrated in Figure 10–8. The angulation required to do this varies ac-

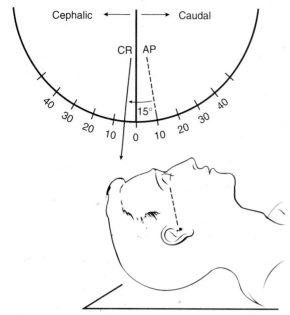

Cephalic ← → Caudal

CR | AP

15°

40 30 20 10 0 10 20 30 40

Figure 10–8. Determining central ray (CR) angulation for trauma AP (Caldwell) cranial radiograph. AP, anteroposterior projection. (Reproduced with permission from Martensen K: Trauma Skulls. (In-Service Reviews in Radiologic Technology, vol 15, no 5.) Birmingham, AL: Educational Reviews, 1991.)

cording to the chin elevation provided by the cervical collar, but is most often between 10 and 15 degrees caudad. From this angulation, adjust the central ray 15 degrees cephalad (a cephalic angulation is used instead of a caudal angle because the patient is now in an AP projection) to align the angle 15 degrees from the OML, as demonstrated in Figure 10–8. For example, if a 10-degree caudal angle was needed to position the central ray parallel with OML, a 5-degree cephalic angulation would be required for the AP (Caldwell) projection; this is 15 degrees cephalad from OML.

- ***Correcting the Central Ray Angulation for a Trauma AP (Caldwell) Projection:*** For the trauma AP (Caldwell) projection, the central ray angulation determines the relationship of the petrous ridges and the orbits. For an AP (Caldwell) cranial radiograph that demonstrates a poor petrous ridge and orbital relationship, adjust the central ray angulation

in the direction that you want the orbits to move. If the petrous ridges are demonstrated inferior to the infraorbital rims, the central ray was angled too cephalically and should be adjusted caudally. (The petrous ridge and orbital relationship obtained would be similar to that shown in Radiograph 7.) If the petrous ridges are demonstrated in the superior half of the orbits, the central ray was angled too caudally and should be adjusted cephalically. (The petrous ridge and orbital relationship obtained would be similar to that shown in Radiograph 8.)

The crista galli and nasal septum are aligned with the long axis of the film, and the supraorbital rims are visualized on the same horizontal plane.

- Aligning the head's midsagittal plane with the long axis of the film ensures that the patient's cranium is demonstrated without tilting. Slight tilting does not change any anatomical relationships for this position, although it does prevent tight collimation and makes viewing the radiograph slightly more awkward.

The ethmoid sinuses are centered within the collimated field. *When the radiograph is taken for the cranium,* **the outer cranial cortex and the ethmoid sinuses are included within the field.** *When the radiograph is taken for facial bones or sinuses,* **the frontal and ethmoid sinuses and the lateral cranial cortices are included within the field.**

- Centering the central ray to the nasion—the area located on the midsagittal plane at a level 0.75 inch (2 cm) inferior to the eyebrows—places the ethmoid sinuses in the center of the collimated field. A slightly higher centering may be needed if the entire cranial cortex is required on the radiograph.)
- Open the longitudinal and transverse collimation to the head skin-line, or use a circle diaphragm, when the radiograph is taken for the cranium.
- Open the longitudinal and transverse collimation to within 1 inch (2.5 cm) of the sinus cavities, or use a circle diaphragm when a radiograph is taken for facial bones or sinuses.
- A 10 × 12 inch (24 × 30 cm) film placed lengthwise should be adequate to include all required anatomical structures when the cranium is radiographed.
- An 8 × 10 inch (18 × 24 cm) film placed lengthwise is sufficient when facial bones or sinuses are radiographed.

Critiquing Radiographs

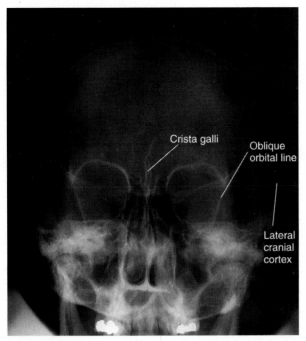

Radiograph 6.

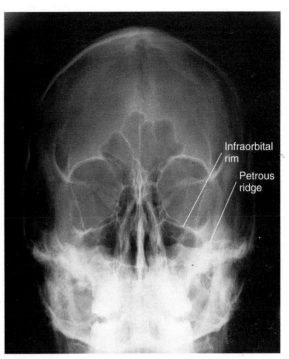

Radiograph 7.

Critique: The distances from the oblique orbital line to the lateral cranial cortex and from the crista galli to the lateral cranial cortex on the left side are greater than on the right side. The patient's face was rotated toward the right side.

Correction: Place an extended flat palm next to each lateral parietal bone. Rotate the patient's face toward the left side until your hands are positioned perpendicular to the film.

Critique: The petrous ridges are demonstrated inferior to the infraorbital rims. The patient's chin was not tucked enough to position the OML perpendicular to the film.

If this anatomical relationship was obtained on a trauma AP (Caldwell) projection radiograph, the central ray angulation was angled too cephalically.

Correction: Tuck the chin toward the chest until the OML is aligned perpendicular to the film. The amount of movement needed is the full distance demonstrated between where the petrous ridges are located on this radiograph and where they should be located on an accurately positioned PA (Caldwell) projection radiograph. If the patient is unable to tuck the chin any farther, leave the chin positioned as is, and angle the central ray cephalically about 5 degrees for every 0.25 inch (0.6 cm) of distance demonstrated between where the petrous ridges are located on this radiograph and where they should be on an accurately positioned PA (Caldwell) projection radiograph. This angulation adjustment is based on a 40-inch (102-cm) source–image distance, as described for Radiograph 2.

If this is a trauma AP (Caldwell) projection radiograph, angle the central ray caudally about 5 degrees for every 0.25 inch (0.6 cm) of distance demonstrated between where the petrous ridges are located on this radiograph and where they should be located on an accurately positioned AP (Caldwell) projection radiograph.

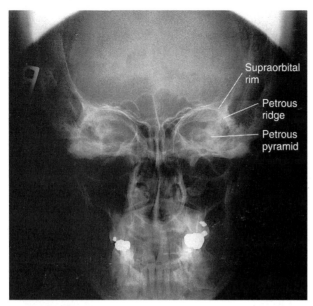

Radiograph 8.

Critique: The petrous ridges and pyramids are demonstrated in the superior half of the orbits. The patient's chin was tucked more than needed to position the OML perpendicular to the film.

If this anatomical relationship was obtained on a trauma AP (Caldwell) projection radiograph, the central ray angulation was angled too caudally.

Correction: Elevate the chin until the OML is perpendicular to the film. The amount of movement needed is the full distance demonstrated between where the petrous ridges are located on this radiograph and where they should be located on an accurately positioned PA (Caldwell) projection radiograph.

If this is a trauma AP (Caldwell) projection radiograph, angle the central ray cephalically about 5 degrees for every 0.25 inch (0.6 cm) of distance demonstrated between where the petrous ridges are located on this radiograph and where they should be located on an accurately positioned AP (Caldwell) projection radiograph.

CRANIUM/MASTOIDS

Anteroposterior Axial Projection (Towne Position)

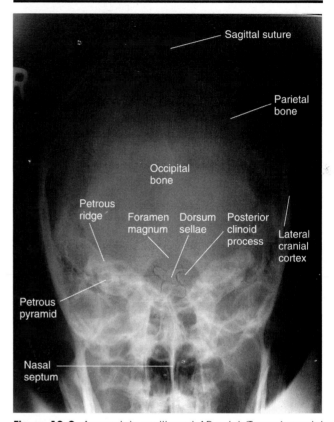

Figure 10-9. Accurately positioned AP axial (Towne) cranial radiograph.

Radiographic Evaluation

Facility's patient identification requirements are visible on radiograph.

- These requirements usually are facility name, patient name, age, and hospital number, and exam time and date.
- Patient ID plate is positioned so as not to obscure anatomy of interest.

A right or left marker, identifying the correct side of the patient, is present on the radiograph and does not superimpose anatomy of interest.

- Place the marker laterally within the collimated light field so it does not superimpose any portion of the cranium.

There is no evidence of preventable artifacts, such as hairpins, hair ornaments, removable dental structures, earrings, and hearing aids.

- These structures might overlap needed information.

Contrast and density are adequate to demonstrate the mastoid air cells and the bony structures of the cranium. Penetration is sufficient to visualize the bony

trabecular patterns and cortical outlines of the parietal bones, occipital bone, petrous pyramids, foramen magnum, dorsum sellae, and posterior clinoids.

- An optimal 70 to 80 kVp technique sufficiently penetrates the soft tissue and bony structures of the cranium.
- Use a high-ratio grid and tight collimation to reduce the amount of scattered radiation that reaches the film, providing a high-contrast radiograph and improving visibility of recorded details.

The bony trabecular patterns and cortical outlines of the cranium, foramen magnum, and dorsum sellae are sharply defined.

- Sharply defined recorded details are obtained when patient motion is controlled, respiration is halted, a small focal spot is used, and a short object–image distance (OID) is maintained.

The cranium is demonstrated without rotation. The distances from the posterior clinoid process to the lateral borders of the foramen magnum on either side are equal, the petrous ridges are symmetrical, and the dorsum sellae is centered within the foramen magnum.

- An AP axial (Towne) projection of the cranium is obtained by positioning the patient in an upright AP projection or supine position with the posterior head resting against the upright film holder or tabletop (Fig. 10–10). Position the midsagittal plane perpendicular to the film to prevent cranial rotation. The best method of accomplishing this goal is to place an extended flat palm next to each lateral parietal bone, and then to adjust patient head rotation until your hands are perpendicular to the film and parallel with each other.
- **Detecting Head Rotation:** Radiographically, head rotation was present if the distance from the posterior clinoid process to the lateral border of the foramen magnum is greater on one side than the other side and if the dorsum sellae is demonstrated closer to one side of the foramen magnum. The patient's

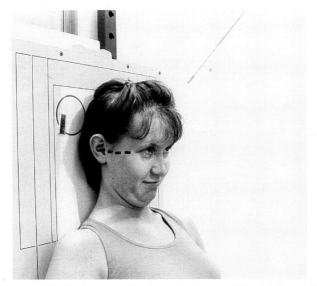

Figure 10–10. Proper patient positioning for AP axial (Towne) cranial radiograph.

face was rotated toward the side demonstrating less distance from the posterior clinoid process to the lateral foramen magnum (Rad. 9).

- **Positioning for Trauma:** For a trauma AP axial (Towne) projection of the cranium, the patient is positioned supine on the radiographic table. If a cervical vertebral injury is suspected, do not adjust the patient head rotation. Take the radiograph with the head positioned as is. If a cervical vertebral injury is not in question, adjust the patient's head until the midsagittal plane is positioned perpendicular to the film, to prevent rotation.

The dorsum sellae and posterior clinoids are demonstrated within the foramen magnum without foreshortening or superimposition of the atlas's posterior arch.

- A combination of patient positioning and central ray angulation accurately demonstrates the dorsum sellae and posterior clinoids within the foramen magnum. To accomplish proper patient positioning, tuck the chin until the orbitomeatal line (OML; imaginary line connecting the outer eye canthus and the external auditory opening) is aligned perpendicular to the film. This positioning aligns an imaginary line connecting the dorsum sellae and foramen magnum at a 30-degree angle with the film and the OML. The central ray needs to be aligned parallel with this line to project the dorsum sellae into the foramen magnum. This explains the need for a 30-degree caudal angulation for the AP axial (Towne) projection of the cranium.
- **Adjusting the Central Ray for Poor OML Alignment:** For a patient who is unable to tuck the chin adequately to position the OML perpendicular to the film, the central ray angulation may be adjusted to compensate. Instruct the patient to tuck the chin to position the OML as close as possible to perpendicular to the film. Angle the central ray parallel with the OML (this is easily accomplished by aligning the collimator's transverse light line with the patient's OML), then adjust the central ray 30 degrees caudally from the angle obtained when the central ray was parallel with the OML (Fig. 10–11).
- **Effect of OML–Central Ray Misalignment:** If the patient's chin is not adequately tucked to bring the OML perpendicular to the film or if the central ray was not angled enough to place it at a 30-degree angle with the OML, the dorsum sellae and posterior clinoids are projected superior to the foramen magnum (see Rad. 10). If the chin was tucked more than needed to bring the OML perpendicular to the film, or if the central ray was angled more than 30 degrees with the OML, the dorsum sellae is foreshortened and superimposes the posterior arch of the atlas (see Rad. 11).
- **Central Ray Angulation for Trauma:** For an AP trauma axial (Towne) radiograph of the cranium, if a cervical vertebrae injury is not suspected, adjust the patient's head as described. If a cervical vertebral injury is suspected, do not adjust the patient's head position, or further cervical injury may result. Instead, begin by angling the central ray parallel with the OML. The angulation required to do this varies ac-

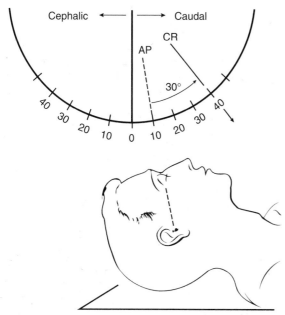

Cephalic ← → Caudal

Figure 10-11. Determinine central ray (CR) angulation for AP axial cranial radiograph in a trauma patient. AP, anteroposterior projection. (Reproduced with permission from Martensen K: Trauma Skulls. (In-Service Reviews in Radiologic Technology, vol 15, no 5.) Birmingham, AL: Educational Reviews, 1991.)

cording to the chin elevation provided by the cervical collar, but is most often between 10 and 15 degrees caudad. From this angulation, adjust the central ray 30 degrees caudally to align it 30 degrees with the OML, as demonstrated in Figure 10–11. For example, if a 10-degree caudal angulation was needed to position the central ray parallel with OML, a 40-degree caudal angulation is the required angle for the AP axial (Towne) projection; this is a 30-degree angle from the OML. The angle used for this projection should not exceed 45 degrees, or excessive distortion will result.

The sagittal suture and nasal septum are aligned with the long axis of the collimated field.

- Aligning the head's midsagittal plane with the long axis of the collimator's longitudinal light line ensures that the patient's cranium is demonstrated without tilting. Head tilting changes the alignment of the central ray, dorsum sellae, and foramen magnum by positioning the dorsum sellae laterally to the central ray and foramen magnum.

The inferior occipital bone is centered within the collimated field. The outer cranial cortex, petrous ridges, dorsum sellae, and foramen magnum are included within the field.

- Center the central ray to the midsagittal plane at a level 2.5 inches (6 cm) above the patient's eyebrows.
- Open the longitudinally and transversely collimated field to the head skin-line, or use a circle diaphragm.
- A 10 × 12 inch (24 × 30 cm) film placed lengthwise should be adequate to include all the required anatomical structures.

Critiquing Radiographs

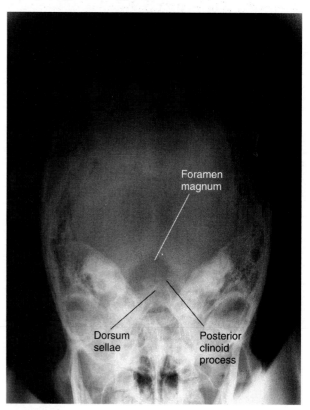

Foramen magnum

Dorsum sellae

Posterior clinoid process

Radiograph 9.

Critique: The distance from the posterior clinoid process to the lateral foramen magnum is less on the patient's left side than on the right side. The patient's face was rotated toward the left side.

Correction: Place an extended flat palm next to each lateral parietal bone. Rotate the patient's face toward the right side until your hands are perpendicular to the film and parallel with each other.

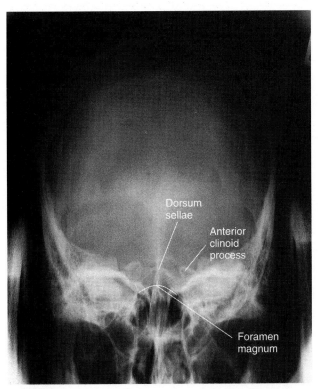

Radiograph 10.

Critique: The dorsum sellae and anterior clinoids are demonstrated superior to the foramen magnum. Either the patient's chin was not tucked enough or the central ray was not angled caudally enough to form a 30-degree angle with the OML.

Correction: Tuck the patient's chin until the OML is perpendicular to the film. The amount of movement needed is the full distance demonstrated between where the foramen magnum is located and where it should be located on an accurately positioned AP axial (Towne) projection. If the patient is unable to tuck the chin any farther, or if this is a trauma AP axial (Towne) projection, leave the patient's chin positioned as is, and angle the central ray caudally about 5 degrees for every 0.25 inch (0.6 cm) of distance demonstrated between where the foramen magnum is located on this radiograph and where it should be on an accurately positioned AP axial (Towne) projection. This angulation adjustment is based on a 40-inch (102-cm) source–image distance, as described for Radiograph 2.

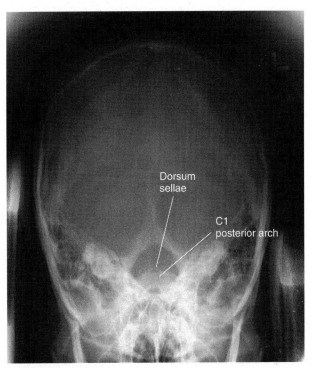

Radiograph 11.

Critique: The dorsum sellae is foreshortened and is superimposing the atlas's posterior arch. Either the patient's chin was tucked more than needed to bring the OML perpendicular to the film or the central ray was angled more caudally than needed to form a 30-degree angle with the OML.

Correction: Elevate the patient's chin until the OML is perpendicular to the film. The amount of movement needed is the full distance needed to position the posterior arch inferior to the dorsum sellae. If this is a trauma AP axial (Towne) projection, angle the central ray cephalically about 5 degrees for every 0.25 inch (0.6 cm) of the posterior arch that is demonstrated.

CRANIUM/FACIAL BONES/SINUSES

Lateral Position

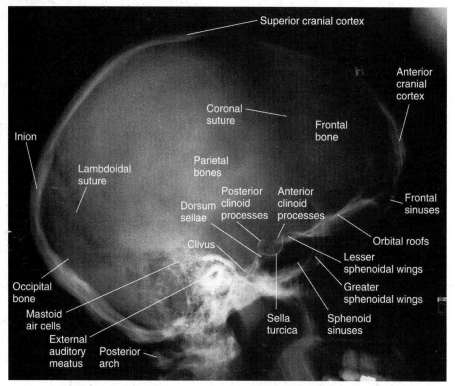

Figure 10-12. Accurately positioned lateral cranial radiograph.

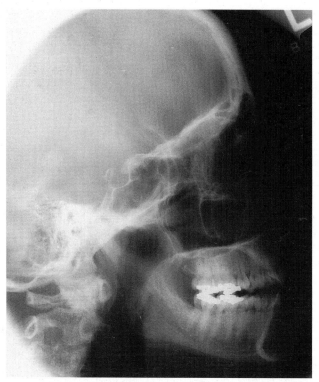

Figure 10-13. Accurately positioned lateral facial bones and sinuses radiograph.

Radiographic Evaluation

Facility's patient identification requirements are visible on radiograph.
- These requirements usually are facility name, patient name, age, and hospital number, and exam time and date.
- Patient ID plate is positioned so as not to obscure anatomy of interest.

A right or left marker, identifying the side of the patient positioned closer to the film, is present on the radiograph and does not superimpose anatomy of interest.
- Place the marker anteriorly within the collimated light field so it does not superimpose any portion of the cranium.

There is no evidence of preventable artifacts, such as hairpins, hair ornaments, earrings, removable dental structures, and hearing aids.
- These structures might overlap needed information.

Contrast and density are adequate to demonstrate the air-filled cavities of the sphenoid sinuses and the superimposed ethmoid, frontal, and maxillary sinuses as well as the bony structures of the cranium. Penetration is sufficient to visualize the bony trabecular patterns and cortical outlines of the cranium, sella turcica, anterior and posterior clinoids, dorsum sellae, clivus, greater and lesser wings of the sphenoid, and orbital roofs.
- An optimal 70 to 75 kVp technique sufficiently penetrates the soft tissue and bony structures of the cranium.
- Use a high-ratio grid and tight collimation to reduce the amount of scattered radiation that reaches the film, providing a high-contrast radiograph and improving visibility of recorded details.

The bony trabecular patterns and cortical outlines of the cranium, sella turcica, clivus, dorsum sellae, greater and lesser wings of the sphenoid, and orbital roofs are sharply defined.
- Sharply defined recorded details are obtained when patient motion is controlled, respiration is halted, a small focal spot is used, and a short object–image distance (OID) is maintained.

The cranium is in a lateral position. The sella turcica is demonstrated in profile, and the orbital roofs, mandibular rami, greater wings of the sphenoid, external auditory canals, and cranial cortices are superimposed.
- Obtain a lateral position of the cranium by placing the patient in an upright PA projection or recumbent prone position, with the affected side of head against the upright film holder or tabletop.
  To demonstrate air-fluid levels within the sinus cavities, this projection should be taken in an upright position. In this position the thick, gelatinlike sinus fluid settles to the lowest position, creating an air-fluid line that shows the reviewer the amount of fluid present.
  Rotate the patient's head and body as needed to place the head in a true lateral position, with the head's midsagittal plane parallel with the film and the

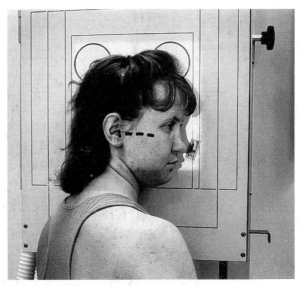

Figure 10-14. Proper patient positioning for lateral cranial radiograph.

interpupillary line (imaginary line connecting the outer corners of the eyelids) perpendicular to the film (Fig. 10–14). It may be necessary to position a sponge beneath the patient's chin or head to help maintain precise positioning.
- ***Positioning for Trauma:*** A trauma lateral cranial radiograph is accomplished by placing a crosswise film vertically against the patient's shoulder and directing a horizontal beam to a point 2 inches (5 cm) superior to the external auditory meatus (EAM). For a patient whose head position can be manipulated, elevate the occiput on a radiolucent sponge and adjust the head until the midsagittal plane is parallel with the film. If a cervical vertebral injury is suspected, do not adjust the patient's head; take the radiograph with the head positioned as is, and position the cassette 1 inch (2.5 cm) below the occipital bone.
- ***Detecting Rotation:*** Accurate positioning of the head's midsagittal plane is essential to prevent rotation and tilting of the cranium. If the patient's head was not adequately turned to position the midsagittal plane parallel with the film, rotation of the cranium results. Radiographically cranial rotation results in distortion of the sella turcica and situates one of the mandibular rami, greater wings of the sphenoid, external auditory canals, and anterior cranial cortices anterior to the other (see Rad. 12).
- ***Distinguishing Tilting from Rotation:*** If the patient's head was tilted toward or away from the film, preventing the midsagittal plane from aligning parallel with the film or the interpupillary line from aligning perpendicular to the film, tilting of the cranium results. Tilting can be radiographically distinguished from rotation by studying the superimposition of the orbital roofs, the greater wings of the sphenoid, the external auditory canals, and the inferior cranial cortices. If the patient's head was tilted, one of each corresponding structure is demonstrated superior to the other (see Rad. 13). Because the two sides of the cranium are mirror images, it is very difficult to

determine which way the face was rotated or the head tilted when studying poorly positioned lateral cranial radiographs. Paying close attention to initial positioning may give you an idea as to which way the patient has a tendency to lean. Routinely, patients tend to rotate their faces and lean the tops of their heads toward the film.

The posteroinferior occipital bone and posterior arch of the atlas are free of superimposition.
- Adjusting the chin to bring the infraorbitomeatal line (imaginary line connecting the lower orbital outline and the EAM) perpendicular to the front edge of the cassette positions the posteroinferior cranium superior to the posterior arch of the atlas, preventing their superimposition.

LATERAL RADIOGRAPH OF THE CRANIUM

An area 2 inches (5 cm) superior to the external auditory meatus (EAM) is centered within the collimated field. The outer cranial cortex is included within the field.
- Centering a perpendicular central ray to a point 2

inches (5 cm) superior to the EAM positions the cranium in the center of the collimated field.
- Open the longitudinally and transversely collimated field to the patient's head skin-line, or use a circle diaphragm.
- A 10 × 12 inch (24 × 30 cm) film placed crosswise should be adequate to include all the required anatomical structures.

LATERAL RADIOGRAPH OF THE FACIAL BONES OR SINUSES

The greater wings of the sphenoid are centered within the collimated field. Included within the field are the frontal, ethmoid, sphenoid and maxillary sinuses, and the mandible.
- Centering a perpendicular central ray halfway between the outer canthus (outer corner of the eyelids) and the EAM positions the greater wings of the sphenoid in the center of the collimated field.
- Open the longitudinally and transversely collimated field to within 1 inch (2.5 cm) from the sinuses, or use a circle diaphragm.
- An 8 × 10 inch (18 × 24 cm) film placed lengthwise should be adequate to include all the required anatomical structures.

Critiquing Radiographs

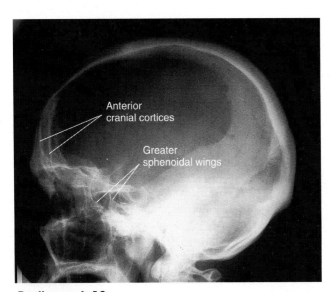

Radiograph 12.

Critique: The greater wings of the sphenoid and the anterior cranial cortices are demonstrated without superimposition. One of each corresponding structure is visualized anterior to the other. The patient's head was rotated.
Correction: Position the cranium's midsagittal plane parallel with the film.

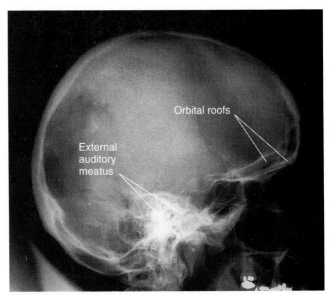

Radiograph 13.

Critique: The orbital roofs, the external auditory meatus, and the inferior cranial cortices are demonstrated without superimposition. One of each corresponding structure is visualized superior to the other. The patient's head was tilted.
Correction: Position the cranium's midsagittal plane parallel with the film and the interpupillary line perpendicular to the film.

Cranium/Facial Bones/Sinuses:
Submentovertex Projection (Basilar Position)

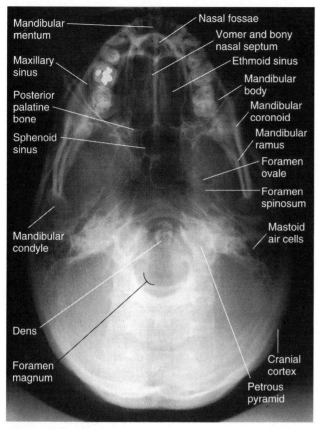

Figure 10-15. Accurately positioned submentovertex (basilar) cranial radiograph.

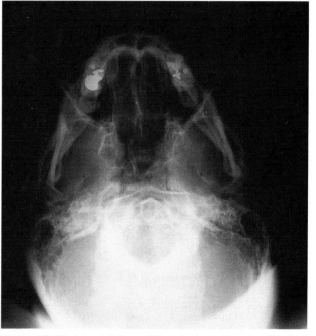

Figure 10-16. Accurately positioned submentovertex (basilar) facial bones and sinuses radiograph.

Radiographic Evaluation

Facility's patient identification requirements are visible on radiograph.

- These requirements usually are facility name, patient name, age, and hospital number, and exam time and date.
- Patient ID plate is positioned so as not to obscure anatomy of interest.

A right or left marker, identifying the correct side of the patient, is present on the radiograph and does not superimpose anatomy of interest.

- Place the marker laterally within the collimated light field so it does not superimpose any portion of the cranium.
- Hang a submentovertex (basiliar) cranial radiograph on the viewbox with the anterior surface facing upward.

There is no evidence of preventable artifacts, such as hairpins, hair ornaments, earrings, hearing aids, necklaces, and removable dental structures.

- These structures might overlap needed information.

Contrast and density are adequate to demonstrate the air-filled cavities of the sphenoid and ethmoid sinuses, nasal fossae, and mastoid processes as well as the bony structures of the cranium. Penetration is sufficient to visualize the bony trabecular patterns and cortical outlines of the foramen ovale and spinosum, mandible, petrous pyramids, foramen magnum, and occipital bone.

- An optimal 70 to 80 kVp technique sufficiently penetrates the soft tissue and bony structures of the cranium.
- Use a high-ratio grid and tight collimation to reduce the amount of scattered radiation that reaches the film, providing a high-contrast radiograph and improving visibility of recorded details.

The bony trabecular patterns and cortical outlines of the cranium, mandible, and foramen magnum are sharply defined.

- Sharply defined recorded details are obtained when patient motion is controlled, respiration is halted, a small focal spot is used, and a short object–image distance (OID) is maintained.

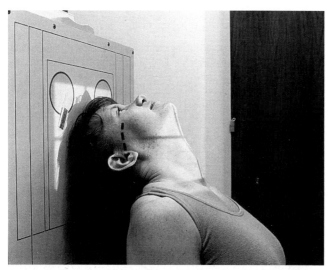

Figure 10-17. Proper patient positioning for submentovertex (basilar) cranial radiograph.

The mandibular mentum and nasal fossae are demonstrated just anterior to the ethmoid sinuses.

- The submentovertex projection (basilar position) is accomplished by placing the patient in an upright AP projection with the cranial vertex resting against the upright film holder or tabletop. Continue to elevate the chin and hyperextend the patient's neck until the infraorbitomeatal line (IOML; imaginary line connecting the palpable lower orbital rim and the external auditory opening) is parallel to the upright film holder or tabletop (Fig. 10–17). For a patient with a retracted jaw, it may be necessary to raise the chin and extend the patient's neck beyond the IOML to position the mandibular mentum anterior to the frontal bone.

   If the patient is unable to align the IOML parallel with the tabletop, extend the patient's neck as far as possible, and angle the central ray cephalad until it is aligned perpendicular to the IOML.

- **Effect of Mispositioning IOML:** Mispositioning of the mandibular mentum and ethmoid sinuses on a submentovertex (basilar) position obscures the nasal fossae, ethmoid sinuses, and foramen ovale and spinosum. If the patient's neck was overextended, the mandibular mentum is demonstrated too far anterior to the ethmoid sinuses (see Rad. 14). If the patient's neck was underextended, the mandibular mentum is demonstrated posterior to the ethmoid sinuses (see Rad. 15).

The distances from the mandibular ramus and body to the lateral cranial cortex on either side are equal.

- Positioning the cranium's midsagittal plane perpendicular to the film prevents cranial tilting.
- **Detecting Head Tilting:** Cranial tilting can be identified on a submentovertex projection (basilar position) of the head by comparing the distances from the mandibular ramus and body to the corresponding lateral cranial cortex on either side. If the head was not tilted, the distances are equal. If the head was tilted the distance is greater on the side the cranial vertex was tilted toward (see Rad. 16).

The vomer, bony nasal septum, and dens are aligned with the long axis of the collimated field.

- Turning the patient's face until the midsagittal plane is aligned with the long axis of the collimator's longitudinal light line ensures that the patient's head is not rotated. Rotation does not change any anatomical relationships for this position, although it does prevent tight collimation and makes viewing of the radiograph slightly more awkward.

SUBMENTOVERTEX PROJECTION (BASILAR POSITION) OF THE CRANIUM

The dens is centered within the collimated field. The mandible and the outer cranial cortices are included within the field.

- Centering a perpendicular central ray to the midsagittal plane at a level 0.50 inch (1.25 cm) posterior to the palpable mandibular angles places the dens in the center of the collimated field.
- Open the longitudinally and transversely collimated field to the patient's lateral head skin-line and mandibular mentum, or use a circle diaphragm.
- A 10 × 12 inch (24 × 30 cm) film placed lengthwise should be adequate to include all the required anatomical structures.

SUBMENTOVERTEX PROJECTION (BASILAR POSITION) OF THE FACIAL BONES OR SINUSES

The sphenoid sinuses are centered within the collimated field. The mandible, lateral cranial cortices, and mastoid air cells are included within the field.

- Centering a perpendicular central ray to the midsagittal plane at a level 1.5 inch (4 cm) posterior to the palpable mandibular mentum places the ethmoid sinuses in the center of the collimated field.
- Open the longitudinally and transversely collimated field to the patient's lateral head skin-line and mandibular mentum, or use a circle diaphragm.
- An 8 × 10 inch (18 × 24 cm) film placed lengthwise should be adequate to include all the required anatomical structures.

Critiquing Radiographs

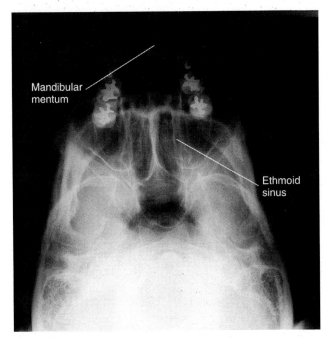

Radiograph 14.

Critique: The mandibular mentum is demonstrated too far anterior to the ethmoid sinuses. The patient's neck was overextended, preventing the IOML from being positioned parallel with the film. If the central ray was angled to accomplish this radiograph, it was angled too cephalically.

Correction: Depress the patient's chin until the IOML is aligned parallel with the film. The amount of movement needed is half the distance demonstrated between the mandibular mentum and the ethmoid sinuses. If the central ray was angled, adjust the angulation 5 degrees caudally for every 0.25 inch (0.6 cm) of distance demonstrated between the mandibular mentum and anterior ethmoid sinuses. This angulation adjustment is based on a 40-inch (102-cm) source–image distance.

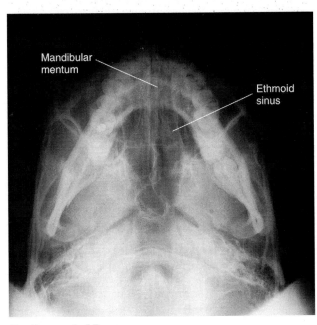

Radiograph 15.

Critique: The mandibular mentum is demonstrated posterior to the ethmoid sinuses. The patient's neck was underextended, preventing the IOML from being positioned parallel with the film.

Correction: Elevate the patient's chin until the IOML is aligned parallel with the film. The amount of movement needed is half the distance demonstrated between the mandibular mentum and the ethmoid sinuses. If the patient is unable to elevate the chin or hyperextend the neck any farther, leave the position as is, and angle the central ray cephalad either until it is perpendicular to the IOML or 5 degrees cephalad for every 0.25 inch (0.6 cm) of distance demonstrated between the mandibular mentum and the anterior ethmoid sinuses.

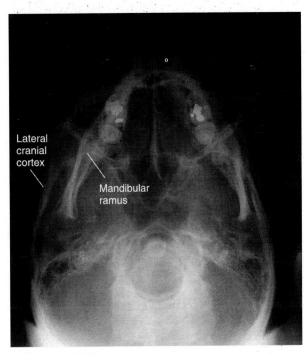

Radiograph 16.

Critique: The distance from the right mandibular ramus and body to its corresponding lateral cranial cortex is greater than the distance from the left mandibular ramus and body to its corresponding lateral cranial cortex. The patient's cranial vertex was tilted toward the right side.

Correction: Tilt the patient's cranial vertex toward the left side until the cranium's midsagittal plane is perpendicular to the film.

FACIAL BONES/SINUSES

Parietoacanthal Projection (Waters and Open-Mouth Waters Position) and Trauma Acanthoparietal Projection

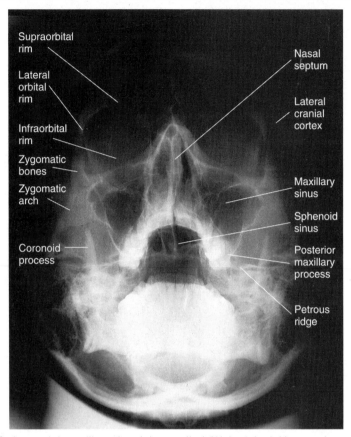

Figure 10-18. Accurately positioned parietoacanthal (Waters) facial bones–sinuses radiograph.

Radiographic Evaluation

Facility's patient identification requirements are visible on radiograph.

- These requirements usually are facility name, patient name, age, and hospital number, and exam time and date.
- Patient ID plate is positioned so as not to obscure anatomy of interest.

A right or left marker, identifying the correct side of the patient, is present on the radiograph and does not superimpose anatomy of interest.

- Place the marker laterally within the collimated light field so it does not superimpose any portion of the cranium.
- PA projection radiographs are hung on the viewbox as if you are facing the patient; therefore, the marker appears backward when the radiograph is correctly hung.

There is no evidence of preventable artifacts, such as earrings, hairpins, hair ornaments, removable dental structures, and hearing aids.

- These structures might overlap needed information.

Contrast and density are adequate to demonstrate the air-filled cavities of the nasal fossae and maxillary (and sphenoid on the open-mouth position) sinuses, as well as the bony structures of the cranium. Penetration is sufficient to visualize the bony trabecular patterns and cortical outlines of the orbital rims, maxillae, nasal septum, zygomatic bones, and arches and petrous ridges.

- An optimal 70 to 80 kVp technique sufficiently penetrates the soft tissue and bony structures of the cranium.
- Use a high-ratio grid and tight collimation to reduce the amount of scattered radiation that reaches the film, providing a high-contrast radiograph and improving visibility of recorded details.

The bony trabecular patterns and cortical outlines of the cranium as well as the soft tissue structures of the maxillary sinuses are sharply defined.

- Sharply defined recorded details are obtained when patient motion is controlled, a small focal spot is used, and a short object–image distance (OID) is maintained.

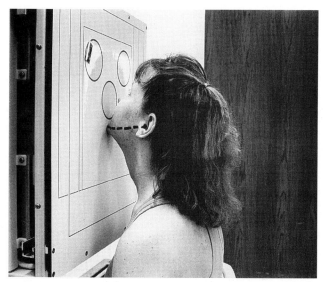

Figure 10-19. Proper patient positioning for parietoacanthal (Waters) facial bones–sinuses radiograph.

The cranium is demonstrated without rotation: The distances from the lateral orbital rim to the lateral cranial cortex and the distance from the bony nasal septum to the lateral cranial cortex on either side are equal.

- The parietoacanthal (Waters) projection of the cranium is obtained by positioning the patient in an upright or recumbent prone position with the neck extended and the chin resting against the upright film holder or tabletop (Fig. 10–19).
- To demonstrate air-fluid levels within the maxillary sinus cavities, this projection should be taken in an upright position. The thick, gelatinlike sinus fluid then settles to the lowest level in the sinus cavity, creating an air-fluid line that shows the reviewer the amount of fluid present.
- To prevent cranial rotation, position an extended flat palm next to each lateral parietal bone. Then adjust the head rotation until your hands are perpendicular to the film and parallel with each other.
- ***Detecting Head Rotation:*** Radiographically, head rotation was present if the distance from the lateral orbital rim to the lateral cranial cortex on one side is greater than on the other side and if the distance from the bony nasal septum to the lateral cranial cortex on one side is greater than on the other side (see Rad. 17). The patient's face was rotated away from the side demonstrating the greater distance.
- ***Positioning for Trauma Acanthoparietal (Waters) Projection:*** For the trauma acanthoparietal (Waters) projection of the cranium, the patient is supine on the radiographic table. If a cervical vertebral injury is suspected do not adjust the patient's head rotation, but take the radiograph with the head positioned as is. If a cervical vertebral injury is not in question, adjust the patient's head to prevent rotation.

An acanthoparietal projection radiograph should meet all the requirements listed for a parietoacanthal projection radiograph, although some features of the cranium appear different. The acanthoparietal

projection demonstrates greater orbital magnification and less distance from the lateral orbital rim to the lateral cranial cortices than does the parietoacanthal projection (Compare Fig. 10–18 and Rad. 20). These differences result from greater magnification of the anatomy situated farther from the film. In the acanthoparietal projection, the orbits are situated farther from the film than the parietal bones, whereas in the parietoacanthial projection, the parietal bones are positioned farther from the film.

The petrous ridges are visualized inferior to the maxillary sinuses and extend laterally from the posterior maxillary alveolar process.

- To accurately position the petrous ridges inferior to the maxillary sinuses, elevate the patient's chin until the orbitomeatal line (OML; imaginary line connecting the outer eye canthus to the external auditory opening) is at a 37-degree angle with the perpendicular central ray. Chin elevation moves the maxillary sinuses superior to the petrous ridges. This is best accomplished by positioning the mentomeatal line (MML; imaginary line connecting the chin with the external ear opening) perpendicular to the film. If an open-mouth Waters position is required, do not have patient drop jaw until *after* the MML has been positioned perpendicular to the film (Fig. 10–20).
- ***Adjusting the Central Ray for Poor MML Alignment:*** For a patient who is unable to elevate the chin adequately to position the MML perpendicular to the film, the central ray may be adjusted to compensate. Instruct the patient to elevate the chin to position the MML as close as possible to perpendicular to the film. Then angle the central ray until it is parallel with the MML. This method should not be used if the maxillary sinuses are being evaluated for air-fluid levels. Unless the central ray remains horizontal, the air-fluid level is obscured or appears higher.

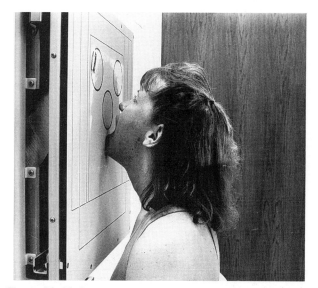

Figure 10-20. Proper patient positioning for open-mouth parietoacanthal (Waters) facial bones–sinuses radiograph.

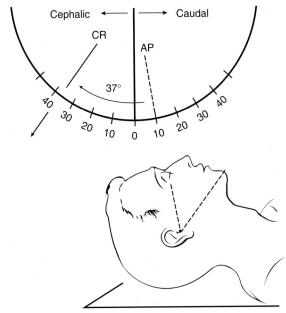

Figure 10-21. Determining central ray *(CR)* angle for acanthoparietal (Waters) facial bones–sinuses radiograph in a trauma patient. *AP,* AP projection.

- **Detecting Poor MML Positioning:** Poor MML positioning can be detected radiographically by evaluating the position of the petrous ridges and posterior maxillary alveolar process. If the patient's chin was not adequately elevated to bring the MML perpendicular to the film, the petrous ridges are demonstrated superior to the posterior maxillary alveolar process superimposing the maxillary sinuses (see Rads. 17 and 18). If the patient's chin was elevated more than needed to position the MML perpendicular to the film, the petrous ridges are demonstrated inferior to the maxillary sinuses and posterior maxillary alveolar process, and the maxillary sinuses superimpose the posterior molars and alveolar process (see Rad. 19).

- **Central Ray Angulation for Acanthoparietal Projection:** For the acanthoparietal projection of the cranium, if a cervical vertebrae injury is not suspected, adjust the patient's head as described for the parietoacanthial projection. If a cervical vertebrae injury is suspected, do not adjust the patient's head position, or increased cervical injury might result. Instead, angle the central ray cephalically until it is aligned parallel with the MML. If the MML is difficult to use or if the patient's mouth is open, the central

ray may also be adjusted 37 degrees cephalically from the OML to obtain identical anatomical relationships (Fig. 10–21).

- **Correcting the Central Ray Angulation for a Trauma Acanthoparietal Projection:** For the trauma acanthoparietal projection, the central ray angulation determines the relationship of the petrous ridges to the maxillary sinuses and posterior maxillary alveolar process. For an acanthoparietal radiograph that demonstrates poor petrous ridge positioning, adjust the central ray angulation in the direction that you want the maxillary sinuses and posterior maxillary alveolar process to move. Because they are situated farther from the film than the maxillary sinuses, their position is most affected by an angulation change. If the petrous ridges are demonstrated within the maxillary sinuses and superior to the posterior maxillary alveolar process, the central ray was angled too caudally (see Rad. 20). If the petrous ridges are demonstrated inferior to the maxillary sinuses and posterior maxillary alveolar process, and the posterior molars and maxillary alveolar process superimpose the maxillary sinuses, the central ray was angled too cephalically. (The petrous ridge and posterior maxillary alveolar relationship would be similar to that shown in Radiograph 19.)

The bony nasal septum is aligned with the long axis of the collimated field, and the infraorbital rims are visualized on the same horizontal plane.

- Aligning the cranium's midsagittal plane with the collimator's longitudinal light line controls tilting of the patient's head. Tilting does not change any anatomical relationships for this projection, but it does prevent tight collimation and makes viewing the radiograph slightly more awkward.

The anterior nasal spine is at the center of the collimated field. The frontal and maxillary (and sphenoid on the open-mouth position) sinuses and the lateral cranial cortices are included within the field.

- Centering a perpendicular central ray to the acanthion (area located at the midsagittal plane where the nose and upper lip meet) places the anterior nasal spine in the center of the collimated field.
- Open the longitudinally and transversely collimated fields to within 1 inch (2.5 cm) of palpable orbits and zygomatic arches, or use a circle diaphragm.
- An 8 × 10 inch (18 × 24 cm) film placed lengthwise should be adequate to include all required anatomical structures.

Critiquing Radiographs

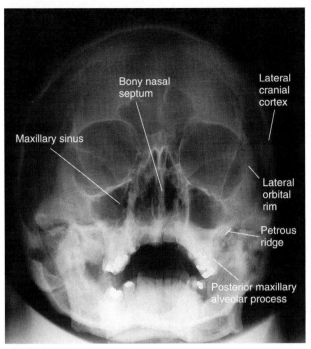

Radiograph 17.

Critique: The distances from the lateral orbital rim to the lateral cranial cortex and from the bony nasal septum to the lateral cranial cortex on the right side of the patient are greater than the same distances on the left side. The petrous ridges are demonstrated within the maxillary sinuses and superior to the posterior maxillary alveolar process. The patient's face was rotated toward the left side, and the chin was not elevated enough to position the MML perpendicular to the film.

Correction: Place an extended flat palm next to each lateral parietal bone. Rotate the patient's face toward the right side until your hands are perpendicular to the film. Elevate the patient's chin until the MML is perpendicular to the film. The amount of movement needed is the full distance demonstrated between the petrous ridges and the posterior maxillary alveolar process. If the patient is unable to elevate the chin any farther, leave the chin positioned as is, and angle the central ray caudally about 5 degrees for every 0.25 inch (0.6 cm) of distance demonstrated between the petrous ridges and the posterior maxillary alveolar process. This should align the central ray parallel with the MML when the patient's mouth is closed.

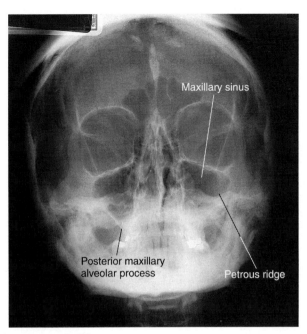

Radiograph 18.

Critique: The petrous ridges are demonstrated within the maxillary sinuses and superior to the posterior maxillary alveolar process. The patient's chin was not elevated enough to position the MML perpendicular to the film.

If this petrous ridge and posterior maxillary alveolar process relationship was obtained on a trauma acanthoparietal projection radiograph, the central ray was angled too caudally.

Correction: Elevate the patient's chin until the MML is perpendicular to the film. The amount of movement needed is the full distance between the petrous ridges and the posterior maxillary alveolar process. If the patient is unable to elevate the chin any farther, leave the patient's chin positioned as is, and angle the central ray caudally about 5 degrees for every 0.25 inch (0.6 cm) of distance demonstrated between the petrous ridges and the posterior maxillary alveolar process. This should align the central ray parallel with the MML when the patient's mouth is closed. If this is a trauma acanthoparietal projection radiograph, adjust the central ray angulation cephalically about 5 degrees for every 0.25 inch (0.6 cm) of distance demonstrated between the petrous ridges and the posterior maxillary alveolar process.

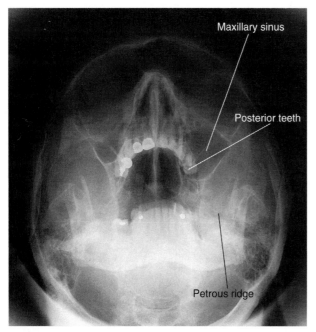

Radiograph 19.

Critique: The petrous ridges are inferior to the maxillary sinuses and the posterior maxillary alveolar process. The patient's chin was elevated more than needed to align the MML perpendicular to the film.

If this petrous ridge and posterior maxillary alveolar process relationship was obtained on a trauma acanthoparietal projection radiograph, the central ray was angled too cephalically.

Correction: Depress the patient's chin until the MML is perpendicular to the film. The amount of movement needed is the full distance demonstrated between the petrous ridges and the posterior maxillary alveolar process.

If this is a trauma acanthoparietal projection radiograph, adjust the central ray angulation caudally about 5 degrees for every 0.25 inch (0.6 cm) of distance demonstrated between the petrous ridges and the posterior maxillary alveolar process.

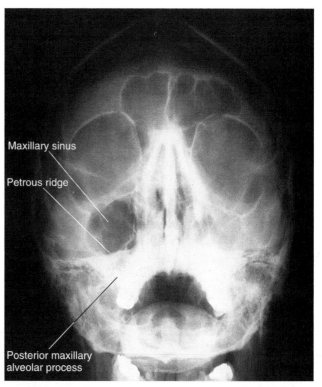

Radiograph 20.

Critique: This is a trauma acanthoparietal projection radiograph. The petrous ridges are demonstrated within the maxillary sinuses and superior to the posterior maxillary alveolar process. Either the patient's chin was not elevated enough to position the MML perpendicular to the film, or the central ray was angled too caudally.

Correction: Elevate the patient's chin until the MML is perpendicular to the film. The amount of movement needed is the full distance demonstrated between the petrous ridges and the posterior maxillary alveolar process. If the patient is unable to elevate the chin any farther, leave the patient's chin positioned as is, and angle the central ray cephalically about 5 degrees for every 0.25 inch (0.6 cm) of distance demonstrated between the petrous ridges and the posterior maxillary alveolar process.

BIBLIOGRAPHY

Anagnostakos NP, Tortora GJ. Principles of Anatomy and Physiology, ed 6. New York: Harper & Row, 1990.

Ballinger PW. Merrill's Atlas of Radiographic Positions and Radiologic Procedures, ed 7. St Louis: CV Mosby, 1991.

Berquist TH. Imaging of Orthopedic Trauma and Surgery. Philadelphia: WB Saunders, 1986.

Bontrager KL. Textbook of Radiographic Positioning and Related Anatomy, ed 3. St Louis: CV Mosby, 1993.

Bushong SC. Radiologic Science for Technologists, ed 5. St Louis: CV Mosby, 1993.

Carroll QB. Fuch's Principles of Radiographic Exposure, Processing and Quality Control, ed 4. Springfield, IL: Charles C Thomas, 1990.

Clemente CD. Gray's Anatomy, ed 30. Philadelphia: Lea & Febiger, 1984.

Draves DJ. Anatomy of the Lower Extremity. Baltimore: Williams & Wilkins, 1986.

O'Toole M (ed). Miller-Keane Encyclopedia and Dictionary of Medicine, Nursing, and Allied Health, ed 5. Philadelphia: WB Saunders, 1992.

Phillips MW. Ensuring Image Quality, Slide/Tape Series. St Louis: CV Mosby, 1987.

Rogers LF. Radiology of Skeletal Trauma. New York: Churchill Livingstone, 1982.

Statkiewicz MA, Viconti PJ, Ritenour RE. Radiation Protection in Medical Radiography, ed 2. St Louis: CV Mosby, 1993.

Warwick R, Williams PL. Gray's Anatomy, ed 36. Philadelphia: WB Saunders, 1980.

INDEX

Note: Page numbers in *italics* refer to illustrations.

Abdominal radiograph(s), anteroposterior, 65–72, *65–72*
   accurate positioning of, *65–66*
   anatomic landmarks on, 66–67
   collimation of, 69
   excess abdominal soft tissue on, 67
   excess bowel gas on, 67, *70*
   film size for, 69–70
   gonadal shielding for, 69, *70*
   in supine position, 69, *71*
   in upright position, 69–70, *72*
   intraperitoneal air on, 68
   kidneys on, 67
   lumbar vertebrae on, 68
   motion artifacts on, 67
   patient positioning for, 67–68, *67–68*
   placement of markers on, 66
   position of diaphragm on, 68–69, *72*
   psoas muscle on, 66–67
   rotation on, 68–69, *70–71*
   underexposure of, *70*
  left lateral decubitus, 72, *72–76,* 74–76
   accurate positioning of, *72*
   anatomic landmarks on, 73
   collimation of, 75, *76*
   compensating filters for, 73
   excess bowel gas on, 73
   film size for, 75
   gonadal shielding for, 75
   intraperitoneal air on, 74
   lumbar vertebrae on, 75, *76*
   patient positioning for, 73–74, *74*
   placement of markers on, 73
   position of diaphragm on, 74–75
   rotation on, 74, *75*
   use of wedge-compensating filter on, 73
Abdominal soft tissue, excess, radiographs with, anteroposterior, 67
Abduct, definition of, 2
AC (acromioclavicular) joint. See *Acromioclavicular (AC) joint radiograph(s).*
Acromioclavicular (AC) joint radiograph(s), anteroposterior, 189–192, *189–192*
   accurate positioning of, *189*
   collimation of, *191,* 191–192
   foreshortening on, 191, *192*
   kyphosis on, 191
   patient positioning for, 190, *190*
   rotation on, 191, *192*
   weight-bearing, *190,* 190–191
Adduct, definition of, 2
Air-fluid level(s), on chest radiographs, anteroposterior, 53
  lateral decubitus, 57
Align, definition of, 2
Anatomical alignment, 11–15, *12–15,* 24, *26*
Anatomical artifact(s), 19, *21,* 33, *33*
Ankle radiograph(s), anteroposterior, 232–235, *232–235*
   accurate positioning of, *232*
   collimation of, 233–234
   patient positioning for, 233, *233–235*
   rotation on, 233, *233–235*
   tibiotalar joint on, *233,* 233–234, *235*

Ankle radiograph(s) *(Continued)*
  internal. See *Ankle radiograph(s), medial oblique.*
  lateral, 239–243, *239–243*
   accurate positioning of, *239*
   collimation of, *241,* 241–242
   fat pads on, 239, *239*
   joint spaces on, 240, *242*
   patient positioning for, 239–241, *239–242*
   position of foot on, 241, *241–242*
   position of lower leg on, 240, *240, 242*
   talar domes on, 240–241, *240–242*
   tibiotalar joint on, 240, *242*
  medial oblique, 236–238, *236–238*
   accurate positioning of, *236*
   collimation of, 237
   joint spaces on, 237, *237–238*
   patient positioning for, 236–237, *236–238*
   rotation on, 236–237, *236–238*
   tarsal sinus on, 237, *238*
  mediolateral. See *Ankle radiograph(s), lateral.*
  oblique, poorly positioned, *14*
Anode-heel effect, on femoral radiographs, anteroposterior, 278–279
   lateral, 283
  on forearm radiographs, anteroposterior, 126
   lateral, 131
  on humeral radiographs, anteroposterior, 154
   lateral, 158–160, *159–160, 162*
  on lower leg radiographs, anteroposterior, 244
   lateral, 248
  on thoracic vertebral radiographs, anteroposterior, 342
Anterior, definition of, 1
Anteroposterior (AP) projection(s). See also under specific structures.
  gonadal shielding for, 18, *18–20*
  hanging technique for, 3, *4*
  markers for, placement of, 8
AP (anteroposterior). See *Anteroposterior (AP) projection(s).*
Arch, longitudinal, low vs. high, *211–212,* 215–216
Articulation(s), definition of, 2
Artifact(s), 32–36, *33–37*
  anatomical, 19, *21,* 33, *33*
  definition of, 2
  equipment-related, 34, *35–36,* 36
  external, 33–34, *33–34*
  from improper film processing, 36, *36–37*
  internal, 34, *34–35*
  on chest radiographs, anteroposterior, 53, 55, *55*
   lateral decubitus, 59, *59*
  on finger radiographs, lateral, 84, *86*
   oblique, 81
   posteroanterior, 77
  on thumb radiographs, anteroposterior, 87
Asthenic body type, 24, *25*
Atlantoaxial radiograph(s), collimation of, 323
  open mouth, 321–325, *321–325*
   accurate positioning of, *321*
   collimation of, *322,* 322–323, *324–325*
   joint spaces on, 323
   patient positioning for, 321–322, *322, 324*
   with trauma, 322–323, *323, 325*
   rotation on, 321–322, *324*

Atlantoaxial radiograph(s) *(Continued)*
upper incisors on, 322–323, *322–325*
position of head on, 323, *324*
Automatic exposure radiograph(s), density and penetration of, 29–31, *30*

Bladder, on coccygeal radiographs, anteroposterior, 371, *373*
Body plane(s), 2
Body type(s), 24, *25*
Bony cortical outline(s), definition of, 2, 20–22, *21–24*
Bowel gas, excess, on abdominal radiographs, anteroposterior, 67, *70*
left lateral decubitus, 73
Breathing technique, for sternal radiographs, right anterior oblique, 377, *378*
for thoracic vertebral radiographs, lateral, 346, *348*

Calcaneal radiograph(s), axial, 224, *224–232*, 226–232
accurate positioning of, *224*
collimation of, 224, *225–227*, 226
dorsiflexion on, 224, *225–227*
joint space on, 224, *224–226*
patient positioning for, 224, *224–227*, 226
plantar flexion on, 224, *225–227*
rotation on, 226, *227*
lateral, 228–232, *228–232*
accurate positioning of, *228*
collimation of, 230, *230*
joint spaces on, 229, *229–230*
patient positioning for, 228–230, *228–231*
plantar flexion on, 230, *232*
talar domes on, 229–230, *229–231*
plantar flexion on, 230, *232*
plantodorsal. See *Calcaneal radiograph(s), axial.*
Caldwell cranial radiograph(s). See *Cranial radiograph(s), Caldwell.*
Capitulum, on elbow radiographs, 151–153, *151–153*
Carpal bone(s), on wrist radiographs, lateral, 116
Carpometacarpal joint(s), on thumb radiographs, anteroposterior, 88, *89*
lateral oblique, 93–94, *94*
on wrist radiographs, medial oblique, 112, *113–115*
posteroanterior, *104, 106*, 106–107, *109–110*
Caudal, definition of, 2
Central ray, and anatomical alignment, *13*
placement of. See *Collimation.*
Cephalic, definition of, 2
Cephalic angulation, on clavicle radiographs, anteroposterior axial, 188, *188–189*
Cervical vertebral radiograph(s), anterior oblique, 332–337, *332–337*
accurate positioning of, *332*
collimation of, 333–335, *336–337*
intervertebral disk spaces on, 333–334, *336*
patient positioning for, 332–334, *332–336*
with kyphosis, 334, *336*
with trauma, 333, *333–334*
position of cranial cortices on, 334, *336–337*
position of head on, 334–335, *337*
position of mandibular cortices on, 334, *336–337*
rotation on, 333, *335*
anteroposterior, 316–321, *316–321*
accurate positioning of, *316*
collimation of, *317–321*, 318
head tilting on, 334–335, *337*
of atlas and axis, open mouth. See *Atlantoaxial radiograph(s), open mouth.*
patient positioning for, 317, *317*
with trauma, 317
position of occiput on, 318, *320*
rotation on, 317, *319*
lateral, 326–331, *326–331*
accurate positioning of, *326*
collimation of, 328–329, *331*
cranial cortices on, 327–328, *329–330*
fat stripe on, prevertebral, 326, *326*
first thoracic vertebra on, 329, *331*

Cervical vertebral radiograph(s) *(Continued)*
head positioning on, and mandibular demonstration, 328, *329–330*
intervertebral disk spaces on, 327–328, *329–330*
mandibular cortices on, 327–328, *329–330*
patient positioning for, 326–328, *327–330*
for evaluation of anteroposterior mobility, 328, *328, 330–331*
with trauma, 327, *327*
rotation on, 327, *327, 329*
seventh cervical vertebra on, 329, *331*
swimmer's position for, 329, 337–341, *337–341*
posterior oblique, 332–337, *332–337*
accurate positioning of, *332*
collimation of, 333–335, *336–337*
head tilting and, 334–335, *337*
intervertebral disk spaces on, 333–334, *336*
patient positioning for, 332–333, *332–335*
with kyphosis, 334, *336*
with trauma, 333, *333–334*
position of cranial cortices on, 334, *336–337*
position of mandibular cortices on, 334, *336–337*
rotation on, 333, *335*
Cervicothoracic vertebral radiograph(s), swimmer's lateral view, 337–341, *337–341*
accurate positioning of, *337*
collimation of, 339
intervertebral disk spaces on, 339, *341*
patient positioning for, *338–340*, 338–339
with trauma, 338–339, *339*
position of shoulder on, 339
rotation on, 338, *340*
Chest radiograph(s), anterior oblique, 62–65, *62–65*
accurate positioning of, *62*
collimation of, 63
lung markings on, 63
patient positioning for, 63–64, *63–65*
rotation on, 64, *65*
anteroposterior, 52–56, *52–56*
accurate positioning of, *52*
air-fluid levels on, 53
artifacts on, 53, 55, *55*
collimation of, 53–54, *55–56*
lung aeration on, 55
lung markings on, 53, *56*
patient positioning for, 54, *54–55*
portable, film size for, 53–54, *54*
rotation on, 53–54, *54–55*
thoracic vertebrae on, 53
anteroposterior lordotic, 60–62, *60–62*
accurate positioning of, *60*
collimation of, 61, *62*
foreshortening on, 62, *62*
lung markings on, 60
rotation on, 61
during expiration, 43, *45*
lateral decubitus, 56–60, *56–60*
accurate positioning of, *56*
air-fluid levels on, 57
anteroposterior vs. posteroanterior, 58–59, *58–60*
artifacts on, 59, *59*
lung markings on, 57
patient positioning for, 57–60, *57–60*
placement of markers on, 56
rotation on, 57–58, *59*
thoracic vertebrae on, 57, 58, *60*
left lateral, 45–52, *45–52*
accurate positioning of, *45*
collimation of, 46
foreshortening on, 47–48, *48*
heart shadow on, 46–47, 48, *50, 52*
lung markings on, 46
midsagittal plane positioning on, 48, *48, 51*
patient positioning for, 48, *48–49, 51–52*
right vs. left lung on, 46–47, *47, 49–50*
rotation on, 46, *46, 49–50*
thoracic vertebrae on, 48–49, *49*
vs. right lateral, 48, *51*

Chest radiograph(s) *(Continued)*
  posterior oblique, lung aeration on, 64
  posteroanterior, accurate positioning of, *40*
    collimation of, 41
    film size for, 41
    foreshortening on, 42, *42–43*
    lung aeration on, 43
    patient positioning for, *41,* 41–42, *42–44*
    position of clavicle on, 42, *44*
    rotation on, 42, *43*
    thoracic vertebrae on, 41
Clavicle, position of, on chest radiographs, posteroanterior, 42, *44*
Clavicle radiograph(s), anteroposterior, 184–186, *184–186*
    accurate positioning of, *184*
    collimation of, 186
    foreshortening on, 185–186, *186*
    kyphosis on, 185
    patient positioning for, 185, *185*
    rotation on, 185, *186*
    thoracic cavity on, 185, *185–186*
  anteroposterior axial, 187–189, *187–189*
    accurate positioning of, *187*
    cephalic angulation on, 188, *188–189*
    collimation of, 188, *188–189*
    patient positioning for, 187–188, *188*
    position of scapula on, 188, *188–189*
    rotation on, 187–188
Clipping, prevention of, 17, *17*
Coccygeal radiograph(s), anteroposterior, 371–373, *371–373*
    accurate positioning of, *371*
    bladder on, 371, *373*
    collimation of, 373, *373*
    gonadal shielding for, 372
    patient positioning for, 372, *372*
    rotation on, 372, *373*
  lateral, 373–375, *373–375*
    accurate positioning of, *373*
    collimation of, 374, *375*
    gonadal shielding for, 374
    patient positioning for, 374, *374*
    rotation on, 374, *375*
Collimation, accuracy of, 15–17, *15–17*
  of abdominal radiographs, anteroposterior, 69
    left lateral decubitus, 75, *76*
  of acromioclavicular joint radiographs, anteroposterior, *191,* 191–192
  of ankle radiographs, anteroposterior, 233–234
    lateral, 241–242, *242*
    medial oblique, 237
  of atlantoaxial radiographs, *322,* 322–323, *324–325*
  of calcaneal radiographs, axial, 224, *225–227,* 226
    lateral, 230, *230*
  of cervical vertebral radiographs, anterior oblique, 333–335, *336–337*
    anteroposterior, 317–318, *317–321*
    lateral, 328–329, *331*
    posterior oblique, 333–335, *336–337*
  of cervicothoracic vertebral radiographs, swimmer's lateral view, 339
  of chest radiographs, anterior oblique, 63
    anteroposterior, 53–54, *55–56*
    anteroposterior lordotic, 61, *62*
    left lateral, 46
    posteroanterior, 41
  of clavicle radiographs, anteroposterior, 186
    anteroposterior axial, 188, *188–189*
  of coccygeal radiographs, anteroposterior, 373, *373*
    lateral, 374, *375*
  of cranial radiographs, anteroposterior, 395, *395, 397*
    with trauma, 395, *395, 397*
    Caldwell, 399–400, *401–402*
    lateral, 408
    posteroanterior, 395
    submentovertex, 410
    Towne, 403–404, *404–405*
  of elbow radiographs, anteroposterior, 138
    lateral, 148
    medial/lateral oblique, 142
    radial head/capitulum view of, 152

Collimation *(Continued)*
  of ethmoid sinus radiographs, 400
  of facial bone/sinus radiographs, 414, *414, 416*
  of femoral radiographs, distal anteroposterior, 279
    distal lateral, 284–285
    proximal anteroposterior, 281
    proximal lateral, 286, *286*
  of finger radiographs, lateral, 85
    oblique, 82
    posteroanterior, 78, *78, 80*
  of foot radiographs, anteroposterior, 211–212
    lateral, 221, *223*
    medial oblique, 217
  of forearm radiographs, anteroposterior, 126–127, *127*
    lateral, 131
  of hand radiographs, lateral, 102
    medial oblique, 99
    posteroanterior, 96
  of hip radiographs, anteroposterior, 292
    axiolateral, *299–300,* 300
    frogleg, 296
  of humeral radiographs, anteroposterior, 155–156, *156*
    lateral, 161–162
  of knee radiographs, anteroposterior, 254
    axial, 271
    lateral, 264, 266, *267*
    medial oblique, 258, *258, 261*
  of lower leg radiographs, anteroposterior, 245, *245*
    lateral, 249
  of lumbar vertebral radiographs, anteroposterior, *352,* 352–353
    lateral, *360,* 360–361
    L5–S1 spot lateral, 364
    posterior oblique, 356
  of patellar radiographs, tangential, 275, *276–277*
  of pelvic radiographs, anteroposterior, 305
    frogleg, 309
  of rib radiographs, anterior/posterior oblique, above diaphragm, 389
      below diaphragm, 390
    anteroposterior/posteroanterior, above diaphragm, 385
      below diaphragm, 385
  of sacral radiographs, anteroposterior, 367, *368*
    lateral, 370
  of sacroiliac joint radiographs, anteroposterior, 312
    posterior oblique, 314
  of scapular radiographs, lateral, 199
  of shoulder radiographs, anterior oblique, 182
    anteroposterior, 167, *167*
    axial, 172–173, *172–174*
    Grashey, 177, *179*
  of sinus radiographs, parietocanthal, 414, *414, 416*
  of sternal radiographs, lateral, 381
    right anterior oblique, 377
  of thoracic vertebral radiographs, anteroposterior, 344
    lateral, 347
  of thumb radiographs, anteroposterior, 88, *89*
    lateral, 91
    lateral oblique, 94, *94*
  of toe radiographs, anteroposterior, 203
    lateral, 209, *209*
    oblique, 206, *207*
  of wrist radiographs, lateral, 117, *119–120*
    medial oblique, 112–113, *114*
    posteroanterior, 107, *107*
Collimator guide(s), 7
Compensating filter(s), for abdominal radiographs, left lateral decubitus, 73
  for foot radiographs, anteroposterior, 210, *211*
  for hip radiographs, axiolateral, 299
  for shoulder radiographs, anteroposterior, 166, *166*
  use of, *30,* 30–31
Concave, definition of, 2
Condyle(s), definition of, 2
Contact shield(s), use of, 32, *32*
Contrast, adequacy of, 31–32, *31–32*
Convex, definition of, 2
Coracoid, anatomy of, *167*

Coronal plane, 2

Cortical outline, definition of, 2, 20–22, *21–24*

Cranial cortices, on cervical vertebral radiographs, anterior oblique, 334, *336–337*
    lateral, 327–328, *329–330*
    posterior oblique, 334, *336–337*
  on cranial radiographs, Caldwell, 398–399, *398–399, 401*

Cranial radiograph(s), anteroposterior, with trauma, 393–397, *393–397, 398–402, 398–402.* See also *Cranial radiograph(s), Caldwell.*
    accurate positioning of, *393*
    collimation of, 395, *395, 397*
    patient positioning for, 394–395, *395–397*
  anteroposterior axial, 402–405, *402–405.* See also *Cranial radiograph(s), Towne.*
  basilar. See *Cranial radiograph(s), submentovertex.*
  Caldwell, alignment of orbitomental line on, 399–400, *401–402*
    collimation of, 395, *395, 397,* 399–400, *401–402*
    cranial cortices on, 398–399, *398–399, 401*
    patient positioning for, 398–399, *399, 401*
    petrous ridges on, 399, *401–402*
    rotation on, 394, *395,* 399, *401*
  lateral, 406–408, *406–408*
    accurate positioning of, *406*
    collimation of, 408
    patient positioning for, 407–408, *407–408*
    rotation on, 407, *408*
  posteroanterior, 393–397, *393–397,* 398–402, *398–402.* See also *Cranial radiograph(s), Caldwell.*
    accurate positioning of, *393*
    collimation of, 395
    orbitomental line on, 394–395, *395–397*
    patient positioning for, 394, *394*
    rotation on, 394, *395*
  submentovertex, 409–411, *409–411*
    accurate positioning of, *409*
    collimation of, 410
    mandibular mentum on, 410, *411*
    patient positioning for, 410, *410–411*
  Towne, 402–405, *402–405*
    accurate positioning of, *402*
    collimation of, 403–404, *404–405*
    foreshortening on, 403, *405*
    orbitomental line on, 403–404, *404–405*
    patient positioning for, 403, *403–405*
    rotation on, 403, *404*

Cranium, lateral positions of, hanging technique for, 3–4, *4*

Cross-table radiograph(s), femoral, distal lateral, 284, *284*
    proximal lateral, *285,* 286
  lateral, markers for, placement of, 9–10, *10*

Density, adequacy of, 26–31, *27–30*

Detail screen(s), use of, 22, *23*

Diaphragm, position of, on abdominal radiographs, anteroposterior, 68–69, *72*
    left lateral decubitus, 74–75

Distal, definition of, I

Distortion, prevention of, 24

Dorsiflexion, definition of, 2
  on calcaneal radiographs, axial, 224, *225–227*

Double exposure, 22, *23*

Elbow(s), flexion of, on forearm radiographs, lateral, 132

Elbow radiograph(s), anteroposterior, 136–140, *136–140*
    accurate positioning of, *136*
    collimation of, 138
    foreshortening on, *139–140*
    joint spaces on, 137, *139*
    patient positioning for, 136–137, *136–138*
    radial tuberosity on, 137, *139*
    rotation on, 136–137, *138*
    with nonextendable elbow, 137–138, *137–140*

Elbow radiograph(s) *(Continued)*
  lateral, 145–150, *145–150*
    collimation of, 148
    fat pads on, 145–146, *145–146, 148*
    patient positioning for, 146–148, *146–150*
    position of forearm on, 147–148, *147–150*
    position of humerus on, 146–147, *147–149*
    radial tuberosity on, 148, *148, 150*
  medial/lateral oblique, 141–144, *141–144*
    accurate positioning of, *141*
    collimation of, 142
    foreshortening on, 141–142, *143*
    joint spaces on, 141–142, *143*
    patient positioning for, 142–143, *142–144*
    with nonextendable elbow, 142, *142*
  radial head/capitulum, 151–153, *151–153*

Elongate, definition of, 2

Equipment-related artifact(s), 34, *35–36,* 36

Ethmoid sinus radiograph(s), collimation of, 400

Expiration, chest radiographs during, 43, *45*
  vs. inspiration, during thoracic vertebral radiographs, 342–343, *344*

Exposure(s), double, 22, *23*

Extension, definition of, 3
  degree of, 12, *13*

External artifact(s), 33–34, *33–34*

External rotation, 3

Extremity(ies), extension of, degree of, 12, *13*
  flexion of, degree of, 12, *13*
  hanging technique for, 4, *5*
  markers for, placement of, 9, *9–10*
  upper. See specific body parts.

Facial bone radiograph(s), 398–402, *398–402.* See also *Cranial radiograph(s).*
  acanthoparietal, with trauma. See *Facial bone radiograph(s), parietocanthal.*
  parietocanthal, 412–416, *412–416*
    accurate positioning of, *412*
    collimation of, 413–414, *414, 416*
    mentomeatal line on, 413–414, *415*
    patient positioning for, 413, *413–416*
    rotation on, 413, *415*

Fat pad(s), on ankle radiographs, lateral, 239, *239*
  on elbow radiographs, lateral, 145–146, *145–146, 148*
  on foot radiographs, lateral, 219, *219*
  suprapatellar, on knee radiographs, lateral, 262, *263*

Fat plane(s), on hip radiographs, anteroposterior, 290, *291*
  on pelvic radiographs, anteroposterior, 303, *304*

Fat stripe, prevertebral, on cervical vertebral radiographs, lateral, 326, *326*
  pronator, on wrist radiographs, lateral, 115–116, *116*
  scaphoid. See *Scaphoid fat stripe.*

Feet. See *Foot.*

Femoral condyle(s), on patellar radiographs, tangential, 273, *276*
  superimposition of, on lateral knee radiographs, 263–264, *263–266, 267–269*

Femoral epicondyle(s), on femoral radiographs, distal anteroposterior, 254, 279, *279*
  distal lateral, 283–284, *287*

Femoral neck, localization of, on axiolateral hip radiographs, 299, *299–300*

Femoral radiograph(s), anteroposterior, 278–282, *278–282*
    accurate positioning of, *278*
    anode-heel effect on, 278–279
    gonadal shielding for, 281
  distal anteroposterior, collimation of, 279
    epicondyles on, 254, 279, *279*
    joint spaces on, 279
    patient positioning for, 279, *279*
    for fractures, 279
  distal lateral, accurate positioning of, *282*
    anode-heel effect on, 283
    collimation of, 284–285
    cross-table, 284, *284*

Femoral radiograph(s) *(Continued)*
  epicondyles on, 283–284, *287*
  patient positioning for, 283–284, *284, 287*
  lateral, 282–288, *282–288*
    gonadal shielding for, 286
  mediolateral. See *Femoral radiograph(s), lateral.*
  proximal anteroposterior, collimation of, 281
    foot rotation on, *278,* 280–281, *280–281*
    foreshortening on, 280–281, *281–282*
    leg rotation on, 280, *280–282*
    patient positioning for, *278,* 280–281, *280–282*
    pelvic rotation on, 280
  proximal lateral, collimation of, 286, *286*
    cross-table, *285,* 286
    flexion on, *285, 288*
    foreshortening on, *285,* 285–286, *288*
    patient positioning for, 284–286, *285–286, 288*
      with fractures, *283, 285,* 286
Femorotibial joint(s), on femoral radiographs, distal anteroposterior, 279
  on knee radiographs, anteroposterior, *252,* 252–253, *254–256*
    lateral, *263–264,* 263–266, *268*
  on lower leg radiographs, anteroposterior, 245, *245*
Femur, dislocation of, on hip radiographs, 292, 300, *302*
  fractures of. See *Fracture(s), femoral.*
  position of, on hip radiographs, frogleg, 295, *295, 297*
    on knee radiographs, posteroanterior axial, 270–271, *270–272*
    on pelvic radiographs, frogleg, 308, *308,* 309
Film, processing of, artifacts from, 36, *36–37*
Film size, for abdominal radiographs, anteroposterior, 69–70
  left lateral decubitus, 75
  for chest radiographs, portable anteroposterior, 53–54, *54*
    posteroanterior, 41
  for forearm radiographs, anteroposterior, 126
    lateral, 131
  for humeral radiographs, anteroposterior, 156
    lateral, 161
  for lumbar vertebral radiographs, anteroposterior, 352–353
    lateral, 360–361
  for sternal radiographs, right anterior oblique, 377
  selection of, 24, *25–26*
Film-screen contact, evidence of, 22, *24*
Filter(s), compensating. See *Compensating filter(s).*
Finger radiograph(s), lateral, *84,* 84–86, *86*
  accurate positioning of, *84*
  artifacts on, 84, *86*
  collimation of, 85
  flexion on, 86, *86*
  patient positioning for, 84, *84*
  placement of markers on, 81
  vs. rotated position, *84,* 84–85, *86*
  oblique, 81–83, *81–83*
    accurate positioning of, *81*
    artifacts on, 81
    patient positioning for, 81, *81,* 82, *82–83*
  posteroanterior, 77–80, *77–80*
    accurate positioning of, *77*
    artifacts on, 77
    collimation of, 78, *78, 80*
    flexion on, 79, *79–80*
    joint space on, 78, *78, 80*
    of unextendable finger, 79, *79*
    patient positioning for, 77, *78*
    placement of markers on, 77
    rotation on, 77–78, *78, 80*
Flexion, definition of, 3
  degree of, 12, *13*
  plantar, 3
Focal spot(s), use of, 20–22, *23–24*
Foot, longitudinal arch of, low vs. high, 211–212
  position of, for knee radiographs, posteroanterior axial, 270, *271*
    for lateral ankle radiographs, 241, *241–242*
    for pelvic radiographs, anteroposterior, 305, *305–306*
    on proximal femoral radiographs, anteroposterior, *278,* 280–281, *280–281*
Foot radiograph(s), anteroposterior, 210–213, *210–213*
  accurate positioning of, *210*

Foot radiograph(s) *(Continued)*
  collimation of, 211–212
  compensating filter for, 210, *211*
  joint spaces on, 211, *211–213*
  patient positioning for, 210–211, *211–213*
  rotation on, 211, *212–213*
  standing, 211
  tarsometatarsal joints on, 211, *211–213*
  dorsoplantar. See *Foot radiograph(s), anteroposterior.*
  internal. See *Foot radiograph(s), medial oblique.*
  lateral, 218–223, *218–223*
    accurate positioning of, *218*
    collimation of, 221, *223*
    fat pads on, 219, *219*
    joint spaces on, 220, *222*
    patient positioning for, 219–221, *219–223*
    plantar flexion on, 221, *223*
    poor positioning for, *220–221*
    talar domes on, 220–221, *220–222*
  lateromedial, standing, *221,* 222, *223*
    patient positioning for, 221–222, *222*
  medial oblique, 214–215, *214–218,* 217
    accurate positioning of, *214*
    collimation of, 217
    degree of obliquity on, 215, *215–216,* 217
    joint spaces on, 215, 217, *217–218*
    patient positioning for, 214–215, *215–218,* 217
    rotation on, 217, *217–218*
Forearm, position of, on elbow radiographs, lateral, 147–148, *147–150*
    radial head/capitulum view, 152, *152–153*
  on radiographs of humeral fracture, 155, *155–157*
  on wrist radiographs, anteroposterior, 106
    lateral, 117, *117*
    oblique, 113
Forearm radiograph(s), anteroposterior, 126–130, *126–130*
  accurate positioning of, *126*
  anode-heel effect on, 126
  collimation of, 126–127, *127*
  distal forearm position for, *127,* 127–128
  film size for, 126
  fractures on, 127–128, *129*
  joint spaces on, *127,* 128–129, *129–130*
  position of styloid on, *129–130*
  proximal forearm positioning for, *127,* 128–129, *129*
  rotation on, 127–128, *129*
  lateral, 130–135, *130–135*
    accurate position of, *130*
    anode-heel effect on, 131
    collimation of, 131
    distal forearm positioning for, 132, *132, 134*
    distal humerus positioning for, 132–133, *132–135*
    elbow flexion on, 132
    film size for, 131
    fractures on, 132–133, *134*
    position of humerus on, 133, *133–135*
    position of styloid on, 132
    proximal forearm positioning for, 132–133, *132–135*
    radial tuberosity on, 132
    soft tissue structures on, 131, *131–132*
Foreshortening, definition of, 3
  on acromioclavicular joint radiographs, anteroposterior, 191, *192*
  on chest radiographs, anteroposterior, lordotic, 62, *62*
    left lateral, 47–48, *48*
    posteroanterior, 42, *42–43*
  on clavicle radiographs, anteroposterior, 185–186, *186*
  on cranial radiographs, Towne, 403, *405*
  on elbow radiographs, anteroposterior, *139–140*
    medial/lateral oblique, 142, *143*
  on femoral radiographs, proximal anteroposterior, 280–281, *281–282*
    proximal lateral, *285,* 285–286, *288*
  on hand radiographs, lateral, 102, *103*
    medial oblique, *100*
    posteroanterior, *97*
  on hip radiographs, anteroposterior, 291, *291, 293*
    axiolateral, 299–300, *302*
    frogleg, 294, 296, *296–297*

Foreshortening *(Continued)*
  on pelvic radiographs, anteroposterior, *303*, 305, *305–307*
    frogleg, *307*, 308–309, *309–310*
  on sacral radiographs, anteroposterior, 366, *367–368*
  on sacroiliac joint radiographs, anteroposterior, 312, *312*
  on scapular radiographs, anteroposterior, 194, *195*
  on shoulder radiographs, anterior oblique, 181–182, *184*
    anteroposterior, 167, *169–170*
    axial, 173, *175*
    Grashey, *178–179*
  on thumb radiographs, anteroposterior, *90*
  on wrist radiographs, medial oblique, 112–113, *114*
    posteroanterior, 105–106, *109–111*
      ulnar-flexed, 123
Fracture(s), femoral, patient positioning for, 279, *279*, 283–284, *284, 287*
    for lateral view, *283, 285*, 286
    on anteroposterior pelvic radiographs, 292, *294*, 305
    on axiolateral hip radiographs, 300, *302*
  humeral, 155, *155–157*, 160–161, *160–161, 163–164*
  of forearm, on anteroposterior radiographs, 127–128, *129*
    on lateral radiographs, 132–133, *134*
  of hip, patient positioning for, 292, *294*
  of lower leg, patient positioning for, for anteroposterior radiographs, 245, *247*
    for lateral knee radiographs, 248–249
  of patella, patient positioning with, for lateral knee radiographs, 263
  of scaphoid, on posteroanterior, ulnar-flexed radiographs, 123–124, *123–124*

Glenohumeral joint space, on shoulder radiographs, Grashey, 177, *178–179*
Glenoid fossa, position of, on scapular radiographs, anteroposterior, 193–194, *195*
  on shoulder radiographs, axial, 172–173, *172–174*
    Grashey, 177, *179*
Gonadal shielding, 17–20, *18–21*
  for abdominal radiographs, anteroposterior, 69, 70
    left lateral decubitus, 75
  for anteroposterior projections, 18, *18–20*
  for coccygeal radiographs, anteroposterior, 372
    lateral, 374
  for femoral radiographs, anteroposterior, 281
    lateral, 286
  for hip radiographs, frogleg, 296
  for lateral positions, 18–19, *20*
  for lumbar vertebral radiographs, anteroposterior, 353
    lateral, 361
    L5–S1 spot lateral, 364
    posterior oblique, 356
  for pelvic radiographs, anteroposterior, 305
    frogleg, 309
  for sacral radiographs, anteroposterior, 367
    lateral, 370
  for sacroiliac joint radiographs, anteroposterior, 312
    posterior oblique, 314
  of female patient, 18, *18*
  of male patient, 18
Grid(s), artifacts from, 34, *35*

Hand radiograph(s), "fan" position. See *Hand radiograph(s), lateral.*
  lateral, 101–104, *101–104*
    accurate positioning of, *101*
    collimation of, 102
    foreshortening on, 102, *103*
    in extension, 102, *103*
    in flexion, 102, *104*
    patient positioning for, 101–102, *101–103*
  medial oblique, 98–100, *98–100*
    accurate positioning of, *98*
    collimation of, 99
    foreshortening on, *100*

Hand radiograph(s) *(Continued)*
    joint spaces on, 99, *99–100*
    patient positioning for, 98–99, *99–100*
    placement of markers on, 98
    vs. posteroanterior, 96, 97
  posteroanterior, 95–97, *95–97*
    accurate positioning of, *95*
    collimation of, 96
    foreshortening on, 97
    joint spaces on, 96, 97
    patient positioning for, 96, *96*
    rotation on, 97
    vs. medial oblique, 96, 97
Hanging technique(s), 3–4, *4–5*
Head, position of, on atlantoaxial radiographs, 323, *324*
    on cervical vertebral radiographs, anterior oblique, 334–335, *337*
    lateral, for visualization of mandible, 328, *329–330*
    posterior oblique, 334–335, *337*
Heart shadow, on chest radiographs, left lateral, 46–48, *50, 52*
High-contrast radiograph(s), 31, *31*
Hip(s), flexion of, for pelvic radiographs, frogleg, *307–310*, 308–309
  markers for, placement of, 9, *10*
  mobility of, evaluation of, by anteroposterior pelvic radiographs, 305
    by frogleg pelvic radiographs, 309
Hip radiograph(s), anteroposterior, 290–294, *290–294*
    accurate positioning of, *290*
    collimation of, 292
    fat planes on, 290, *291*
    foreshortening on, 291, *291, 293*
    patient positioning for, 290–292, *291–294*
      for fractures, 292, *294*
      with dislocated femur, 292
    position of leg on, 290, 291–292, *292*
    rotation on, 291–292, *292–294*
  anteroposterior axial. See *Hip radiograph(s), frogleg.*
  axiolateral, 298–302, *298–302*
    accurate positioning of, *298*
    collimation of, *299–300*, 300
    compensating filters for, 299
    film placement for, 299–300, *299–301*
    foreshortening on, 299–300, *302*
    localization of femoral neck on, 299, *299–300*
    locating symphysis pubis for, 300
    patient positioning for, 299, *299–300, 301–302*
      for dislocated femur, 300, *302*
      for fractured femur, 300, *302*
    rotation on, 300, *300, 302*
  frogleg, 294–298, *294–298*
    accurate positioning of, *294*
    collimation of, 296
    distal femur elevation on, 295
    foreshortening on, 294, 296, *296–297*
    gonadal shielding for, 296
    hip rotation on, 295, *297*
    leg abduction on, 294, 296, *296–298*
    patient positioning for, 295–296, *295–297*
    position of femur on, 295, *295, 297*
    rotation on, 295, *297*
  inferosuperior. See *Hip radiograph(s), axiolateral.*
Holmblad knee radiograph(s). See *Knee radiograph(s), posteroanterior axial.*
Horizontal plane, 2
Humeral radiograph(s), anteroposterior, 154–157, *154–157*
    accurate position of, *154*
    anode-heel effect on, 154
    collimation of, 155–156, *156*
    film size for, 156
    patient positioning for, 154–155, *155–157*
    rotation on, 155, *156–157*
  lateral, 158–164, *158–164*
    accurate positioning of, *158*
    anode-heel effect on, 158–160, *159–160, 162*
    collimation of, 161–162
    film size for, 161
    rotation on, *162*
    patient positioning for, *158–160, 162*

Humerus, distal, anatomy of, *146*
    fractures of, 155, *155–157*, 160–161, *160–161, 163–164*
    position of, on elbow radiographs, 146–147, *147–149*
        on forearm radiographs, 132–133, *133–135*
            on scapular radiographs, anteroposterior, 194, *196*
                lateral, 198–199, *198–199, 201*
            on shoulder radiographs, anteroposterior, 165–166, 167–168, *168, 170–171*
                axial, 173–174, *174–175*
Hypersthenic body type, 24, *25*
Hysterosalpingography, gonadal shielding for, 18, *18*

Identification information, 5
Image receptor system(s), choice of, 26
Incisor(s), upper, on atlantoaxial radiographs, 322–323, *322–325*
Inferior, definition of, 1
Inspiration, and lung dimensions, 41
    vs. expiration, during thoracic vertebral radiographs, 342–343, *344*
Internal artifact(s), 34, *34–35*
Internal rotation, 3
Interphalangeal (IP) joint(s), on hand radiographs, medial oblique, 99, *99–100*
    on lateral radiographs, 85
    on oblique radiographs, 82, *83*
    on posteroanterior radiographs, 78, *78,* 80
    on thumb radiographs, anteroposterior, 88, *89*
        lateral oblique, 93–94, *94*
    on toe radiographs, anteroposterior, 203, *204*
        lateral, 209
        oblique, 206, *207*
Intervertebral disk space(s), on cervical vertebral radiographs, anterior oblique, 333–334, *336*
    lateral, 327–328, *329–330*
    posterior oblique, 333–334, *336*
    on cervicothoracic vertebral radiographs, swimmer's lateral view, 339, *341*
    on lumbar vertebral radiographs, anteroposterior, 352, *352*
    lateral, *359,* 359–360, *361*
    L5–S1 spot lateral, *363,* 364, *365*
    on sacral radiographs, lateral, *369,* 370
    on thoracic vertebral radiographs, anteroposterior, 343–344, *345*
    lateral, *346,* 347, *347,* 349
Intraperitoneal air, on abdominal radiographs, anteroposterior, 68
    left lateral decubitus, 74

Joint(s), extension of, degree of, 12, *13*
    flexion of, degree of, 12, *13*
Joint space(s), on ankle radiographs, lateral, 240, *242*
        medial oblique, 237, *237–238*
    on atlantoaxial radiographs, open mouth, 323
    on calcaneal radiographs, axial, 224, *224–226*
        lateral, 229, *229–230*
    on elbow radiographs, anteroposterior, 137, *139*
        medial/lateral oblique, 141–142, *143*
    on femoral radiographs, distal anteroposterior, 279
    on finger radiographs, posteroanterior, 78, *78,* 80
    on foot radiographs, anteroposterior, 211, *211–213*
        medial oblique, 215, 217, *217–218*
    on forearm radiographs, anteroposterior, *127,* 128–129, *129–130*
    on hand radiographs, medial oblique, 99, *99–100*
        posteroanterior, 96, *97*
    on knee radiographs, anteroposterior, 252–253, *252–256*
        lateral, *263–264,* 263–266, *268*
        medial oblique, 257–258
    on lower leg radiographs, anteroposterior, 245, *245*
    on lumbar vertebral radiographs, posterior oblique, 355–356, *355–357*
    on patellar radiographs, tangential, 274–275, *274–277*
    on sacroiliac joint radiographs, posterior oblique, 313, *314–315*
    on shoulder radiographs, Grashey, 177, *178–179*
    on thumb radiographs, anteroposterior, 88, *89*
        lateral, 91
        lateral oblique, 93–94, *94*

Joint space(s) *(Continued)*
    on toe radiographs, anteroposterior, 203, *204*
        lateral, 209
        oblique, 206, *207*
    on wrist radiographs, medial oblique, 112, *113–115*
        posteroanterior, *104, 106,* 106–107, *109–110*
            ulnar-flexed, *121–125,* 122–124

Kidney(s), on abdominal radiographs, anteroposterior, 67
Kilovoltage peak (kVp), and adequacy of penetration, 26
Knee(s), flexion of, for pelvic radiographs, frogleg, *307–310,* 308–309
    lateral view of, poorly positioned, *14*
Knee radiograph(s), anteroposterior, 251–256, *251–256*
    accurate positioning of, *251*
    collimation of, 252–254, *252–255*
    joint spaces on, 252, *252–253,* *254–256*
    patellar subluxation on, 253–254, *256*
    patient positioning for, *251,* 251–252, 254
        for nonextendable knee, 253, *256*
    position of patella on, knee flexion and, 253, *253, 256*
    rotation on, 252, *254*
    axial, collimation of, 271
        flexion on, 270–271, *272*
    Holmblad. See *Knee radiograph(s), posteroanterior axial.*
    joint spaces on, narrowing of, 253, *254–255*
    lateral, 262–269, *262–269*
        accurate positioning of, *262*
        collimation of, 264, 266, *267*
        joint spaces on, *263–264,* 263–266, *268*
        lateral vs. medial condyles on, 264
        patellar position on, flexion and, 263, *266*
        patient positioning for, 263–266, *263–269*
            supine, 264
            with fractures, 263
        rotation on, 265–266, *265–266, 268–269*
        superimposition of femoral condyles on, *263–264,* 263–266, *267–269*
        suprapatellar fat pads on, *262,* 263
    lateral oblique, 257–261, *257–261.* See also *Knee radiograph(s), medial oblique.*
    medial oblique, 257–261, *257–261*
        accurate positioning of, *257*
        angulation of central ray for, 258, *258, 261*
        collimation of, 258, *258, 261*
        joint spaces on, 257–258
        patient positioning for, 257–259, *258, 260–261*
        rotation on, 258–259, *258–260*
    mediolateral. See *Knee radiograph(s),lateral.*
    posteroanterior axial, 269–272, *269–272*
        accurate positioning of, *269*
        knee thickness and, 269–270
        mispositioning of foot on, 270, *271*
        patient positioning for, 270–271, *270–271*
        position of femur on, 270–271, *270–272*
        position of patella on, 270–271, *270–272*
kVp (kilovoltage peak), and adequacy of penetration, 26
Kyphosis, patient positioning for, on acromioclavicular joint radiographs, anteroposterior, 191
    on cervical vertebral radiographs, anterior oblique, 334, *336*
        posterior oblique, 334, *336*
    on chest radiographs, anteroposterior, 54, *55*
    on clavicle radiographs, anteroposterior, 185
    on scapular radiographs, anteroposterior, 194
    on shoulder radiographs, anterior oblique, 182, *184*
        anteroposterior, 166, *170*
        Grashey, 177, *179*
    on thoracic vertebral radiographs, anteroposterior, 344

Lateral, definition of, 1
Lateral cross-table radiography, markers for, placement of, 9–10, *10*
Lateral decubitus position(s), markers for, placement of, 9, *9*
Lateral position(s), gonadal shielding for, 18–19, *20*

Lateral position(s) *(Continued)*
  hanging technique for, 3–4, *4*
  markers for, placement of, 8, *8*
Lateral rotation, 3
Leg(s), lower, position of, on lateral ankle radiographs, 240, *240, 242*
  position of, on femoral radiographs, 280, *280–282*
    on hip radiographs, anteroposterior, 290, 291–292, *292*
      axiolateral, 299, *301*
        frogleg, *294*, 296, *296–298*
    on pelvic radiographs, anteroposterior, *303*, 305, *305*
      frogleg, *307*, 309, *309–310*
    on sacral radiographs, anteroposterior, 366–367, *368*
Leg radiograph(s), lower. See *Lower leg radiograph(s).*
Longitudinal arch, of foot, low vs. high, *211–212*
Longitudinal plane, 2
Lordosis, on lumbar vertebral radiographs, anteroposterior, 352, *354*
Low-contrast radiograph(s), 31, *31*
Lower leg radiograph(s), anteroposterior, 244–246, *244–246*
  accurate positioning of, *244*
  anode-heel effect on, 244
  collimation of, 245, *245*
  joint spaces on, 245, *245*
  patient positioning for, 244–245, *245–247*
    with fracture, 245, *247*
  positioning of tibia for, 245, *245*
  rotation on, 244–245, *246*
  lateral, 247–250, *247–250*
    accurate positioning of, *247*
    anode-heel effect on, 248
    collimation of, 249
    patient positioning for, *247–250*, 248–249
      with fracture, 248–249
    rotation on, 248, *250*
Lumbar vertebra(e), on abdominal radiographs, anteroposterior, 68
  left lateral decubitus, 75, *76*
Lumbar vertebral radiograph(s), anteroposterior, 350–354, *350–354*
  accurate positioning of, *350*
  collimation of, *352*, 352–353
  film size for, 352–353
  gonadal shielding for, 353
  intervertebral disk spaces on, 352, *352*
  lordosis on, 352, *354*
  patient positioning for, *351*, 351–352, *353–354*
  psoas muscle on, 351
  rotation on, 351–352, *353–354*
  lateral, 358–362, *358–362*
    accurate positioning of, *358*
    collimation of, *360*, 360–361
    film size for, 360–361
    gonadal shielding for, 361
    intervertebral disk spaces on, *359*, 359–360, *361*
    patient positioning for, 358–359, *359, 361*
      for anteroposterior mobility evaluation, 360, *360, 362*
    rotation on, 358–359, *359, 361*
    supplemental views of, 361, *361*
  L5–S1 spot lateral, 363–365, *363–365*
    accurate positioning of, *363*
    collimation of, 364
    gonadal shielding for, 364
    intervertebral disk spaces on, 363, 364, *365*
    patient positioning for, 363–364, *363–364*
    rotation on, 363–364, *364*
  posterior oblique, 355–357, *355–357*
    accurate positioning of, *355*
    collimation of, 356
    gonadal shielding for, 356
    joint spaces on, 355–356, *355–357*
    patient positioning for, 355–356, *355–357*
    rotation on, 355–356, *355–357*
    "Scottie dogs" on, 356, *356–356*
Lung(s), aeration of, on anterior/posterior oblique rib radiographs, above diaphragm, 389
    below diaphragm, 390
  on anteroposterior/posteroanterior rib radiographs, above diaphragm, 385
    below diaphragm, 385, *387*

Lung(s) *(Continued)*
    on chest radiographs, anteroposterior, 55
      posterior oblique, 64
      posteroanterior, 43
    on thoracic vertebral radiographs, anteroposterior, 343–344, *345*
  air in, 40–41
  dimensions of, inspiration and, 41
  fluid levels in, 40–41
  right vs. left, on chest radiographs, left lateral, 46–47, *47, 49–50*
Lung marking(s), on chest radiographs, anterior oblique, 63
    anteroposterior, 53, *56*
    anteroposterior lordotic, 60
    lateral decubitus, 57
    left lateral, 46
    vascular, 40–41

Magnification, definition of, 3
  prevention of, 22
Mandible, visualization of, head position for, on lateral cervical vertebral radiographs, 328, *329–330*
Mandibular cortices, on cervical vertebral radiographs, anterior oblique, 334, *336–337*
    lateral, 327–328, *329–330*
    posterior oblique, 334, *336–337*
Mandibular mentum, on cranial radiographs, submentovertex, 410, *411*
Manually set radiograph(s), density and penetration of, 28–29, *28–29*
Marker(s), distortion of, *7*
  magnification of, *7*
  placement of, 7–11, *7–11*
    on abdominal radiographs, anteroposterior, 66
      left lateral decubitus, 73
    on chest radiographs, lateral decubitus, 56
    on extremity radiographs, 9, *9–10*
    on finger radiographs, lateral, 84
      oblique, 81
      posteroanterior, 77
    on hand radiographs, medial oblique, 98
    on hip radiographs, 9, *10*
    on posteroanterior projections, 8
    on thumb radiographs, anteroposterior, 87
mAs (milliampere-seconds), and adequacy of density, 26
Mastoid radiograph(s), 402–405, *402–405*. See also *Cranial radiograph(s), Towne.*
Medial, definition of, 2
Medial rotation, 3
Median plane, 2
Mentomeatal line, on facial bone/sinus radiographs, parietocanthal, 413–414, *415*
Merchant method. See *Patellar radiograph(s), tangential.*
Metacarpophalangeal (MP) joint(s), on hand radiographs, medial oblique, 99, *99–100*
  on oblique radiographs, 82, *83*
  on posteroanterior radiographs, 78, *78, 80*
  on thumb radiographs, anteroposterior, 88, *89*
    lateral, 91, *92*
    lateral oblique, 93–94, *94*
Metatarsophalangeal (MP) joint(s), on toe radiographs, anteroposterior, 203, *204*
    lateral, 209
    oblique, 206, *207*
Midcoronal plane, 2
Midsagittal plane, 2
  positioning of, on left lateral chest radiographs, 48, *48, 51*
Milliampere-seconds (mAs), and adequacy of density, 26
Motion artifact(s), 21–22, *22*
  on abdominal radiographs, anteroposterior, 67
  on finger radiographs, posteroanterior, 77

Navicular-cuneiform joint(s), on foot radiographs, anteroposterior, 211, *211–213*

Object-image distance (OID), 3
  on finger radiographs, lateral, 84

Object-image distance (OID) *(Continued)*
    oblique, 81
    posteroanterior, 77
Oblique position(s), definition of, 2
    hanging technique for, 3, *4*
    markers for, placement of, 8, *8–9*
Obliquity, degree of, 12, *12*
    for rib radiographs, anterior/posterior oblique, 389, *389, 391–392*
    for sternal radiographs, right anterior oblique, 377, *378–379*
    on foot radiographs, medial oblique, 215, *215–216*, 217
    on sacroiliac joint radiographs, posterior oblique, 313–314, *314–315*
    on scapular radiographs, lateral, 197
    on shoulder radiographs, anterior oblique, *181*, 181–182, *183*
        Grashey, 177, *177–179*
Occiput, position of, on atlantoaxial radiographs, 322–323, *322–325*
    on cervical vertebral radiographs, anteroposterior, 318, *320*
OID (object-image distance), 3. See also *Object-image distance (OID).*
Open mouth radiograph(s). See *Atlantoaxial radiograph(s), open mouth.*
Orbitomental line, on cranial radiographs, Caldwell, 399–400, *401–402*
    posteroanterior, 394–395, *395–397*
    Towne, 403–404, *404–405*
Overexposure, 26–27, *27*
Overpenetration, 27, *27*

PA (posteroanterior). See *Posteroanterior (PA) projections.*
Patella, fractures of, patient positioning with, for lateral knee radiographs, 263
    position of, on knee radiographs, anteroposterior, *256*
        lateral, flexion and, 263, *266*
        posteroanterior axial, 270–271, *270–272*
    subluxation of, on knee radiographs, anteroposterior, 253–254, *256*
Patellar radiograph(s), merchant method. See *Patellar radiograph(s), tangential.*
    tangential, 272–277, *272–277*
        accurate positioning of, *272*
        collimation of, with large calves, 275, *276–277*
        femoral condyles on, 273, *276*
        joint spaces on, 274–275, *274–277*
        patient positioning for, 273, *273–274, 276–277*
        rotation on, 273–274, *276*
        subluxation on, 274
Patellofemoral joint(s), on patellar radiographs, tangential, 274–275, *274–277*
Patient positioning. See under specific projection(s).
Pelvic radiograph(s), anteroposterior, 303–306, *303–306*
        accurate positioning of, *303–304*, 304–305
        collimation of, 305
        fat planes on, 303, *304*
        for evaluation of hip joint mobility, 305
        foreshortening on, *303*, 305, *305–307*
        gonadal shielding for, 305
        patient positioning for, *303–304*, 303–305, *306*
            with femoral fracture, 305
        position of foot for, 305, *305–306*
        position of leg for, *303*, 305, *305*
        rotation on, 304, *306*
    anteroposterior axial. See *Pelvic radiograph(s), frogleg.*
    frogleg, 307–310, *307–310*
        accurate positioning of, *307*
        collimation of, 309
        femoral abduction for, 309
        flexion of knees and hips for, *307–310*, 308–309
        for evaluation of hip mobility, 309
        foreshortening on, *307*, 308–309, *309–310*
        gonadal shielding for, 309
        leg abduction for, *307*, 309, *309–310*
        patient positioning for, 308–309, *308–310*
        position of femur for, 308, *308*
        rotation on, 308, *310*
Penetration, adequacy of, 26–31, *27–30*
Petrous ridge(s), on cranial radiographs, Caldwell, 399, *401–402*
    on facial bone/sinus radiographs, parietocanthal, 413–414, *413–416*
Phototimed radiograph(s), density and penetration of, 29–31, *30*

Physicians' order(s), fulfillment of, 36–37, *38*
PIP (proximal interphalangeal joints). See *Proximal interphalangeal joint(s) (PIP).*
Plane(s), body, 2
Plantar flexion, 3
    on calcaneal radiographs, axial, 224, *225–227*, 226
        lateral, 230, *232*
    on foot radiographs, lateral, 221, *223*
Portable chest radiograph(s), film size for, 53–54, *54*
Position(s), relationship with anatomical structures, 11–15, *12–15*
Positioning. See also under specific projections.
    terms used in, 1–2
Posterior, definition of, 2
Posteroanterior (PA) projection(s), hanging technique for, 3, *4*
    markers for, placement of, 8
Prevertebral fat stripe, on cervical vertebral radiographs, lateral, 326, *326*
Projection(s), definition of, 3
    relationship with anatomical structures, 11–15, *12–15*
Pronate, definition of, 3
Pronator fat stripe, on wrist radiographs, lateral, 115–116, *116*
Prosthesis (prostheses), artifacts from, *34*
Protract, definition of, 3
Proximal, definition of, 2
Proximal interphalangeal (PIP) joint(s), on lateral radiographs, 86
    on oblique radiographs, 82
    on posteroanterior radiographs, 79
Psoas muscle, on abdominal radiographs, anteroposterior, 66–67
    on lumbar vertebral radiographs, anteroposterior, 351

Radial head, on elbow radiographs, 151–153, *151–153*
Radial tuberosity, on elbow radiographs, anteroposterior, 137, *139*
    lateral, 148, *148, 150*
    on forearm radiographs, lateral, 132
Radiation, scattered, and adequacy of contrast, 31–32, *32*
Radiation protection, 17–20, *18–21*
Radiograph(s), hanging technique for, 3–4, *4–5*
Radiographic contrast, adequacy of, 31–32, *31–32*
Radiographic critique, form for, *6*
Radiolucent, definition of, 3
Radiopaque, definition of, 3
Radioscaphoid joint space, on posteroanterior, ulnar flexed radiographs, 124, *125*
Radiosensitive cell(s), shielding of, 19
Radioulnar articulation, distal, on wrist radiographs, posteroanterior, 105–106, *108–109*
Repeat/reject analysis, completion of, 37, *39*, 39
Requisition(s), completion of, 37, *38–39*, 39
Respiration, and scapular radiographs, anteroposterior, 193
Respiration artifact(s), 21–22
Retract, definition of, 3
Rib radiograph(s), anterior/posterior oblique, 388–392, *388–392*
    above diaphragm, 389–390
        collimation of, 389
    accurate positioning of, *388*
    below diaphragm, 390
        collimation of, 390
    degree of obliquity for, 389, *389, 391–392*
    patient positioning for, 389, *389*
    soft tissue on, 388–389
    anteroposterior/posteroanterior, 383–387, *383–387*
        above diaphragm, collimation of, 385
            lung aeration on, 385
            patient positioning for, 384–385, *387*
        accurate positoning of, *383*
        below diaphragm, collimation of, 385
            lung aeration on, 385, *387*
        patient positioning for, 384, *384*
        rotation on, 384, *386*
        rotation vs. scoliosis on, 384
        soft tissue on, 383–384
Rotation, external, 3
    internal, 3
    lateral, 3

Rotation (*Continued*)
  medial, 3
  on abdominal radiographs, anteroposterior, 68–69, *70–71*
    left lateral decubitus, 74, *75*
  on acromioclavicular joint radiographs, anteroposterior, 191, *192*
  on ankle radiographs, anteroposterior, 233, *233–235*
    medial oblique, 236–237, *236–238*
  on atlantoaxial radiographs, open mouth, 321–322, *324*
  on calcaneal radiographs, axial, 226, *227*
  on cervical vertebral radiographs, anterior oblique, 333, *335*
    anteroposterior, 317, *319*
    lateral, 327, *327, 329*
    posterior oblique, 333, *335*
  on cervicothoracic vertebral radiographs, swimmer's lateral view, 338, *340*
  on chest radiographs, anterior oblique, 64, *65*
    anteroposterior, 53–54, *54–55*
    anteroposterior lordotic, 61
    lateral decubitus, 57–58, *59*
    left lateral, 46, *46, 49–50*
    posteroanterior, 42, *43*
  on clavicle radiographs, anteroposterior, 185, *186*
    anteroposterior axial, 187–188
  on coccygeal radiographs, anteroposterior, 372, *373*
    lateral, 374, *375*
  on cranial radiographs, Caldwell, 394, *395*, 399, *401*
    lateral, 407, *408*
    posteroanterior, 394, *395*
    Towne, 403, *404*
  on elbow radiographs, anteroposterior, 136–137, *138*
  on facial bone/sinus radiographs, parietocanthal, 413, *415*
  on femoral radiographs, proximal anteroposterior, 278, 280–281, *280–281*
  on finger radiographs, posteroanterior, 77–78, *78, 80*
  on foot radiographs, anteroposterior, 211, *212–213*
    medial oblique, 217, *217–218*
  on forearm radiographs, anteroposterior, 127–128, *129*
  on hand radiographs, posteroanterior, 97
  on hip radiographs, anteroposterior, 291–292, *292–294*
    axiolateral, 300, *300, 302*
    frogleg, 295, *297*
  on humeral radiographs, anteroposterior, 155, *156–157*
    lateral, *162*
  on knee radiographs, anteroposterior, 252, *254*
    lateral, 265–266, *265–266, 268–269*
    medial oblique, 258–259, *258–260*
  on lower leg radiographs, anteroposterior, 244–245, *246*
    lateral, 248, *250*
  on lumbar vertebral radiographs, anteroposterior, 351–352, *353–354*
    lateral, 358–359, *359, 361*
    L5–S1 spot lateral, 363–364, *364*
    posterior oblique, 355–356, *355–357*
  on patellar radiographs, tangential, 273–274, *276*
  on pelvic radiographs, anteroposterior, 304, *306*
    frogleg, 308, *310*
  on rib radiographs, anteroposterior/posteroanterior, 384, *386*
  on sacral radiographs, anteroposterior, 366, *367–368*
    lateral, 369–370, *370*
  on sacroiliac joint radiographs, anteroposterior, 311–312
    posterior oblique, 313–314, *314*
  on scapular radiographs, lateral, 197–198, *200*
  on shoulder radiographs, anteroposterior, 166, *166, 168–170*
  on sinus radiographs, parietocanthal, 413, *415*
  on sternal radiographs, lateral, 380–381, *380–382*
  on thoracic vertebral radiographs, anteroposterior, 343
    lateral, 346–347, *348–349*
  on thumb radiographs, anteroposterior, 87–88, *89*
  on toe radiographs, anteroposterior, 203, *204*
    lateral, 208–209, *208–209*
    oblique, 205–206, *206–207*
  on wrist radiographs, lateral, 116–117, *118–119*
    medial oblique, *113–114*
    posteroanterior, 105, *108–111*
  vs. scoliosis. See *Scoliosis, vs. rotation.*

Sacral radiograph(s), anteroposterior, 365–368, *365–368*
  accurate positioning of, *365*

Sacral radiograph(s) (*Continued*)
    collimation of, 367, *368*
    foreshortening on, 366, *367–368*
    gonadal shielding for, 367
    leg flexion on, 366–367, *368*
    patient positioning for, 366–367, *366–368*
    rotation on, 366, *367–368*
  lateral, 369–371, *369–371*
    accurate positioning of, *369*
    collimation of, 370
    gonadal shielding for, 370
    intervertebral disk spaces on, *369*, 370
    patient positioning for, 369–370, *369–370*
    rotation on, 369–370, *370*
Sacroiliac joint radiograph(s), anteroposterior, 311–312, *311–312*
    accurate positioning of, *311*
    collimation of, 312
    foreshortening on, 312, *312*
    gonadal shielding for, 312
    patient positioning for, 311–312, *312*
    rotation on, 311–312
  posterior oblique, 313–315, *313–315*
    accurate positioning of, *313*
    advantages of, vs. anterior oblique, 313
    collimation of, 314
    degree of obliquity on, 313–314, *314–315*
    gonadal shielding for, 314
    joint space on, 313, *314–315*
    patient positioning for, *313*, 313–314
    rotation on, 313–314, *314*
Sagittal plane, 2
Scaphocarpal joint space(s), repositioning of, on wrist radiographs, posteroanterior ulnar-flexed, *121*, 123, *123, 125*
Scaphoid, fractures of, on posteroanterior ulnar-flexed wrist radiographs, 123–124, *123–124*
Scaphoid fat stripe, on wrist radiographs, medial oblique, 111–112, *112*
    posteroanterior, 105, *105*
    ulnar-flexed, 121–122, *122*
Scaphotrapezius joint(s), on wrist radiographs, medial oblique, 112, *113*
Scapula, on clavicle radiographs, anteroposterior axial, 188, *188–189*
Scapular radiograph(s), anteroposterior, 192–196, *193–196*
    accurate positioning of, *193*
    density of shoulder girdle on, 193, *195*
    foreshortening on, 194, *195*
    kyphosis on, 194
    patient positioning for, 193–194, *194–195*
      in trauma patients, 194–195
    position of glenoid fossa on, 193–194, *195*
    position of humerus on, 194, *196*
    respiration and, 193
    shoulder retraction on, 194, *195*
    thoracic cavity on, 193–195, *195–196*
  lateral, 196–201, *196–201*
    accurate positioning of, *196*
    collimation of, 199
    degree of obliquity on, 197
    patient positioning for, 197–198, *197–198, 200*
      supine, 197, *197*
    position of humerus on, 198–199, *198–199, 201*
    rotation on, 197–198, *200*
Scattered radiation, and adequacy of contrast, 31–32, *32*
Scoliosis, vs. rotation, on abdominal radiographs, anteroposterior, 68–69, *71*
    left lateral decubitus, 74
    on chest radiographs, left lateral, 47, *51*
      posteroanterior, 42, *43*
    on lumbar vertebral radiographs, anteroposterior, 352, *353–354*
    on rib radiographs, anteroposterior/posteroanterior, 384
    on thoracic vertebral radiographs, anteroposterior, 343
      lateral, 346
"Scottie dogs," on lumbar vertebral radiographs, posterior oblique, 356, *356–357*
Shape distortion, 24
Shielding, gonadal, 17–20, *18–21*
Shoulder, dislocation of, anterior oblique view of, 181, *182, 184*
    anteroposterior view of, 166–167, *169*

Shoulder *(Continued)*
markers for, placement of, 9, *10*
position of, on cervicothoracic vertebral radiographs, swimmer's lateral view, 339
retraction of, on scapular radiographs, anteroposterior, 194, *195*
Shoulder girdle, density of, on scapular radiographs, anteroposterior, 193, *195*
Shoulder radiograph(s), anterior oblique, 180–184, *180–184*
accurate positioning of, *180*
collimation of, 182
degree of obliquity on, *181*, 181–182, *183*
dislocations on, 181, *182, 184*
foreshortening on, 181–182, *184*
patient positioning for, 180–182, *181–184*
anteroposterior, 165–171, *165–171*
accurate positioning of, *165*
collimation of, 167, *167*
compensating filters for, 166, *166*
dislocation on, 166–167, *169*
foreshortening on, 167, *169–170*
humeral position on, *165–166*, 167–168, *168, 170–171*
patient positioning for, *166*, 166–167, *170*
rotation on, 166, *166, 168–170*
axial, 171–175, *171–175*
accurate positioning of, *171*
collimation of, 172–173, *172–174*
foreshortening on, 173, *175*
humeral position on, 173–174, *174–175*
patient positioning for, 172–173, *172–174*
position of glenoid fossa on, 172–173, *172–174*
Grashey, 176–179, *176–179*
accurate positioning of, *176*
collimation of, 177, *179*
degree of obliquity on, 177, *177–179*
foreshortening on, *178–179*
glenohumeral joint space on, 177, *178–179*
kyphosis on, 177, *179*
patient positioning for, 176–177, *176–178*
position of glenoid fossa on, 177, *179*
repositioning for, 177
trans-scapular Y. See *Shoulder radiograph(s), anterior oblique.*
SID (source-image distance), 3
Sinus radiograph(s), 398–402, *398–402*. See also *Cranial radiograph(s).*
parietocanthal, 412–416, *412–416*
accurate positioning of, *412*
collimation of, 414, *414, 416*
mentomeatal line on, 413–414, *415*
patient positioning for, 413, *413–416*
petrous ridges on, 413–414, *413–416*
rotation on, 413, *415*
Size distortion, 24
Skin line, collimation to, 16, *16*
Soft tissue, definition of, 20–22, *21–24*
density of, on sternal radiographs, lateral, 379–380, *380*
on forearm radiographs, lateral, 131, *131–132*
on rib radiographs, anterior/posterior oblique, 388–389
anteroposterior/posteroanterior, 383–384
Source-image distance (SID), 3
Sternal radiograph(s), lateral, 379–382, *379–382*
accurate positioning of, *379–380*
collimation of, 381
patient positioning for, 380–381, *380–382*
reduction of scattered radiation on, 380
rotation on, 380–381, *380–382*
soft tissue density and, 379–380, *380*
right anterior oblique, 376–379, *376–379*
accurate positioning of, *376*
blurring of overlying structures on, 376–377, *378*
breathing technique for, 377, *378*
collimation of, 377
degree of obliquity for, 377, *378–379*
film size for, 377
patient positioning for, 377, *377–379*
vs. left anterior oblique, 376, *378*
Sthenic body type, 24, *25*
Styloid, position of, on forearm radiographs, anteroposterior, *129–130*

Styloid *(Continued)*
lateral, 132
on wrist radiographs, lateral, 117, *121*
medial oblique, 113
posteroanterior, 105–106
Superimpose, definition of, 3
Superior, definition of, 2
Supination, definition of, 3
Suprapatellar fat pad(s), on lateral knee radiographs, *262*, 263
Swimmer's position, for cervical vertebral radiographs, lateral, 329, 337–341, *337–341*
for cervicothoracic vertebral radiographs. See *Cervicothoracic vertebral radiograph(s), swimmer's lateral view.*
Symmetrical, definition of, 3
Symphysis pubis, location of, for hip radiographs, axiolateral, 300

Talar dome(s), on ankle radiographs, lateral, 240–241, *240–242*
on calcaneal radiographs, lateral, 229–230, *229–231*
on foot radiographs, lateral, 220–221, *220–222*
Talocalcaneal joint(s), on calcaneal radiographs, axial, 224, *224–227*
Tarsi sinus, on ankle radiographs, medial oblique, 237, *238*
Tarsometatarsal joint(s), on foot radiographs, anteroposterior, 211, *211–213*
Testicle(s), shielding of, 18, *20*
Thoracic cavity, on clavicle radiographs, anteroposterior, 185, *185–186*
on scapular radiographs, anteroposterior, 193–195, *195–196*
Thoracic vertebra(e), first, on cervical vertebral radiographs, lateral, 329, *331*
on chest radiographs, anteroposterior, 53
visualization of, on chest radiographs, lateral decubitus, 57, 58, *60*
left lateral, 48–49, *49*
posteroanterior, 41
Thoracic vertebral radiograph(s), anteroposterior, 341–345, *341–345*
accurate positioning of, *341*
anode-heel effect on, 342
collimation of, 344
expiration vs. inspiration during, 342–343, *344*
intervertebral disk spaces on, 343–344, *345*
lung aeration on, 343–344, *345*
patient positioning for, *342*, 342–343, *344*
with kyphosis, 344
rotation on, 343
wedge-compensating filter for, 342, *342*
lateral, 345–349, *345–349*
accurate positioning of, *345*
breathing technique for, 346, *348*
collimation of, 347
intervertebral disk spaces on, *346*, 347, *347, 349*
patient positioning for, 346–347, *346–348*
rotation on, 346–347, *348–349*
verifying inclusion of all thoracic vertebrae on, 347–348
lateral swimmer's position, 337–341, *337–341*, 348. See also *Cervicothoracic vertebral radiograph(s), swimmer's lateral view.*
Thumb radiograph(s), anteroposterior, 87–90, *87–90*
accurate positioning of, *87*
anatomic landmarks on, 87–88, *89*
artifacts on, 87
carpometacarpal joints on, 88, *89*
collimation of, 88, *89*
foreshortening on, *90*
joint spaces on, 88, *89*
patient positioning on, 88, *89*
placement of markers on, 87
rotation on, 87–88, *89*
lateral, 90–92, *90–92*
accurate positioning of, *90*
collimation of, 91
joint spaces on, 93–94, *94*
metacarpal joints on, 91, *92*
patient positioning on, 91, *91–92*
lateral oblique, 93–95, *93–95*
accurate positioning of, *93*
carpometacarpal joints on, 93–94, *94*
collimation of, 94, *94*

Thumb radiograph(s) *(Continued)*
    patient positioning for, 93, *93–94*
    posteroanterior, 88, *88*
Tibia, positioning of, for lower leg radiographs, anteroposterior, 245, *245*
Tibiotalar joint(s), on ankle radiographs, anteroposterior, *233,* 233–234, *235*
        lateral, 240, *242*
        medial oblique, 237, *237–238*
    on calcaneal radiograph(s), lateral, 229, *229–230*
    on lower leg radiographs, anteroposterior, 245, *245–246*
Toe radiograph(s), anteroposterior, 202–204, *202–204*
        accurate positioning of, *202*
        angulation of central ray on, for unextendable toes, 203
        collimation of, 203
        joint spaces on, 203, *204*
        patient positioning for, 203, *203*
        rotation on, 203, *204*
    lateral, 208–209, *208–209*
    oblique, 205–207, *205–207*
        accurate positioning of, *205*
        collimation of, 206, *207*
        joint spaces on, 206, *207*
        midshaft concavity on, 205
        patient positioning for, 205, *205*
        rotation on, 205–206, *206–207*
Torso radiograph(s), hanging technique for, 3–4, *4*
Towne radiograph(s). See *Cranial radiograph(s), Towne.*
Trabecular pattern, 3
Transverse plane, 2
Trapezium, position of, on wrist radiographs, lateral, 118, *121*
Trauma, positioning with. See under specific structures.

Underexposure, 27, *27*
    of abdominal radiographs, anteroposterior, *70*
Underpenetration, 27–28, *28–29*
Upper extremity(ies). See specific body parts.
Upper incisor(s), on atlantoaxial radiographs, 322–323, *322–325*

Valgus deformity, on knee radiographs, anteroposterior, 253, *254–255*
Varus deformity, on knee radiographs, anteroposterior, 253, *255*
Vascular lung marking(s), 40–41
Vertebra(e), cervical. See *Cervical vertebral radiograph(s);*
    Cervicothoracic vertebral radiograph(s).
    lateral positions of, hanging technique for, 3–4, *4*
    lumbar. See *Lumbar vertebra(e)* and *Lumbar vertebral radiograph(s).*
    oblique positions of, hanging technique for, 3, *4*
    thoracic. See *Thoracic vertebra(e)* and *Thoracic vertebral radio-graph(s).*

Waters radiograph(s). See *Facial bone radiograph(s)* and *Sinus radiograph(s), parietocanthal.*
Wedge-compensating filter, for abdominal radiographs, left lateral decubitus, 73
    for thoracic vertebral radiographs, anteroposterior, 342, *342*
Weight-bearing radiograph(s), of acromioclavicular joint, *190,* 190–191
Wrist(s), position of, on elbow radiographs, radial head/capitulum view of, *151–153,* 152
Wrist radiograph(s), anatomic landmarks on, 107–108, *109–111*
    lateral, 115–121, *115–121*
        accurate positioning of, *115*
        carpal bones on, 116
        collimation of, 117, *119–120*
        patient positioning for, 116–117, *116–119*
        position of styloid on, 117, *121*
        position of trapezium on, 118, *121*
        pronator fat stripe on, 115–116, *116*
        rotation on, 116–117, *118–119*
        with no forearm rotation, 117–118, *118, 120–121*
    medial oblique, 111–115, *111–115*
        accurate positioning of, *111*
        collimation of, 112–113, *114*
        foreshortening on, 112–113, *114*
        joint spaces on, 112, *113–115*
        patient positioning for, 112–113, *112–115*
        position of styloid on, 113
        rotation on, *113–114*
        scaphoid fat stripe on, 111–112, *112*
    mediolateral, 117, *119*
    posteroanterior, 104–111, *104–111*
        accurate positioning of, *104*
        collimation of, 107, *107*
        distal radioulnar articulation on, 105–106, *108–109*
        foreshortening on, 105–106, *109–111*, 123
        joint spaces on, *104, 106,* 106–107, *109–110*
        patient positioning for, 105, *105, 108–111*
        position of styloid on, 105–106
        rotation on, 105, *108–111*
        scaphoid fat stripe on, 105, *105*
        ulnar-flexed, 121–125, *121–125*
            accurate positioning of, *121*
            foreshortening on, 123
            joint spaces on, *121–125,* 122–124
            patient positioning for, 122–123, *122–123*
            scaphoid fat stripe on, 121–122, *122*
            scaphoid fractures on, 123–124, *123–124*

Zygapophyseal joint(s), on lumbar vertebral radiographs, posterior oblique, 355–356, *355–357*